TRANSCULTURAL NURSING
Assessment & Intervention

TRANSCULTURAL NURSING
Assessment & Intervention
THIRD EDITION

Joyce Newman Giger, EdD, RN, CS, FAAN

Professor, Graduate Studies
University of Alabama at Birmingham
School of Nursing
Birmingham, Alabama

Ruth Elaine Davidhizar, DNS, RN, CS, FAAN

Dean and Professor
Division of Nursing
Bethel College
Mishawaka, Indiana

With 22 illustrations

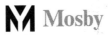

Mosby

St. Louis Baltimore Boston Carlsbad Chicago Minneapolis New York Philadelphia Portland
London Milan Sydney Tokyo Toronto

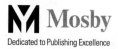

Mosby

Dedicated to Publishing Excellence

Publisher Sally Schrefer
Editor Michael S. Ledbetter
Developmental Editor Lisa P. Newton
Project Manager Dana Peick
Production Editor Dan Begley
Manuscript Editor Carl Masthay
Designer Amy Buxton

Third Edition

Printed in the United States of America

Composition by The Clarinda Company
Printing/Binding by Maple-Vail Book Manufacturing Group
Cover by Coral Graphics

Mosby, Inc.
11830 Westline Industrial Drive
St. Louis, Missouri 63146

ISBN 0-3230-0287-0

99 00 01 02 03 / 9 8 7 6 5 4 3 2 1

Karen Chang, MS, RN
Doctoral Student
University of Illinois
Chicago, Illinois

Brenda Cherry, MSN, RN, CCRN
Assistant Professor
DeKalb College
Clarkson, Georgia

Robert Cosgray, MA, BSN, RNC
Director of Nursing
Logansport State Hospital
Logansport, Indiana

Ruth Elaine Davidhizar, DNS, RN, CS, FAAN
Professor and Dean of Nursing
Division of Nursing
Bethel College
Mishawaka, Indiana

Jai Bun Earp, PhD, RN
Associate Professor
Florida A&M University
Tallahassee, Florida

Joyce Newman Giger, EdD, RN, CS, FAAN
Professor, Graduate Studies
University of Alabama at Birmingham
School of Nursing
Birmingham, Alabama

Jill Nerala Goodin, BSN, RN
Cardiac Rehabilitation
Mercy Hospital
Merced, California

Catherine E. Hanley, MSN, RN, FAAN, FACHE
Chief Executive Officer
Carl Albert Indian Hospital
Ada, Oklahoma

Jillian Inouye, PhD, APRN
Associate Professor
School of Nursing
University of Hawaii
Honolulu, Hawaii

Dianne Ishida, MS, APRN
Associate Professor
University of Hawaii
Honolulu, Hawaii

Joan Kuipers, MSN, RN
Associate Professor
Purdue University School of Nursing
West Lafayette, Indiana

Dolly Lefever, MS, RN, ANP
Nurse Midwife and Nurse Practitioner
Anchorage, Alaska

Cheryl Martin, PhD, RNC
Associate Professor and Coordinator of Programs at Ancilla College
Bethel College
Mishawaka, Indiana

Scott Wilson Miller, PhD
Candidate, RN, CPAN
Predoctoral Fellowship for the Institute of Health Studies
UCSF School of Medicine
University of California
San Francisco, California

Mary Reidy, RN, BN, MEC (App.)
Associate Professor
Faculty of Nursing
University of Montreal
Montreal, Quebec

Enid A. Schwartz, MS, RNC
Instructor of Nursing
Cochise College
Douglas, Arizona

Cynthia C. Small, MSN, RN
Instructor, Medical-Surgical Nursing
Lake Michigan College
Benton Harbor, Michigan

Linda S. Smith, DNS, RN
US Department of Health and Human Services/FDA
Special Government Employee and Staff Nurse at St. Mary's Hospital
Rogers, Arkansas

Ruth Yoder Stauffer, MSN, RN
Home Health Care Nurse
Virginia Mennonite Retirement Community
Harrisonburg, Virginia

Marie-Elizabeth Taggart, PhD, RN
Full Professor, Retired
Faculty of Nursing
University of Montreal
Montreal, Quebec

Anna Rambharose Vance, PhD, RN
Assistant Professor
East Carolina University
Greensville, North Carolina

To Our Parents
The late Ionia Holmes Newman
Lucille & Ralph Holderman
and the late Naomi Holderman

To Our Husbands
Argusta Giger, Jr. and Ronald Davidhizar

To Our Mentors
Richmond Calvin, EdD; Frances P. Dixon, BS; and
Angela Barron McBride, PhD, RN, FAAN

To the students of Bethel College, past, present, and future,
and all nurses and students who seek a better way
to render culturally appropriate care

FOREWORD

Caring has long been regarded as the foundation of nursing practice (Benner and Wrubel, 1988; Watson, 1985). The American Nurses' Association has gone on record as describing the profession as being "committed to the care and nurturing of sick and well people, individually and in groups" (1980, p. 9). Fry (1989) has argued that the central value of nursing ethics is caring that protects and enhances the human dignity of patients. A 1989 Wingspread Conference on *Knowledge about Care and Caring: State of the Art and Future Development,* cosponsored by the American Academy of Nursing and Sigma Theta Tau International in collaboration with the Johnson Foundation and select nursing schools, discussed care and caring as core representations of elaborating on the characteristics of the need for care, agents of care, recipients of care, context of care, methods of care, and goals of care in the range of specific clinical situations (McBride, 1989). Today's discussions of professional practice include an emphasis on the integrity and ethics of caring (Crigger, 1997). They also urge the development of critical thinking, so necessary to clinical problem solving (Carmack, 1997; Copp, 1996). To provide culturally competent care in the next millennium, nurses must then be able to combine the art of caring with the analytic skills of critical thinking but must do so in a way that recognizes transcultural health care as essential to the promotion of efficacious health care behaviors in a diverse global society.

This volume on transcultural nursing, edited by Giger and Davidhizar, addresses aspects of that agenda by elaborating in great detail on what constitutes culturally appropriate care. In proposing a framework for assessment that focuses on six key cultural phenomena believed to shape care—communication, space, social organization, time, environmental control, and biological variations—the authors provide students and practitioners with a template for systematically exploring how caregivers' responses, recipients of care, contexts of care, and goals of care may vary, given the cultural diversity in the United States. Not only do the many chapters specifying how a particular cultural group (for example, African Americans, Appalachians, Navajos, Eskimos, or Mexican Americans) may vary in these six areas and provide rich information that heightens awareness of the special perspectives that must be taken into account in planning care, but these chapters also provide a model for looking at the experience of other populations not included in this book.

It has become commonplace for nurse educators to advocate culturally appropriate care, but what that really means is not clear, other than some general admonition to be aware that not all patients with the same medical diagnosis are likely to have the same experience. Indeed, the notion that patients make choices based on the unique meaning of their illness experience is often discounted on a day-to-day basis when the emphasis seems to be more on the importance of routine, procedures, and covering the unit than it is on providing individualized attention. Yet this volume forces the reader to confront the many ways in which an individual's experience is likely to vary in ways that go well beyond the patterning of medical diagnosis: Is this man one who responds well to frequent touching? Does this woman need considerable personal space? Will an effective intervention necessarily have to involve the client's extended family? Does this patient have little future orientation? What are this person's beliefs about the nature of illness? What does well-oxygenated skin color look like when the infant being rated on the Apgar Scale is not White?

This volume, which draws on the clinical experience of many individuals, speaks to the needs of our pluralistic society by providing a wealth of insights about how cultural assessment is that part of the nursing process that considers the meaning of behaviors that might, if not understood within the context of ethnic values, be regarded as puzzling or even negative. The details make us sensitive to the concerns of various population groups; the framework provides a general approach to cultural thinking on this broad topic. In the final analysis, this volume is a part of the growing health care revolution that is critical of the professional who paternalistically sets out to do what is best for the patient and that emphasizes, instead, the importance of the patient's concept of his or her own good for directing the professional's caregiving.

Angela Barron McBride, PhD, RN, FAAN
Professor and Dean,
Indiana University School of Nursing
Indianapolis, Indiana

References

American Nurses' Association (1980). *Nursing—a social policy statement.* Kansas City, Mo.: Author.

Benner, P.E., & Wrubel, J. (1988). *The primacy of caring.* Reading, Mass.: Addison-Wesley.

Carmack, B. (1997). Balancing engagement and detachment in caregiving. *Image: Journal of Nursing Scholarship, 29*(2), 139-144.

Copp, L. (1996, March-April). Critical caring: can faculty do it? *Journal of Professional Nursing, 12*(2), 63-64.

Crigger, N.J. (1997, July-Aug.). The trouble with caring: a review of eight arguments against an ethic of care. *Journal of Professional Nursing, 13*(4), 217-221.

Fry, S.T. (1989). The role of caring in a theory of nursing ethics. *Hypatia, 4*(2), 88-103.

Leininger, M. (Ed.). (1988). *Care: the essence of nursing and health.* Thorofare, N.J.: Slack.

McBride, A.B. (1989). Knowledge about care and caring: state of the art and future development. *Reflections, 15*(2), 5-7.

Watson, J. (1985). *Nursing: the philosophy and science of caring.* Boulder, Colorado: University Press of Colorado.

PREFACE

The concept of transcultural nursing is relatively new to the nursing literature. In fact, it has been only in the last three decades that nurses have begun to develop an appreciation for the need to incorporate culturally appropriate clinical approaches into the daily routine of client care. Although nurses have begun to recognize the need for culturally appropriate clinical approaches, the literature on the subject is either scanty or does not provide a systematic method for comprehensive assessment and intervention. However, a good foundation in transcultural nursing is essential for the nurse because it can provide a conceptual framework for holistic client care in a variety of clinical settings and assist the nurse throughout a nursing career.

When we were challenged several years ago by the nursing students at Bethel College to develop a systematic approach to client assessment for use with individuals from diverse cultural backgrounds, we had no idea how profoundly important this topic would become for all health care providers. The United States is rapidly becoming a multicultural, heterogeneous, pluralistic society. With changing demographics, it is imperative that nurses develop not only sensitivity but also cultural competence to render safe, effective care to all clients.

When we were first challenged by the students at Bethel College, we discovered that the students had difficulty finding adequate literature to assist in planning for clients from diverse cultural backgrounds. We, like our students, had identified a similar need by virtue of our own diverse cultural backgrounds: one of us is African American and was raised in the South, and the other is White and was raised in an Eskimo setting in Alaska. Thus, in response to both a personal interest and the need identified by our students, we set about to synthesize a body of literature that would assist students in developing the theoretical knowledge necessary to provide culturally appropriate care. Although the literature has vastly improved since the initial release of this text, there is still much work to be done in this area.

This text, like the two previous editions, is divided into two parts. The first part, which focuses on theory, includes an introduction and six chapters describing the six cultural phenomena that make up our transcultural conceptual theory of assessment. The six cultural phenomena that we have identified as being evidenced in all cultural groups are (1) communication, (2) space, (3) social organization, (4) time, (5) environmental control, and (6) biological variations. The chapters in Part One describe how these phenomena vary with application and utilization across cultures.

Part Two contains chapters by contributing authors in which the six cultural phenomena are systematically applied to the assessment and care of individuals in specific cultures. The cultures selected for inclusion represent those most likely to be encountered by a nurse practicing in the United States.

In the third edition, we have once again selected contributing authors with expertise and clinical backgrounds in the care of selected cultural groups. As in our first and second editions, many of our chapters were written by contributing authors who actually represent, by ethnic heritage, the cultural group described. Not only are unique and diverse cultures represented, but also the contributing authors span the North American continent with representation truly from coast to coast and from California to Alaska and Hawaii. Thus the assessment model is applied to persons in diverse cultural settings by nurses who have expertise and sensitivity in the cultural group and in the unique care strategies that a nurse should use in providing culturally appropriate and competent care.

Because our first edition was translated into French, we perceived a need to incorporate some of the cultural uniqueness of our neighbors to the north (the people of Quebec in Canada). This perceived need led to a new book, *Canadian Transcultural Nursing,* published in 1998, which we urge our readers to review. Once again, in this third edition we have tried to select cultural groups who by virtual numbers reflect the greater percentage of our current population. We recognize and value the diversity of all the cultural groups found in the United States, but because of space and fiscal consideration, we have selected the most populous groups.

Since publication of the first edition, we have developed a quick reference, user-friendly assessment tool for use with clients in diverse clinical settings. Our model has either been cited, excerpted, or modified for inclusion in approximately 200 new nursing textbooks. Our model has shown great applicability across clinical disciplines. As such, the text was included in the library of the Education Testing Service (ETS) for many years as the only text of its kind to validate test items developed for the former RN-NCLEX and the current RN-CAT.

This book was written primarily for all nurses and nursing students who are interested in developing a knowledge of transcultural concepts to apply to client-centered care. However, we believe our new edition also will be applicable across other disciplines, such as psychology, sociology, medicine, and anthropology, because it provides not only a nursing perspective but also a historical and biotechnological approach to transcultural health care.

In our commitment to transcultural nursing, we have once again made every effort, through extensive research, to be as culturally sensitive as possible and not offend our readers or specific racial, cultural, ethnic, or religious groups. Despite our careful attention to detail to prevent this from happening, we realize that the presentation of literature and research findings are often interpreted differently by individuals. We apologize for any content that our readers may find insensitive and assure our readers that as nurse researchers, clinicians, and academicians, we have as our only intent the presentation of factual information.

ACKNOWLEDGMENTS

We would like to acknowledge and thank our former editors: Linda Duncan, whose vision of the future allowed this project to come to fruition; Darlene Como, who took up the challenge to continue this project; Loren Wilson, who continued to challenge us to provide the best-referenced text on this subject; and Michael Ledbetter, who has worked diligently to bring this project to fruition. A special thanks to Lisa Newton and Laura Selkirk for being available for our many questions and to Carl Masthay and Dan Begley for their diligence in bringing the most culturally and linguistically accurate text to American health care providers.

We would like to thank Dr. Clyde Root, director of Library Services, Bethel College, for the multitude of computer searches conducted on our behalf. A special recognition goes to the people who by their religious affiliation proved to be invaluable content experts in providing advice, counsel, and information on special religious groups. These individuals include Judy Mason, a member of the staff, University of Alabama at Birmingham, School of Nursing, whose expert advice on Jehovah's Witnesses proved to be invaluable. Similarly, we would like to thank Tamra Walters, a former baccalaureate nursing student at the University of Tulsa, Tulsa, Oklahoma, who read our first edition and graciously provided in-depth insight on the Church of Jesus Christ of Latter Day Saints (Mormons).

We wish to thank the many persons who took the photos and provided them for use in this textbook and all the individuals who posed for these pictures. A special thanks to Dottie Kauffman, our photographer, who has labored on this project for some ten years. We thank our chapter contributors who believed in this project. Each of you has made invaluable contributions. Finally, we would like to acknowledge the friendship and respect that has grown over these 20 years. We believe that the diversity of our heritages (one African American and one White American) and our ability to complement each other is a testimonial to the achievement of racial, ethnic, and cultural harmony across the United States, Canada, and countries throughout the world in this century. As we close this millennium and look toward the new millennium, we are hopeful that all health care providers will continue to strive to achieve cultural competence.

Joyce Newman Giger
Ruth Elaine Davidhizar

SPECIAL ACKNOWLEDGMENTS

A special acknowledgment is made to Dr. Joyce Newman Giger, my friend and colleague who in 1996 was diagnosed with breast cancer. In 1997, Dr. Giger was diagnosed with what was believed to be terminal breast cancer or some other mysterious illness. I would like to take this opportunity to say the following:

Joyce: During the writing of this book you have struggled with endless diagnostic procedures, the traumatic misdiagnosis of a terminal illness, and then a series of changing diagnoses and recommended treatments as doctors sought to unravel inconsistent diagnostic reports. Through all of this, you maintained your steadfast faith in the goodness of God and your trust that his will would be done. Your hope in life and your knowledge that your life has a special plan not only saw us through this book but will also see us through as we plan the next one. Just as you stood by me in support as I recovered from my automobile accident, I stand by you in support through the unchartered waters of your battle with the new mysterious disease and breast cancer. I hope for a new and challenging treatment for breast cancer in our lifetime. On your behalf and on behalf of your friends at Mosby, Inc., I dedicate this book to all the women of the world who are breast-cancer survivors. May each and every woman with breast cancer continue to rise to enjoy all the precious moments of life.

With Love, Ruth

CONTENTS

PART ONE

Framework for Cultural Assessment and Intervention Techniques

CHAPTER 1 · Introduction to Transcultural Nursing

Theories of transcultural nursing with established clinical approaches to clients from varying cultures are relatively new. According to Madeleine Leininger (1987), founder of the field of transcultural nursing in the mid-1960s, the education of nursing students in this field is only now beginning to yield significant results. Today, nurses with a deeper appreciation of human life and values are developing cultural sensitivity for appropriate, individualized clinical approaches. Transcultural nursing concepts are being incorporated into the curricula for student nurses in the United States and Canada.

The Transcultural Nursing Society, founded in 1974, is promoting interest in transcultural concepts and the education of transcultural nurses at the graduate level (Giger & Davidhizar, 1990; Wenger, 1989). Since its inception, the society has promoted such efforts at annual transcultural nursing conferences in different worldwide locations. The society also implemented the first certification plan in transcultural nursing. Through the efforts of the society, a number of United States and Canadian nurses have received certification. Other international conferences such as those supported by the Rockefeller Foundation in October 1988 in Bellagio, Italy, have sought to promote international health care management. The society also publishes the *Transcultural Nursing Society Newsletter,* international nursing journals, the *International Journal of Nursing Studies,* and the *International Nursing Review.* Although the literature on patient approaches in culturally diverse situations is mushrooming and nurses are beginning to do transcultural research studies, relatively few theories on transcultural nursing up to now have provided a systematic method for comprehensive nursing assessment (Brink, 1990a, 1990b; Leininger, 1991, 1985a, 1985b; Spector, 1996; Tripp-Reimer, 1984a, 1984b; Tripp-Reimer & Dougherty, 1985; Tripp-Reimer & Friedl, 1977).

CULTURE DEFINED

Culture is a patterned behavioral response that develops over time as a result of imprinting the mind through social and religious structures and intellectual and artistic manifestations. Culture is also the result of acquired mechanisms that may have innate influences but are primarily affected by internal and external environmental stimuli. Culture is shaped by values, beliefs, norms, and practices that are shared by members of the same cultural group. Culture guides our thinking, doing, and being and becomes patterned expressions of who we are. These patterned expressions are passed down from one generation to the next. Other definitions of culture have been offered by Leininger (1991, 1985a, 1985b), Spector (1996), and Andrews and Boyle (1996). According to Leininger (1991, 1985a, 1985b) culture is the values, beliefs, norms, and practices of a particular group that are learned and shared and that guide thinking, decisions, and actions in a patterned way. Spector (1996) contends that culture is a metacommunication system based on nonphysical traits such as values, beliefs, attitudes, customs, language, and behaviors that are shared by a group of people and are passed down from one generation to the next. According to Andrews and Boyle (1996), culture represents a unique way of perceiving, behaving, and evaluating the external environment and as such provides a blueprint for determining values, beliefs, and practices. Regardless of the definition chosen, the term "culture" implies a dynamic, ever-changing, active, or passive process.

Cultural values are unique expressions of a particular culture that have been accepted as appropriate over time. They guide actions and decision making that facilitate self-worth and self-esteem. Leininger (1985a) postulates that cultural values develop as a direct result of an individual's desirable or preferred way of acting or knowing something that is often sustained by a culture over time and that governs actions or decisions.

THE NEED FOR TRANSCULTURAL NURSING KNOWLEDGE

It is believed that demography is destiny, demographic change is reality, and demographic sensitivity is imperative. The United States is rapidly becoming a multicultural, pluralistic society. In 1998, 70.9% of the population in the United States were White of European descent, 12.9% were African American, 11.4% were Hispanic American, 4.1% were Asian American, and 0.9% were Native American Indian (U.S. Department of Commerce, Bureau of the Census, 1998). It is projected that by the year 2020 only 53% of the U.S. population will be White of European descent. It is further projected that by the year 2021 the number of Asian Americans and Hispanic Americans will triple, while the number of African Americans will double (U.S. Department of Commerce, Bureau of the Census, 1998).

If the 1990 census data on fertility, birth, and mortalities are correct, it is conceivable that it will be virtually impossible to isolate and identify a "pure" race of Whites of European descent by the year 2070 (U.S. Department of Commerce, Bureau of the Census, 1998). In light of these statistical data, it is imperative that "Nursing Workforce 2000" rapidly adapt itself to a changing heterogeneous society.

Providing culturally appropriate and thus competent care in the year 2000 and beyond will be a complex and difficult task for many nurses. In many professional health career programs such as nursing, medicine, and respiratory therapy, students are rarely taught culturally appropriate and competent care techniques. Thus, when these individuals encounter clients from culturally diverse backgrounds in the clinical setting, they are often unable to accurately assess and provide the kind of interventions that are culturally appropriate.

The burden of teaching nurses culturally competent care techniques will rest not only with the individual programs of practice development, but also with the health care agency itself. Regardless of who is responsible for this task, nurses must develop an understanding about culture and its relevance to competent care.

A nurse who does not recognize the value and importance of culturally appropriate care cannot possibly be an effective care agent in this changing demographic society. If nurses do not recognize that the intervention strategies planned for an African-American client with diabetes are uniquely different from those planned for a Vietnamese American, Italian American, etc., they cannot possibly hope to change the health-seeking behaviors or actively encourage the wellness behaviors of this client or any client. When nurses consider race, ethnicity, culture, and cultural heritage, they become more sensitive to clients. This is not to suggest that there is a cookbook approach to delivering care to clients by virtue of race, ethnicity, or culture. There is as much variation within certain races, cultures, or ethnic groups as there is across cultural groups. When the informed nurse considers the significance of culture, clients are approached with a more informed perspective.

The time to learn differing perspectives about culture is at hand. As professional health care providers, nurses will be asked to step forward to provide the leadership to ensure that all people have equal access to quality, culturally appropriate, and culturally competent health care. This task can be accomplished only through culturally diverse nursing care.

CULTURAL ASSESSMENT
Using nonnursing models

In a pluralistic society nurse practitioners need to be prepared to provide culturally appropriate nursing care for each client, regardless of that client's cultural background. To provide culturally appropriate nursing care, nurses must understand specific factors that influence individual health and illness behaviors (Tripp-Reimer, Brink, & Saunders, 1984). According to Affonso (1979), cultural assessment can give meaning to behaviors that might otherwise be judged negatively. If cultural behaviors are not appropriately identified, their significance will be confusing to the nurse.

Although transcultural nursing theories have appeared in the literature (Affonso, 1979; Leininger, 1985a, 1985b), adequate nursing assessment methods to accompany these theories have not been consistently provided. One of the most comprehensive tools used for nursing cultural assessment is the

Outline of Cultural Materials by Murdock et al. (1971); however, this tool was developed primarily for anthropologists who were concerned with ethnographic descriptions of cultural groups. Although the tool is well developed and contains 88 major categories, it was not designed for nurse practitioners and thus does not provide for systematic use of the nursing process. Another assessment tool is found in Brownlee's (1978) *Community, Culture, and Care: A Cross-Cultural Guide for Health Workers.* Brownlee's work is devoted to the process of practical assessment of a community, with specific attention given to health areas. The work deals with three aspects of assessment: what to find out, why it is important, and how to do it. Brownlee's assessment tool has been criticized as being too comprehensive, too difficult, and too detailed for use with individual clients. Although this tool was developed for use by health care practitioners, it is not exclusively a nursing assessment tool.

Using nursing-specific models

Transcultural nursing as defined by Leininger (1991) is a "humanistic and scientific area of formal study and practice which is focused upon differences and similarities among cultures with respect to human care, health (or well-being), and illness based upon the people's cultural values, beliefs, and practices." According to Leininger (1991), the ultimate goal of transcultural nursing is use of relevant knowledge to provide culturally specific and culturally congruent nursing care to people. From this theoretical perspective, Leininger (1985a, 1985b) provides a comprehensive transcultural theory and assessment model. For over 30 years, this model has helped nurses discover and understand what health care means to various cultures. Leininger's sunrise model symbolizes the rising of the sun (care). The model depicts a full sun with four levels of foci. Within the circle in the upper portion of the model are components of the social structure and world view factors that influence care and health through language and environment. These factors influence the folk, professional, and nursing systems or subsystems located in the lower half of the model. Also included in the model are levels of abstraction and analysis from which care can be studied at each level. Various cul-

tural phenomena are studied from the micro, middle, and macro perspectives (Leininger, 1985a, 1985b). Leininger's model has served as the prototype for the development of other culturally specific nursing models and tools (Bloch, 1983; Branch & Paxton, 1976; Orque, 1983; Rund & Krause, 1978).

An analysis of culturally specific models and tools

Tripp-Reimer, Brink, and Saunders (1984) analyzed selected culturally appropriate models and tools to determine if significant differences existed among the models. They concluded that most cultural assessment guides are similar because they all seek to identify major cultural domains that are important variables if culturally appropriate care is to be rendered. Nine culturally appropriate models or guides were analyzed, including Aamodt (1978), Bloch (1983), Branch and Paxton (1976), Brownlee (1978), Kay (1978), Leininger (1977), Orque (1983), Rund and Krause (1978), and Tripp-Reimer (1984b). In analyzing the models, Tripp-Reimer, Brink, and Saunders (1984) concluded that the same two limitations existed in each guide. The first limitation was the tendency to include too much cultural content, ultimately negating the "heart of the matter," which is the process itself. The second limitation was that it is often impossible to separate client-specific data from normative data.

Using nursing diagnoses

The relative significance of culturally appropriate health care cannot be understood if the nurse does not understand the value of culturally relevant nursing diagnoses. Geissler (1991) reports a study to determine the applicability of the North American Nursing Diagnosis Association (NANDA) taxonomy as a culturally appropriate assessment tool for use with diverse populations. In the study, three nursing diagnoses were analyzed to validate their cultural appropriateness: (1) impaired verbal communication, (2) social isolation, and (3) noncompliance in culturally diverse situations. Participants in the study (n = 245 nurses) were experts in the field of transcultural nursing and were members of either the Transcultural Nursing Society or the American Nurses Association Council on Cultural Diversity

(Geissler, 1991). Findings from this study also indicate that nursing diagnoses tend to (1) be client focused rather than provider focused and therefore do not acknowledge the existence of other culturally relevant viewpoints (such as those expressed by the provider); (2) be generalized, and as a result increase the likelihood, when applied in diverse cultural settings, for stereotyping and victimization because so-called non-Western medical models are believed to be "abnormal" and thus require necessary interventions; and (3) involve mislabeling phenomena, which in actuality arise as expressions of cultural dissonance rather than expressions of political, social, psychological, or economic factors.

In the study reported by Geissler (1991), the NANDA nursing diagnosis, "impaired communication, verbal, related to cultural differences," is an excellent example of a client-oriented diagnosis that does not recognize linguistic cultural differences. The study concludes that the NANDA diagnosis of "impaired verbal communication" connotes that the client's verbal communication and ability to understand and use language is impaired in some way. This diagnosis does not consider the causative factors creating the impairment (Giger, Davidhizar, Evers, & Ingram, 1994). It is apparent that individuals who speak a language different from that used by health care providers or nurses may be very capable of both use and comprehension of a specific language when interacting with persons fluent in that language (Giger, Davidhizar, Evers, & Ingram, 1994). According to Geissler (1991), if the client in this situation is "verbally impaired," the nurse is equally impaired. Geissler also concludes that the NANDA diagnosis of "impaired verbal communication" does not adequately address the issue of nonverbal communication, which was identified in the earlier nursing literature as an essential assessment factor (Giger & Davidhizar, 1990, 1991).

According to Geissler (1991), nursing diagnoses related to social isolation and noncompliance need further defining characteristics for use with culturally diverse populations. Rather than use the term "noncompliance," Geissler (1991) suggests that the term "nonadherence" may be more appropriate because this term may more accurately reflect behavior resulting from cultural dissonance. At the same time, the use of "nonadherence" may remove the stigma of guilt experienced by the health care recipient who is inappropriately labeled "noncompliant."

GIGER AND DAVIDHIZAR'S TRANSCULTURAL ASSESSMENT MODEL

In response to the need for a practical assessment tool for evaluating cultural variables and their effects on health and illness behaviors, a transcultural assessment model is offered that greatly minimizes the time needed to conduct a comprehensive assessment in an effort to provide culturally competent care. The metaparadigm for the Giger and Davidhizar Transcultural Assessment Model includes (1) transcultural nursing and culturally diverse nursing, (2) culturally competent care, (3) culturally unique individuals, (4) culturally sensitive environments, and (5) health and health status based on culturally specific illness and wellness behaviors.

Transcultural nursing defined

In the context of Giger and Davidhizar's Transcultural Assessment Model (1990, 1995), transcultural nursing is viewed as a culturally competent practice field that is client centered and research focused. Although transcultural nursing is viewed as client centered, it is important for nurses to remember that culture can and does influence how clients are viewed and the care that is rendered.

Every individual is culturally unique, and nurses are no exception to this premise. Nonetheless, nurses must use caution to avoid projecting on the client their own "cultural uniqueness" and "world views" if culturally appropriate care is to be provided. Nurses must carefully discern personal cultural beliefs and values to separate them from the client's beliefs and values. To deliver culturally sensitive care, the nurse must remember that each individual is unique and a product of past experiences, beliefs, and values that have been learned and passed down from one generation to the next.

According to Stokes (1991), nursing as a profession is not "culturally free" but rather is "culturally determined." Nurses must recognize and understand this fact to avoid becoming grossly ethnocentric

(Stokes, 1991). Because there is a contingent relationship between cultural determination and the delivery of culturally sensitive care, the transcultural nurse must be guided by acquired knowledge in the assessment, diagnosis, planning, implementation, and evaluation of the client's needs based on culturally relevant information. This ideology does not presuppose that all individuals within a specific cultural group will think and behave in a similar manner with relative predictability. The astute nurse must remember that there is as much diversity within a cultural group as there is across cultural groups. Nonetheless, the goal of transcultural nursing is the discovery of culturally relevant facts about the client to provide culturally appropriate and competent care.

Although transcultural nursing is becoming a highly specialized field of specially educated individuals, every nurse regardless of academic or experiential background must use transcultural knowledge to facilitate culturally appropriate care. Regardless of preparation in the field of transcultural nursing, every nurse who is entrusted with care of clients must make every effort to deliver culturally sensitive care that is free of inherent biases based on gender, race, or religion.

Culturally diverse nursing care

Culturally diverse nursing care refers to the variability in nursing approaches needed to provide culturally appropriate and competent care. By the year 2000 and beyond, it will be necessary for nurses to utilize transcultural knowledge in a skillful and artful manner to render culturally appropriate and competent care to a rapidly changing, heterogeneous client population. Culturally diverse nursing care must take into account six cultural phenomena that vary with application and use yet are evident in all cultural groups: (1) communication, (2) space, (3) social organization, (4) time, (5) environmental control, and (6) biological variations (Fig. 1-1 and Fig. 1-2).

Cultural competent care defined

As a heightened awareness of transcultural health care has been espoused, so too has been the widened

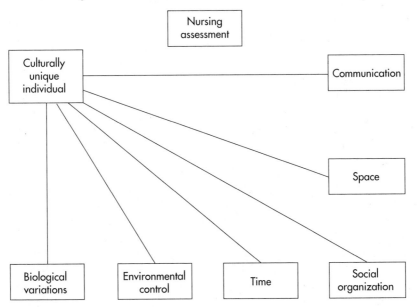

Figure 1-1   Application of cultural phenomena to nursing care and nursing practice.

use of the term "cultural competence." There are as many varying definitions for the term "cultural competence" as there are for the term "culture." Purnell and Paulanka (1998) note that the term "cultural competence" is the act whereby a health care professional develops an awareness of one's existence, sensations, thoughts, and environment without letting these factors have an undue effect on those for whom care is provided. Further, they conclude that cultural competence is the adaptation of care in a matter that is congruent with the client's culture. In this sense, cultural competence is a conscious process, and such cannot be necessarily viewed as linear (Purnell & Paulanka, 1998).

According to Smith (1998b), cultural competence is a continuous process of awareness, knowledge, skill, interaction, and sensitivity that is demonstrated among those who render care and the services they provide. Smith concludes that cultural competence requires continuous seeking of skills,

practices, and attitudes that enables nurses to transform interventions into positive health outcomes such as improved client morbidity and mortality, as well as augmenting client and professional levels of satisfaction.

Cultural competence is a dynamic, fluid, continuous process whereby an individual, system, or health care agency finds meaningful and useful care-delivery strategies based on knowledge of the cultural heritage, beliefs, attitudes, and behaviors of those to whom they render care. To develop cultural competence, it is essential for the health care professional to utilize knowledge gained from conceptual and theoretical models of culturally appropriate care. In addition, cultural competence connotes a higher, more sophisticated level of refinement of cognitive skills and psychomotor skills, attitudes, and personal beliefs. Attainment of cultural competence can assist the astute nurse to devise meaningful interventions to promote optimal health among

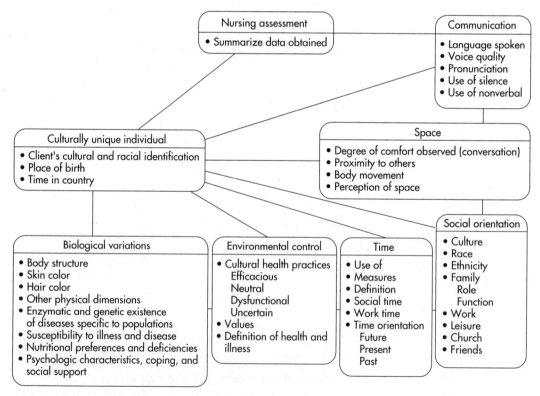

Figure 1-2 Giger and Davidhizar's transcultural assessment model.

individuals regardless of race, ethnicity, gender identity, sexual identity, or cultural heritage.

Culturally unique individuals

To provide culturally appropriate and competent care, it is important to remember that each individual is culturally unique and as such is a product of past experiences, cultural beliefs, and cultural norms. Cultural expressions become patterned responses and as such give each individual a unique identity (see Fig. 1-2). Although there is as much diversity within cultural and racial groups as there is across and among cultural and racial groups, knowledge of general baseline data relative to the specific cultural group is an excellent starting point to provide culturally appropriate care.

Culturally sensitive environments

Culturally diverse health care can and should be rendered in a variety of clinical settings. Regardless of the level of care—primary, secondary, or tertiary—knowledge of culturally relevant information will assist the nurse in planning and implementing a treatment regimen that is unique for each client.

In response to the apparent lack of practical assessment tools available in nursing for evaluating cultural variables and their effects on health and illness behaviors, this text provides a systematic approach to evaluating the six essential cultural phenomena to assist the nurse in providing culturally appropriate nursing care. Although the six cultural phenomena are evident in all cultural groups, they vary in application across cultures. Thus an individualized assessment of these areas is necessary when working with clients from diverse cultural groups (Fig. 1-3).

DEVELOPMENT AND REFINEMENT OF THE GIGER AND DAVIDHIZAR TRANSCULTURAL ASSESSMENT MODEL
Clinical application

Since its introduction in 1991, the Giger and Davidhizar Transcultural Assessment Model has been applied to the care of clients in a variety of clinical specialties: the maternity client (Giger, Davidhizar, & Wieczorek, 1993), the operating room client (Bowen & Davidhizar, 1991), and the psychiatric client (Giger, Davidhizar, Evers, & Ingram, 1994).

In 1993, Spector illustrated the model's utility by combining it with the Cultural Heritage Model. The combination of these two models (Fig. 1-4), which appears in Potter and Perry's *Fundamentals of Nursing* textbook, is unique because it provides a holistic method of providing culturally competent care. In addition, using Giger and Davidhizar's six cultural phenomena, though in a different hierarchical arrangement, Spector (1996) created a unique quick reference guide for cultural assessment of people from a variety of racial and cultural groups (Table 1-1).

In 1993, Kozier, Erb, Blaise, Johnson, and Smith-Temple used the model to provide a mechanism by which cultural behaviors relevant to health assessment could easily be identified across cultural groups. Their work relative to Giger and Davidhizar's Transcultural Assessment Model compiles basic culturally relevant information (Table 1-2). This work was further utilized in 1995 by Kozier, Erb, Blaise, and Williamson. In addition, in 1992, the editors at Editions Lamarre translated the model into French for use by French and French Canadian nurses. In 1998, Giger and Davidhizar's work was further expanded on the international horizon to include a method for assessing select cultural groups in Canada.

In 1993, the National League for Nursing published *Nursing Management Skills: A Modular Self-Assessment Series, Module IV, Transcultural Nursing* (Sheridan & Zimbler, 1993). Included in this publication are numerous articles on the application of the model in a variety of clinical situations to be used by nurses to learn and refine managerial skills. In 1994, the Nashville-based production company Envision, Inc., produced a half-inch VHS-format video titled "Cultural Diversity in Healthcare: A Different Point of View," utilizing Giger and Davidhizar's Transcultural Assessment Model as the overarching framework for the video.

In 1994, the fourth edition of Mosby's *Medical, Nursing, and Allied Health Dictionary* was published. Included in the new edition is Guidelines for Relating to Patients from Different Cultures, which was excerpted from the work of Giger and Davidhizar.

In 1995, Burk, Wieser, and Keegan proposed a method for analyzing the cultural beliefs and health

Giger and Davidhizar's Transcultural Assessment Model

CULTURALLY UNIQUE INDIVIDUAL

1. Place of birth
2. Cultural definition
   What is . . .
3. Race
   What is . . .
4. Length of time in country (if appropriate)

COMMUNICATION

1. Voice quality
   A. Strong, resonant
   B. Soft
   C. Average
   D. Shrill
2. Pronunciation and enunciation
   A. Clear
   B. Slurred
   C. Dialect (geographical)
3. Use of silence
   A. Infrequent
   B. Often
   C. Length
      (1) Brief
      (2) Moderate
      (3) Long
      (4) Not observed
4. Use of nonverbal
   A. Hand movement
   B. Eye movement
   C. Entire body movement
   D. Kinesics (gestures, expression, or stances)
5. Touch
   A. Startles or withdraws when touched
   B. Accepts touch without difficulty
   C. Touches others without difficulty
6. Ask these and similar questions:
   A. How do you get your point across to others?
   B. Do you like communicating with friends, family, and acquaintances?
   C. When asked a question, do you usually respond (in words or body movement, or both)?

D. If you have something important to discuss with your family, how would you approach them?

SPACE

1. Degree of comfort
   A. Moves when space invaded
   B. Does not move when space invaded
2. Distance in conversations
   A. 0 to 18 inches
   B. 18 inches to 3 feet
   C. 3 feet or more
3. Definition of space
   A. Describe degree of comfort with closeness when talking with or standing near others
   B. How do objects (e.g., furniture) in the environment affect your sense of space?
4. Ask these and similar questions:
   A. When you talk with family members, how close do you stand?
   B. When you communicate with coworkers and other acquaintances, how close do you stand?
   C. If a stranger touches you, how do you react or feel?
   D. If a loved one touches you, how do you react or feel?
   E. Are you comfortable with the distance between us now?

SOCIAL ORGANIZATION

1. Normal state of health
   A. Poor
   B. Fair
   C. Good
   D. Excellent
2. Marital status
3. Number of children
4. Parents living or deceased?
5. Ask these and similar questions:
   A. How do you define social activities?
   B. What are some activities that you enjoy?
   C. What are your hobbies, or what do you do when you have free time?

Figure 1-3 Giger and Davidhizar's transcultural assessment model.

Giger and Davidhizar's Transcultural Assessment Model–cont'd

D. Do you believe in a Supreme Being?
E. How do you worship that Supreme Being?
F. What is your function (what do you do) in your family unit/system?
G. What is your role in your family unit/system (father, mother, child, advisor)?
H. When you were a child, what or who influenced you most?
I. What is/was your relationship with your siblings and parents?
J. What does work mean to you?
K. Describe your past, present, and future jobs.
L. What are your political views?
M. How have your political views influenced your attitude toward health and illness?

TIME

1. Orientation to time
   A. Past-oriented
   B. Present-oriented
   C. Future-oriented
2. View of time
   A. Social time
   B. Clock-oriented
3. Physiochemical reaction to time
   A. Sleeps at least 8 hours a night
   B. Goes to sleep and wakes on a consistent schedule
   C. Understands the importance of taking medication and other treatments on schedule
4. Ask these and similar questions:
   A. What kind of timepiece do you wear daily?
   B. If you have an appointment at 2 PM, what time is acceptable to arrive?
   C. If a nurse tells you that you will receive a medication in "about a half hour," realistically, how much time will you allow before calling the nurses' station?

ENVIRONMENTAL CONTROL

1. Locus-of-control
   A. Internal locus-of-control (believes that the power to affect change lies within)
   B. External locus-of-control (believes that fate, luck, and chance have a great deal to do with how things turn out)
2. Value orientation
   A. Believes in supernatural forces
   B. Relies on magic, witchcraft, and prayer to affect change
   C. Does not believe in supernatural forces
   D. Does not rely on magic, witchcraft, or prayer to affect change
3. Ask these and similar questions:
   A. How often do you have visitors at your home?
   B. Is it acceptable to you for visitors to drop in unexpectedly?
   C. Name some ways your parents or other persons treated your illnesses when you were a child.
   D. Have you or someone else in your immediate surroundings ever used a home remedy that made you sick?
   E. What home remedies have you used that worked? Will you use them in the future?
   F. What is your definition of "good health"?
   G. What is your definition of illness or "poor health"?

BIOLOGICAL VARIATIONS

1. Conduct a complete physical assessment noting:
   A. Body structure (small, medium, or large frame)
   B. Skin color
   C. Unusual skin discolorations
   D. Hair color and distribution
   E. Other visible physical characteristics (e.g., keloids, chloasma)
   F. Weight
   G. Height
   H. Check lab work for variances in hemoglobin, hematocrit, and sickle cell phenomena if Black or Mediterranean
2. Ask these and similar questions:
   A. What diseases or illnesses are common in your family?

Figure 1-3, cont'd   Giger and Davidhizar's transcultural assessment model.

Continued

GIGER AND DAVIDHIZAR'S TRANSCULTURAL
ASSESSMENT MODEL–cont'd

B. Has anyone in your family been told that there is a possible genetic susceptibility for a particular disease?

C. Describe your family's typical behavior when a family member is ill.

D. How do you respond when you are angry?

E. Who (or what) usually helps you to cope during a difficult time?

F. What foods do you and your family like to eat?

G. Have you ever had any unusual cravings for:
   (1) White or red clay dirt?
   (2) Laundry starch?

H. When you were a child what types of foods did you eat?

I. What foods are family favorites or are considered traditional?

NURSING ASSESSMENT

1. Note whether the client has become culturally assimilated or observes own cultural practices.

2. Incorporate data into plan of nursing care:
   A. Encourage the client to discuss cultural differences; people from diverse cultures who hold different world views can enlighten nurses.
   B. Make efforts to accept and understand methods of communication.
   C. Respect the individual's personal need for space.
   D. Respect the rights of clients to honor and worship the Supreme Being of their choice.

E. Identify a clerical or spiritual person to contact.

F. Determine whether spiritual practices have implications for health, life, and well-being (e.g., Jehovah's Witnesses may refuse blood and blood derivatives; an Orthodox Jew may eat only kosher food high in sodium and may not drink milk when meat is served).

G. Identify hobbies, especially when devising interventions for a short or extended convalescence or for rehabilitation.

H. Honor time and value orientations and differences in these areas. Allay anxiety and apprehension if adherence to time is necessary.

I. Provide privacy according to personal need and health status of the client (NOTE: the perception of and reaction to pain may be culturally related).

J. Note cultural health practices.
   (1) Identify and encourage efficacious practices.
   (2) Identify and discourage dysfunctional practices.
   (3) Identify and determine whether neutral practices will have a long-term ill effect.

K. Note food preferences.
   (1) Make as many adjustments in diet as health status and long-term benefits will allow and that dietary department can provide.
   (2) Note dietary practices that may have serious implications for the client.

Figure 1-3, cont'd   Giger and Davidhizar's transcultural assessment model.

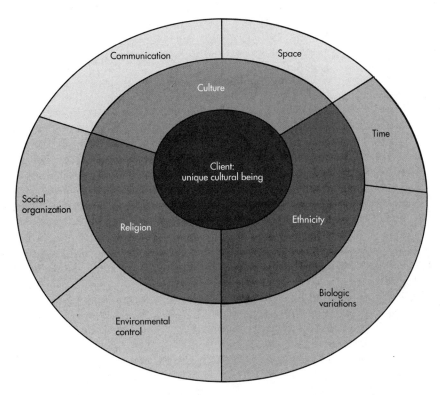

Figure 1-4 Model of the client within a culturally unique heritage and the cultural phenomena that have a profound effect on nursing care. (Compiled from Spector R.E. [1991] *Cultural diversity in health and illness,* ed. 3, Norwalk, Conn.: Appleton & Lange and Giger J., & Davidhizar, R. [1995] *Transcultural Nursing,* ed.2, St. Louis: Mosby.)

behaviors of pregnant Mexican-American women utilizing the Giger and Davidhizar Transcultural Assessment Model as an underpinning for assessment.

Application to other disciplines

The model is broad enough in scope to be recognized for applicability by many other healthcare professions (i.e., medical imaging, dentistry, education and training departments, and hospital administration) (Dowd, Giger, & Davidhizar, 1998). This model has had numerous applications in medical imaging: one a description of its use in dealing with diversity in radiology departments (Davidhizar, Dowd, Giger, 1997a); one a proposal of its use in the theory base of the profession of radiography (Davidhizar, Dowd, & Giger, 1997b); and another describing how to deal with cultural differences affecting pain response

(Davidhizar, Dowd, & Giger, 1997c). Dental hygienists are also involved with clients from diverse cultures. "Transcultural patient assessment, a method of advancing dental care", published in *Dental Assistant* (Davidhizar & Giger, 1998, 1999, in press) illuminates how awareness of the behavior of clients in the dental office is often culturally motivated. The model is also described in journals that cross health care professionals such as *Hospital Topics,* (Davidhizar & Giger, 1996), *Community Health Education and Promotion Manual* (Giger, Davidhizar, Johnson, & Poole, 1996), *Health Care Traveler* (Giger, Davidhizar, Johnson, & Poole, 1997). Application of the Giger and Davidhizar model to diverse clinical settings is quickly producing a way for staff across disciplines to understand cultural diversity and to learn techniques of culturally competent care. In addition,

Table 1-1 Cross-cultural examples of cultural phenomena impacting on nursing care

Nations of origin	Communication	Space	Time orientation	Social organization	Environmental control	Biological variations
Asian China Hawaii Philippines Korea Japan Southeast Asia (Laos, Cambodia, Vietnam)	National language preference Dialects, written characters Use of silence Nonverbal and contextual cuing	Noncontact people	Present	Family: hierarchical structure, loyalty Devotion to tradition Many religions, including Taoism, Buddhism, Islam, and Christianity Community social organizations	Traditional health and illness beliefs Use of traditional medicines Traditional practitioners: Chinese doctors and herbalists	Liver cancer Stomach cancer Coccidioidomycosis Hypertension Lactose intolerance
African West Coast (as slaves) Many African countries West Indian Islands Dominican Republic Haiti Jamaica	National languages Dialect: pidgin, creole, Spanish, and French	Close personal space	Present over future	Family: many female, single parent Large, extended family networks Strong church affiliation within community Community social organizations	Traditional health and illness beliefs Folk medicine tradition Traditional healer: root-worker	Sickle cell anemia Hypertension Cancer of the esophagus Stomach cancer Coccidioidomycosis Lactose intolerance
Europe Germany England Italy Ireland Other European countries	National languages Many learn English immediately	Noncontact people Aloof Distant Southern countries: closer contact and touch	Future over present	Nuclear families Extended families Judeo-Christian religions Community social organizations	Primary reliance on modern health care system Traditional health and illness beliefs Some remaining folk medicine traditions	Breast cancer Heart disease Diabetes mellitus Thalassemia
Native American 500 Native American tribes Aleuts Eskimos	Tribal languages Use of silence and body language	Space very important and has no boundaries	Present	Extremely family oriented Biological and extended families Children taught to respect traditions Community social organizations	Traditional health and illness beliefs Folk medicine tradition Traditional healer: medicine man	Accidents Heart disease Cirrhosis of the liver Diabetes mellitus
Hispanic countries Spain Cuba Mexico Central and South America	Spanish or Portuguese primary language	Tactile relationships Touch Handshakes Embracing Value physical presence	Present	Nuclear family Extended families Compadrazzo: godparents Community social organizations	Traditional health and illness beliefs Folk medicine tradition Traditional healers: curandero, espiritista, partera, señora	Diabetes mellitus Parasites Coccidioidomycosis Lactose intolerance

Compiled by Rachel Spector, RN, PhD. In Potter, P.A., & Perry, A. G. (1997). Fundamentals of nursing: concepts, process, and practice (ed. 4). St Louis: Mosby.

Table 1-2   Cultural behaviors relevant to health assessment

Cultural group	Cultural variations (common belief/practice)	Nursing implications
African Americans	Dialect and slang terms require careful communication to prevent error (i.e., "bad" may mean "good").	Question the client's meaning or intent.
Mexican Americans	Eye behavior is important. An individual who looks at and admires a child without touching the child has given the child the "evil eye."	Always touch the child you are examining or admiring.
Native Americans	Eye contact is considered a sign of disrespect and is thus avoided.	Recognize that the client may be attentive and interested even though eye contact is avoided.
Appalachians	Eye contact is considered impolite or a sign of hostility. Verbal patter may be confusing.	Avoid excessive eye contact. Clarify statements.
American Eskimos	Body language is very important. The individual seldom disagrees publicly with others. Client may nod yes to be polite, even if not in agreement.	Monitor own body language closely as well as client's to detect meaning.
Jewish Americans	Orthodox Jews consider excess touching, particularly from members of the opposite sex, offensive.	Establish whether client is an Orthodox Jew and avoid excessive touch.
Chinese Americans	Individual may nod head to indicate yes or shake head to indicate no. Excessive eye contact indicates rudeness. Excessive touch is offensive.	Ask questions carefully and clarify responses. Avoid excessive eye contact and touch.
Filipino Americans	Offending people is to be avoided at all cost. Nonverbal behavior is very important.	Monitor nonverbal behaviors of self and client, being sensitive to physical and emotional discomfort or concerns of the client.
Haitian Americans	Touch is used in conversation. Direct eye contact is used to gain attention and respect during communication.	Use direct eye contact when communicating.
East Indian Hindu Americans	Women avoid eye contact as a sign of respect.	Be aware that men may view eye contact by women as offensive. Avoid eye contact.
Vietnamese Americans	Avoidance of eye contact is a sign of respect. The head is considered sacred; it is not polite to pat the head. An upturned palm is offensive in communication.	Limit eye contact. Touch the head only when mandated and explain clearly before proceeding to do so. Avoid hand gesturing.

From Giger, J., & Davidhizar, R. (1995) *Transcultural Nursing*, ed. 2, St. Louis: Mosby; also appears in Kozier, B., Erb, G., Blaise, K., Johnson, J. Y., & Smith-Temple, J. (1993). *Techniques in clinical nursing* (ed. 2). Menlo Park, Calif.: Addison-Wesley.

Giger and Davidhizar's Transcultural Assessment Model has also been shown to be applicable to the analysis of current trends in multiculturalism in health care (Smith, 1998a).

Refinement through research

Refinement of the Giger and Davidhizar's Transcultural Assessment Model is also being enhanced through research efforts of various individuals. For example, in 1992, a graduate student from the University of Kansas completed a master's thesis titled "Utilizing Giger and Davidhizar's Transcultural Assessment Model for the Cultural Assessment of Farm Families" (Daugherty, 1992). In 1993, a graduate student at Georgia Southern University at Statesboro conducted a research study on the health beliefs and self-care practices of hypertensive African-American women using Giger and Davidhizar's Transcultural Assessment Model as a theoretical framework to guide and evaluate research findings (Walthour, 1993). In addition to these master's theses, several doctoral dissertations have been completed using the model. In 1995, a group of interdisciplinary researchers (nursing, behavioral medicine, lipoprotein research, human genetics, preventive medicine, nutrition, biostatistics) at the University of Alabama at Birmingham and Emory University received $750,000 from the Uniformed Health Sciences, University of the Health Sciences, Tri-Services Nursing Military Research Group, Department of Defense, to identify behavioral risk-reduction strategies and chronic indicators for premenopausal African-American women with coronary heart disease or associated risk factors. The model served as the overarching theoretical framework to test its usefulness as an educational tool to enhance and promote compliance. The study is titled "Culturally Appropriate Behavioral Risk Reduction Strategies and Chronic Indicators and High Risk Factors for Premenopausal African-American Women (25-45) with Coronary Heart Disease" (Giger & Strickland, 1995).

In 1998, Linda Smith, a doctoral student at the University of Alabama at Birmingham, completed a pilot study utilizing Giger and Davidhizar's Transcultural Assessment Model as the overarching theoretical framework to guide the study. The primary purpose of this descriptive correlational study was to describe the relationship among scores and subscores on scales measuring concepts of cultural competence. A secondary purpose of this study was to develop reliability and validity data on each of three cultural scales for a population (n = 51) of hospital-based registered nurses. These three scales include (1) the Cultural Attitude Scale (CAS) originally developed by Bonaparte (1977, 1979) and modified by Rooda (1992, 1990); (2) the Cultural Self-Efficacy Scale (CSES) developed by Bernal and Froman (1987); and (3) knowledge-base questions (Rooda, 1990). Each of the scales had previously reported reliability and validity data but were administered to populations potentially different from hospital-employed RNs. The Giger and Davidhizar Transcultural Assessment Model served as the theoretical foundation, and the Cultural Self-Efficacy Scale (CSES), the Cultural Attitude Scale (CAS), and knowledge base questions were the chosen instruments. The analysis of the data indicates that for this study population, the reliability analysis scale (al-

pha) for the 58-item CSES was 0.9778, was 0.6038 for the 22 knowledge base questions, and was 0.6412 for the 40-item CAS. Canonical correlation analysis was performed between a set of attitude variables and a set of self-efficacy variables. Both sets of variables demonstrated statistically significant relationships (at an a priori alpha of 0.05) to each other (with an approximate eta-squared value for practical significance of 0.365), providing sufficient evidence to reject the nonrelationship null hypothesis. For this sample and for these data, cultural self-efficacy toward Asian, African-American, and Hispanic clients and self-efficacy regarding nursing skills when caring for diverse clients related to cultural attitudes and cultural self-efficacy. Nursing care, cultural health beliefs, and cultural health attitudes are related to attitudes toward care of diverse clients. Both sets of variables relate to each other as qualities of culturally competent nursing care (Smith, 1998b).

In 1998, Dr. Sharon S. Mullen and Dr. Carla G. Phillips, Ohio University, School of Nursing, Athens, Ohio, also utilized Giger and Davidhizar's Transcultural Assessment Model as the overarching theoretical framework to explore the cultural beliefs of Southeastern Ohio Appalachians. The primary purpose of the qualitative ethnographic study was to identify cultural beliefs of Southeastern Ohio Appalachians as a means of providing culturally competent nursing care. Giger and Davidhizar's Transcultural Assessment Model was used to identify cultural beliefs from six phenomena of interest, which include (1) communication, (2) space, (3) social organization, (4) time, (5) environmental control, and (6) biological variations. Subjects were 14 adults who were native to southeasern Ohio and who had resided in the area their entire life. Giger and Davidhizar's Transcultural Assessment Model, which also included interview questions and observational guidelines, was used for structured interviews. Findings from this study suggest that these individuals were more socially inclined, communicate more openly, have more of an internal locus of control, have fewer personal space needs, are more future oriented, use no significant home remedies, are more conscientious about getting to appointments on time, and are more likely to follow medical protocols than Appalachians in general. However, findings also suggest that these individuals still resembled the mainstream Appalachian population in that they tended to have a strong character, tended to be stoic and nonassertive, and also tended to have a strong belief in a Supreme Being.

ORGANIZATION OF THE TEXT

In this book the six cultural phenomena (communication, space, social organization, time, environmental control, and biological variations) are presented in individual chapters with areas that must be assessed when working with clients from multicultural populations. In addition, these six phenomena are applied to the care and management of clients in 15 subcultural groups found in the United States and throughout the world. A comprehensive nursing assessment is necessary for both the nurse practitioner and the researcher to provide culturally appropriate nursing care.

References

Aamodt, A.M. (1978). The care component in a health and healing system. In Bauwens, E. (Ed.), *The anthropology of health,* St. Louis: Mosby.

Affonso, D. (1979). Framework for cultural assessment. In Clark, A.L. (Ed.), *Childbearing: a nursing perspective* (ed. 2) (pp. 107-119). Philadelphia: F.A. Davis.

Andrews, M., & Boyle, J. (1996). *Transcultural concepts in nursing care.* Glenview, Ill.: Scott, Foresman.

Bernal, H., & Froman, R. (1987). The confidence of community health nurses in caring for ethnically diverse populations. *Image: Journal of Nursing Scholarship, 19*(4), 201-203.

Bloch, B. (1983). Bloch's assessment guide for ethnic/cultural variations. In Orque, M.S., & Bloch, B., & Monrroy, L.S.A. (Eds.), *Ethnic nursing care: a multicultural approach* (pp. 49-75). St. Louis: Mosby.

Bonaparte, B.H.G. (1977). *An investigation of the relation between ego defensiveness and open-closed mindedness of female registered professional nurses and their attitude toward culturally different patients.* Unpublished doctoral dissertation, New York, New York.

Bonaparte, B.H.G. (1979). Ego defensiveness, open-closed mindedness, and nurses' attitude toward culturally different patients. *Nursing Research, 28*(3), 166-172.

Bowen, M., & Davidhizar, R. (1991). Communication with the client in the OR. *Today's OR Nurse, 1,* 11-14.

Branch, M.F., & Paxton, P.P. (Eds.). (1976). *Providing safe nursing care for ethnic people of color.* Englewood Cliffs, N.J.: Prentice-Hall.

Brink, P.J. (1990a). *Transcultural nursing: a book of readings.* Prospect Heights, Ill.: Waveland Press.

Brink, P.J. (1990b). Cultural diversity in nursing: How much can we tolerate? In McClusky, J., & Grace, H. (Eds.), *Current issues in nursing* (ed. 3). St. Louis: Mosby.

Brownlee, A.T. (1978). *Community, culture, and care: a cross-cultural guide for health workers.* St. Louis: Mosby.

Daugherty, B. (1992). *Utilizing Giger and Davidhizar's transcultural assessment model for the cultural assessment of farm families.* Unpublished master's thesis, University of Kansas, Lawrence, Kansas.

Davidhizar, R., & Giger, J. (1998 Nov/Dec). Transcultural patient assessment: a method of advancing dental care. *The Dental Assistant 39(1),* 40-43.

Davidhizar, R., & Giger, J. (1998). Caring for the patient from another culture. *Journal of the Canadian Dental Association, 39*(1), 24-27.

Davidhizar, R., & Giger, J. (1996, Summer). Reflections on the minority elderly in health care. *Hospital Topics, 74*(3), 20-24.

Davidhizar, R., Dowd, S., & Giger, J. (1997a, Jan./Feb.). Managing a multicultural radiology staff. *Radiology Management, 19*(1), 50-55.

Davidhizar, R., Dowd, S., & Giger, J. (1997b, Jan./Feb.). Model for cultural diversity in the radiology department. *Radiologic Technology, 68*(3), 233-238.

Davidhizar, R., Dowd, S., & Giger, J. (1997c, March/April). Cultural differences in pain management. *Radiologic Technology, 68*(4), 345-348.

Dowd, S., Giger, J. & Davidhizar, R. (1998, July/Aug.). Use of the Giger and Davidhizar Model by other Health Professions: contributions of nursing science. *International Nursing Review, 45*(4)119-203.

Geissler, E.M. (1991). Transcultural nursing and nursing diagnosis. *Nursing and Health Care, 12*(4), 190-203.

Giger, J., Davidhizar, R., Johnson, J., & Poole, V. (1997, January). The changing faces of America: using cultural phenomena to improve care. *The Health Care Traveler, 4*(4), 10-40.

Giger, J., Davidhizar, R., Johnson, J., & Poole, V. (1996). Health promotion in minority populations. In Schust, C.S. (Ed.), *Community health: education and promotion manual.* Gaithersburg, Md.: Aspen Publishers.

Giger, J., & Strickland, O. (1995). Behavioral risk reduction strategies for chronic indicators and high risk factors for premenopausal African-American women (25-45) with coronary heart disease, Grant Number N95-019, Department of Defense, Uniformed Health Services, University of the Health Sciences, Tri-Service Nursing Research, Bethesda, Md.

Giger, J., Davidhizar, R., Evers, S., & Ingram, C. (1994). Cultural factors influencing mental health and mental illness. In Taylor, C.M. (Ed.), *Merness' essentials of psychiatric nursing* (ed. 14) (pp. 217-236). St. Louis: Mosby.

Giger, J. Davidhizar, R., & Wieczorek, S. (1993). Culture and ethnicity. In Bobak, I., & Jensen, M. (Eds.), *Maternity and gynecological care* (ed. 5) (pp. 43-67). St. Louis: Mosby.

Giger, J. & Davidhizar, R. (1990). Transcultural nursing assessment: a method for advancing practice. *International Nursing Review, 37*(1), 199-203.

Kay, M. (1978). Clinical anthropology. In Bauwens, E.E. (Ed.), *The anthropology of health* (pp. 3-11). St. Louis: Mosby.

Kozier, B., Erb, G., Blaise, K., Johnson, J., & Smith-Temple, J. (1993). *Techniques in clinical nursing* (ed. 2). Reading, Mass.: Addison-Wesley.

Kozier, B., Erb, G., Blaise, K., & Wilkinson, J. (1995). *Fundamentals of nursing* (ed. 2). Reading, Mass.: Addison-Wesley.

Leininger, M. (1977). Transcultural nursing and a proposed conceptual framework. In Leininger, M. (Ed.), *Transcultural nursing care of infants and children: proceedings from the first transcultural conference.* Salt Lake City: University of Utah.

Leininger, M. (1985a). *Qualitative research methods in nursing.* Orlando, Fla.: Grune & Stratton.

Leininger, M. (1985b). Transcultural care, diversity and universality: a theory of nursing. *Nursing and Health Care, 6*(4), 209-212.

Leininger, M. (1991). Transcultural nursing: the study and practice field. *Imprint, 38*(2), 55-66.

Mosby's medical, nursing, and allied health dictionary. (1994) (ed. 4). St. Louis: Mosby.

Murdock, G.P, et al. (1971). *Outline of cultural materials* (ed. 4). New Haven, Conn.: Human Relations Area Files.

Mullens, S., Phillips, C. (1998). Cultural beliefs of Southeastern Ohio Appalachians. *Proceedings of the Fourth International and Interdisciplinary Health Reasearch Symposium 1998 Health Care and Culture.* School of Nursing, West Virginia University, Morgantown, Va. 65 pp. 57.

Orque, M.S. (1983). Orque's ethnic/cultural system: a framework for ethnic nursing care. In Orque, M.S., & Bloch, B., Monrroy, L.S.A. (Eds.), *Ethnic nursing care: a multi-cultural approach* (pp. 5-48). St. Louis: Mosby.

Purnell, L.D., & Paulanka, B.J. (Eds.) (1998). Transcultural health care. Philadelphia: F.A. Davis.

Rooda, L. (1990). *Knowledge and attitudes of nurses toward culturally diverse patients.* Unpublished doctoral dissertation, Purdue University, West Lafayette, Indiana.

Rooda, L. (1992). Attitudes of nurses toward culturally diverse patients: an examination of the social contact theory. *Journal of the National Black Nurses Association, 6*(1), 48-56.

Rund, N., & Krause, L. (1978). Health attitudes and your health programs. In Bauwens, E.E. (Eds.), *The anthropology of health* (pp. 73-78). St. Louis: Mosby.

Sheridan, D., & Zimbler, E. (1993). *Nursing management skills: a modular self-assessment series, module IV, transcultural nursing.* New York: National League for Nursing.

Smith, L. (1998a). Trends in multiculturalism in health care. *Hospital Material Management Quarterly, 20*(1), 61-69.

Smith, L. (1998b). Concept analysis: culture competence. *Journal of Cultural Diversity, 5*(1), 4-10.

Smith, L. (1998c). Cultural competence for nurses: canonical correlation of two culture scales. Unpublished.

Spector, R. (1996). *Cultural diversity in health and illness* (ed. 3). Norwalk, Conn.: Appleton & Lange.

Spector, R. (1993). Culture, ethnicity, and nursing. In Potter, P., & Perry, A. (Eds.), *Fundamentals of nursing: concepts, process, and practice* (ed. 3). St. Louis: Mosby.

Stokes, G. (1991). A transcultural nurse is about. *Senior Nurse, 11*(1), 40-42.

Tripp-Reimer, T. (1984a). Research in cultural diversity. *Western Journal of Nursing Research, 6*(3), 353-355.

Tripp-Reimer, T. (1984b). Cultural assessment. In Bellack, J.P., & Bamford, P.A. (Eds.), *Nursing assessment: a multidimensional approach* (pp. 226-246). Monterey, Calif.: Wadsworth.

Tripp-Reimer, T., Brink, P., & Saunders, J. (1984). Cultural assessment: content and process. *Nursing Outlook, 32*(2), 78-82.

Tripp-Reimer, T., & Dougherty, M.C. (1985). Cross-cultural nursing research. *Annual Review of Nursing Research, 3,* 77-104.

Tripp-Reimer, T., & Friedl, M. (1977). Appalachians: a neglected minority. *Nursing Clinics of North America, 12*(1), 41-54.

United States Department of Commerce, Bureau of Census (1998). *Population projection of the United States by age, sex, race, and Hispanic Origins:* 1990 to 2050. Washington, D.C.: U.S. Government Printing Office. Internet update.

Walthour, E. (1993). *Health beliefs and self-care practices of hypertensive African-Americans.* Unpublished master's thesis, Georgia Southern University, Statesboro, Ga.

Wenger, F. (1989). President's address. *Transcultural Nursing Society Newsletter, 9*(1), 3.

CHAPTER 2 Communication

BEHAVIORAL OBJECTIVES

After reading this chapter, the nurse will be able to:

1. Describe the importance of communication as it relates to transcultural nursing assessment.
2. Delineate barriers to communication that hinder the development of a nurse-client relationship in transcultural settings.
3. Understand the importance of dialect, style, volume, use of touch, context of speech, and kinesics and their relationship to transcultural nursing assessment and care.
4. Describe appropriate nursing intervention techniques to develop positive communication in the nurse-client relationship.
5. Understand the significance of nonverbal communication and the use of silence and their relationship to transcultural nursing assessment and care.
6. Explain the significance of the structure and format of names in various cultural groups.
7. Explain the significance of variations in word meanings across and within various cultural and ethnic groups.

The word "communication" comes from the Latin verb *communicāre:* 'to make common, share, participate, or impart' (Guralnik, 1984). Communication, however, goes further than this definition implies and embraces the entire realm of human interaction and behavior. All behavior, whether verbal or nonverbal, in the presence of another individual is communication (Potter & Perry, 1996; Watzlawich, Beavin, & Jackson, 1967; Haber, 1997).

As the matrix of all thought and relationships among people, communication provides the means by which people connect. It establishes a sense of commonality with others and permits the sharing of information, signals, or messages in the form of ideas and feelings. Communication is a continuous process by which one person may affect another through written or oral language, gestures, facial expressions, body language, space, or other symbols.

Nurses have long recognized the importance of communication in the healing process (Reakes, 1997; Buckett, 1995). Communication is the core of most nursing curricula. Despite this, communication frequently presents barriers between nurses and clients, especially when the nurses and the clients are from different cultural backgrounds. If the nurse and the client do not speak the same language, or if communication styles and patterns differ, both the nurse and the client may feel alienated and helpless. A client who does not understand what is happening or who feels misunderstood may appear angry, noncompliant, or withdrawn. When communication is impaired, often the physical healing process may be impaired. Nurses may also feel angry and helpless if their communication is not understood or if they cannot understand the client. Without the ability to communicate, care will be inadequate. Nurses need to have not only a working knowledge of communication with clients of the same culture, but also a thorough awareness of racial, cultural, and social factors that may affect communication with persons from other cultures. Health care settings must have an organizational climate for multiculturalism (Bruhn, 1996; Giger & Davidhizar, 1996). Fielding and Llewelyn (1987) related that although communication skills are needed in nursing curricula, the more important issue is the broader understanding of the client from a cultural perspective.

Nurses must have an awareness of how an individual, though speaking the same language, may differ in communication patterns and understandings as a result of cultural orientation. Nurses must also have communication skills in relating to individuals who do not speak a familiar language (Kasch, 1984; Knowles, 1983; Taylor, Malone, & Kavanagh, 1997; Buttaglia, 1992). Most nurses generally assume that their perceptions and assessment of the client's health status are accurate and congruent with those of the client. Despite the client education process, however, there is evidence that discrepancies in perceptions persist. These discrepancies should be of particular concern to the nurse when providing transcultural nursing care because they may interfere with the provision of that care. Many factors obstruct quality client care, including poor communication, noncompliance with the treatment regimen, inadequate or unnecessary treatment, and ethical problems. All these factors combine to create discrepancies in perceptions between nurse and client (Molzahn & Northcott, 1989; Andrews & Boyle, 1995).

COMMUNICATION AND CULTURE

Communication and culture are closely intertwined. Communication is the means by which culture is transmitted and preserved (Delgado, 1983). Culture influences how feelings are expressed and what verbal and nonverbal expressions are appropriate. Americans may be more likely to conceal feelings, and the United States is generally considered a low-touch culture, whereas a member of an Eastern culture may be open and loud with expressions of grief, anger, or joy and may use touch more (Hall, 1966; Thayer, 1988; Cheng & Barlas; 1992). Other cultural variables, such as the perception of time, bodily contact, and territorial rights, also influence communication. The cultural differences in contact can be quite dramatic. Sidney Jourard (1971) reported that when touch between pairs of people in coffee shops around the world was studied, there was more touch in certain cities. For example, it was reported that touch occurred as frequently as 180 times an hour between couples in San Juan, Puerto Rico, and 110 times an hour in Paris, France. In other cities there was less touch; specifically, touch occurred two times an hour between couples in Gainesville, Florida, and zero times an hour in London, England.

Cultural patterns of communication are embedded early and are found in childrearing practices (Capirci, Iverson, Pizzuto & Volterra, 1996). Gibson (1984) studied the playgrounds and beaches of Greece, the Soviet Union, and the United States and compared the frequency and nature of touch between caregivers and children ranging from 2 to 5 years of age. The analysis of data indicates that although rates of touching for retrieving or punishing the children were similar, rates of touching for soothing, holding, and playing were dissimilar. American children were less likely to be touched than children from other cultures. The communication practices of persons in individual cultural groups affect the expression of ideas and feelings, decision making, and communication strategies. The communication of an individual reflects, determines, and consequently molds the culture (Hedlund, 1992; Kretch, Crutchfield, & Ballachey, 1962). In other words, a culture may be limited and molded by its communication practices. Sapir (1929) proposed that individuals are at the mercy of the particular language that has become the medium of expression of their society. Experiences are determined by language habits that predispose the individual to certain conceptions of the world and choices of interpretation. Kayser (1996) noted that educational programming that is provided to children of different cultural and linguistic backgrounds is critical for the successful implementation of language interventions. Focusing on English language development while minimizing learning opportunities limits children who do not speak English as their first language from development of higher-level cognitive skills. However, despite the costly surge in bilingual courses in the United States, there is opposition: 35% of voters say bilingual education programs slow down learning English and should be eliminated (Headden, 1995).

Variations in communication may be limited to specific meanings for a few individuals in a small group, for example, a family group. On the other hand, unique communication patterns are frequently found among persons from the same ethnic and cultural group such as the Gypsies or the Amish (Banks and Banks, 1995; Nolt, 1992). Some persons consider the deaf a cultural group. In any case, persons who are deaf have a unique language and communication patterns that require special communication approaches to be utilized by the nurse (McLeod & Bently, 1996). However, the nurse must be cautious about assuming that a certain communication pattern can be generalized to all persons in a designated cultural group because communication patterns are often unique. In assessing the client, the nurse should keep in mind common cultural patterns and approach the client as an individual who should not be categorized because of cultural heritage.

LINGUISTICS

Because communication is a broad concept and encompasses all human behavior, it has been conceptualized in many ways. One way is to consider the structure of communication, as in linguistics. The major focus on the structure of communication has been developed within the fields of ethnomethodology in sociology and of linguistics in anthropology. Structure may be perceived as a form of language and the use of words and behaviors to construct messages. The role of ethnomethodologists is to consider the structure and effects of communication and to look at rules of communication and the consequences of breaking these rules. Ethnomethodologists not only have emphasized the study of the structure and rules of language, but also have studied the structure and

rules of nonverbal communication (Sudnow, 1967). Linguistics is the area within anthropology concerned with the study of the structure of language. Linguistic patterns represent more than the use of grammatically nonequivalent words; these patterns can create real disparity in social treatment.

FUNCTIONS OF COMMUNICATION

Another way to think about communication is to consider what it achieves or accomplishes in human interaction. Consideration of the functions of communication refers to examining what the communication accomplishes rather than how the communication is structured. A relationship exists between communication structure and communication function in the sense that structure does affect function.

As a part of human interaction, communication discloses information or provides a specific message. Messages can be sent with no expectation of a response. Included in the disclosure of information may be an element of self-disclosure. Communication may or may not be intended as a method of self-disclosure or a means to provide information about the self or the individual's perception of self (Hedlund, 1992; Luft & Ingham, 1984). Perceptions of self include acts that describe the self and estimations of self-worth. In some situations self-awareness may be achieved through communication. This function of communication involves interaction with people. Through communication with others, an individual may become more aware of personal feelings.

PROCESS OF COMMUNICATION

Communication may be conceptualized as a process that includes a sender, a transmitting device, signals, a receiver, and feedback (Murray & Zentner, 1993). A sender attempts to relay a message, an idea, or information to another person or group through the use of signals or symbols. Many factors influence how the message is given and how it is received. For example, physical health, emotional well-being, the situation being discussed and the meaning it has, other distractions, knowledge of the matter being discussed, skill at communicating, and attitudes toward the other person and the subject being discussed may all affect the communication that

---

Box 2-1

FACTORS INFLUENCING COMMUNICATION

1. Physical health and emotional well-being
2. The situation being discussed and its meaning
3. Distractions to the communication process
4. Knowledge of the matter being discussed
5. Skill at communicating
6. Attitudes toward the other person and toward the subject being discussed
7. Personal needs and interests
8. Background, including cultural, social, and philosophical values
9. The senses involved and their functional ability
10. Personal tendency to make judgments and be judgmental of others
11. The environment in which the communication occurs
12. Past experiences that relate to the current situation

---

takes place (Box 2-1). In addition, personal needs and interests; background, including cultural, social, and philosophical values; the senses and their functional ability; personal tendency to make judgments and be judgmental of others; the environment in which the communication takes place; and past experiences that relate or are related to the present situation, all may affect the message that is received. The receiver then interprets the message. Feedback is given to the sender about the message, and more communication may occur. If no feedback is given, there may be no reciprocal interaction.

Although the process of communication is universal, nurses should be aware that styles and types of feedback may be unique to certain cultural groups. For example, before the assimilation of the Alaskan Eskimo into the American culture, the Alaskan Eskimo would indicate a message was received by blinking rather than making a verbal response (Davidhizar, 1988c). Nonverbal responses are also found in the Vietnamese. Vietnamese persons may smile, but the smile may not indicate understanding. A Vietnamese person may say yes simply to avoid confrontation or out of a desire to please. A smile may cover up disturbed feelings. Nodding, which

nurses commonly interpret as understanding and compliance, may, for a Vietnamese individual, simply indicate respect for the person talking (Hoang & Erickson, 1982; Rocereto, 1981). The nurse may be surprised later when the Vietnamese client who smiled and nodded does not follow through with the instructions given.

Uchida (1997) has proposed a model of women's intercultural communication and suggests that this culture-building model can guide the analysis of intercultural communication events. Uchida (1997) has suggested that through events such as international wives' support groups, participants can attempt to create a shared personhood using gendered practices as resources of culture building.

In today's health care system, optimal communication must also involve modern technology. E-mail, cell phones, and voice mail have greatly improved timeliness in communication. The infamous and often frustrating "telephone tag" has been significantly reduced. E-mail messages can be printed off to provide hard copy for documentation purposes. Notebook computers with cell-phone modem connections to access clinical information can be used in a client's home in a rural setting to give clients more efficient service. The nurse needs to be able to use the Internet and do website searches to keep up to date on health care information (Gunderson, 1996; Treger, 1996).

VERBAL AND NONVERBAL COMMUNICATION

Another way to conceptualize communication is in terms of verbal and nonverbal behavior (Box 2-2). Communication first of all involves language or verbal communication, including vocabulary or a repertoire of words and grammatical structure (Barkauskas, 1994).

Although foreign persons presently need to demonstrate English proficiency to obtain United States citizenship, many persons the nurse will encounter in the United States may not be fluent in English. In 1994 23 million (9%) of the U.S. population was foreign born. Among the foreign born in 1998, 68% were White, 7% were Black, and 21% were Asians and Pacific Islanders. Nearly half (46%) of all immi-

---

Box 2-2

VERBAL AND NONVERBAL COMMUNICATION

LANGUAGE OR VERBAL COMMUNICATION
1. Vocabulary
2. Grammatical structure
3. Voice qualities
4. Intonation
5. Rhythm
6. Speed
7. Pronunciation
8. Silence

NONVERBAL COMMUNICATION
1. Touch
2. Facial expression
3. Eye movement
4. Body posture

COMMUNICATIONS THAT COMBINE VERBAL AND NONVERBAL ELEMENTS
1. Warmth
2. Humor

---

grants were Hispanics and Asians, with Mexicans (6 million) making up the largest group and Filipinos making up the second largest (1 million) (Information Please Almanac, 1998). California was the state with the largest immigrant population in 1998 (8 million) with these immigrants comprising over one third of all immigrants to the United States (Information Please Almanac, 1998). The *Statistical Abstract of the United States* (1997) reports that according to the 1990 census, persons speaking English in home over 5 years of age accounted for 198,601,000 persons, with 17,339,000 speaking Spanish, 1,702,000 French, 1,547,000 Italian, 1,249,000 Chinese, 843,000 Tagalog, and 723,000 Polish. Vietnamese was spoken by 507,000, Portugese by 430,000, Japanese by 428,000, Greek by 388,000, Arabic by 355,000, and Hindi by 331,000. Russian, Yiddish, Thai, Persian, French Creole, Armenian, Navaho, Hungarian, Hebrew, Dutch, Khmer (Cambodian), and Gujarathi were all spoken by over 100,000 people. In addition to these persons registered as living in households, many other non–English speaking persons are in the United States as

visitors, on temporary visas, or illegally. Approximately one sixth (31,845,000) persons reported they spoke another language besides English in the home, yet only a small minority of caregivers speak a language another than English (Statistical Abstract of the United States, 1997).

It is important to appreciate that along with language, significant communication cues are received from voice quality, intonation, rhythm, and speed as well as from the pronunciation used. Dialect may differ significantly among persons both across and within cultures. Silence during communication may itself be a significant part of the message.

Communication involves nonverbal messages, which include touch, facial expressions, eye behavior, body posture, and the use of space (Giger & Davidhizar, 1990a). Spatial behavior also affects communication and encompasses a variety of behaviors, including proximity to others and to objects in the environment and movement (see Chapter 3). Although nonverbal communication is powerful and honest, its importance and meaning vary among and within cultures; therefore it is essential that the nurse have an awareness and appreciation of the role that body language may have in the communication process. In addition, some communications combine nonverbal and verbal components in the message that is sent. Two examples of combination messages are warmth and humor.

Language, or verbal communication

Language is basic to communication. Without language the higher-order cognitive processes of thinking, reasoning, and generalizing cannot be attained. Words are tools or symbols used to express ideas and feelings or to identify or describe objects. Words shape experiences and influence cultural perceptions. Words convey interpretations and influence relationships (Murray & Zentner, 1993; Pirandello 1970; Talbot, 1996). Although words provide a special way of looking at the world, the same words often have different meanings for different individuals within cultural groups. In addition, word meanings change over time and in different situations. It is important to ascertain that the message is received and understood as the sender intended. As early as 1954,

Sullivan emphasized the importance of ongoing validation in a therapeutic relationship to verify interpretations made on the behavior and words of another. Even today, this validation remains relevant in a nurse-client relationship in which many experiential, educational, and cultural differences are present. Smith and Cantrell (1988) reported a study comparing the effect of personal questions and physical distance on anxiety rates. Pulse rates were found to be higher when the investigator asked personal questions, regardless of the physical distance from subjects. Although the data from this study indicate that the most important part of a message may be verbal, the opposite has also been found to be true. Thus both verbal and nonverbal communication must be considered before a conclusion about the true meaning of a message can be determined.

To provide culturally appropriate nursing care, nurses must separate values based on their own cultural background from the values of the clients to whom care is given. Transcultural communication and understanding break down when caregivers project their own culturally specific values and behaviors onto the client. Thiederman (1986) has suggested that projection of values as well as hindering care may actually contribute to noncompliance.

Vocabulary Even though people may speak the same language, establishing communication is often difficult because word meanings for both the sender and the receiver vary based on past experiences and learning. Words have both denotative and connotative meanings. A denotative meaning is one that is in general use by most persons who share a common language. A connotative meaning usually arises from a person's personal experience. For example, although all Americans are likely to share the same general denotative meaning for the word "pig," depending on the occupation and cultural perception of the person, the connotation may be entirely different and may precipitate completely different reactions. The word "pig" will invoke either negative or positive reactions from certain people based on occupation and culture. For example, an Orthodox Jew's reactions will differ from those of a pig farmer. For an Orthodox Jew the word "pig" is synonymous with the word "unclean" or "unholy" and thus

should be avoided. On the other hand, for a pig farmer the word "pig" implies a clean, wholesome means of making a living. Numerous conflicts resulting from differences in word meaning among various ethnic and racial groups are reported in the literature. Among her many famous cultural studies, Margaret Mead (1947) reported on the different meanings that the word "compromise" carries for an Englishman and an American:

In Britain, the word "compromise" is a good word, and one may speak approvingly of any arrangement which has been a compromise, including, very often one in which the other side has gained more than fifty per cent of the points at issue. Where, in Britain, to compromise means to work out a good solution, in America it usually means to work out a bad one, a solution in which all the points of importance are lost.

Often people who have learned a language have learned the meaning for the word in only one context. For example, Díaz-Duque (1982) reported that a Hispanic person who was told he was going "to be discharged tomorrow" somehow interpreted this to mean that he was going to develop "a discharge from below." Díaz-Duque also indicated that for Hispanics problems arise with cognates such as constipation because for Hispanics this term generally refers to nasal congestion rather than intestinal constipation.

Although barriers exist when people speak the same language, more profound barriers are present when different languages are spoken. Each language has a whole set of unconscious assumptions about the world and life. Understanding differences in the meaning of words can provide insight into people of different cultures. For example, many English-speaking Americans are puzzled by what seems to be a different time orientation among Hispanic peoples. An understanding of the meaning of the word "time" helps provide insight into this different orientation. In Spanish, time is defined as "passing"—a clock "passes time" or "moves," whereas in English a clock "runs." If time is moving rapidly, as English usage declares, we must hurry. On the other hand, the Spanish definition allows for a more leisurely attitude (Randall-David, 1989). Such cultural understandings can provide insight into the reasons why Spanish individuals are often late for health care appointments.

Language reflects the dominant concerns and interests of a people, which can be noted in the number of words for certain things. Some classic studies have reported that certain cultures use many words to describe a particular object of importance. Boas (1938) pointed out that Eskimos have 20 or so words for snow depending on consistency and texture. The language of a people is a key that unlocks their culture. A nurse who is familiar with the language of clients will have the best chance of gaining insight into their culture.

Names Names have a special psychological and cultural significance. All people have names, and in every culture naming a newborn is considered important. The considerations that go into the naming process vary greatly from culture to culture. For example, in Roman tradition there is a given name for boys; a family name, which is second; and a third name that specifies an extended family unit. The name Caius Julius Caesar illustrates the importance of tribal connections as well as male chauvinism (Clemmens, 1988). In Roman times girls had only one name, the female version of the family name; for example, Caesar's sister was Julia, as was his aunt, father's sister, and so on. During the early Roman times women lacked individuality and thus in Roman society were not worth being named.

The Hebrew tradition has a patrilineal way of looking at names, that is, a given name plus "son of." Mothers' names are not included. A spiritual and traditional continuity is evidenced in this system of naming. The Hebrew tradition can be seen today in Iceland, where all males have their given names, followed by their father's given name, ending in "son." In contemporary Western society, as well, there are systems of naming. The most common one in the dominant culture in the United States is a patrilineal succession plus one or more given names. In the United States the middle name is often one that relates to the family, such as the mother's maiden name.

The Russian system of naming provides a clue to the significance placed on relating son and father, as well as daughter and father. The mother is left out, with Russians habitually addressing each other by the individual's given name together with the patronymic. The family name is omitted. Spaniards and Latin Americans include women more than other cultures, with children carrying their father's name first and their mother's name second. The mother's name usually appears only on documents and for formal occasions because the addition of the mother's name makes the name quite long. Another variation is seen in the Dutch, who have the option of using both the husband's and the wife's family names jointly. Among the various cultures the most common theme of naming is pride in lineage (Clemmens, 1985, 1988).

Grammatical structure Cultural differences are reflected in grammatical structure and the use and meaning of phrases. "That's all right" is a phrase frequently used by African Americans when they actually mean, "I have some plans, but I am not telling you what they are" (Mitchell, 1978). In another example, for some Hispanic-American women, having a stillborn child or a miscarriage does not equate with a pregnancy. For some Hispanic-American women, a pregnancy is equated only with a successful live birth (Haffner, 1992). It is important for nurses to keep in mind that there is little validity in generalizations about the meaning of phrases by persons in varying cultures.

Length of sentence and speech forms may vary not only with culture, but also with social class. For example, Argyle (1992) noted that persons from the lower class commonly use short, simple sentences and are more direct than are persons with more education. Word choice, grammatical structure, speech fluency, and articulation provide cues to social status and class. Jargon is also a speech variation that may prove to be a barrier to communication. Nurses frequently have difficulty expressing things in simple jargon-free language (without medical terms) that clients can understand. On the other hand, a nurse who does not know the jargon used by the clients served may have a difficult time relating to them.

For some cultures, patterns of social amenities can create communication problems. Small talk, social chitchat, and discussion of mundane topics that may appear to "kill time" are necessary as preliminaries for more purposeful discussion. Yet the busy nurse seeking short, succinct answers to questions may be annoyed by the amount of anecdotal information that a Hispanic-American client gives. Many clients tend to add irrelevant material because it lessens embarrassment. They may be more comfortable if attention is not focused on their medical problem, and so they may intersperse actual symptoms with other biographical data. Cultural factors may also play a role in what seems to be verbal rambling. Patients who are used to folk healers believe that information on the weather, the environment, and eating habits are really important pieces of information for the health professional.

Voice qualities Paralinguistics, or paralanguage, refers to something beyond the words themselves. Voice quality, which includes pitch and range, can add an important element to communication. The commonly used phrase, "Don't speak to me in that tone of voice," provides an indication of the significance of this aspect of the communication message.

The softer volume of Asian-American or Native-American speech may be interpreted by the nurse as shyness. On the other hand, the nurse's behavior may be viewed as loud and boisterous if the volume is loud and if there is a deliberate attempt to accent particular words. Sometimes people who speak softly, slowly, and without emphasis on particular words are viewed as "wishy-washy." When the nurse cannot hear what the client is saying, there is a tendency for the nurse to speak louder. It is important to remember that amplifying the volume does not necessarily equate with being understood or understanding (Spector, 1993). Nurses must remember that paralinguistic behavior is an important cultural consideration when they are assessing the client. The nurse can recognize this behavior by listening to nonword vocalizations such as sobbing, laughing, and grunting; tone of voice; and quality of voice.

Intonation Intonation is an important aspect of the communication message. When people say they feel "fine," they may mean they genuinely do or they do not feel fine but do not wish to discuss it. If said sarcastically, it may also mean they feel just the opposite of fine. There is often a latent or hidden

meaning in what a person is saying, and intonation frequently provides the clue that is needed to interpret the true message.

Techniques of intonation vary among cultures. For example, Americans put commands in the form of suggestions and often as questions, whereas Arabic speech contains much emphasis and exaggeration (Argyle, 1992). Some cultures value indirectness and subtlety in speech and may be alienated by the frankness of Western health care professionals. Asian clients, for example, may interpret this method of communication as rude, immature, and lacking finesse. On the other hand, health care professionals may label Asian clients as evasive, fearful, and unable to confront problems (Sue & Sue, 1990).

Rhythm Rhythm also varies from culture to culture; some people have a melodic rhythm to their verbal communication, whereas others appear to lack rhythm. Rhythm may also vary among persons within a culture. For example, some U.S. African-American ministers use a singsong rhythm to deliver fiery sermons.

Speed Rate and volume of speech frequently provide a clue to an individual's mood. A depressed person will tend to talk slowly and quietly, whereas an aggressive, dominating person is more apt to talk rapidly and loudly.

Pronunciation Persons from some cultural groups may be identified by their dialect, such as Black dialect or Black English, Irish brogue, or Brooklyn accent. Black English includes words and expressions not commonly found in Standard English and is presently spoken by African Americans. It ranges on a continuum from being more to less Africanized, with the mild end of the continuum being much like Standard English (Taylor, 1976). However, even persons with dialects at the mild end of the continuum may have a "Black sound" that identifies them as African American. A person may hear a boil called a "raisin," or difficult breathing called "the smothers" (Snow, 1976); dentures may be called "racks" (Dillard, 1973). Some African Americans speak in dialect when they do not want others to understand what is being said. One function of the Black dialect may be to enhance the in-group solidarity of African Americans (Taylor, 1976).

"Ahs," "ers," and grunts also provide important dimensions to communication. Although hesitations may indicate a person who is unsure of self and slow to make a commitment, for some cultures this can have the opposite meaning.

Silence The meaning of silence varies among cultural groups. Silences may be thoughtful, or they may be blank and empty when the individual has nothing to say. A silence in a conversation may also indicate stubbornness and resistiveness, or apprehension or discomfort. Silence may be viewed by some cultural groups as extremely uncomfortable; therefore, attempts may be made to fill every gap with conversation. Persons in other cultural groups value silence and view it as essential to understanding a person's needs. Many Native Americans have this latter view of silence just as some traditional Chinese and Japanese persons have. Therefore, when one of these persons is speaking and suddenly stops, what may be implied is that the person wants the nurse to consider the content of what has been said before continuing. Other cultures may use silence in yet other ways. For example, English and Arabic persons use silence for privacy, whereas Russian, French, and Spanish persons may use silence to indicate agreement between parties. Some persons in Asian cultures may view silence as a sign of respect, particularly to an elder. Mexicans may use silence when instructions are given by a person in authority rather than showing the disrespect of disagreement (de Paula, Lagana, & González-Ramírez, 1996).

Nurses need to be aware of possible meanings of silence so that personal anxiety does not promote the silence to be interrupted prematurely or to be nontherapeutic. A nurse who understands the therapeutic value of silence can use this understanding to enhance care of clients from other cultures.

Nonverbal communication

In his early and classic work, Hall (1966) suggested that 65% of the message received in communication is nonverbal. Through body language or motions (kinetic behavior), the person conveys what cannot or may not be said in words. For a message to be accurately interpreted, not only must words be translated, but also the meaning held by nuances, intonation patterns, and facial expressions. Just as verbal behavior may undo nonverbal behavior, nonverbal behavior may repeat, clarify, contradict, modify, emphasize, or regulate the flow of communication. Nonverbal behavior is less significant as an isolated behavior, but it does add to the whole communication message. To understand the client, the nurse may wish to validate impressions with other health team members, since nonverbal behavior is often interpreted differently by different people. It is important for the nurse to be aware not only of the client's nonverbal behavior, but also of personal nonverbal behavior that may add to, undo, or contradict verbal communication (Reusch, 1961).

Touch Touch, or tactile sensation, is a powerful form of communication that can be used to bridge distances between nurse and client (Davidhizar & Giger, 1988; Giger, Davidhizar, & Wieczorek, 1993; Bronstein, 1996). Touch has many meanings (Box 2-3). It can connect people, provide affirmation, be reassuring, decrease loneliness, share warmth, provide stimulation, and increase self-concept. Being touched can be highly valued and sought after. On the other hand, touch can also communicate frustration, anger, aggression, and punishment; invade personal space and privacy; and convey a negative (such as a subservient) type of relationship with another. In certain situations touch can be disconcerting because it signals power. In a study reported by Thayer (1988), higher-status individuals were found to enjoy more liberties concerning touch than their lower-status associates. It is generally considered improper for individuals to put their hands on superiors.

Touching or lack of touch has cultural significance and symbolism and is a learned behavior. Cultural uses of touch vary. Each culture trains its children to develop different kinds of thresholds to tactile contacts and stimulation so that their organic, constitutional, and temperamental characteristics are accentuated or reduced. Some cultures are characterized by a "do not touch me" way of life. These persons may view fondling and kissing as embarrassing. Some cultures include every possible variation on the theme of tactility. In some countries in North America, the dominant culture generally tolerates hugs and embraces among intimates and a pat

---

Box 2-3

MEANINGS OF TOUCH

Touch may:

1. Connect one individual with another both literally and figuratively by indicating availability
2. Provide affirmation and approval
3. Be reassuring by providing empathy, interest, encouragement, nurturance, caring, trust, concern, gentleness, and protection
4. Decrease loneliness by indicating a relationship with another
5. Share warmth, rapport, love, intimacy, excitement, and happiness
6. Provide stimulation by being a mode of sensation, perception, and experience
7. Increase self-concept
8. Communicate frustration, anger, aggression, or punishment
9. Invade personal space and privacy by physical and psychological assault or intrusion
10. Convey a negative type of relationship with another
11. Cause sexual arousal
12. Allow a person to perform a functional or professional role, such as a physician, barber, or tailor, and be devoid of personal message
13. Reflect cordiality, such as a handshake by business associates and among strangers and acquaintances

---

on the shoulder as a gesture of camaraderie. The firm, hearty handshake is symbolic of good character and a sign of strength. In some Native American groups, however, the hand is offered in some interpersonal interactions but the expectation is different. Rather than a firm handshake, there is a light touch or grasp or even just a passing of hands. Some Native Americans interpret vigorous handshaking as an aggressive action and are offended by a firm, lengthy handshake (Montagu, 1971).

Americans often give a lingering touch a sexual connotation. For some Americans, even casual touching is considered taboo and may be a result of residual Victorian sexual prudence (DeThomaso, 1971). Other cultures also consider touching taboo; the English and Germans carry untouchability further than Americans do. On the other hand, highly tactile cultures do exist, such as the Spanish, Italians,

French, Jews, and South Americans (Montagu, 1971). However, generalizations about different national or ethnic groups in the area of touch can be problematic. For example, Shuter (1976) reported on studies of touch in Costa Rica, Columbia, and Panama. Findings from this study indicate that Latin Americans are commonly high contact oriented individuals. Thayer (1988) also compared couples in Costa Rica, Columbia, and Panama and found that partners in Costa Rica were touched and held more often than partners in the other two countries.

Most cultures give touch different rules and meanings depending on the sex of the persons involved. Whitcher and Fisher (1979) reported that women in a hospital study had a strikingly positive reaction to being touched, with subsequent lowering of blood pressure and anxiety before surgery, whereas men found the same experience upsetting, with a subsequent increase in blood pressure and anxiety. Thayer (1988) reported on a study at the Kansas City International Airport in which it was found that women greeted women and men more physically, with lip kisses, embraces, and more kinds of touch and holding and for longer periods than did men. For men a more common greeting was to shake hands. Regardless of sex, some research has been reported showing that people who are most uncomfortable with touch are also uncomfortable with communicating through other means and have lower self-esteem (Thayer, 1988). Other studies have shown that people who touch more are less afraid and suspicious of other people's motives and intentions and have less anxiety and tension in their everyday lives. In some cultures, leaning back, showing the palm of the hand, and fussing with the other person's collar may be perceived as possible courting behaviors because they may convey an invitation for closeness or affiliation. Touching behaviors such as reaching out during conversation to poke the other person in the chest may be viewed as domineering behavior. However, laughing while being poked may be a way to submit to and at the same time trivialize or eliminate the other person's aggressive intent (Scheflen, 1972).

In some cultures touch is considered magical and healing (Mackey, 1995). For example, some Mexican

Americans and Native Americans view touch as symbolic of "undoing" an evil spell, as a means for prevention of harm, or as a means for healing (Montagu, 1971). On the other hand, Vietnamese Americans may find touching shoulders with another to be anxiety producing, since they believe that the soul can leave the body on physical contact and health problems may result (Rocereto, 1981). The Vietnamese regard the human head as the seat of life and therefore highly personal. Procedures that invade the surface or any orifice of the head can frighten the Vietnamese, who fear that these procedures could provide an escape for the essence of life (Stauffer, 1997).

Nurses must be alert to the rules of touch for individuals encountered in the work role. Lane (1989) found that nurses perceive male clients as being less receptive to touch and closeness than their female counterparts, which could be attributed to the fact that males generally have a larger personal space than females have. Thus it is believed that people generally maintain a greater distance from males (Insel, 1978; Sommer, 1959). Lane concluded that there may be a double standard concerning touch because of societal norms and expectations: male clients may be more receptive to touch than female nurses, but female nurses are perhaps more comfortable with the closeness and touch of female clients.

Although the rules of touch may be unspoken and unwritten, they are usually visible to the observer. A nurse should stay within the rules of touch that are culturally prescribed. It is essential that the nurse use touch judiciously and avoid forcing touch on anyone. Nurses must keep in mind that the message conveyed through touch depends on the attitude of the person involved and on the meaning of touch both to the person touching and to the person being touched. Generally, the need for intimacy and touch is so strong that the satisfaction of that need is a greater influence on behavior than the fears about its inappropriateness (Johnson, 1965). A momentary and seemingly incidental touch can establish a positive, temporary bond between strangers, making them more compliant, helpful, positive, and giving. In all cases touch needs to be applied deliberately, with empathy, and with close attention given to the person's particular needs. All cultural groups have rules, often unspoken, about who touches whom, when, and where. The astute nurse must be mindful of the client's reaction to touch to avoid being perceived as intrusive.

Facial expression Facial expression is commonly used as a guide to a person's feelings. Research shows that generally in Americans, facial expression is used as a part of the communication message. A constant stare with immobile facial muscles indicates coldness. During fear, the eyes open wide, the eyebrows raise, and the mouth becomes tense with the lips drawn back. When a person is angry, the eyes become fixed in a hard stare with the upper lids lowered and the eyebrows drawn down. An angry person's lips are often tightly compressed. Eyes rolled upward may be related to tiredness or may show disapproval. Narrowed eyes, upper lip curled up, and a moving nose commonly signal disgust. A person who is embarrassed or self-conscious may turn the eyes away or down; have a flushed face; pretend to smile; rub the eyes, nose, or face; or twitch the hair or beard or mustache. A direct gaze with raised eyebrows shows surprise (Ekiman & Friesen, 1975; Polhemus, 1978).

Facial expression also varies with culture. Italian, Jewish, African-American, and Hispanic persons smile readily and use many facial expressions, along with gestures and words, to communicate feelings of happiness, pain, or displeasure. Irish, English, and northern European persons tend to have less facial expression and are generally less responsive, especially to strangers. Facial expression can also be used to convey an opposite meaning of the one that is felt; for example, in the Orient, negative emotions may be concealed with a smile (Sue & Sue, 1990).

Eye movement Research on eye movement has vastly increased as a result of the development of computer-based data collection and analysis routines. Eye movement-recording techniques provide a vast array of data to the researcher (Rayner, 1992; Shapiro, 1991; Grainger, 1992).

Eye movement is an important aspect of interpersonal communication. Generally, during social interaction, most people look each other in the eye for short periods (Argyle & Dean, 1965; Davidhizar, 1988a). People use more eye contact while they are listening and may use glances of about 3 to 10 seconds. When glances are longer than this, anxiety is aroused.

Eye contact is an important tool in transcultural nursing assessment and is used both for observation and to initiate interaction. In the United States, those of the dominant culture (predominately Whites) value eye contact as symbolic of a positive self-concept, openness, interest in others, attentiveness, and honesty. Eye contact can communicate warmth and bridge interpersonal gaps between people. A nurse who wears glasses and wants to make a point may increase the intensity of eye contact by taking the glasses off. The removal of glasses has also been cited as a technique that can humanize an individual's face, since barriers to eye contact are removed (Giger & Davidhizar, 1990b; Personal Report for the Executive, 1987).

Lack of eye contact may be interpreted as a sign of shyness, lack of interest, subordination, humility, guilt, embarrassment, low self-esteem, rudeness, thoughtfulness, or dishonesty. In social interaction the speaker glances away from the listener to indicate collecting thoughts or planning what is to be said. If contact is not resumed, disinterest may be interpreted. Pupil dilation and constriction can also be a clue to anxiety level and positive response (Hess, 1965, 1975).

Most Mexican-American and African-American clients are comfortable with eye contact (Murray & Huelskoetter, 1991; Guruge & Donner, 1996). In contrast to this view, others have suggested that through a process of socialization in a "minority status" of relative powerlessness, some African-Americans have learned to deliberately avoid eye contact with others (Giger, Davidhizar, Evers, & Ingram, 1994). In fact, in the United States avoidance of eye contact is sometimes considered rude, an indication of lack of attention, or a sign of mental illness (Bigham, 1964; Giger & Davidhizar, 1990b; Paynich, 1964). On the other hand, McKenzie and Chrisman (1977) reported that for some Filipinos, eye contact that turns away is associated with the possibility of being a witch. Other groups who find eye contact difficult include some Oriental people and some Native Americans who relate eye contact to impoliteness and an invasion of privacy. Many

Native Americans regard eye contact as disrespectful because it is believed that "looking in an individual's eyes" is "looking into an individual's soul" (Henderson & Primeaux, 1981; McRae, 1994).

Persons in certain Indian cultures avoid eye contact with persons of a higher or lower socioeconomic class. The Vietnamese generally practice less eye contact (Giger & Davidhizar, 1990b; Rocereto, 1981), and prolonged eye contact is also avoided by some African Americans (Giger & Davidhizar, 1990b). In some Indian cultures eye contact is given a special sexual significance. Some Orthodox Jews also attribute a sexual significance to eye contact by an elderly man with a woman other than his wife (Sue & Sue, 1990). Some Appalachian people tend to avert their eyes because for them eye contact is related to hostility and aggressiveness (Tripp-Reimer & Friedl, 1977). Certain cultures place more focus on the eyes than others; for example, in India and Greece the use of the eyes is all important (Eibl-Eibesfelt, 1972).

Body posture Communication is also affected by body posture. A nurse can bridge distance in an interaction by placing the forearms on the table, palms up. In Western culture, palms up can send a message of acquiescence even while disagreeing. However, the nurse should also recognize that palms up in other cultures may have a sexual implication. Therefore, the decision to use this gesture should be weighed carefully.

Body posture can provide important messages about receptivity. In some Western cultures such as among Whites in the United States, the closer a listener's overall posturing matches the posture of the speaker, the higher is the likelihood of receptivity. If the individuals' unconscious gestures differ, probably their perspective on the matter at hand is also different. Matching body movements to those of another person can communicate a sense of solidarity even if solidarity is not present. Body posture can also communicate attitude toward a person. For example, within the dominant culture of Whites in the United States, an attentive posture is indicated by leaning toward a person. Attentive posture is used toward people of higher stature and toward people who are liked (Mehrabian, 1968, 1981). An American man may indicate sexual attraction by placing his arms in front of his body with his legs closed. An American woman, on the other hand, indicates attraction by a more open posture, that is, arms down at the side (Hall, 1966). Physical pain is communicated by rigid muscles, flexed body, and cautious movements. Argyle et al. (1970) reported that in England dominance is communicated when the dominant person stands or sits more erect than the compliant or submissive person. Knowledge of sociocultural heritage is essential in interpreting body language, since various body parts are used differently in different cultures.

Communications that combine verbal and nonverbal elements

Many interpersonal communications combine both verbal and nonverbal elements. The communications of warmth and humor are two of these.

Warmth Warmth is a quality or state that promotes feelings of friendship, well-being, or pleasure. Warmth can be communicated verbally ("You really laid still during the procedure, and that surely helped us to do it as quickly as possible") and may also be communicated nonverbally, as by a pat on the shoulder or a gentle smile.

Although warmth is also a matter of perception, communication that focuses on human needs is more likely to be related to warmth in the speaker. Statements that show respect, address the human need to be needed, and promote self-acceptance will usually be interpreted positively and can increase motivation, morale, and cooperation. Personal recognition and concern also communicate warmth. Verbal recognition (for example, a hello on meeting) or a statement of genuine concern (for example, "How are you feeling?") can convey interest and may facilitate a positive relationship between client and family and the nurse (Davidhizar, 1989).

The nurse's communication of warmth is an important and dynamic aspect of a therapeutic nurse-client relationship. If the client is from another culture and is having difficulty with understanding communication, the nurse's warmth may be vital to promoting a positive relationship. Graham-Dickerson (1996) suggests that the healing process is promoted by the interrelation between the nurse and the client, and without this relationship

the client from another culture may not be engaged in the healing process.

Humor Humor is a powerful component of verbal and nonverbal communication. Humor can create a bond of shared pleasure between people, decrease anxiety and tension, build relationships, promote problem solving and learning, provide motivation, and enable personal survival. As a healthy and constructive coping mechanism, humor can provide a discharge for aggressive feelings in a more or less acceptable way and can enable stressful situations to be managed (Davidhizar, 1988b). Humor that is therapeutic does not ridicule and rarely uses cynicism (Huckaby, 1987). Personality, culture, background, and levels of stress and pain may influence reactions to humor. When people are from a different culture, humor must be used in limited and well-thought out situations because humor can be an obstacle to a relationship if it is misunderstood. The nurse must carefully assess the individual client and the situation to decide if humor is appropriate. Humor not only can improve communication when used appropriately, but may also affect the immune system by promoting the body's ability to combat such problems as cancer and diseases of the connective tissue such as arthritis and lupus (Simonton & Matthews-Simonton, 1978).

When the individual spoken with does not have a full grasp of the language and the nuances and puns that are often involved in humor, jokes and statements meant as humorous may not be understood or may be misinterpreted. It is also important for an individual who tries to speak in another language to be prepared to precipitate laughter. A statement meant to be serious may be perceived as comical. The ability to laugh at oneself and with others can ease the anxiety that may be present in an intercultural situation.

IMPLICATIONS FOR NURSING CARE
Guidelines for relating to patients from different cultures

Nurses commonly relate to clients in an interview setting. The nurse may also relate during the process of client care or at a more informal level on the hospital unit or in the clinic. Although cultural issues may cause the client to interpret the nurse's behavior

---

Box 2-4

GUIDELINES FOR RELATING TO PATIENTS FROM DIFFERENT CULTURES

1. Assess your personal beliefs surrounding persons from different culture.
   - Review your personal beliefs and past experiences.
   - Set aside any values, biases, ideas, and attitudes that are judgmental and may negatively affect care.
2. Assess communication variables from a cultural perspective.
   - Determine the ethnic identity of the patient, including generation in America.
   - Use the patient as a source of information when possible.
   - Assess cultural factors that may affect your relationship with the patient and respond appropriately.
3. Plan care based on the communicated needs and cultural background.
   - Learn as much as possible about the patient's cultural customs and beliefs.
   - Encourage the patient to reveal cultural interpretation of health, illness, and health care.
   - Be sensitive to the uniqueness of the patient.
   - Identify sources of discrepancy between the patient's and your own concepts of health and illness.
   - Communicate at the patient's personal level of functioning.
   - Evaluate effectiveness of nursing actions and modify nursing care plan when necessary.
4. Modify communication approaches to meet cultural needs.
   - Be attentive to signs of fear, anxiety, and confusion in the patient.
   - Respond in a reassuring manner in keeping with the patient's cultural orientation.
   - Be aware that in some cultural groups discussion concerning the patient with others may be offensive and may impede the nursing process.
5. Understand that respect for the patient and communicated needs is central to the therapeutic relationship.
   - Communicate respect by using a kind and attentive approach.
   - Learn how listening is communicated in the patient's culture.
   - Use appropriate active listening techniques.
   - Adopt an attitude of flexibility, respect, and interest to help bridge barriers imposed by culture.
6. Communicate in a nonthreatening manner.
   - Conduct the interview in an unhurried manner.
   - Follow acceptable social and cultural amenities.
   - Ask general questions during the information-gathering stage.
   - Be patient with a respondent who gives information that may seem unrelated to the patient's health problem.
   - Develop a trusting relationship by listening carefully, allowing time, and giving the patient your full attention.
7. Use validating techniques in communication.
   - Be alert for feedback that the patient is not understanding.
   - Do not assume meaning is interpreted without distortion.
8. Be considerate of reluctance to talk when the subject involves sexual matters.
   - Be aware that in some cultures sexual matters are not discussed freely with members of the opposite sex.
9. Adopt special approaches when the patient speaks a different language.
   - Use a caring tone of voice and facial expression to help alleviate the patient's fears.
   - Speak slowly and distinctly, but not loudly.
   - Use gestures, pictures, and play acting to help the patient understand.
   - Repeat the message in different ways if necessary.
   - Be alert to words the patient seems to understand and use them frequently.
   - Keep messages simple and repeat them frequently.
   - Avoid using medical terms and abbreviations that the patient may not understand.
   - Use an appropriate language dictionary.
10. Use interpreters to improve communication.
    - Ask the interpreter to translate the message, not just the individual words.
    - Obtain feedback to confirm understanding.
    - Use an interpreter who is culturally sensitive.

---

from a unique perspective, adherence to the following guidelines will increase the likelihood that the nurse-client relationship will be positive (Box 2-4).

1. Assess personal beliefs of persons from different cultures. Awareness of the nurse's personal be-

liefs is vital in relating to clients from diverse cultural backgrounds (Carpio & Majumdar, 1991). A nurse working with a client from another background should carefully review personal beliefs and past experiences to determine conscious and unconscious attitudes. It is important for the nurse to set aside personal values, biases, ideas, and attitudes that are judgmental and may negatively affect care. The nurse can learn to control personal reactions by a broadened understanding of others' beliefs and behaviors (Winans-Orr & McIntosh, 1996). Leininger (1989) contends that "there is a major crisis in nursing in that most nurses are unprepared to function effectively with migrants and cultural strangers." Understanding cultural diversity occurs best through student or nurse exchange programs (Levine, 1997). Newly developed cultural assessment tools provide a method to assess personal attitude (Anthony, 1997). Answers can provide direction in interventions to promote a positive attitude.

2. Assess communication variables from a cultural perspective. To communicate with a client from another culture, it is essential to assess each client receiving care from a cultural perspective (College of Nurses of Ontario, 1990; Rosenbaum, 1991). A nurse who is reluctant to admit lack of understanding can significantly hinder the provision of adequate care (Burner, Cunningham, & Hattar, 1990). Each individual has a dominant culture and also belongs to a subculture. The cultural phenomena of communication cannot be minimized when providing culturally appropriate nursing care. The nurse who understands differences in communication variables can attempt to transcend communication barriers to provide quality client care.

It is important to realize that cultural assessment does not require information on every aspect of a specific culture. However, data should elicit ethnic identity, including generation in the United States (that is, first or second generation); the beliefs of a first-generation immigrant, regardless of ethnic heritage, may differ from those of a second-generation person. Whenever possible, the client should be used as the primary informant, since others, even though close to the client, may have different ideas and beliefs.

After a careful assessment of cultural factors that may enter into a relationship, the nurse must respond appropriately. For example, for African and Mexican Americans who tend to value eye contact, it is important for the nurse to use eye contact (Kendall, 1996). On the other hand, when relating to Filipino Americans who are afraid of eye contact, the nurse should avoid eye contact. When relating to Southeast Asians, it is important to remember that persons from this cultural background usually are very formal in language. It is essential that courtesy be shown by use of the family name or a title until one is given permission to address the client by a given name. Asians also use an indirect approach to obtaining information and so direct questions are not received well; it is considered rude, and the interviewer is not likely to receive the information sought (Hagen, 1988; Mattson, 1995; Stauffer, 1997). If communication is to be effective in today's multicultural society, relating in a culturally sensitive manner is essential (Campinha-Bacote, 1995).

3. Plan care based on the communicated needs and cultural background. When planning care for persons from other cultures, care must be consistent with the life-style and unique needs of the client that have been communicated by the client to the nurse and mutually agreed on (Geissler, 1991; Grossman, 1996). To establish an appropriate plan, it is essential to improve personal knowledge about the customs and beliefs of the culture of the clients receiving care. The nurse should encourage the client to communicate cultural interpretations of health, illness, and health care. A client's perception of illness will affect not only communication, but also the care that is planned. Sensitivity to the uniqueness of each client is required if the nurse is to work effectively, particularly with clients from different cultures. This sensitivity can be gained only through appropriate communication techniques. Additionally, nurses who cannot communicate and correctly interpret cultural behavior will feel inadequate and helpless and quickly experience stress and burnout (Scholz, 1990). It is important to remember that the best teacher in learning about culture is people themselves. Individuals must be communicated with at their personal level of functioning. Values and beliefs of persons from different cultures may affect the way care is delivered. Many cultures have similar idiosyncrasies that must be considered. Finally, it is important to evaluate the effectiveness of nursing actions with clients from diverse culture groups. It may be necessary to modify the plan of care to provide an effective intervention based on communicated needs.

4. Modify communication approaches to meet cultural needs. A factor that commonly interferes with care delivery to a person from another culture is confusion and fear about the treatment process. The fact that a non-English speaking or a French-speaking client is ill and receiving treatment can interfere with the client's ability to communicate. The nurse must be attentive to signs of anxiety and respond in a reassuring manner in keeping with the person's cultural orientation.

Some cultures are primarily oral and do not rely on a written form of communication. In such a society, the spoken word holds greater meaning and power. For example, Hmongs are considered an oral cultural group. For these individuals, the formation of and acceptance in a social group is primarily dependent on the spoken word (Shadick, 1993). When interacting with individuals from an oral culture, the nurse must remember that if the teaching-learning process is to be effective, instruction must be oral.

When working with persons from diverse cultural backgrounds, the astute nurse must recognize that the communication process may be impeded by hesitancy to speak to Westerners about health concerns. Some Native Americans are becoming more confident and willing to speak out about their personal needs. However, Hagey and Buller (1983) noted that the Ojibway people traditionally avoided direct oral questioning by health care workers and viewed it as a form of violation of dignity and thus inappropriate. Such questions could be met with complete silence and meaningless answers. For some Ojibway, in response to a question, it would be entirely acceptable for an answer to be given in a few days or weeks. It is critical that the nurse serve as a client advocate to provide culturally sensitive care. It is also essential that the nurse learn to appreciate a value held by some Ojibways that espouses deep-rooted ideals of noninterference, which may be found among some Native and ethnic groups (Grypma, 1993). Regardless of cultural background, listening is one of the most effective therapeutic techniques (Potter & Perry, 1996).

5. Understand that respect for the client and communicated needs is central to the therapeutic relationship. The need to communicate respect for the client is a nursing concept that crosses all cultural boundaries. Regardless of the language spoken or the cultural orientation, communication is increased and interpersonal distance is reduced by the nurse whose approach focuses on individuals and their emotional and physical needs. Communication of respect is central to a focus on emotional needs. Respect for clients is communicated by a kind and attentive approach where the client is heard. Active listening techniques are used, such as encouraging clients to share thoughts and feelings by reflecting back what has been heard. The nurse should be attentive to how listening is communicated in the client's culture. For example, for some persons, listening may be indicated by eye contact, whereas for others listening may mean having the listener turn a listening "ear." Predictions about what the client is trying to express may be made to encourage elaboration. At the heart of the task of hearing is the art of listening (Martin, 1995). Listening communicates genuine interest and caring. The feeling of being heard is powerful, reducing distance and drawing people together into positive interpersonal interactions. An attitude of flexibility, respect, and interest can bridge artificial barriers of distance imposed by culture and role.

6. Communicate in a nonthreatening manner. The interview should be started in an unhurried manner with adherence to acceptable social and cultural amenities. It is usually wise to start with general social topics. During the information-gathering stage, general rather than specific questions should be asked. The interviewer should allow time for the respondent to give what appears to be unrelated information. For many persons a direct approach appears rude and uncaring. For example, persons of European background and Hispanic individuals often value "small talk" and will not relate optimally to the nurse who talks only about illness-related matters. Many persons, specifically Oriental and Spanish-speaking persons, respond better to a nondirective approach with open-ended questions than to direct questions and answers (Giger & Davidhizar, 1990b).

When personal matters are discussed, it is important to allow time for the development of a relationship. For example, Mexican Americans tend to be hesitant to discuss personal affairs quickly. For such individuals it is important to first communicate a positive attitude and to develop trust. Bonaparte (1979) found that the nurse's positive attitude was strongly correlated with lower ego defensiveness and with open-mindedness.

The appearances of being too busy, of not having time to listen, of not giving sufficient time for an answer, and of not really wanting to hear are equally effective in "cutting off" the client. Patients will be encouraged to talk by a nurse who "wants" to hear.

7. Use validating techniques in communication. Although validating techniques are always important, they are especially important when the client is from a different culture. The nurse should be alert for feedback that the client is not understanding and should use restating and validating techniques such as, "Did I hear and understand you correctly?" When the nurse had difficulty understanding, it may help to find out precisely what the topic is, such as, "Are you telling me where you're having pain?" By determining the topic the number of words can be decreased. If the message is not understood, it may be helpful to have the client try to convey the message in another way; for example, through pointing or imitation. The nurse should never pretend to understand a message. People usually know when they are understood. By pretending, the nurse conveys that the message is not really important (Pore, 1995).

Even if an interpreter is used, the nurse should not assume that the meaning has been transmitted without some distortion. It is difficult to transmit exact meaning when both persons speak the same language and even more so when both persons do not.

8. Be considerate of reluctance to talk when the subject involves sexual matters. Hispanic and Indian clients, who tend to be hesitant to talk about sexually related matters, may talk more freely to a nurse of the same sex. When talking about sexual matters with a male child from certain cultures (such as Spanish, Pakistani, or Arabic), it is important to have the father rather than the mother present.

9. Adopt special approaches when the client speaks a different language. A client who enters the health care system without being able to speak to the caregivers enters a frightening and frustrating world. Without the availability of words, the nurse must relate to a client at an affective level. A tone and facial expression of caring can be vital in alleviating a client's fear.

The nurse should guard against the common assumption that the client will understand better if the nurse talks loudly. If an interpreter is not available and the client seems to have some understanding of the language, speaking slowly and distinctly, using a lot of gestures, acting out, using pictures, and repeating the message several times in different ways may enable the client to understand what is being said. The nurse should be alert for words that the client seems to understand so that these words can be used more frequently. Messages should be kept simple and stated sentence by sentence, not paragraph by paragraph.

It is especially necessary to avoid using medical terms and jargon when speaking to a client with only partial understanding of the language. Abbreviations such as TPR and BP should be avoided. An individual usually first understands standard words and picks up slang expressions and professional terms at a much later stage of language acquisition.

The nurse should select a dictionary that has both the language the nurse speaks and the language the client speaks, such as a Spanish-English, English-Spanish dictionary. In addition, standard nursing references such as *Taber's Cyclopedic Medical Dictionary* (Taber, 1993) and *Mosby's Medical, Nursing, and Allied Health Dictionary* (1997) have sections that give common medical statements and questions in several languages. Translation of health information pamphlets from English to the language of the client is very important in providing adequate teaching. When a hospital serves a particular cultural group, other pieces of important information such as orientation to the services of the hospital and consent forms need to be in the language of the client. The nurse should keep in mind that for clients who do not speak English, even the most basic procedures such as registering at the emergency desk may be seen as an insurmountable barrier.

The cultural orientation of the client also affects such factors as assignment of caregivers. For example, for conservative Arab clients, females giving instructions to males may not be effective. If a male nurse is providing services to a female Arab client, strict rules would require that a family member always be present. Older Arab clients may not comply with direct instructions given by a young staff member; with these clients, indirect requests and suggestions are the desired methods (Nellum-Davis, 1993; Wilson, 1996).

10. Use interpreters to improve communication. Assessment tools are available for Spanish-speaking immigrants and refugee communities at minimal or no cost (Urrutia-Rojas & Aday, 1991). The nurse should be alert for the client who pretends to understand to please the caregiver and gain acceptance. This patient will usually say yes to all questions. When a client does not speak the nurse's language, an interpreter, who may be either a family member or a person from an agency or the community, should be included. The nurse should evaluate if having a family member interpret is satisfactory to the client because some clients may have information that will not be confided in a family member (Clark, 1995). The interpreter should be able to translate not only the literal meaning of the words, but also the nonverbal messages that accompany the communication. Interpreters who "act out" their message through intonation, facial expression, or gestures are more likely to be effective in getting the message across. Even when every effort is made to ensure effective translations, neither the nurse nor the interpreter can be completely sure that accurate communication has been accomplished; therefore, obtaining feedback remains essential. Communication through a third party compounds the problem of sending a message clearly. Interpreters often face the difficulty of interpreting versus translating. Although a message may be translated into another language, helping another understand is much more complex and involves interpreting the message into understandable terms. An interpreter must have transcultural sensitivity, understand how to impart knowledge, and understand how to be a client advocate to represent the client's needs to the nurse. Interpreting with cultural sensitivity is much more complex than simply putting the words into another language (Díaz-Duque, 1982; Wolfson, 1996). Monolingualism in multicultural practices frequently presents ethnical dilemmas. If the nurse, the interpreter, and the client's views on the ethical principles regarding care differ, problems can be compounded (Kaufert & Putsch, 1997). Learning a second language is an important tool in lowering cultural barriers. A nurse who learns the language of the clients who are served will find this profoundly affects communication (Stoltzfus, 1993). Boston (1993) conducted a study in Montreal of Italian immigrant families to determine if they had a perception of frustration with their caregivers because of language barriers. Findings from this study indicated that respondents expressed fear and helplessness about their treatment because of the language barriers. Even when a interpreter was provided, family members believed that their own deeper concerns and fears were not adequately communicated.

Case Study

A 35- to 37-year-old Black woman who has been recently diagnosed as having hypertension is admitted for a medical workup examination. Her history reveals that she has recently moved from New Orleans to New York. The nurse is having difficulty communicating with the client because she not only speaks in Black English but also has a heavy Southern drawl and tends to speak in pidgin English. Another factor complicating the development of the nurse-client relationship is that not only does the client not understand the hospital jargon and medical terms, but also word meanings for the nurse and the client vary. For example, when the nurse asks if the client likes her physician, she

---

Case Study—cont'd

responds, "He's bad." Only later does the nurse discover that the client was speaking in an argot that is a special linguistic code for some Blacks. The client appears very fearful and anxious about being in the hospital. When questioning the client, the nurse finds that the fear and anxiety are related to the connotative and denotative meanings of the word "hospital." In this case the client believes that hospitals are associated with death and that she may not leave the hospital alive. When the nurse communicates with the client, she speaks very loudly and repeats the same words again and again.

STUDY QUESTIONS

1. Describe at least two problems encountered by the nurse when giving nursing care to persons who do not speak English as their primary language.

2. Describe four communication approaches that the nurse can use to give culturally appropriate care.

3. Describe approaches the nurse can use when relating to a client whose primary language is not English.

4. Describe at least two nonverbal indicators of anxiety the nurse may encounter when dealing with a client who does not speak English.

5. List at least two problems encountered by the nurse who assumes that speaking louder will improve communication.

References

Andrews, M.M., & Boyle, J.S. (1995). *Transcultural nursing.* Philadelphia: Lippincott-Raven.

Anthony, M. (1997). A cultural values assessment tool. *Journal of Cultural Diversity, 4*(2), 49-52.

Argyle, M. (1992). *The social psychology of everyday life.* New York: Routledge.

Argyle, M., & Dean, J. (1965). Eye-contact, distance, and affiliation. *Sociometry, 28,* 289-304.

Argyle, M., Salter, H., Nicholson, N., et al. (1970). The communication of inferior and superior attitudes by verbal and nonverbal signals. *British Journal of Social and Clinical Psychology, 9,* 221-231.

Banks, A., & Banks, S. (1995, Nov.). Cultural identity, resistance, and "good theory": implications for intercultural communication theory from Gypsy culture. *The Howard Journal of Communication, 6*(3), 146-163.

Barkauskas, P. (1994). *Quick reference to cultural assessment.* St. Louis: Mosby.

Bigham, C. (1964). To communicate with Negro patients. *American Journal of Nursing, 64*(9), 113-115.

Boas, F., (Ed.) (1938). *General anthropology.* Boston: D.C. Heath.

Bonaparte, B.H. (1979, May/June). Ego defensiveness, open-closed mindedness, and nurses' attitude toward culturally different patients. *Nursing Research, 28*(3), 166-172.

Boston, P. (1993). Culture and cancer: the relevance of cultural orientation within cancer education programmes. *European Journal of Cancer Care, 2,* 72-76.

Bronstein, M. (1996,). Healing hands. *The Canadian Nurse, 92*(1), 32-34.

Bruhn, J. (1996). Creating an organizational climate for multiculturalism. *Health Care Supervisor, 14*(4), 16-20.

Buckett, H. (1995, Sept./Oct.). Tales from the road. *HealthTraveler, 3*(2), 48.

Burner, O.Y., Cunningham, P., & Hattar, H.S. (1990). Managing a multicultural nurse staff in a multicultural environment. *Journal of Nursing Administration, 20*(6), 30-34.

Buttaglia, B. (1992). Skills for managing multicultural teams. *Cultural Diversity at Work, 4*(3), 4.

Campinha-Bacote, J. (1995, October/December). The quest for cultural competence in nursing care. *Nursing Forum, 30*(4), 19-24.

Capirci, O., Iverson, J., Pizzuto, E., & Volterra, V. (1996). Gestures and words during the transition in two-word speech. *Journal of Child Language, 23,* 645-673.

Carpio, B., & Majumdar, B. (1991, Aug.). Putting culture into curricula. *The Canadian Nurse, 87*(7),32-33.

Cheng, P., & Barlas, R. (1992). *Culture shock.* Portland, Oreg.: Graphic Arts Publishing Company.

Clark, C. (1995, Sept./Oct.). Enhancing communication with families. *Health Traveler, 3*(2), 34.

Clemmens, E. (1985). An analyst looks at languages, cultures, and translations. *American Journal of Psychoanalysis, 45*(4), 310-321.

Clemmens, E. (1988). Some psychological functions of language. *American Journal of Psychoanalysis, 43*(4), 294-304.

College of Nurses of Ontario. (1990). *Standards of nursing practice for registered nurses and registered nursing assistants.* Toronto: Author.

Davidhizar, R. (1988a). Distance in managerial encounters. *Today's OR Nurse, 10*(10), 23-29.

Davidhizar, R. (1988b). Humor—No nurse should be without it. *Today's OR Nurse, 10*(1), 18-20.

Davidhizar, R. (1988c). Personal communication.

Davidhizar, R. (1989). Developing managerial warmth. *Dimensions of Critical Care, 8*(1), 28-34.

Davidhizar, R., & Giger, J. (1988). Managerial touch. *Today's OR Nurse, 10*(7), 18-23.

Delgado, M. (1983). Hispanics and psychotherapeutic groups. *International Journal of Psychotherapy, 33*(4), 507-520.

de Paula, T., Lagana, K, & González-Ramírez, L. (1996). Mexican Americans. In Lipson, J., Dibble, S., & Mirarik, P. (Eds.), *Culture and Nursing Care.* School of Nursing, University of California, San Francisco, Calif.: UCSF Nursing Press.

DeThomaso, M. (1971). Touch power and the screen of loneliness. *Perspectives in Psychiatric Care, 9*(3), 112-117.

Díaz-Duque, O.F. (1982). Overcoming the language barrier: advice from an interpreter. *American Journal of Nursing, 82*(9), 1380-1382.

Dillard, J. (1973). *Black English.* New York: Vintage Books.

Eibl-Eibesfelt, I. (1972). Similarities and differences between cultures in expressive movements. In Hinde, R.A. (Ed.), *Nonverbal communication* (pp. 297-312). Cambridge, England: Cambridge University Press.

Ekiman, P., & Friesen, W. (1975). *Unmasking the face.* Englewood Cliffs, N.J.: Prentice Hall.

Fielding, R., & Llewelyn, S. (1987). Communication training in nursing may damage your health and enthusiasm: some warnings. *Journal of Advanced Nursing, 12*(3), 281-290.

Geissler, E. (1991). Transcultural nursing and nursing diagnosis. *Nursing and Health Care, 12*(4), 190-192.

Gibson, J. (1984, Jan.). As they grow: 1 year olds. *Parents,* p. 128.

Giger, J., & Davidhizar, R. (1990a). Culture and space. *Advancing Clinical Care, 6*(6), 8-10.

Giger, J., & Davidhizar, R. (1990b). Transcultural nursing assessment: a method for advancing nursing practice. *International Nursing Review, 37*(1), 199-202.

Giger, J. & Davidhizar, R. (1996). When the operating room has a multicultural team. *Today's Surgical Nurse, 18*(5), 26-32.

Giger, J., Davidhizar, R., Evers, S., Ingram, C. (1994). Cultural factors influencing mental health and mental illness. In Taylor, C. (Ed.), *Mereness' Essentials of psychiatric nursing* (pp. 214-238). St. Louis: Mosby.

Giger, J., Davidhizar, R., & Wieczorek, S. (1993). Culture and ethnicity. In Bobak, I.M., & Jensen, M. (Eds.), *Maternity and gynecological care* (ed. 5) (pp. 43-67). St. Louis: Mosby.

Graham-Dickerson, P. (1996, Summer). Healing through discourse for culturally diverse people within the health care system. *The Journal of Multicultural Nursing and Health, 2*(3), 33-37.

Grainger, R. (1992). Eye movements: a new psychotherapeutic tool. *American Journal of Nursing, 92*(5), 18.

Grossman, D. (1996, July). Cultural dimensions in home health care nursing. *American Journal of Nursing, 96*(7), 33-36.

Grypma, S. (1993, Sept.). Culture shock. *The Canadian Nurse,* 33-36.

Gunderson, J. (1996, Feb.). Progress in building communication links. *The Canadian Nurse,* 8-9.

Guralnik, D. (Ed.) (1984). *Webster's new world dictionary* (ed. 3). New York: William Collins & World Publishing.

Guruge, S., & Donner, G. (1996, Sept.). Transcultural nursing in Canada. *The Canadian Nurse,* 34-39.

Haber, J. (1997). Therapeutic communication. In Haber, J., Krainovich-Miller, B., McMahon, A., & Price-Hoskins, P. (Eds.), *Comprehensive Psychiatric Nursing* (ed. 5) (pp. 122-142). St. Louis: Mosby.

Haffner, L. (1992). Translation is not enough: interpreting in a medical setting. *Western Journal of Medicine, 157*(3), 248-254.

Hagen, E. (1988, July 8). *Southeast Asians in the United States: an overview of belief systems, and the refugee experience.* Paper presented at the seminar Working with the Southeast Asian Health Consumer, St. Mary Medical Center, Long Beach, Calif.

Hagey, R., & Buller, E. (1983). Drumming and dancing: a new rhythm in nursing care. *The Canadian Nurse, 79*(4), 28-31.

Hall, E.T. (1966). *The silent language.* New York: Doubleday.

Headden, S. (1995, Jan.). Favor aliens with job skills. *U.S. News and World Report, 123*(25), 83-85.

Hedlund, N. (1992). Communication. In Beck, C.K., Rawlins, R.P., & Williams, S. (Eds.), *Mental health-psychiatric nursing: a holistic life approach* (ed. 3). St. Louis: Mosby.

Henderson, G., & Primeaux, M. (1981). *Transcultural health care.* Menlo Park, Calif.: Addison-Westley Publishing Company.

Hess, E.H. (1965). Attitude and pupil size. *Scientific American, 212,* 46-54.

Hess, E.H. (1975). The role of pupil size in communication. *Scientific American, 233*(5), 110-119.

Hoang, G., & Erickson, R. (1982). Guidelines for providing medical care to Southeast Asian refugees. *Journal of the American Medical Association, 248*(6), 710-714.

Huckaby, D. (1987). Take time to laugh. *Nursing 87,* 17, 81.

Information Please Almanac (1998). Boston: Houghton Mifflin Company.

Insel, P.M. (1978). *Too close for comfort: the psychology of crowding.* Englewood Cliffs, N.J.: Prentice Hall.

Johnson, B. (1965). The meaning of touch in nursing. *Nursing Outlook, 13*(2), 59-60.

Jourard, S. (1971). *The transparent self.* New York: D. Van Nostrand.

Kasch, C. (1984). Interpersonal competence and communication in the delivery of nursing care. *Advances in Nursing Science, 62,* 71-88.

Kaufert, J., & Putsch, R. (1997, Spring). Communication through interpreters in healthcare: ethical dilemmas arising from differences in class, culture, language, and power. *The Journal of Clinical Ethics, 8*(1), 71-87.

Kayser, H. (1996, October). Cultural/linguistic variations in the United States and its implications for assessment and intervention in speech-language pathology: an epilogue. *Language, Speech and Hearing Services in Schools, 27*(4), 385-387.

Kendall, J. (1996, June). Creating a culturally responsive psychotherapeutic environment for African American youths: a critical analysis. *Advances in Nursing Science, 18*(4), 11-28.

Knowles, R. (1983). Building rapport through neurolinguistic programming. *American Journal of Nursing, 83,* 1011-1014.

Kretch, D., Crutchfield, R., & Ballachey, E. (1962). *Individual in society.* New York: McGraw-Hill.

Lane, P. (1989). Nurse-client perceptions: the double standard of touch. *Issues in Mental Health Nursing, 10,* 1-13.

Levine, M. (1997, Summer). Exploring cultural diversity. *Journal of Cultural Diversity, 4*(2), 53-56.

Luft, J., & Ingham, H. (1984). The Johari window: a graphic model of awareness in interpersonal relations. In Luft, J. (Ed.), *Group processes: an introduction to group dynamics* (ed. 3). Palo Alto, Calif.: National Press Books.

Mackey, R. (1995, Apr.). Discover the health power of therapeutic touch. *American Journal of Nursing, 95,* 27-32.

Martin, B. (1995, Dec. 12). The difficult art of listening. *Gospel Herald, 88*(48), 1-2.

Mattson, S. (1995, May). Culturally sensitive perinatal care for Southeast Asians. *Journal of Obstetric and Gynecological Neonatal Nursing, 24*(4), 335-341.

McKenzie, J., & Chrisman, N. (1977). Healing herbs, gods, and magic folk health beliefs among Filipino-Americans. *Nursing Outlook, 25*(5), 326.

McLeod, R., & Bently, C. (1996, Fall). Understanding deafness as a culture with a unique language. *Advanced Practice Nursing Quarterly, 2*(2), 50-58.

McRae, L. (1994). Cultural sensitivity in rehabilitation related to Native clients. *Canadian Journal of Rehabilitation, 7*(4), 251-256.

Mead, M. (1947). The application of anthropological technique to cross-national communication. *Transcultural New York Academy of Science, Series II, 9,* 4.

Mehrabian, A. (1968). The influence of attitudes from the posture, orientation, and distance of a communicator. *Journal of Consulting Clinical Psychology, 32,* 296-308.

Mehrabian, A. (1981). *Silent messages: implicit communication of emotion and attitude.* Belmont, Calif.: Wadsworth.

Mitchell, A. (1978). Barriers to therapeutic communication with Black clients. *Nursing Outlook, 26,* 109-112.

Molzahn, A., & Northcott, H. (1989). The social bases of discrepancies in health/illness perceptions. *Journal of Advanced Nursing, 14*(2), 132-140.

Montagu, A. (1971). *Touching: the human significance of skin.* New York: Columbia University Press.

Mosby's medical, nursing, and allied health dictionary. (1997). (ed. 5). St. Louis: Mosby.

Murray, R., & Huelskoetter, N. (1991). *Psychiatric/mental health nursing: giving emotional care* (ed. 2). Norwalk, Conn.: Appleton & Lange.

Murray, R., & Zentner, J. (1993). *Nursing assessment and health promotion strategies through the life span* (ed. 5). Norwalk, Conn.: Appleton & Lange.

Nellum-Davis, P. (1993). Clinical practice issues. In Battle, D.E., (Ed.), *Communication Disorders in Multicultural Populations.* Boston: Andover Medical Publishers.

Nolt, S. (1992). *A history of the Amish.* Intercourse, Penn.: Good Books.

Paynich, M. (1964). Cultural barriers to nurse communication. *American Journal of Nursing, 64* (2), 87-90.

Personal Report for the Executive. (1987). New York: National Institute of Business Management.

Pirandello, L. (1970). Language and thought. *Perspectives in Psychiatric Care, 8*(5), 230.

Polhemus, T. (Ed.) (1978). *The body reader: social aspects of the human body.* New York: Pantheon Books.

Pore, S. (1995, July). I can't understand what my patient is saying. *Advance for Nurse Practitioners, 3,* 47-48.

Potter, R., & Perry, A. (1996). *Fundamentals of nursing: Concepts, process, and practice* (ed. 4). St. Louis: Mosby.

Randall-David, E. (1989). *Strategies for working with culturally diverse communities and clients* [Brochure]. Washington, D.C.: U.S. Department of Health and Human Services.

Rayner, K. (1992). *Eye movements and visual cognition.* New York: Springer-Verlag.

Reakes, J. (1997). Communication. In Johnson, B. (Ed.), *Psychiatric-mental health nursing* (ed. 4). Philadelphia: Lippincott.

Reusch, J. (1961). *Therapeutic communication.* New York: W.W. Norton.

Rocereto, L. (1981). Selected health beliefs of Vietnamese refugees. *Journal of School Health, 51*(1), 63-64.

Rosenbaum, J. (1991, April). A cultural assessment guide. *The Canadian Nurse,* 32-33.

Sapir, E. (1929). The status of linguistics as a science. *Language 5,* 207-214.

Scheflen, A. (1972). *Body language and social order.* Englewood Cliffs, N.J.: Prentice Hall.

Scholz, J. (1990). Cultural expressions affecting patient care. *Dimensions in Oncology Nursing, IV*(1), 16-20.

Shadick, K. (1993). Development of a transcultural health education program for the Hmong. *Clinical Nurse Specialist, 7*(2), 48-53.

Shapiro, F. (1991, May). Eye movement desensitization and reprocessing procedure: from EMD to EMD/R—a new treatment model for anxiety and related traumata. *The Behavioral Therapist,* pp. 133-135.

Shuter, R. (1976). Proxemics and tactility in Latin America. *Journal of Communication, 26*(3), 46-52.

Simonton, O.C., & Matthews-Simonton, S. (1978). *Getting well again.* Los Angeles: Jeremy P. Tarcher.

Smith, B., & Cantrell, P. (1988). Distance in nurse-patient encounters. *Journal of Psychosocial Nursing, 26*(2), 22-26.

Snow, L. (1976, June). "High blood" is not "high blood pressure," *Urban Health,* 54-56.

Sommer, R. (1959). Studies in personal space. *Sociometry,22,* 247-260.

Spector, R. (1993). Cultural, ethnicity, and nursing. In Potter, P., & Perry, A. (Eds.), *Fundamentals of Nursing: concepts, process, and practice* (ed. 3). St. Louis: Mosby.

Stauffer, R. (1997). Personal communication. Harrisburg, Virginia.

Stoltzfus, V. (1993, May). Language and culture. *Goshen College Bulletin,* p. 32.

Sudnow, D. (1967). *Passing on.* Englewood Cliffs, N.J.: Prentice Hall.

Sue, D.W., & Sue, D. (1990). *Counseling the culturally different: theory and practice* (ed. 2). New York: John Wiley & Sons.

Sullivan, H. (1954). *The interpersonal theory of psychiatry* New York: W.W. Norton.

Taber, C. (1993). *Taber's cyclopedic medical dictionary* (ed. 17). Philadelphia: FA Davis.

Talbot, L.R. (1996). The power of words. *Canadian Journal of Nursing Research, 28*(1), 9-15.

Taylor, C. (1976). Soul talk: a key to Black cultural attitudes. In Luckroft, D. (Ed.), *Black awareness: implications for Black patient care.* New York: American Journal of Nursing Company.

Taylor, C., Malone, B., & Kavanagh, K. (1997). Sociocultural aspects of love. In Johnson, B.S. (Ed.), *Psychiatric–Mental Health Nursing* (ed. 4). Philadelphia: Lippincott-Raven.

Thayer, S. (1988, March). Close encounters. *Psychology Today,* pp. 31-36.

Thiederman, S. (1986). Ethnocentrism: a barrier to effective health care. *Nurse Practitioner, 11*(8), 52-59.

Thomas, W.I. (1937). *Primitive behavior: an introduction to the social sciences.* New York: McGraw-Hill.

Treger, C. (1996, January). The missing communication link. *The Canadian Nurse,* 53-54.

Tripp-Reimer, T., & Friedl, M. (1977). Appalachians: a neglected minority. *Nursing Outlook, 32*(2), 41-45.

Uchida, A. (1997). Doing gender and building culture: toward a model of women's intercultural communication. *The Howard Journal of Communication, 8,* 41-76.

Urrutia-Rojas, X., & Aday, L.A. (1991). A framework for community assessment: designing and conducting a survey in a Hispanic immigrant and refugee community. *Public Health Nursing, 8*(1), 20-26.

U.S. Department of Commerce. (1996). *Statistical Abstract of the United States* (ed. 116). Washington D.C.: U.S. Department of Commerce.

Watzlawich, P., Beavin, J., & Jackson, D. (1967). *Pragmatics of human communication.* New York: W.W. Norton.

Whitcher, S.J., & Fisher, J.D. (1979). Multidimensional reaction to therapeutic touch in hospital setting. *Journal of Personality, Sociology, and Psychology, 37*(1), 87-96.

Wilson, M. (1996, August). Arabic speakers: language and culture, here and abroad. *Topics in Language Disorders, 18*(4), 65-80.

Winans-Orr, P., & McIntosh, M. (1996, April). Putting control theory to work. *The Canadian Nurse,* 51.

Wolfson, L. (1996, January). Breaking the language barrier. *Hemispheres,* 37-38.

Space

Personal space is the area that surrounds a person's body; it includes the space and the objects within the space. Personal space is an extension of the body and is also referred to as "outer space"; inner space refers to the personal state of consciousness or awareness (Sideleau, 1992; Sommer, 1969). Personal space can also describe inner space that filters incoming stimuli that a person receives (Scott & Dumas, 1995). Scott (1988) defines inner personal space as dynamic, invisible lines of demarcation that can be divided into four concentric areas of space. These four areas include: (1) the inner spirit core, (2) an area of thoughts and feelings perceived as unacceptable, (3) an area of thoughts and feelings perceived as acceptable, and (4) an area of superficial public image. An individual's comfort level is related to both inner and outer personal space, and discomfort is experienced when personal space is invaded. Although personal space is an individual matter and varies with the situation, dimensions of the personal space comfort zone also vary from culture to culture.

Spatial behavior is an important consideration in measuring distance in relationships. Since spatial behavior is usually judged to be spontaneous and unintentional, individuals are typically more likely to trust the accuracy of actions rather than words as a reflection of true feelings. Although a large percentage of spatial behaviors are spontaneous and unintentional, communication in this domain can be managed to promote favorable and desired impressions. For example, a nurse may choose to stand when greeting a client to show respect.

To understand human behavior, one must understand something of the nature of our receptor systems and how the information received by these systems is modified by culture. Because spatial behavior is a response to sensory stimulation in the internal and external environment, the phenomenon of space can be understood only as an integral part of the sensory systems, that is, sight, sound, touch, and smell. Spatial behavior encompasses a variety of behaviors, including proximity to others, objects in the environment, and movement.

PERCEPTION OF SPACE

Sensory apparatuses fall into two categories:

1. *Distance receptors* are those apparatuses that are concerned with the examination of distant objects. The sensory receptors for distance include the eyes, ears, and nose.
2. *Immediate receptors* are those apparatuses that are used to examine the world up close. Sensory receptors used to examine the world up close include touch, which is the sensation received from the skin membranes (Hall, 1969, 1977).

These two classifications can be broken down even further to facilitate the nurse's understanding of the phenomenon of space. For example, the skin is the chief organ of touch and is sensitive to heat gain and heat loss—both radiant and conducted heat are detected by the skin. Therefore the skin must be perceived as both an immediate receptor and a distance receptor. In general, there is a relationship between the evolutionary age of the receptor system and the amount and quality of information it can convey to the central nervous system. Many psychologists estimate that the touch system is as old as life itself (Hall, 1966). Because the ability to respond to stimuli is based on touch, the response to touch is one of the basic criteria for the maintenance of life. In comparison, sight is believed to be the last and most specialized sense to be developed in humans. From an anthropological view, vision became more important than olfactory response when our ancestors left the ground and took to trees in search of food and safety. Stereoscopic vision became essential for primitive man because without it jumping from branch to branch was difficult and dangerous.

Distance receptors

Distance receptors include sensory apparatuses for visual, auditory, and olfactory perception. It is essential that the nurse understand the relationship between sight, touch, and smell and how the reaction to these stimuli can be modified by culture.

Visual and auditory perception As indicated earlier, vision was the last of the senses to evolve. However, it is by far the most complex. Seemingly, more data are fed to the nervous system through the eyes at a much greater rate than through the senses of touch or hearing. For example, the information that can be gathered by a blind person outdoors is limited to a circle of 20 to 100 feet because a blind person can perceive by way of auditory or olfactory stimuli only what is immediately surrounding him or her. However, with sight a person can see the stars if they are out. Even very talented blind persons are limited to an average speed of perception of 2 to 3 miles an hour over familiar territory. In contrast, with sight a person has to fly faster than sound before additional visual aids are needed to avoid bumping into things. The amount of information that can be gathered by the eyes as contrasted to the ears cannot be precisely calculated. If such a calculation were possible, it would require not only a translation process but also the ability on the part of scientists to know precisely what to count. A general notion held by most scientists is that the relative complexities of the two systems, visual and auditory, can be obtained by comparison of the size of the nerves connecting the eyes and the ears to the centers of the brain (Brown, Leavitt, & Graham, 1977).

The optic nerve contains roughly 18 times as many neurons as the cochlear nerve; therefore, one might assume that it transmits at least that much more information. The eyes may act as a defense mechanism because they normally alert us to danger; the eyes may be as much as a thousand times as effective as the ears in gathering information to protect us from harmful stimuli. The area that the unaided ear can effectively cover in the course of daily living is quite limited. The ear is very efficient, but only up to a distance of 20 feet. At about 100 feet one-way vocal communication is possible, but at a somewhat slower rate than at a conversational distance. Although two-way conversation is also possible at this distance, it is considerably altered. Beyond this distance the auditory cues begin to break down rapidly. The unaided eye, on the other hand, can gather an extraordinary amount of information within a 100-yard radius and is efficient for human interaction at up to a mile (Hall, 1969).

The impulses that activate the eyes and the ears differ in speed and quality. For example, at a temperature of 0° C (32° F) at sea level, sound waves can travel 1100 feet per second and be heard in frequencies of 50 to 1500 cycles per second (Hertz). On the other hand, light rays can travel 186,000 miles (300,000 km) per second and thus are visible at a maximal frequency of 500 trillion at yellow-green (Hall, 1969).

Many complex and remarkable instruments have been invented to extend the eyes and ears. Radio and television have revolutionized the perception of space and shortened distances between people worldwide. During World War II, radio was relied on quite extensively to bring news from the occupied countries to parts of the free world. Perhaps one of the most famous broadcasts of this period was done by Tokyo Rose, whose broadcasts, which were reported to be untrue, influenced many people in the listening audience about the nature and direction of World War II. However, radio lacked the visual stimuli offered later by television, which filled in perception gaps left by radio. Television came of age in the 1960s, when for the first time, brighter, clearer, and bolder pictures were offered to viewers. The addition of color filled another perception gap and enhanced our receptor fields. For the first time in history, from their living rooms, the people of the United States could view their president doing the ordinary, the extraordinary, and the unusual. For example, the people of the United States were informed about the Cuban missile crisis by the U.S. President Kennedy on television. They were also able to see this president playing with his children in the Oval Office. In 1963, when President Kennedy was assassinated, nothing was left to the imagination of the people of the United States, who were mesmerized by complete television coverage from assassination to burial. Because of television, the nation and the world at large experienced grief still present today and mourned collectively. In 1997, when Princess Diana (formerly Her Royal Highness Diana of Great Britain) was killed in a tragic automobile accident, it was estimated that more than 2 billion people mourned throughout the world collectively through the modern medium of television. It is believed that her legend, though admirable, was largely created and captured imaginatively by the media. In

1998, the media "hype" surrounding the impeachment of the United States president, William Jefferson Clinton for possible perjury in a sex-related scandal once again clearly illuminated the modern medium of television. President Clinton was sued in a civil rights sexual harassment trial in 1997, brought by Paula Corbin Jones, the plaintiff. On January 17, 1998, during a civil deposition, Clinton allegedly gave perjurious information about his relationship with an intern, Monica Lewinsky, who was 22 years old at the time of the alleged affair. In April of 1998, Judge Susan Webber Wright dismissed the suit, citing the failure of the plaintiff to provide substantial and credible evidence. Nonetheless, on December 19, 1998, President William Jefferson Clinton became the first duly elected President of the United States to be impeached by the United States House of Representatives. He was impeached on two counts, including (1) providing perjurious testimony to a grand jury, and (2) obstruction of justice. Like the coverage of the life and death of Princess Diana, news related to President Clinton was telecast throughout the world.

In summary, visual space has an entirely different character from that of auditory space. The overriding quality that differentiates visual space from auditory space is that visual information tends to be less ambiguous and more focused than auditory information. Therefore visual information is less subject to external manipulation than is auditory information. One major exception to this rule is the blind person who has learned to understand selectively the higher audio frequencies, which can assist him or her in locating objects within a familiar or unfamiliar room. For example, a blind person may know where the door is in a room by the relationship of the sound that comes from that direction.

Even today it is not known what effects the incongruencies between auditory and visual space have on individuals. Some data indicate that auditory space is a factor in performance. J.W. Black, a phonetician, demonstrated that the size and reverberation (vibrations of external sounds) of a room can affect an individual's reading rate. In a classic study, Black (1950) found that people read more slowly in larger rooms, where the reverberation time, or circulation of sound, is slower than that in smaller rooms. Hall (1966, 1969) interviewed subjects in regard to the slowing of reverberation time in a larger room. Among the interviewees was a gifted English architect who improved the performance of a malfunctioning committee by simply blending the auditory and visual worlds of the conference chamber where the committee met. The complaint the architect had received was that the chairman was inadequate and was about to be replaced. However, the architect had reason to believe that the difficulties encountered by this committee were caused by more in the environment than just the chairman. In this situation the meeting room was next to a busy street where traffic noises were intensified by reverberations from the hard walls and rugless floors inside the building and particularly in the meeting room. The architect was able to readjust the room by adding an acoustic ceiling, carpet, and soundproof walls. Once interferences were reduced, the chairman was able to conduct the meeting without undue strain, and complaints about the chairman ceased.

People who are brought up in different cultures learn unknowingly to screen out various information and to sort information into relevant or irrelevant categories, and once set, these perceptual patterns remain stable throughout life. For example, Japanese people screen visually in a variety of ways and are more perceptive to visual stimuli. Japanese people are therefore perfectly content with paper walls as acoustic screens. A Westerner who finds himself in a Japanese inn where a party is going on next door may be in for a new sensory experience, since only paper-thin walls separate each room. In contrast, German and Dutch people depend on double doors and thick walls to screen out sound and may have difficulty if they must rely on their own powers of concentration to screen out sound. If two rooms are the same size and one screens out sound and the other one does not, a sensitive German or Dutch person who is trying to concentrate will feel less intruded on in the former and thus less crowded (Hall, 1966, 1969).

Olfactory perception Some cultures place more importance on olfactory perceptions than do others. For example, Hall (1966, 1969) found Americans culturally underdeveloped in the use of their olfactory apparatus. Hall (1966) contended that the deprivations of the olfactory stimulus are a result of the extensive use of deodorants and the suppression of odors in public places, which has resulted in a land of olfactory blandness and sameness that is difficult to duplicate anywhere else in the world.

People in the United States are continuously bombarded with commercials for room deodorizers, antiperspirants, mouthwashes, carpet deodorizers, and so on. All of these factors result in bland, undifferentiated spaces and deprive many people in the United States of the richness and variety of life. For example, if one is cooking with garlic, a room deodorizer may be used during the cooking process, causing the garlic smell to be eliminated. It is this type of behavior on the part of people of the United States that obscures memories. It is believed that smells evoke much deeper memories than either vision or sound; when the sound or the sight of what has happened has passed, the memory of the smell lingers on. Even today many United States citizens equate certain holidays, such as Christmas, with certain smells. For example, because Christmas is traditionally equated with the smell of baked goods, holly, pine, and fruit, today many people in the United States try to reproduce these smells at Christmas. An individual who has an artificial Christmas tree may buy a pine-scented spray to create the effects of a fresh tree. Another old-fashioned scent for many United States citizens is country potpourri, which has now been simulated in aerosol cans for easy dispensing. A new car can be simulated by a car spray that smells like new leather. Soap may be purchased to recreate a desired feeling; for example, the soap Mother used at home may create a feeling of hominess. Smells may also create a negative reaction; for example, an individual who washes with lye soap may be thought to have body odor because the smell is unusually strong and medicinal. A medicinal smell is perceived by most individuals in the United States to be appropriate for a hospital room but not in a non–health care setting.

Odor is perhaps one of the most basic methods of communication. It is primarily chemical in nature and is therefore referred to in a chemical sense. The olfactory sense has diverse functions and not only differentiates individuals, but also makes it possible to identify the emotional state of others. Even an infant can learn to identify his or her parents through the sense of smell. Although the young infant has not learned to see and discriminate patterns well, the infant can distinguish identity through the olfactory sense.

In a hospital setting an employee who has an unpleasant odor creates a real management dilemma. The supervisor may counsel and even reprimand the employee for poor hygiene. Employees who have the smell of alcohol may be sent home. It is important that the nurse appreciate that odors may be pathological, as in certain diabetic states, or the result of certain mouthwashes or soaps. If a client has an unpleasant odor, the nurse should first assess whether some pathological condition is present, such as an inflammatory process. In a psychiatric hospital a client's odor could be associated with a condition such as schizophrenia, and although there is some thought that such an odor may be pathological, it is more likely to be related to a lack of motivation for self-care skills.

Immediate receptors

Immediate receptors are those that examine the world up close and include tactile stimuli received by way of the skin membranes. It is important that the nurse appreciate the effect culture may have on an individual's reaction to these stimuli and how these stimuli can be modified by cultural influences.

Skin membranes Human beings receive a tremendous amount of information from the distance receptors, which include the eyes, ears, and nose. Because of the vast amount of information that is received from the distance receptors, few people think of the skin as a major sense organ. However, if we humans lacked the ability to perceive heat and cold, we would soon perish. Without the ability to perceive heat and cold or to react appropriately to these stimuli, we would freeze in the winter and become overheated in the summer. The skin, as a major sense organ, is so grossly overlooked that even some of its subtle sensing and communicating qualities are overlooked. Nerves called "proprioceptors" keep us in-

formed as to exactly what is happening as we work our muscles. These nerves provide the feedback that enables us to move our bodies smoothly; thus they occupy a key position in kinesthetic space perception. The body also has another set of nerves called "exteroceptors," which are located in the skin and convey the sensations of heat, cold, touch, and pain to the central nervous system. In light of the fact that two different systems of nerves are employed in the perception of space, kinesthetic space is considered qualitatively different from thermal space. However, nurses must remember that these two systems work together and are mutually reinforcing most of the time.

It has been only in modern scientific times that some remarkable thermal characteristics of the skin have been discovered. The capacity of the skin for emitting and detecting radiant or infrared heat is extraordinarily high. One might assume that because the capacity of the skin to emit and detect radiant or infrared heat is so highly developed, it was important to survival in the past and most certainly had a significant function in early human beings. Although the discovery of the thermal characteristics of the skin has been only within recent times, the importance of the skin as an immediate receptor should not be overlooked by the nurse.

Humans are well equipped to send and receive messages concerning emotional states based on changes in skin temperature. Skin temperature can give very important clues to the emotional state of the individual. A common indicator of embarrassment or anger in fair-skinned individuals is blushing. However, dark-skinned people also blush. Therefore blushing cannot be perceived as simply a matter of change in skin coloration. The nurse must carefully observe dark-skinned persons when looking for changes in emotional state such as embarrassment or anger by noting a swelling of regions of the forehead. The additional blood to these areas will raise the temperature, and these areas will appear flushed. Therefore, even if there is no significant change in color to these areas in dark-skinned individuals, these areas will appear warm to the touch.

Many novel instruments have been developed to make it possible to study heat emission. These instruments should make it possible to study the thermal details of interpersonal communication, an area not previously accessible to direct observation. Thermographic devices (infrared-detection devices and cameras) that were originally developed for satellites and homing missiles have been developed for recording subvisual phenomena. Photographs taken in the dark using radiant heat of the human body have shown that an inflamed area of the body actually emits more heat than the surrounding areas. Diagnosis of cancer is also possible with thermographic devices that measure blocked circulation of blood. Thermographic devices have been useful in health care delivery because skin color does not affect the amount of heat delivered; dark skin does not emit more or less heat than light skin. Thus the observable phenomenon in all individuals regarding heat emission is the blood supply in a given area of the body.

Increased heat on the surface is detected in three ways:

1. Thermal detectors in the skin, particularly if two individuals are close enough to each other.
2. Intensified olfactory interactions, which are augmented when skin temperature rises. Perfumes or body or face lotions may be smelled at a greater distance when the body temperature is increased.
3. Visual examination, which can give clues to an increase or decrease in body temperature. For example, an individual who is pale may have a decrease in body temperature, whereas a person who appears flushed may have an increase in body temperature.

Certain individuals or racial groups are more aware of subtle changes in skin temperature. In addition, some persons accentuate or take advantage of this medium of communication. For example, an individual knowledgeable about variations in skin temperature according to location may apply perfume to certain parts of the body. The phenomenon of crowding is a chain reaction set in motion when there is not enough space to dissipate the heat within a crowd and the heat becomes more intense. A hot crowd will require more room than a cool crowd if they are to maintain the same degree of comfort and lack of involvement. It is important for the nurse to

remember that when thermal spaces overlap and people can smell each other, they become more involved and may even be under the chemical influences of each other's emotions. Some individuals by virtue of cultural heritage have trouble with the phenomenon of crowding. These individuals are more likely to be unable to sit in a chair soon after someone else has vacated it. An example of this phenomenon is often given by sailors on submarines who are forced to participate in "hot bunking," the practice of sharing a bunk as soon as someone gets out of it. It is not understood why one's own heat is not objectionable whereas a stranger's may be. It may be attributable in part to the fact that humans have a great sensitivity to small differences; therefore individuals respond negatively to a heat pattern that is not familiar (Hall, 1966, 1969).

Body-heat regulation lies deep in the brain and is controlled by the hypothalamus. Culture affects attitudes in regard to the perception of skin temperature changes. Human beings exert little or no conscious control over the heat system of the body. Many cultural groups tend to stress phenomena that can be controlled and deny those that cannot. In other words, because some individuals by virtue of their cultural heritage have been taught to ignore certain uncontrollable stimuli, they experience body heat as a highly personal stimulus. Body heat is therefore linked to intimacy as well as to the experiences of childhood. An adult who as a child was used to close personal contact with parents and other loved ones may have a pleasant association when in a crowded environment where heat and warmth are radiated. On the other hand, an adult who was subjected to discomfort in close relationships or who was not exposed to closeness as a child may experience a great deal of difficulty and anxiety when in a close environment, for example, an overcrowded bus.

A person born in a heavily populated country where closeness was necessitated by overcrowding may experience conscious discomfort in moving to another locality where closeness is not the norm. On the other hand, persons born in thinly populated countries may have a conscious feeling of overcrowding in a country where closeness is the norm. For example, a tourist from the United States visiting a country such as Hong Kong, Jamaica, or China, all of which are extremely overpopulated, may quickly react to the experience of closeness and associate the country with unpleasantness. This experience is not limited to different cultures but may also be noted when a rural person visits an urban setting, such as a person from rural Mississippi visiting New York City.

The English language is full of expressions that relate to skin sensation and body temperature changes. For example, it is not uncommon in the United States to hear individuals say that another person made them hot under the collar, gave them a cold stare, involved them in a heated argument, or warmed them up. These expressions may be more than just a figure of speech; they may be a way of recognizing the changes in body temperature that occur both personally and in other people. Thus these common experiences have been incorporated into language in the United States.

Relationship between tactile space and visual space

Touch and visual spatial experiences are so interwoven with one another that they cannot be separated easily. Young children and infants learn to reach, grasp, fondle, and mouth everything in the environment. Teaching children the relationship between tactile and visual space is a difficult task that requires many years of training for children to subordinate the world of touch to the visual world. Visual and tactile space can be distinguished by the fact that tactile space separates the viewer from the object, whereas visual space separates objects from each other. As early as 1945, Michael Baliant described two different perceptual worlds: sight oriented and touch oriented. According to Baliant, the touch-oriented world is both immediate and friendlier than the sight-oriented world, in which space is friendly but filled with dangerous and unpredictable objects, namely, people. Using Baliant's definition of tactile space, it is difficult to conceive that designers and engineers have failed to grasp in all of their scientific research the deep significance of touch, particularly active touch (actually contacting others or objects). Individuals incorporate both tactile and vi-

sual stimuli in relating to the world. For example, although automakers tend to rely heavily on visual perception when designing a particular automobile, they are also concerned with tactile perception, as evidenced by their giving attention to such things such as luxury upholstery, automatic windows, doors, gas-cap locks, ornate trimmings, and carpeting. In response to this stimuli, prospective buyers touch both the car's interior and exterior before making a purchase.

Some objects in the environment are appraised and appreciated almost entirely by touch, even when these objects are visually presented, such as objects made from wood, cloth, or ceramics. The Japanese are very conscious of the significance of texture. Emphasis is placed on the smoothness of the item being crafted. It may be perceived that it requires more time to make a smooth-textured item than a rough-textured item and that the time spent on the crafted item is related to the care and concern of the craftsman. The objects that are produced by Japanese people may be perceived as being made by caring craftsmen.

Touch is the most personal of all the sensations. Touch is sometimes described as the most important sense because it confirms the reality perceived through the other senses (Montagu, 1971). Touch is central to the human communication process and is often used to communicate messages. Beyond general communication, touch is associated with breaking down the distance between individuals. Most people associate life's most intimate moments with touch. For example, during lovemaking or in a loving relationship, touch takes on a private and special meaning. Nurses have long appreciated touch as an important component of the nurse-client interaction (Clement, 1987; Giger, Davidhizar, Johnson, & Poole, 1997). Nurses face the challenge of developing trust, creating a humanistic and responsive atmosphere, and effectively exchanging information in a system energized by high technology and concern for cost effectiveness. Most nursing literature focuses on touch as a communication behavior and describes using touch to communicate caring (Geldard, 1960; Leininger, 1977; Mintz, 1969; Montagu, 1971), the physiological and psychological dynamics of touch (Davidhizar & Giger, 1989; Giger & Davidhizar, 1995; Spector, 1996; Goodykoontz, 1980; Hedlund & Jeffrey, 1992; Heidt, 1981; Krieger, 1975; Lynch, 1978; West, 1981), and the components of touch behavior. Research also supports the belief that using touch appropriately with clients can result in positive physiological and psychological responses (Day, 1973; Seaman, 1982; Ujhely, 1979). Nurses need to be aware of the characteristics of touch and how they can affect the entire communication process.

In contrast to tactile space is the phenomenon of visual space. To understand visual space, the nurse must understand that no persons see exactly the same thing when actively using their eyes in a natural situation; people do not relate to the world around them in exactly the same way. For example, different persons will visually notice different objects because of perceptual differences (Davidhizar, Dowd, & Giger, 1997). It is important for the nurse to recognize these differences and at the same time be able to translate from one perceptual world to another. The distance between the perceptual worlds of two persons of the same culture may be considerably less than the distance between the perceptual worlds of two persons of different cultures. There is significant evidence that people brought up in different cultures live in different perceptual worlds. North Americans tend to have a more linear perceptual field. This difference is demonstrated in art and architectural design. American artists prefer designs that are linear, whereas Chinese and Japanese artists prefer depth and maintaining constancy in a design.

Relationship of space-time and illness

Gilman and Knox (1995) examined childhood cancers for evidence of space-time interactions within three distinct sets of dates and places (at birth, at diagnosis, and at death). Birth clustering and diagnosis clustering occurred. It was concluded that two types of clustering must be regarded as separate and statistically independent phenomena. This suggests the involvement of multiple time-space localized exposures to hazards with short and constant latent intervals; probably an infectious agent or an environmental toxin. Silman et al. (1997) also examined

whether new cases of rheumatoid arthritis cluster in time or space. Although a viral cause is the strongest candidate for rheumatoid arthritis, no evidence of a localized event in time was associated with disease development in the population studied.

SPATIAL BEHAVIOR

Spatial behavior is often described in nursing literature in relation to the universal need for territoriality (Allekian, 1973; Davidhizar, 1988; Hayter, 1981; Hedlund & Jeffrey, 1992; Oland, 1978; Reakes, 1997; Brant, 1983). People by nature are territorial. Territoriality refers to a state characterized by possessiveness, control, and authority over an area of physical space. If the need for territoriality is to be met, the person must be in control of some space and must be able to establish rules for that space. The need for territoriality cannot be fully met unless individuals can defend their space against invasion or misuse by others (Roberts, 1978). Hayter (1981) has suggested three important aspects of territoriality to consider when planning nursing care: a physical space of one's own, a personal space, and the territory of expertise or role. One can also relate territoriality needs to spatial behaviors of or proximity to others, to objects in the environment, and to body movement or position. Territoriality serves to achieve diverse functions for individuals, including meeting needs for security, privacy, autonomy, and self-identity. A variety of factors may influence needs for territoriality, including culture, age, sex, and health status. It is important for the nurse to understand the effect such variables may have on spatial behavior and the ethical implications (Piaschenko, 1997).

Proximity to others

Proxemics is the term for the study of human use and perception of social and personal space (Hall, 1974). Individuals tend to divide surrounding space into regions of front, back, right, and left (Franklin, Henkel, & Zangas, 1995). The front region is considered the most important, largest, recalled with the greatest precision, and to be described with the greatest detail. Proxemics has been shown to allow one to predict self-esteem and self-evaluative moods even after controlling for the contributing of the personality dimensions of neuroticism, extroversion, and agreeableness (Hart, Field, Garfinkle, & Singer, 1997). Physical distancing from others varies with setting and is culturally learned (Murray & Huelskoetter, 1991). Generally, in Western culture there are three primary dimensions of space: the intimate zone (0 to 18 inches), the personal zone (18 inches to 3 feet), and the social or public zone (3 to 6 feet) (Hall, 1966). The intimate zone may be used for comforting, protecting, and counseling and is reserved for people who feel close. The personal zone usually is maintained with friends or in some counseling interactions. Touch can occur in the intimate and personal zones. The social zone is usually used when impersonal business is conducted or with people who are working together. Sensory involvement and communication are often less intense in the social zone. Wide variations to these general dimensions do occur and are often influenced by cultural background (Giger & Davidhizar, 1990). Montagu (1971) has suggested that childrearing practices affecting sleep behavior may have an effect on the use of space, especially as it determines acceptable interaction distance. He reported on varying cultural approaches apparently related to family group sleeping arrangements and the Western middle-class practice of separating the child from parents for sleep. According to Oland (1978), the Western practice of putting small children in a room of their own, which separates them from other family members, may enculturate children to desire isolation and separation and cause or facilitate a desire for more extensive territory.

Among the Eskimos and northern Indians of Canada, the practice of separate bedrooms varies dramatically because living quarters are often small with all persons sleeping in the same room (Burke, Maloney, Pothaar, & Baumgart, 1988; Giger and Davidhizar, 1998; Young, 1988; Giger & Davidhizar, 1990). For these individuals, proximity to others in small living quarters is often a necessity for survival since staying inside and the body heat of others may be necessary to avoid freezing in the frigid arctic temperatures. The need for space also varies for many Southeast Asian immigrants who have come to the United States as refugees. These individuals are also accustomed to living in crowded living situations. Therefore, for some South east Asian Americans, spacious living accommodations may cause discomfort (Van Esterik, 1980).

Spatial needs and the desire for a certain proximity to certain people continue through life and have been studied in the elderly. In nursing homes elderly clients may have certain chairs identified as theirs and become upset when a stranger sits in their chair or in the seat nearby that is reserved for a special friend. Moving from household to household to stay with children on a rotating basis, rather than being viewed as a pleasant variation, is also likely to be upsetting. Since the elderly are more likely to experience separation from others through the death of a spouse and the moving away of offspring, their spatial needs may appear to change; that is, they may withdraw or may reach out more for others (Ittelson, Proshansky, Rivlin, & Winkel, 1974).

Interpersonal messages are communicated not only by body proximity but also by the location and availability of the nurse during the day. A client who knows that the nurse will answer when the call bell is pressed feels differently from the client who does not understand how the call bell works or feels that it is an imposition to ask for help and waits for the nurse to ask what can be done (Schuster & Ashburn, 1986).

Individuals have different requirements for sensory stimulation. Either overstimulation, as by crowding, or understimulation, as by isolation, may cause an untoward reaction. For example, in times of disaster overstimulation induced by crowding can be so extreme that it can result in insanity or death. In this example, a person is perceived as being in a little black box and unable to move about freely, which causes the person to jostle, push, and shove. How the individual responds to jostling and therefore to the enclosed space depends on how he or she feels about being touched by strangers. It is this constant touching and being touched that may result in widespread panic and "freezing" in disaster situations (Hall, 1966).

An enclosed space requirement can also be overstimulating. For example, a client who must remain in a hospital room in bed and in isolation for a lengthy period can be overstimulated because of the spatial limits presented by the boundaries, including bed rest and the four walls of the room. Nursing interventions for this client include opening curtains, calling by intercom frequently to check on the client, and stopping by to see the client as often as possible. A client in isolation can suffer from understimulation in regard to tactile stimulation. The few people who do enter the room may hesitate to touch the client out of fear of contracting the illness. One of the greatest problems expressed by clients with acquired immunodeficiency syndrome (AIDS) is the isolation they experience because of physical distances from others. Family members afraid of catching AIDS may hesitate to touch, hug, or kiss the AIDS victim. Caregivers also may show their fear by standing a greater distance from the client, wearing gloves, and having less frequent encounters with the client (Zook & Davidhizar, 1989). The strong link between curing, the major focus of health care, and caring by health care practitioners has been emphasized by Leininger (1977), who cites touch as one of the special constructs of the caring process. As a therapeutic element of human interaction, touch can help the nurse to show caring.

Today, the image of the nurse as someone standing close to the bedside and having physical proximity is changing. Within the wider discourse of fiscal restraint on health care spending, professional nurses need not be in physical proximity for meanings to be generated, to be acted upon, and to have effects in the present. Modern technology is redefining the need for physical proximity. The needs of modern health care are redefining where the nurse's presence needs to be to accomplish the needs of professional nursing (Purkis, 1996).

Cultural implications

Watson (1980) noted that although there are variations in spatial requirements from person to person, individuals in the same cultural group tend to act similarly. For example, nomads do not seem to desire a permanent territory but are content with establishing a temporary territory and then moving on. Because individuals are usually not consciously aware of their personal space requirements, they frequently

have difficulty understanding a different cultural pattern. What may be considered an act of friendliness by one person (such as standing close to another person) may be perceived by the other as a threatening invasion of personal space. A person who wishes to maintain distance will indicate this by body language. Clients who step back, do not face the nurse directly, or pull their chair back from the nurse are sending messages indicating additional space requirements. The nurse's responsiveness to the client's spatial requirements is an important factor in the client's emotional comfort. It is important that the nurse be cognizant of the effects of culture on the client's spatial needs and use sensitivity in responding to the client's need for personal territory. Subtle cultural variations in the use of nonverbal signals often lead to misunderstanding; thus, to meet the client needs, it is essential that the nurse have knowledge of cultural variations in spatial requirements.

Nurses and clients from the population groups of Native Americans, Appalachians, Japanese Americans, and Mexican Americans often find a comfortable position between the personal and social distance (Tripp-Reimer & Lively, 1993). Watson (1980) studied cultural differences in the use of personal space. He compiled a range of space by nationality and found that persons in the United States, Canadians, and the British require the most personal space, whereas Latin Americans, Japanese, and Arabic persons need the least. These latter groups seemingly have a much higher tolerance for crowding in public spaces than some other cultural groups, such as North Americans and northern Europeans have, but they also appear to be more concerned about their own requirements for the space they live in. In particular, the Japanese tend to devote more time and attention to the proper organization of their living space for perception by all the senses (Hall, 1966). Asians are generally more sensitive to personal space and are more likely to feel comfortable conversing from a distance of 5 or 6 feet. Maintaining distance in relationships for some Asian Americans is an indication of respect. Therefore, it important to remember to avoid invading the personal space of these individuals. Some West Indians maintain little space between friends when communicating. For some West Indians, an outsider is expected to maintain some distance when interacting (Carson & Arnold, 1996).

A White American female nurse from a nontactile culture may experience discomfort when a male client from a tactile culture, such as the Latin American, African-American, or Indonesian-cultures, stands in the intimate zone while describing symptoms (Rawlins, Williams, & Beck, 1993; Tripp-Reimer & Friedl, 1977). Touching between persons of the same sex, including men, is more common among Arabic persons than it is among Americans. However, among some Asian cultures touch between women is less common. For example, in some Asian cultures women do not shake hands with each other or with men (Randall-David, 1989). In the United States the kind of familiarity common among Arabs may be considered a homosexual pass (Hall, 1966). Hall and Whyte (1990) note that a handshake in Latin America, particularly between two men, is seen as cold and impersonal. For some Latins, the "doble abrazo" in which two men embrace by placing their arms around each other's shoulders is the accepted form of greeting. On the other hand, touching the shoulders of a Japanese man is seen as a humiliation and an unpardonable breach of traditional etiquette. Argyle and Dean (1965) reported that members of primitive societies in Africa and Indonesia also came closer and maintained body contact during conversation.

In the Thai and Vietnamese cultures, the head is sacred and patting the head of a small child is considered offensive. For these individuals the head is considered to be the "seat of life." When the head is touched, it is believed that the spirit leaves through this channel. Therefore, when the head needs to be touched for medical reasons, it is important to explain the reason and to ask permission of the adults (Carson & Arnold, 1996; Randall-David, 1989).

In the United States a person who stands at a slight angle to another person indicates body position of readiness to communicate. A desire to exclude a third person can be shown by two persons who face each other directly and have ongoing eye contact. Rejection is also communicated by a person who stands at a right angle to another (Scheflen,

1972). The position of the toes can create distance by communicating rank. A person who feels subordinate will usually stand with the toes inward, whereas a person who feels superior will stand with the toes facing out (Personal Report, 1987). A comparison of the movie shown in the United States *Three Men and a Baby* and the French comedy on which it was based *Three Men and a Cradle* illustrates the differences in responses in the two cultures. In the French version when the natural father returns to the two bachelors who have been inconvenienced by the care of the baby, icy silence occurs. The two men sit stiffly in their chairs and refuse to answer their friend's questions or even acknowledge his presence. In the version seen in the United States, when the natural father returns, he is pummeled and a loud scene occurs (Grosvenor, 1989).

Territoriality influences relationships between people. Some German people tend to need a larger space and are less flexible in their spatial behavior than some American, French, and Arabic people. Differences in spatial patterns between persons in different cultures apply not only to their body proximity, but also to such behavior as changing geographic location. For example, Germans often live in the same house their entire lives, whereas Americans tend to change houses approximately every 5 years, and nomads are content with temporary territories rather than permanent ones. According to Evans and Howard (1973), some Puerto Ricans and African Americans may have different perspectives about space. Some African Americans have more eye contact when they speak, have greater body activity, and have a closer personal space (Sue & Sue, 1990). However, as indicated in Chapter 2, some African Americans have been socialized through a long history of hostile, punitive interactions with Whites to avoid direct eye contact. This behavior may also influence personal space zones (Giger, Davidhizar, Evers, & Ingram, 1994).

OBJECTS IN THE ENVIRONMENT

Objects in the environment offer additional dimensions to communication and can provide both positive and negative qualifiers to verbal communication. Easily movable chairs in a waiting room or office can be pulled together to provide physical closeness or separated to provide distance. Positioning chairs at a 90-degree angle can communicate a cooperative stance, whereas a side-by-side arrangement of chairs can decrease communication. Discomfort and consequently emotional distance can be created by uncomfortable furniture. The nurse's position during the conversation (such as being behind a desk or leaning against the corner of the desk looking down on the client seated at a lower level) can also promote the perception of psychological distance. The nurse must be aware of the effect culture may play on the client's reaction to objects in the environment and should respond in a way that client comfort will be increased (Pearlin, 1982). The nurse dealing with Eskimos should appreciate the value Eskimos place on objects they possess. These individuals tend to highly value generosity and a sense of sharing, "What is mine is here for all." For some of these people, only what is needed for the present is taken and used. This can be a problem for the Eskimo who is diabetic because, if food is available, it will be shared with anyone, regardless of the special health needs (McRae, 1994).

Cleanliness in the environment may also be a significant factor in creating a healthy and comfortable milieu. This is particularly true in surgical areas where space is used in designing a physical layout that will allow for maintaining aseptic technique (Fox, 1997). Comfortable air conditioning in a client waiting room on a hot day can facilitate a client's ease and decrease anxiety. On the other hand, when the air conditioning is absent or malfunctioning on a hospital ward on a hot day, client and staff anxiety can escalate.

When the nurse is interacting with some Eskimos living in rural Alaska, it is important to be aware that their life-style may be substandard by the nurse's standards. For some Eskimos, living standards are substandard and homes are often poorly heated, have no indoor plumbing, have unsafe water supplies, and lack telephones. A lack of vehicles and the presence of poor roads limit accessibility to facilities for food, clothing, and health service for many of these people. The environment can be profoundly important when ongoing health care is needed to monitor a chronic illness or to prevent recurrence of an acute illness (McRae, 1994).

Structural boundaries

The term "personal boundaries" is sometimes used to describe the use of structural boundaries in the environment. A boundary separates a person from others and also helps define a person's space. Fences, doors, curtains, walls, desks, chairs, and other objects may create boundaries between persons (Scott, 1988). The purpose of a boundary is to facilitate individuation or separation from the environment. Developmentally this concept begins at approximately 6 months of age. Mahler, Pine, and Bergman (1975) described an infant's first attempts at separation or individuation as consisting in behaviors such as pulling at the parent's hair, ears, or nose, and pushing the body away from the parent to get a better look at him or her. At 7 to 8 months of age the infant begins to differentiate self from the parent. The child may examine the parent's jewelry or glasses and is anxious around others. These crucial developmental steps are indicative of the child's beginning formation of boundary, which continues through the toddler stage. By 3 years of age the toddler has a fairly stable sense of identity and self-boundaries.

Doors, walls, glass panels, and waist-high partitions serve as structural boundaries for nurses' territories in health care settings. Doors, curtains, and furniture arrangements may define client territories. Structural boundaries can help the individual adapt to both internal and external stresses. On the other hand, when structural boundaries are violated, anxiety may increase. The nurse needs to assess whether the client has rigid or flexible boundaries. If a client has open boundaries, less anxiety will be encountered in interactions with health professionals that may violate personal boundaries. If the client has rigid boundaries, the nurse should guard against approaches that may be perceived as threatening.

The use of restraints with agitated clients involves physical invasion of both intimate space and body boundaries. Patients who resist restraints and become aggressive and combative may be viewed as resisting this personal invasion.

Just as individuals can be described by personal boundaries that determine comfort levels in relation to others, territoriality also describes an interpersonal phenomenon in the environment. As indicated earlier, territoriality is a state characterized by possessiveness, control, and authority over an area of physical space (Hayter, 1981). For the need for territoriality to be met fully, the person must be in control of some space, be able to establish rules for that space, and be able to defend it against invasion or misuse by others. In addition, the person's right to do things in the space must be acknowledged by others (Roberts, 1978). For example, a hospitalized client needs not only a personal sleeping area, but also a place to put and arrange personal belongings without fear that they will be bothered by others. There should also be freedom to do things in the personal space, such as taking a nap.

For clients who have chronic disability with difficulty moving it is important that space in the living environment be arranged to maximize power and use of resources (Moss, 1997). Access and ability to negotiate space in the living environment can be critical to quality of life and maximum independence.

The nursing staff also have professional territorial imperatives. Nurses' stations and lounges may be designated as staff territory. When a psychiatric unit is renovated and the staff are asked by administration to move from a locked-nursing-station concept to an open-nursing-station concept wherein clients may come to an open half wall to interact openly with staff who may be inside, the staff may find this very intrusive of "their" territory and object to this invasion of their space. Nursing staff may also fear personal assault (Croker & Cummings, 1995; Roberts, 1991, 1989). McMahon (1994) noted that, for psychiatric staff, space in the ward office serves several significant functions including the opportunity for informal contact between nurses and the opportunity to have a liaison with visiting professionals, to store possessions, to provide a "patient-free" zone, and to serve as a communication center. Staff needs for territory must be considered when unit staff and clients' areas are designed. Restricting certain staff from certain hospital areas (such as the mailroom or the copy machine room) may be seen as punitive

and dehumanizing. Thus it is essential that explanations given for this restriction be clearly understood to avoid paranoid interpretations of this action.

Cultural implications

Color is a phenomena with cultural implications. In many North American cultures, warm colors such as yellow, red, and orange tend to stimulate creative and happy responses. In some Asian countries, white is associated with a funeral. In many African countries, red symbolizes witchcraft and death (Carson & Arnold, 1996). In the dominant culture in the United States, good mental health is often associated with the ability to coordinate the color of one's wardrobe (Ramírez, 1991). In contrast, in some countries including Africa, the Caribbean, and the South Pacific, bright, multiple colors are the accepted norm of dress (Carson & Arnold, 1996). Leff and Isaacs (1981) noted that a scarf tied around the forehead may not indicate "royalty" or schizophrenia but may be a cultural response by a West Indian to a headache. In Western culture, cool colors such as blue, green, and gray tend to encourage meditation and deliberation and thus may have a dampening effect on communication. The nurse should plan color in the environment to be therapeutic in an effort to enhance communication (Bartholet, 1968; Mufford, 1992).

BODY MOVEMENT OR POSITION

Body movement or position can also communicate a message to others. This concept has been well documented by the pioneering work of Efron (1941), Birdwhistell (1970), Scheflen (1972), Ekman and Friesen (1975), and Ekman (1985) and by recent reviews of the state of the art in this field (Bull, 1983; Davis, 1975; Davis & Skupien, 1982; Hickson & Stacks, 1985; Wolfgang, 1984; Leathers, 1992). This information has also been applied to counseling and psychotherapeutic techniques through the work of Moreno (1946); Gendlin (1969); Steere (1982); Marcus (1985); and Perls, Hefferline, and Goodman (1983), all of whom made body movement and awareness central aspects of their therapeutic approach. Thus, a broad body of knowledge supports the premise that through body movement a person may convey what is not verbalized.

It is well known that body movements may be of particular importance during periods of stress. Expressions of self through movement are learned before speech; therefore, when stress is experienced, a person may revert to a form of expression used at an earlier level. Attention to body movement can facilitate understanding of a person experiencing stress. There are endless expressions of body movement, such as finger pointing, head nodding, smiles, slaps on the back, head and general body movements, and even body sounds, including belching, knuckle cracking, and laughing. A seemingly insignificant act such as how a door bell is rung may bear the stamp of an individual's personality, as well as emotional state. For example, the door bell may be rung loudly, impatiently, repetitively, tentatively, feebly, or aggressively (Bendich, 1988).

The nurse must also consider the effect of slow versus fast movements (Newman, 1976). In an emergency rapid movements are essential. On the other hand, a young child in the hospital for the first time may be frightened by a health professional who enters the room quickly, approaches the child rapidly, and picks the child up. In another situation an agitated psychiatric client who is approached slowly and with a quiet voice may be calmed by the slow movements of the nurse, which are seen as reassuring.

Nurses are also exploring movement as a therapeutic medium, such as movement therapy for the aged (Goldberg & Fitzpatrick, 1980; Stevenson, 1989), movement therapy after inactivity or infection (Folta, 1989; Kasper, 1989), dance and movement therapy, and exercise to music. It has been thought that movement therapy can provide a way to communicate when the ability to communicate feelings is limited. Movement therapy has also been used for relaxation and to provide relief of blocked emotion.

Body motions, or kinetic behaviors, can be categorized as follows (Knapp & Hall, 1992).

1. *Emblems.* Nonverbal actions that have a verbal translation into a word, phrase, or symbol. This includes sign language used in the operating room or the gesture of thumb and forefinger to form a circle to say "A-OK" in the United States or to indicate an obscenity in Brazil.

2. *Affect displays.* Facial expressions such as a frown, a smile, or lips pulled down at the corners.
3. *Illustrations.* Nonverbal acts accompanying speech. Examples of this include an upturned thumb to indicate that a ride is desired or pointing a finger to indicate a direction.
4. *Adapters.* Nonverbal behavior that modifies or adds to what is being said. For example, folded arms may indicate disgust or that a person is feeling closed to others; a wave may be used as a friendly greeting; leg swinging and finger tapping may indicate anxiety.
5. *Regulators.* Movements that maintain interaction and provide feedback. Head nods or changing gaze can indicate that it is the other person's turn to talk. A head nod can also indicate listening.

Cultural implications

Body movement is also related to culture. For example, in the United States head nodding is common, whereas in Africa the torso is frequently moved (Eibl-Eibesfeldt, 1972). Gestures are used by Americans and British to denote activity and by Italian or Jewish persons to emphasize words (Bigham, 1964). In some cultures, certain actions are not considered proper with strangers, such as touching, standing close to, or looking directly at the individual. Some cultures give certain body movements a sexual interpretation. In the Western culture, stroking the hair, adjusting the clothes, or changing position to accent maleness or femaleness may have or be given a sexual connotation (Scheflen, 1972). Although a kiss is often given a sexual connotation in the United States, the Japanese kiss to show deference to superiors (Sue & Sue, 1990). When Brazilian clients were compared to American clients for space and motion discomfort in relation to anxiety disorders, it was noted that there is a country bias. Brazilian clients were more likely than American clients to endorse symptoms, thus showing a transcultural bias (Romas, Jacob, & Lilienfeld, 1997).

IMPLICATIONS FOR NURSING CARE

It is important for the nurse to remember that territoriality, or the need for space, serves four functions: security, privacy, autonomy, and self-identity

(Oland, 1978). The nurse needs an understanding of cultural diversity and culturally appropriate behaviors in relation to these functions (Carson & Arnold, 1996; England, 1986). Security includes actual safety from harm and giving the person a feeling of being safe. The nurse must also remember that if a client is in a place where a feeling of control is experienced, the client will feel safer, less threatened, and less anxious (Giger & Davidhizar, 1994). People generally tend to feel safer in their own territory because it is arranged and equipped in a familiar manner. In addition, most people believe there is a degree of predictability associated with being in one's own personal space and that this degree of predictability is hard to achieve elsewhere. Nurses must also remember that the anxiety level of a client is increased when the client is hospitalized. However, the same client may experience a decrease in anxiety if the client is allowed to return home, even if still sick. Some terminally ill clients request to go home because of the feeling of security experienced in one's own personal space.

In addition to security, personal space provides privacy and at the same time protected communication. Most people believe it is not necessary to be on guard or to keep up pretenses—to be themselves—in the security of one's personal space. The fulfillment of the desire to be oneself contributes to feelings of decreased anxiety and promotes relaxation. Many people may complain of feeling tense and tired after a long day at work but may experience relaxation and ease of tension as soon as they get home. Two factors that contribute to these feelings are (1) activities at home are different from those at work and (2) people experience more relaxation in their personal space (Hayter, 1981). In some instances, hospital staff have a tendency to treat elevators as private space and make inappropriate comments while riding back and forth on the elevator. Hospital employees need to be very careful to consider certain hospital locations such as elevators as public spaces and to guard against violation of client privacy (Ubel et al., 1995). If it becomes necessary to transfer a client from one room to another or from one floor to another, the nurse should remember that the client may experience increased anxiety because of the loss of security and privacy of the room to which the client has become accustomed (Smith, 1976). This feeling of loss of security and privacy can also be related to nursing practice. For example, a nurse manager who returns from vacation to find office furniture rearranged may feel unsettled until the furniture is returned to a familiar arrangement. The nurse should remember that clients may already be experiencing feelings of anxiety that are related to the reasons for seeking health care. Additional anxiety invoked by issues involving territoriality can be minimized by the nurse who develops an understanding of culture and its implications for territoriality or interpersonal space.

Another important aspect of territoriality for nurses is the function of autonomy. Autonomy is the means by which a person controls what happens. In personal territory a person may feel free to ask questions, resist suggested actions, hold out for those things that are most important personally, and share personal feelings. A client, on the other hand, is out of personal territory and lacks control. Therefore it is important for the nurse to determine if the client has an adequate understanding of the treatment regimen and is not submitting to treatment merely because of a lack of control of territory. Statements to the client that maximize feelings of control, such as, "How do you want to arrange the room?" or "Are you concerned about your treatment? We can walk down the hall to the visiting room, where it is private, to discuss your feelings" should promote feelings of security and autonomy for the client. Feelings of autonomy are also evidenced in nursing practice. For example, when a nurse manager needs to counsel an employee, the manager's control will be maximized if the counseling occurs in the manager's office. On the other hand, if the manager is viewed as too controlling, the manager may intentionally select a more neutral territory for the counseling, such as a conference room.

It is essential to remember that having personal space promotes self-identity by affording opportunities for self-expression and that personal well-being is often related to the critical distance a person keeps from others (Wilson & Kneisl, 1995; Reakes, 1997; Giger, Davidhizar, Johnson, & Poole, 1997).

Another way to define self-identity in relation to personal space is to view self-identity as a mode of individuality. The personal space over which a person has jurisdiction often becomes a personal extension of self and a reflection of characteristics, personality, and interest. A nurse may communicate warmth and reduce feelings of anxiety by moving close to a client. On the other hand, rapidly moving toward an anxious client may dramatically increase the client's anxiety. People have a need to organize and arrange personal space so that it maximizes functioning and at the same time meets needs. For example, when a person purchases a new home, it becomes essential for that home to take on the person's identity. This is evidenced by the desire of the new occupants to change such items as the wallpa-

per, colors of the walls, carpet, lighting fixtures, and draperies. Regardless of whether these items are new, each person has a need for self-expression or individuality. When clients set out personal pictures of their family and other personal items from home and wear their own sleepwear, self-identity is enhanced. Therefore changing items to reflect this individuality becomes an essential aspect of personal security and autonomy. Self-identity is also created by the nurse when he or she is negotiating symbolic space. For example, Martin and Hutchinson (1997) describe how nurse practitioners use techniques such as cultivating, bargaining, confronting, and disengaging in order to define the role of the nurse practitioner and to make it part of the national consciousness.

Case Study

Mr. Bernhard Wolfgang, a 56-year-old German immigrant who works as an engineer, is admitted with chest pain and shortness of breath. Mr. Wolfgang is admitted to the coronary care unit to rule out myocardial infarction. Immediately after admission Mr. Wolfgang's wife comes to the coronary care unit with personal items such as family portraits, some roses from the client's garden, and some personal clothing. However, since the coronary care unit is restricted in space, personal items are not allowed, and the wife is instructed to take the items home. On admission, Mr. Wolfgang's vital signs are stable and his color is good. He reports that the chest pain is not debilitating and is more or less an occasional dull ache. After 2 days the diagnosis of myocardial infarction is confirmed, and Mr. Wolfgang remains restricted to bed but is transferred to a semiprivate room in the coronary care step-down unit. After admission to the coronary care step-down unit, the nurse observes that Mr. Wolfgang is anxious, somewhat withdrawn, and unable to express his needs and feelings.

STUDY QUESTIONS

1. When assessing Mr. Wolfgang, the nurse should realize that some German people have specific needs that are related to territoriality and space. Name at least two factors that affect some Germans and their spatial behavior.

2. List ways the nurse could enable Mr. Wolfgang to meet his needs for privacy and autonomy while in a semiprivate room.

3. Identify markers that would indicate Mr. Wolfgang's need for the establishment of a temporary territorial space.

4. Identify ways in which illness and hospitalization could threaten Mr. Wolfgang's personal sense of territoriality.

5. Identify factors present in a coronary care unit that could negatively affect spatial behavior.

6. List two factors related to perceptual and visual stimuli that adversely affect some German clients.

7. List ways the nurse could control perceptual and verbal stimuli that may affect Mr. Wolfgang.

References

Allekian, C.E. (1973). Intrusions of territory and personal space. *Nursing Research, 22,* 236-241.

Argyle, M., & Dean, J. (1965). Eye-contact, distance, and affiliation. *Sociometry, 28,* 289-304.

Baliant, M. (1945). Friendly expanses—hard empty spaces. *International Journal of Psychoanalysis, 1,* 38 46.

Bartholet, M. (1968). Effects of color on dynamics of patient care. *Nursing Outlook, 6*(10), 51-53.

Bendich, S. (1988). Appreciating bodily phenomena in verbally oriented psychotherapy sessions. *Issues in Mental Health Nursing, 9,* 1-7.

Bigham, C. (1964). To communicate with Negro patients. *American Journal of Nursing, 64*(9), 113-115.

Birdwhitstell, R. (1970). Kinesics and context. Philadelphia: University of Pennsylvania Press.

Black, J.W. (1950). The effect of room characteristics on vocalizations and rate. *Journal of Acoustical Society in America, 22,* 174-176.

Brant, C. (1983). Native ethics and rules of behavior. London, Ontario: University of Western Ontario.

Brown, J. W., Leavitt, L., & Graham, F. (1977). Response to auditory stimuli in six- and nine-week-old infants. *Developmental Psychobiology, 10,* 255-266.

Bull, P. (1983). *Body movement and interpersonal communication.* New York: John Wiley & Sons.

Burke, S., Maloney, R., Pothaar, D., & Baumgart, A. (1988). Four views of childbearing and child health care: Northern Indians, urban natives, urban Euro-Canadians and nurses. A report for the National Health Research Development Program, Health and Welfare Canada. Ontario.

Carson, V., & Arnold, E. (1996). *Mental health nursing: the nurse-patient journey.* Philadelphia: W.B. Saunders Co.

Clement, J. (1987). Touch. *Association of Operation Room Nurses, 45*(6), 1429-1439.

Croker, K., & Cummings, A. (1995). Nurses' reactions to physical assault by their patients. *Canadian Journal of Nursing Research, 27*(2), 81-93.

Davidhizar, R. (1988). Distance in managerial encounters. *Today's OR Nurse, 10*(10), 23-30.

Davidhizar, R., & Giger, J. (1989). Managerial touch. *Today's OR Nurse, 10*(7), 18-25.

Davidhizar, R., Dowd, S., & Giger, J. (1997). Model for cultural diversity in the radiology department. *Radiology Technology, 68*(3), 233-240.

Davis, M. (1975). *Towards understanding the intrinsic body movement.* New York: Ayer.

Davis, M., & Skupien, J. (1982). Body movement and nonverbal communication: an annotated bibliography, 1971-1981. Bloomington, Ind.: Indiana University Press.

Day, F. (1973). The patient's perception of touch. In Anderson, E.H., Bergerson, B.S., Duffey, M., Lohr, M., & Rose, M.H. (Eds.), *Current concepts in clinical nursing* (vol. 4) (pp. 266-275). St. Louis: Mosby.

Efron, D. (1941). *Gesture and environment.* New York: King's Crown Press.

Eibl-Eibesfeldt, I. (1972). Similarities and differences between cultures in expressive movements. In Hinde, R.A. (Ed.), *Nonverbal communication* (pp. 297-312). Cambridge, England: Cambridge University Press.

Ekman, P. (1985). *Telling lies.* New York: W.W. Norton.

Ekman, P., & Friesen, W.V. (1975). Unmasking the face. Englewood Cliffs, N.J.: Prentice Hall.

England, J. (1986). Cross-cultural health care. *Canada's Mental Health, 34*(4), 13-15.

Evans, G.W., & Howard, R.B. (1973). Personal space. *Psychological Bulletin, 80,* 335-344.

Folta, A. (1989, April 3). Exercise and functional capacity after myocardial infarction. Paper presented at the 13th Annual Midwest Nursing Research Society Conference, Cincinnati, Ohio.

Franklin, N., Henkel, L., Zangas, T. (1995, July). Parsing surrounding space into regions. *Memory and Cognition, 23*(4), 397-407.

Geldard, F. (1960). Some neglected possibilities of communication. *Science, 131,* 1583-1588.

Gendlin, E.T. (1969). Focusing. *American Journal of Psychotherapy, 1,* 1-18.

Giger, J., & Davidhizar, R. (1990). Culture and space. *Advancing Critical Care, 5*(8), 8-11.

Giger, J., & Davidhizar, R. (1998). *Canadian transcultural nursing.* St. Louis: Mosby.

Giger, J., Davidhizar, R., Evers., & Ingram, C. (1994). Cultural factors influencing mental health and mental illness. In Taylor, C. (Ed.), *Mereness' Essentials of psychiatric nursing* (ed. 14) (pp. 215-238). St. Louis: Mosby.

Giger, J., Davidhizar, R., Johnson, J., & Poole, V. (1997). The changing face of America. *Health care Traveler, 4*(4), 11-17.

Gilman, E., & Knox, E. (1995, April). Childhood cancers: space-time distribution in England. *Journal of Epidemiology in Community Health, 49*(2), 158-163.

Goldberg, W., & Fitzpatrick, J. (1980). Movement therapy with the aged. *Nursing Research, 29,* 339-346.

Goodykoontz, L. (1980). Touch: dynamic aspect of nursing care. *Journal of Nursing Care, 13,* 16-18.

Grosvenor, G.M. (1989, July). Viva la différence [President's editorial]. *National Geographic,* p. 15.

Hall, E., & Whyte, W. (1990). Interpersonal communication: a guide to men of action. In Brink, P.J. (Ed.), *Transcultural nursing: a book of readings.* Prospect Heights, Ill.: Waveland Press.

Hall, E.T. (1977). *Beyond culture.* Garden City, N.Y.: Anchor.

Hall, E.T. (1974). Proxemics. In Weitz, S. (Ed.), *Nonverbal communication* (pp. 205- 229). New York: Oxford Press.

Hall, E.T. (1969). *The hidden dimension.* New York: Doubleday.

Hall, E.T. (1966). *The silent language.* Westport, Conn.: Greenwood Press.

Hart, D., Field, N., Garfinkle, J., & Singer, J. (1997). Representations of self and others: a semantic space model. *Journal of Personality, 65*(1), 77-105.

Hayter, J. (1981). Territoriality as a universal need. *Journal of Advanced Nursing, 6,* 79-85.

Hedlund, N., & Jeffrey, F. (1993). Therapeutic communication. In Rawlins, R., Williams, S., & Beck, C. (Eds.), *Mental health–psychiatric nursing* (ed. 3) (pp. 65-91). St. Louis: Mosby.

Heidt, P. (1981). Effect of therapeutic touch on anxiety level of hospitalized patients. *Nursing Research, 30,* 32-37.

Hickson, M.L., & Stacks, D.W. (1985). *Nonverbal communication studies and applications.* Dubuque, Iowa: W.C. Brown.

Ittelson, W., Proshansky, H., Rivlin, I., & Winkel, H. (1974). *An introduction to environmental psychology.* New York: Holt, Rinehart, & Winston.

Kasper, C. (1989, April 3). Exercise-induced degeneration of skeletal muscle following inactivity. Paper presented at the 13th Annual Midwest Nursing Research Society Conference, Cincinnati, Ohio.

Knapp, M., & Hall, J. (1992). *Nonverbal communication in human interaction* (ed. 3). New York: Holt, Rinehart, & Winston.

Krieger, D. (1975). Therapeutic touch: the imprimatur of nursing. *American Journal of Nursing, 75*(5), 784-787.

Leathers, D.B. (1992). *Successful nonverbal communication principles and applications* (ed. 2). New York: Macmillan.

Leff, J., & Isaacs, A. (1981). *Psychiatric examination in clinical practice.* St. Louis: Mosby.

Leininger, M. (1977, December). Caring: the essence of central focus of nursing. *Nursing Research,* Report I, p. 2.

Lynch, J. (1978). The simple act of touching. *Nursing, 78*(8), 32-36.

Mahler, M., Pine, F., & Bergman, A. (1975). *The psychological birth of the human infant.* New York: Basic Books.

Marcus, N. (1985). Utilization of nonverbal expressive behavior in cognitive therapy. *American Journal of Psychotherapy, 39*(4), 467-478.

Martin, P., & Hutchinson, S. (1997, Jan.). Negotiating symbolic space: strategies to increase NP status and value. *Nurse Practitioner, 22*(1), 89-91.

McMahon, B. (1994). The functions of space. *Journal of Advanced Nursing, 19,* 362-366.

McRae, L. (1994). Cultural sensitivity in rehabilitation related to native clients. *Canadian Journal of Rehabilitation, 7*(4), 251-256.

Mintz, E. (1969). On the rationale of touch in psychotherapy. *Psychotherapy: theory, research, and practice, 6*(4), 232-234.

Montagu, A. (1971). *The significance of the human skin* New York: Columbia University Press.

Moreno, J.L. (1946). *Psychodrama* (vol. 1). New York: Beacon House.

Moss, P. (1997, July). Negotiating spaces in home environments: older women living with arthritis. *Social Science Medicine, 45*(1), 23-33.

Mufford, C. (1992, October). A cure of many colors. *New Physician,* 14-19.

Murray, R., & Huelskoetter, M. (1991). *Psychiatric–mental health nursing* (ed. 3). Norwalk, Conn.: Appleton & Lange.

Newman, M. (1976). Movement therapy and the experience of time. *Nursing Research, 25,* 273-279.

Oland, L. (1978). The need for territoriality. In Yura, H. & Walsh, M.B. (Eds.), *Human needs and the nursing process* (pp. 97-140). New York: Appleton-Century-Crofts.

Pearlin, L. (1982). The social context of stress. In Goldberger L., & Breznitz, S. (Eds.), *Handbook of stress* (pp. 367-379). New York: Free Press.

Perls, F.S., Hefferline, R., & Goodman, P. (1983). *Gestalt therapy.* New York: Dell.

Personal Report for the Executive (1987, July 15). New York: National Institute of Business Management.

Piaschenko, J. (1997). Ethics and the geography of the nurse-patient relationship: spatial vulnerable and gendered space. *Scholarly Inquiry of Nursing Practice, 11*(1), 45-59.

Purkis, M.E. (1996). Nursing in quality space. *Nursing Inquiry, 3*(2), 101-111.

Ramírez, M. (1991). *Psychotherapy and counseling with minorities.* New York: Pergamon Press.

Randall-David, E. (1989). Strategies for working with culturally diverse communities and clients [Brochure]. Washington, D.C.: U.S. Department of Health and Human Services.

Rawlins, R., Williams, S., & Beck, C. (1993). *Mental health–psychiatric nursing* (ed. 3). St. Louis: Mosby.

Reakes, J. (1997). Communication. In Johnson, B. (Ed.), *Psychiatric-mental health nursing* (ed. 4). Philadelphia: J.B. Lippincott.

Roberts, S. (1989). The effects of assault on nurses who have been physically assaulted by their clients. Unpublished master's thesis, University of Toronto, Toronto, Ontario.

Roberts, S. (1991). Nurse abuse: a taboo topic. *The Canadian Nurse, 87*(3)23-25.

Roberts, S.L. (1978). *Behavioral concepts and nursing throughout the life span.* Englewood Cliffs, N.J.: Prentice Hall.

Romas, R.T., Jacob, R.G., Lilienfeld, S.O. (1997). Space and motion discomfort in Brazilian versus American patients with anxiety disorders. *Journal of Anxiety Disorders, 11*(2), 131-139.

Schleflen, A. (1972). *Body language and social order.* Englewood Cliffs, N.J.: Prentice Hall.

Schuster, C., & Ashburn, S. (1986). *The process of human development: a holistic approach* (ed. 2). Boston: Little, Brown & Co.

Scott, A. (1988). Human interaction and personal boundaries. *Journal of Psychosocial Nursing, 26*(8), 23-28.

Scott, A., & Dumas, R. (1995). Personal space boundaries: clinical applications in psychiatric mental health nursing. *Perspectives in Psychiatric Care, 31*(3), 14-19.

Seaman, L. (1982). Affective nursing touch. *Geriatric Nursing, 3,* 162-164.

Sideleau, B.F. (1992). Space and time. Part Two. In Haber, J., Leach-McMahon, A., Price-Hoskins, P., & Sideleau, B. (Eds.), *Comprehensive psychiatric nursing* (ed. 4). St. Louis: Mosby.

Silman, A., Bankhead, C., Rowlingston, et al. (1997). Do new cases of rheumatoid arthritis cluster in time or in space? *International Journal of Epidemiology, 26*(3), 628-634.

Smith, M. (1976). Patient responses to being transferred during hospitalization. *Nursing Research, 25,* 192-196.

Spector, R. (1996). *Cultural diversity in health care* (ed. 4). Stamford, Conn.: Appleton & Lange.

Steere, D.A. (1982). *Bodily expressions in psychotherapy.* New York: Brunner/Mazel.

Stevenson, J. (1989, April 3). Exercise in frail elders: findings and methodological issues. Paper presented at the 13th Annual Midwest Nursing Research Society Conference, Cincinnati, Ohio.

Sue, D.W, & Sue, D. (1990). *Counseling the culturally different: theory and practice* (ed. 2). New York: John Wiley & Sons.

Tripp-Reimer, T., & Friedl, M. (1977). Applachians: a neglected minority. *Nursing Clinics of North America, 12*(41), 41-54.

Tripp-Reimer, T., & Lively, S. (1993). Cultural considerations in mental health–psychiatric nursing. In Rawlins, R., Williams, S., & Beck, C. (Eds.), Mental health–psychiatric nursing (ed. 3). St. Louis: Mosby.

Ubel, P., Zell, M., Miller, D. et al. (1995, August). Elevator talk: observational study of in appropriate comments in a public space. *American Journal of Medicine, 99*(2), l, 190-194.

Ujhely, G. (1979). Touch: reflections and perceptions. *Nursing Forum, 18*(1), 18-32.

Van Esterik, P. (1980). Cultural factors affecting adjustment of Southeast Asian refugees. In Tepper, E. (Ed.), *Southeast Asian exodus: from tradition to resettlement* (pp. 151-172). Ottawa: The Canadian Asian Studies Association.

Watson, O.M. (1980). Proxemic behavior: a crosscultural study. The Hague, The Netherlands: Mouton.

West, B. (1981). Understanding endorphins: our natural pain relief system. *Nursing 81*(2), 11, 50-53.

Wilson, H., & Kneisl, C. (1995). *Psychiatric nursing* (ed. 5). Reading, Mass.: Addison-Wesley.

Wolfgang, A. (Ed.) (1984). *Nonverbal behavior: perspectives, applications, and intercultural insights.* Lewiston, N.Y.: C.J. Hogrete.

Young, T. (1988). *Health care and cultural change: the Indian experience in the central subarctic.* Toronto: University of Toronto Press.

Zook, R., & Davidhizar, R. (1989). Caring for the psychiatric inpatient with AIDS. *Perspectives in Psychiatric Nursing Care, 25*(2), 3-8.

CHAPTER 4

Social Organization

BEHAVIORAL OBJECTIVES

After reading this chapter, the nurse will be able to:

1. Describe how cultural behavior is acquired in a social setting.
2. Define selected terms unique to the concept of social organization, such as culture-bound, ethnocentrism, homogeneity, bicultural, biracial, ethnicity, race, ethnic people of color, minority, and stereotyping.
3. Describe significant social organization groups.
4. Define family groups, including nuclear, nuclear dyad, extended, alternative, blended, single-parent, and special forms of family groups.
5. List at least two primary goals inherent to the American culture in regard to the family as a unit.
6. Describe the significant influence that religion may have on the way individuals relate to health care practitioners.

Cultural behavior, or how one acts in certain situations, is socially acquired, not genetically inherited. Patterns of cultural behavior are learned through a process called "enculturation" (also referred to as "socialization"), which involves acquiring knowledge and internalizing values. Most people achieve competence in their own culture through enculturation. Children learn to behave culturally by watching adults and making inferences about the rules for behavior (Nolt, 1992). Patterns of cultural behavior are important to the nurse because they provide explanations for behavior related to life events. Life events that are significant transculturally include birth, death, puberty, childbearing, childrearing, illness, and disease. Children learn certain beliefs, values, and attitudes about these life events, and the learned behavior that results persists throughout the entire life span unless necessity or forced adaptation compels the learning of different ways. It is important for the nurse to recognize the value of social organizations and their relationship to physiological and psychological growth and maturation (Murray & Huelskoetter, 1991).

CULTURE AS A TOTALITY

Most anthropologists believe that to understand culture and the meaning assigned to culture-specific behavior, one must view culture in the total social context. The concept of holism requires that human behavior not be isolated from the context in which it occurs. Therefore culture must be viewed and analyzed as a totality—a functional, integrated whole whose parts are interrelated and yet interdependent. The components of culture, such as politics, economics, religion, kinship, and health systems, perform separate functions but nevertheless mesh to form an operating whole. Culture is more than the sum of its parts (Goldsby, 1977; Henderson & Primeaux, 1981).

Culture-bound

As children grow and learn a specific culture, they are to some extent imprisoned without knowing it.

Some anthropologists have referred to this existence as "culture-bound." In this context the term culture-bound describes a person living within a certain reality that is considered "the reality." Most people have learned ways to interpret their world based on enculturation. Thus, although certain interpretations are understandable and persuasive to persons brought up to share the same frame of reference, other people may not share these interpretations and therefore may make little sense out of the context. Shipler (1997) who has traveled extensively around the United States notes that connecting across racial lines is among the most difficult things on earth. In a perceptive work, *A Country of Strangers,* it is noted that "even as we look upon each other like strangers from afar, we are trapped in each other's imaginations." Interracial marriages bring subtle issues of discrimination home to the dinner table. For example, a Black child reports being dropped by a White pen pal who discovers her race (Coleman, 1997; Cose, 1997). In *Reaching Beyond Race,* Sleeper (1997) suggests that rather than trying to overcome racism and a color-blind world, individuals should fight for equality on nonracial terms. In fact, polls in America have indicated that most Americans agree that people should be judged for themselves, not for their race (Sniderman & Carmines, 1997). Although Americans generally want persons from all races treated equally, such practices at Dartmouth University where African Americans have a far better chance of being admitted than Whites of equal qualitifications are viewed as giving an unfair advantage (Kantrowitz, 1997; Dickerson, 1997).

Nurses are also culturally bound within the profession because they are likely to bring a unique scientific approach—the nursing process—to determining and resolving health problems. Many nurses are likely to consider the nursing process the best and only means of meeting the needs of all clients regardless of their cultural heritage. However, clients may view this modern scientific approach differently, believing that the nursing process meets their needs in some ways but not in others. The nursing process may not take into consideration alternative health services, such as folk remedies, holistic health care, and spiritual interventions. In these cultures,

medicine is often practiced in unscientific ways based on the Western viewpoint. Therefore desirable outcomes for treatment may occur independently of medical and health care interventions.

Traditionally, American nurses have been socialized to believe that modern Western medicine is the answer to all humanity's health needs. Most illnesses have been attributed to a biological cause (Grypma, 1993). More recently, Americans have been moving toward a more harmonious relationship with nature in which there is a growing sensitivity to the environment. Traditional attitudes toward disease are being reassessed. Today, more attention is being given to the concept of the individual as an organic whole. Many nursing leaders in the United States and Canada are calling for a change in nursing paradigms from scientific to holistic (Grypma, 1993; Thompson, 1993; McRae, 1994; Guruge & Donner, 1996).

Ethnocentrism

For the most part, people look at the world from their own particular cultural viewpoint. Ethnocentrism is the perception that one's own way is best. Even in the nursing profession, there is a tendency to lean toward ethnocentrism. Nurses must remain cognizant of the fact that their ways are not necessarily the best and that other people's ideas are not "ignorant" or "inferior." Nurses must remember that the ideas of lay persons may be valid for them and, more importantly, will influence their health care behavior and consequently their health status. In contrast to the term ethnocentrism is the word "ethnic," which relates to races or to large groups of people classed according to common traits or customs. In populations throughout the world, people are bound by common ties, elements, life patterns, and basic beliefs germane to their particular country of origin.

In general, the medical paradigm used in the Western culture views health, illness, and dying as biophysical realities. However, the meaning a nurse places on life can affect relationships with clients. For example, if the nurse believes there is no relationship between illness and evil, this may be at conflict with the client who believes that illness is a punishment from God or the work of spirits (Gregory, 1988; Grypma, 1993). On one hand, some Puerto

Ricans believe that sickness and suffering is a result of one's evil deeds; on the other hand, many Ugandans believe that an infant's illness or death is the result of a neighbor's curse (Grypma, 1993).

Homogeneity

It is difficult to find a homogeneous culture in the United States. If a homogeneous culture did exist, all individuals would share the same attitudes, interests, and goals—a phenomenon referred to as "ethnic collectivity." People who are reared in ethnic collectivity share a bond that includes common origins, a sense of identity, and a shared standard for behavior. These values are often acquired from experiences that are perceived to be cultural norms and determine the thoughts and behaviors of individual members (Harwood, 1981; Saunders, 1954). The ultimate consequences of enculturation are carried over to health care and become an important influence on activities relative to health and illness behaviors. In the American culture there is a tendency to speak of culture as if it included a set of values shared by everyone. However, even within an ethnic collectivity, intraethnic variations occur and are obvious in health behaviors. For example, intraethnic variations are seen in the concept of mental illness (Guttmacher & Elinson, 1972; Berry, 1988; Beiser, Barwick, Berry, et al., 1988; Sands & Berry, 1993), in cultural definitions of health and illness, in skepticism about medical care and consequently the use or lack of use of health care services (Berkanovic & Reeder, 1973; Spector 1996; Prilleltensky, 1993), and finally in the willingness of the individual to assume a dependent role when ill (Suchman, 1964).

Bicultural

The term "bicultural" is used to describe a person who crosses two cultures, life-styles, and sets of values. To understand biculturalism, the nurse must understand the differences in meaning of ethnicity, race, biracial, and minority.

Ethnicity

Ethnicity is frequently and perhaps erroneously used to mean race, but the term "ethnicity" includes more than the biological identification. Ethnicity in its broadest sense refers to groups whose members share a common social and cultural heritage passed on to each successive generation. The most important characteristic of ethnicity is that members of an ethnic group feel a sense of identity.

Race

In contrast to the term "ethnicity" is the term "race," which is related to biology. Members of a particular race share distinguishing physical features such as skin color, bone structure, or blood group. Ethnic and racial groups can and do overlap because in many cases the biological and cultural similarities reinforce one another (Bullough & Bullough, 1982). A more precise definition of race is a breeding population that primarily mates within itself (Giger, Davidhizar, & Wieczorek, 1994). It is important to remember that there are very few races that still mate largely within the group. There are some pure-blooded lineages found in certain parts of the world. For example, in the United States, some of the descendants of West Africans are of a "pure-blooded lineage" and live along the Georgia and South Carolina seacoasts. These people have protected their lineage because they have refused to intermarry. These individuals are known as the Gullah people, who have not only their own lineage but also their own distinct dialect of English (Wolfram & Clark, 1971). It is important for the nurse to remember that, regardless of race, all people have a cultural heritage that makes them ethnic (Giger, Davidhizar, & Wieczorek, 1994).

Biracial

When an individual crosses two racial and cultural groups, the individual is considered "biracial." To be both biracial and bicultural often creates an almost insurmountable dilemma for an individual. Physical attributes such as color, shape of eyes, or hair may have a profound influence on acceptance of the "biracial" individual by others. One problem associated with biracialism is the inability of the individual to identify or find acceptance in any one of the biologically related racial groups (Giger, Davidhizar, Evers, & Ingram, 1994). It is the total exclusion and the sense of not belonging to either of the racial or cultural groups that often creates the dilemma. For example, an African American who is an "octoroon," a person with one-eighth African-American blood, may have difficulty being accepted as African American because of the lightness of the skin. Conversely, this same individual might be ostracized by some Whites because of the "blackness of the blood lineage." Some refer to the offspring of a French Canadian and an American Indian as a Métis (pronounced /may-tee′/) (Bailey & Bailey, 1995). For some people of color, there is a perception that the belief held by White America is "color is the difference that makes the differences" (Giger, Johnson, Davidhizar, & Fishman, 1993).

Minority

A minority can consist of a particular racial, religious, or occupational group that constitutes less than a numerical majority of the population. Using this definition for the term "minority," it is obvious that all types of people can belong to various kinds of minorities (Bullough & Bullough, 1982). Often a group is designated "minority" because of its lack of power, assumed inferior traits, or supposedly undesirable characteristics. In any society, cultural groups can be arranged in a hierarchical power structure. Dominant groups are considered to be powerful, whereas those in minority groups are considered inferior and lacking in power.

The term "minority" is not synonymous with numbers. For example, until recently, the ruling class in South Africa (only 2% of the population) were White (Gary, 1991). In the United States, people of color (African Americans, Latin Americans, Asian Americans) are considered minorities. However, when the population of the world is considered in its aggregate, it is obvious that people of color are in the majority.

Gender is another example of how the term "minority" is used erroneously. Females in the United States compose a larger numerical percentage (51%) than do males (49%) but are considered to be in the minority because of their underrepresentation in high-level managerial positions in the workplace. In fact, 95% of all top managerial jobs in the corporate

structure in the United States are held by White males (U.S. Deparment of Commerce, Bureau of the Census, 1998).

The significance of the term "minority" cannot be underemphasized. The central defining characteristic of any minority group, according to Gary (1991), is its relative powerlessness and inability to chart its own course to a better way of life.

Ethnic minority

The term "ethnic minority" is often used because it is less offensive to people of color than other terms. Supposedly it takes into account ethnicity, race, and the relative status of the groups of persons included in the category. Were it not for the use of the word "minority," perhaps this terminology would be less culturally offensive to some groups of people (that is, ethnic people of color). According to Gary (1991), use of the term "people of color" might be the preferable option, particularly in situations where sensitivity to racial preferences needs to be heightened. It is estimated that by the year 2050 about half of the total American population will be nonwhite, thus eliminating the meaning of the term "ethnic minority" (U.S. Department of Commerce, Bureau of the Census, 1998; Kunen, 1996).

Stereotyping

Stereotyping is the assumption that all people in a similar cultural, racial, or ethnic group are alike and share the same values and beliefs. For example, stereotyping occurs when an African-American nurse is assigned to care for an African-American client simply because of ethnicity and race. It is stereotypical when the assumption is made that all African Americans are alike and therefore the African-American nurse is more likely to be more sensitive to the needs of the African-American client. Race and ethnicity do not, in and of themselves, make us "resident experts" on the belief and value systems of other persons. Whether we engage in stereotyping as a result of scientifically proved, research-based data or because of past associations and experiences, stereotyping can ultimately lead to faulty data gathering and faulty interpretation.

Role of gender and cultural significance

In traditional Chinese society, women have held subordinate roles to men, a belief that dates back to the first millennium B.C. (Mo, 1992). Traditional Chinese believe that the universe developed from two complementary opposites: *yin* (Cantonese, *yam*), the female, and *yang* (Cantonese, *yeung*), the male. For some traditional Chinese Americans, the *yin* represents the dark, cold, wet, passive, weak feminine aspect of humankind. In stark contrast, the *yang* represents the bright, hot, dry, active, strong masculine aspect of humankind (Mo, 1992). In traditional societies, there are "written" and "unwritten" roles that dictate behavior of girls and women (Strickland & Giger, 1994). Although some countries in North America are highly evolved technologically, traditional beliefs about the role of women in society still exist throughout many regions of America. Peitchinis (1989) noted that discrimination exists for women in the workplace because women are viewed as having a higher absentee rate than their male counterparts. For many women, this creates a barrier to entrance into the workplace and even more importantly places a "glass ceiling" for advancement that their male counterparts need not overcome (Sartorelli, 1994; Misener, Sowell, Phillips, & Harris, 1997). On the other hand, although women have tended to be an oppressed group in the workplace, numerous studies have indicated efforts by industries to implement policies and procedures to prevent discrimination on the basis of sexual orientation. For example, women may have access to benefits such as child-care leaves, alternative working arrangements, child-care arrangements, and special brief leaves to deal with family problems not available to men (Hyland, 1990; Sussman, 1990; York, 1991). For example, Aetna is one of the growing numbers of companies offering their employees free prenatal classes, access to pumping rooms for women who are lactating, and conferences with lactation consultants trained in breast-feeding problems. About 75 employers have similar programs including Eastman Kodak, Cigna, Home Depot, and Georgia's Fulton County government according to Medela Inc., a breast-pump manufacturer that sells programs through its Sanvita division. Another 200 employers offer only breast pumps and a room where they can be used in private (Danyliw, 1997). Because breast-feeding reduces the incidence and severity of diarrhea, ear infections, allergies, and sudden infant death syndrome and lessens the risk of ovarian and breast cancer in mothers, such programs result in significant savings for companies in medical claims (Danyliw, 1997).

Although the United States is a highly evolved technological country, traditional beliefs about the role of women in society still exist. For example, although 14% of the 1.4 million soldiers, sailors, airmen, and marines in the United States are female, women in military service are still not allowed to engage in active combat during wartime (Thompson, 1998). Controversy also continues about how training should occur. Since coeducational training began in 1994, there has been a high frequency of sexual relations between male and female recruits. Consequently, in 1998, the United States Congress empaneled a commission to consider whether men and women should be separated in boot camp (Thompson, 1998; Newman, 1998; Taylor, 1994). Interestingly, women are making inroads into the world of sports. For example, with more women lacing on boxing gloves, women's boxing is fast on its way to becoming a spectator sport enjoyed by both women and men in America (Bierck, 1997).

SOCIAL ORGANIZATION GROUPS AS SYSTEMS

Social organizations are structured in a variety of groups, including family, religious, ethnic, racial, tribal, kinship, clan, and other special interest groups. Groups are dependent on particular persons and are more affected by changes in members than are other systems. In most groups, except for racial and ethnic groups, members may come and go. Thus the formation and the disintegration of groups are more likely to occur during the members' lifetimes than are the formation and the disintegration of other systems.

According to the general systems theory, social organization groups are characterized by a steady state and a sense of balance or equilibrium that is maintained even as the group changes. Most groups form, grow, and reach a state of maturity. Social organization groups begin with a variety of elements that include individuals with unique personalities, needs, ideas, potentials, and limits. In the course of development of the group, a pattern of behavior and a set of norms, beliefs, and values evolve. As the group strives toward maturity, parts become differentiated, and each member assumes special functions.

Family groups

One group of paramount concern for the nurse when working with persons transculturally is the family. In the United States in 1996 55% of men and 52% of women 15 years of age and older were married. Of 100 million households in 1996, 70% contained families. Married couples maintained 77% of all families, whereas women with no husband maintained 18% (World Almanac, 1998). Regardless of cultural background or the nature of the family, the family is the basic unit of society in the United States. From a sociological perspective the family may be defined as a social unit that interacts with a larger society. The discipline of economics may define the family in terms of how it works together to meet material needs. From a psychological perspective the family may be defined as a basic unit for personality development and the development of subgroup relationships, such as parent-child relationships. Still another definition is offered from a biological perspective, which conceptualizes the family as a unit with the biological function of perpetuating the species.

The most predominant family system in the United States is the nuclear family, which is defined as a group consisting of parents (or a parent) and their nonadult children living in a single household (McMahon, 1997). A similar definition views the family as a cluster of people whose relationship is stipulated by law in terms of marriage and descent and whose precise membership varies according to the circumstances. A broader conceptualization of the term "family" portrays the family as a relationship community of two or more persons in which individuals may come from the same or different kinship groups. Mauksch (1974) views the family as a basic human unit with generic properties, including the coexistence of more than one human being involved in continuous, presumably permanent, sharing of living facilities; a perception of reciprocal obligations; a sense of commonality; and a perception of certain obligations toward others. These varying definitions of the family range from viewing the family as having one structure exclusively to perceiving the family as a household unit representative of various types of family structures.

Types of family structures

Traditional nuclear family According to Virginia Satir (1983), the traditional nuclear family consists of one man and one woman of the same race, religion, and age who are of sound mind and body and who marry during their early or middle 20s, are faithful to the other for life, have and raise their own children, retire, and finally die. This definition appears narrow; however, it has maintained popularity over the years and is still seen by many persons as the most desirable family form. Today a more current definition of the nuclear family allows for more variation. This newer definition defines the nuclear family as a family of two generations formed by a married woman and man with their children by birth or adoption (Govaets, 1987). Within this particular family form, as within all identified family forms, the assigned roles and functions performed by each member vary. One example is a common family structure that has the father working outside the home and the mother working at home taking care of the children and household tasks. However, today the traditional nuclear family often finds both mother and father working outside the home. Thus childrearing and child care may be shared by both parents as well as by others outside the family, such as a day care center.

The traditional nuclear American family has become a rarity. In 1983 approximately 6.2% of American families included a breadwinning husband, a full-time housewife, and two children. In 1992, there were 95.7 million family households (U.S. Department of Commerce, Bureau of the Census, 1993a). By 1998, there were 70.9 million family households and 31.6 million nonfamily households, representing 69.1% and 30.9% of all United States households, respectively. The term "family households" is defined as "people who occupy a housing unit," rather than a physical dwelling (U.S. Department of Commerce, Bureau of the Census, 1993a). Of the households in 1992, only 25% were married-couple families with children. Of that number, 65.8% had children between 6 and 17 years of age, and both parents worked away from the home. Similarly, among female-headed households, 69.9% of mothers with children between 6 and 17 years of age worked away from the home (U.S. Department of Commerce, Bureau of the Census, 1993a). By 1998, among female-headed households, 72.4% of women with children between the ages of 6 and 17 years worked away from home (U.S. Department of Commerce, Bureau of the Census, 1998). It is projected that the mix of families and households will change in the coming years. As the population continues to age, relatively fewer families will have children with a projected 41% in 2010, down from 50% in 1994. It is projected that among families with children, a lower proportion will include two married parents, with a projected 72% in 2010, down from 74% in 1994. Meanwhile, households maintained by a person living alone are projected to rise from 24% to 27% (World Almanac, 1998).

Interestingly, although the nuclear family is on the decline, immigration laws still lean toward "family preference." In the interest of keeping families together, United States policy allows an unlimited number of visas to certain relatives of United States citizens and of permanent resident aliens. Thus an illiterate laborer with no skills but with a parent in the United States has a better chance of immigration than a graduate school–educated foreigner with no family or employer in the United States. About 68% of immigrants came to the United States through the family preference in 1995 and about one tenth of them came as adult siblings. Mexicans, who send more legal immigrants—18%—to the United States than does any other country, have responded to family preference in particularly high numbers, and they are more likely to use ties to extended family members than any other group. The result is a family-based immigrant population that, for Mexicans and Central Americans at least, is skewed toward unskilled labor (Headden, 1998).

Nuclear dyad family The nuclear dyad family consists of one generation and is made up of a married couple without children. There are numerous reasons why this particular family remains childless: the family may have chosen not to have children; they may not be able to have children or to adopt them; or the children may have died. In some cultures this family form is frequently thought of as a beginning point for the formation of the family. However, in other cultures the nuclear dyad family is considered a part of the mainstream of the social organization of the family. The number of nuclear dyad families continues to grow and survive as a functioning unit throughout the world.

Extended family The extended family is multigenerational and includes all relatives by birth, marriage, or adoption. The family group is made up of grandparents, aunts, uncles, nieces, nephews, cousins, brothers, sisters, and in-laws. In today's society there is a tendency for children to leave the homes and communities of their parents, which has resulted in a separation of the nuclear family from the extended family. On the other hand, as America is aging, an increase of multigenerational or extended family households is expected (McMahon, 1997). Today, 1 in 8 Americans is over 65. However, by 2005 1 in 5 Americans will be over 65 with many of the elderly being taken care of in the home by their children and grandchildren (Fineman, 1995; McKibbon, Généreux, & Séguin-Roberge, 1996; U.S. Department of Commerce, Bureau of the Census, 1998).

Skip-generation family Grandparents who are taking care of grandchildren are a growing family group. With increasing numbers of parents dying of AIDS and single parents who are not interested in child care, grandparents are finding themselves in the role of primary caregiver (McMahon, 1997).

Alternative family The alternative family consists of adults of a single generation or a combination of adults and children who live together without social sanction of marriage. The alternative family is often either a communal arrangement—composed of roommates who might be either homosexual or heterosexual—or a love relationship between a man and a woman.

Single-parent family The single-parent family consists of two generations and is made up of a mother or a father and children by birth or adoption. The reasons for a single-parent family include electing to be a single parent, divorce, death, separation, or abandonment. The prevalence of the single-parent family is increasing because of factors such as divorce and the acceptability of being a single parent. Of the children born in the 1990s, it is estimated 22% are being born to single mothers. With two thirds of all single mothers in the work force, a substantial amount of parenting is done by someone other than the biological parent (U.S. Department of Commerce, Bureau of the Census, 1990).

Reconstituted or blended family The reconstituted or blended family is a family that is formed by "put-together parts" of previously existing families with the intention of forming a new nuclear family (Satir, 1983). The blended family, like the traditional nuclear family, is two-generational. However, the blended family differs in form and may be made up of a single person who marries a person with children, or a man and a woman, both of whom have children, who marry. This family form may also yield biological children; thus, there may be a composition of "yours," "mine," and "ours" in the family. The blended family can become very complicated because of the composition and blending of family members, which may include stepbrothers, stepsisters, stepparents, and stepgrandparents. The number of children living in step-blended, or reconstituted families is increasing by 3% annually, and it is estimated that by the year 2000, one third of all children will live with a step-parent by age 18 (U.S. Department of Commerce, Bureau of the Census, 1998).

Special forms of families: gay families and communal families In some cultures an even wider array of family forms occurs, particularly if ideas about marriage and the requirement that the nuclear family is essential to family definition are disregarded. These groups do function as families and therefore must be recognized. These special forms of families may be either unigenerational or multigenerational. Two or more adults constitute these special family forms, and they may or may not be of the same sex.

A commune is a group of people that intertwines husband-wife, parent-child, and brother-sister types of relationships of individuals who have elected to live together in one household or in closely adjoining structures. Family members in a commune must express a feeling of commitment to others in the group. Assigned family roles as well as responsibilities are divided among the members of the group. Generally there are specific rules and expectations for each member of the group. A commune may be formed when people have a common goal, such as a religious, philosophical, or political goal, or a common need, such as an economic, social, or physical need. Examples of communes include Israeli kibbutzim, religious cults, retirement homes for the elderly, and households where couples share resources.

Some gay households consist of two persons and generally function as a nuclear dyad. Other gay households may consist of more members, such as a commune. Today, perhaps as a result of the gay rights movement, homosexual couples have openly taken up residence together. Nevertheless, many members of society continue to be nonaccepting of this particular family form. In 1997 a New Jersey gay couple was first allowed to adopt a child jointly. In doing so New Jersey became the first state to explicitly allow lesbian and gay couples to adopt children jointly, just as married couples do. Although most pro-gay legislation has banned job and housing discrimination against gays, the adoption agreement enters more areas fraught with problems. It not only says that homosexual couples must be treated as full equals with heterosexual couples but also does so in the delicate arena of childrearing. Although most Americans oppose discrimination against lesbians and gays, the country has been less certain that these individuals should be allowed to marry and adopt children. In 1996, Congress passed a bill dubbed the "Defense of Marriage Act," which upheld the right of each State to choose whether to recognize gay marriages (Cloud, 1998). Up to now, 25 states have banned such marriages outright (Cloud, 1998). As a whole, nursing has been slow to endorse a position regarding the debate over the issue of discrimination in the workplace based on sexual orientation. In fact, knowledge on the part of health care workers about sexual orientation has been found to be skewed to nonexistent (Misener, Sowell, Phillips, & Harris, 1997). Gays and lesbians report that they have historically been treated with insensitivity, antagonism, and discrimination in their health care encounters (Misener, Sowell, Phillips, & Harris, 1997).

Characteristics of a family system

According to the general systems theory, a system is a group of interrelated parts or units that form a whole. When the general systems theory is applied to the family, the individual family members are those units that make up the identifiable family system. These parts or units act as one or more subsystems within the larger system. Within the family system the subsystems refer to the way in which the members align themselves with one another. For example, in the family system, the parents may be one subsystem, whereas the children may be another subsystem. At the same time, males and females of the family system may be two other subsystems. A subsystem may consist of any number of members who are linked by some common factor. Within the family system, membership in a particular subsystem may be determined by generational considerations, sexual identity, areas of interest, or a specifically designated function. Individual family members may belong to several different subsystems. Family members also belong to external systems, such as the community system, the school system, and career systems. Subsystems may be constructed to ensure that important functions within the family system are carried out to maintain the overall family structure.

Fawcett (1975) studied the family as a living open system and thus viewed family nursing as an emerging conceptual framework for nursing care. Nurses have cared for families for years; however, it is only recently that nurse researchers have begun to study the family as a whole (Murphy, 1986). Nursing studies in family health are increasing, such as qualitative studies in family health by Campbell (1989), Phipps (1989), and Breitmayer, Gallo, Knafl, and Zoeller (1989).

Family as a behavioral system

The family is conceptualized as a behavioral system with unique properties inherent to the system. A close interrelationship exists between the psychosocial functioning of the family as a group and the emotional adaptation of individual family members. A distinguishable link exists between disorders of family living and disorders of family members. This link can best be understood in the context of systems theory. Systems theory is an orientation whereby people are recognized and defined by who they are in the context of their relationship with family, friends, and the society in which they live. Family systems theories were developed in the 1950s on both the East and West coasts of the United States. On the West Coast a group of people that included Jackson, Haley, and their associates in Palo Alto, California, explored the notions of communication theory and homeostasis applied to the family with a schizophrenic member (Bateson, Jackson, Haley, & Weakland, 1968; Satir, 1983). On the East Coast, in Washington, D.C., Bowen (1994) conceptualized a family systems theory based on a biological systems model. In Philadelphia, Minuchin (1974) used a systems model in his research with families with psychosomatic disorders.

Lewis, Beavers, Gossett, and Phillips (1976) and Caplan (1975) explored both disturbed families and healthy families from a systems perspective. A system is a whole that consists of more than the sum of its parts; a system can be divided into subsystems, but the subsystems are not representative pieces of the whole. To study the family from a cultural perspective, one must understand the basic characteristics of a family system and of a living system. Today in nursing the family nursing process is the same whether the focus is on the family as the client or the family as the environment. Therefore the nursing process used in family nursing is the same as that used with individuals, that is, assessment, nursing diagnosis, planning, intervention, and evaluation. According to Friedman (1986), the only distinguishable difference is that both the individual and the family receive care simultaneously. There are some inherent underlying assumptions germane to the family approach to the nursing process, including the beliefs that all individuals must be viewed within their family context, that families have an effect on individuals, and that individuals have an effect on families. As nursing becomes more involved in the delivery of care in the community, it is imperative to strengthen nursing expertise in the delivery of care to the entire family (McMahon, 1997).

Independent units All systems have basic units that make functioning possible. Within the structure of the family system, the basic interdependent units are the individual family members. As with any open system, change within one family member affects the entire family system. For example, when one family member becomes physically or emotionally ill, the entire family system is changed in some way. Additional alterations in the family system occur because of the changing composition of family membership as a result of events such as birth, divorce, death, hospitalization, leaving home for college, or marriage. All these variables, whether positive or negative, may bring about disruption and disequilibrium in the family system. All family systems have dynamic characteristics that must be used when disruption or disequilibrium occurs if the family system is to be permitted to return to equilibrium as matter, energy, and information are exchanged (Lewis, 1979).

The number of adults who are unmarried (never married, currently divorced, or widowed) is dramatically increasing in the United States. In 1994 there were 74 million unmarried adults compared with 38 million in 1970. Unmarried persons represented 39% of all adults (18 years of age and older) in 1994, up from 28% in 1970. Divorced persons were the fastest growing segment of the unmarried population, with their number quadrupling from 4 million in 1970 to 17 million in 1994. Divorced persons who had not remarried represented 9% of all adults in 1994. Never-married persons, who represented the largest segment of the unmarried population in 1994 (59%), more than doubled from 21 million in 1970 to 44 million in 1994. In fact, during this period, the proportion of persons ages 30 to 34 years of age who had never married tripled from 6% to 20% for women and from 9% to 30% for men. Never-married persons represented 23% of all adults in 1994 (Information Please Almanac, 1998).

Environment As with all open systems there is an internal and external environment that controls the direction of growth of the family system. The internal environment involves the social and physical factors within the family boundaries, the quality of which is reflected by such factors as (1) marital relationship, (2) location of power, (3) closeness of family members, (4) communication, (5) problem-solving abilities, (6) free expression of feelings, (7) ability to deal with loss, (8) family values, (9) degree of intimacy, and (10) autonomy of family members. Within the family system, the external environment involves the social and physical world outside of the family, such as church, neighbors, extended family, school, friends, work, health care system, political systems, and recreation.

Boundaries Within the family system the "boundary" is the imaginary line or area of demarcation that keeps the family system separate and unique from its external environment. As with all open systems, energy, in the form of information, material goods, and feeling states, passes among family members and the external environment. Openness and closedness in a family system are governed by the degree of information or energy that is exchanged and the nature of the boundaries. Information coming into the family system provides the family with information about the environment and about family functioning. If the family accepts the information, it may be used to formulate and respond to the environment, to assist the family in coping with disequilibrium, or to rejuvenate the family. Energy coming into the family can also be stored until needed. Finally, energy or information coming into the family can be rejected or ignored (Satir, 1983).

As with all open systems, the amount of energy or information that enters and leaves the system must be balanced within certain limits to maintain a steady state of functioning or homeostasis if proper adaptation of the system is to occur. Any system can become dysfunctional if the system is allowed to become too open or too closed. No truly closed systems exist, except in a theoretical sense. On the other hand, if a family system were totally open, the family system would probably lose its identity as a system separate from other systems to which family members belong. Therefore the family members might suffer from alienation, rootlessness, and a lack of belonging. The opposite extreme, or a theoretically closed family system, would consist of boundaries that were very rigid, and thus family members would become enmeshed, fixed, and unable to move out, grow, or change.

Communication within the family system

The verbal and nonverbal interaction among family members is called "communication." Factors that contribute to the family member's patterns of communication include (1) the pattern of members acknowledging each other's verbal and nonverbal messages; (2) the degree of responsibility taken by each member for expressing individual feelings, thoughts, and reactions in a constructive way; (3) the extent to which the family encourages a clear exchange of words; (4) the extent to which family members are allowed to talk for themselves; and (5) the patterns of spontaneous talking. Bonding among family members occurs as a result of the form of communication patterns that exist.

Roles in the family

Family member roles are patterns of wants, goals, beliefs, feelings, attitudes, and actions that family members have for themselves and others in the family. Roles are both assigned and acquired, and they specify what individuals do in the family. Although they are usually dependent on social class and cultural norms, roles are dynamic and change in response to factors both within the family and without. Roles are reciprocal and complement roles taken by other family members. Family equilibrium is dependent on how well roles in the family are balanced and reciprocated (Duvall and Miller, 1984; Friedman, 1986).

The way in which a family member assumes a particular role is influenced by various factors, including temperament, height, weight, gender, birth order, age, and health status. Certain roles, however, depend solely on the sex of the family member. Females can be sister, daughter, wife, mother, or girl friend, whereas males can be brother, son, father,

husband, or boy friend. Other roles, such as breadwinner, homemaker, cook, handyman, or gardener, are performance roles and depend on the person's ability to perform a certain task. In contrast to performance roles are emotional roles, such as leader, nurturer, scapegoat, caretaker, jester, arbitrator, or martyr, which may be adopted at certain times as a means of adjusting to the demands of a family system, to an extended family crisis such as a long-term family illness, or to long-term family conflict. The functions of emotional roles are to reduce conflict among family members and to promote temporary adaptation among family members. However, consistent use of emotional roles may serve to impair adaptation, thus hindering the growth of the family. An example of this is when one family member, perhaps the oldest child, assumes the role of family caretaker, supporting other members and arbitrating disputes. The role may take on negative characteristics in this instance because the family caretaker may appear outwardly strong and capable but inwardly have unrealistic feelings, such as "I can't fail" or "I can't be weak." In this emotional role this person may function under pressure to be perfect but at the same time have feelings of self-doubt and fear. It is important for the nurse to remember that roles have a significant effect on individual adjustment.

Family organization

To understand family organization, it is important for the nurse to remember that structuring of both functions and goals must be addressed. It is also important for the nurse to remember that most families are dynamic, endlessly adaptable, and continuously evolving in both structure and function. The functional ability of a family depends in part on the individual needs and wants of the members. If the nurse is unable to assist family members in meeting needs within the family structure, pain may be felt and confusion may exist. The nurse must keep in mind that, in the American culture, families are expected to be self-perpetuating and at the same time be the primary system for the transfer of social values and norms.

In the American culture two primary goals are inherent to the family: (1) the encouragement and nurturance of each individual and (2) the production of autonomous, healthy children (O'Brien, 1992). Marital partners are expected to be supportive and protective of each other. Both the husband and the wife are expected to share a sense of meaning and emotional closeness within the boundaries of their relationship, thus fostering the goal of personality development. In families in which supportive relationships do not exist, the achievement of the first goal (the encouragement and nurturance of each individual) is not attainable. The second goal of the family includes encouraging children to develop their own identity and individuality by allowing them to develop ideals, feelings, and life directions. At the same time, children are encouraged to sense both similarities to and differences from others and to be able to initiate activities based on this information (Lewis, 1979). Factors that must be addressed to determine the degree to which the family will accomplish these two primary goals include the patterns of relationship and adaptive mechanisms that are present. There are many reasons why some families fail to accomplish these two primary goals, including psychiatric disturbance among family members, incomplete maturation of children, and disintegration of the family system. When adaptive mechanisms are used by the family, internal equilibrium may result. These adaptive mechanisms are dependent on (1) the level of communication skills within the family; (2) the individual contributions of each family member to the family welfare; (3) the mutual respect and love within the family; (4) the type, kind, and amount of stressors encountered; (5) the response pattern to stressors encountered in the internal and external environment; and (6) the support or resources available and the opportunity to participate in support systems (Ackerman, 1984; Black, 1991). For example, a family that has an alcoholic father may not be able to accomplish goals because this problem may result in psychiatric disturbances in the wife and children, and ultimately the family system may disintegrate. The reasons for the disintegration of this family include not only the individual psychiatric disturbances, but also accompanying difficulties such as incomplete maturation of children and adult members, financial instability, in-

ability to adapt successfully to stressors, and more importantly, the inability of each family member to perceive the family unit as caring and loving (Brown, 1986).

Levels of functioning Four levels of family functioning that have been identified form a continuum in increasingly abstract levels (Box 4-1): (I) family functions and activities, (II) intrafamilial interactions, (III) interpersonal relationships, and (IV) the family system (Averaswald, 1973).

To understand the family from a cultural perspective, it is essential that the nurse recognize that family relationships are stronger among some ethnic or cultural groups than among others. However, the importance of socioeconomic class cannot be overlooked. According to Casavantes (1976), a pattern of strong family relationships exists particularly among poor people, who have few resources and must rely on the support of the family kinship network to meet physical and emotional needs. Middle- or upper-class people often have resources that extend beyond the extended family and are therefore able to avail themselves of physical and emotional support within the community. It is often believed that when people do not have money or other available resources for recreation and social activities in the community, they tend to spend more time together and depend on the family group for recreational and social outlets.

Regardless of socioeconomic class, families must organize and structure themselves. Structure refers to the organization of the family and includes the type of family, such as nuclear or extended. The value system of the family dictates the roles assigned in the family, communication patterns within the family, and power distribution within the family (Friedman, 1986; Schneflen, 1972). The basic beliefs about humankind, nature, the supernatural (fate), time, and family relationships constitute a family's value system. Value systems are often clustered by socioeconomic status or ethnic groups. For example, families from lower socioeconomic groups tend to have a present-time orientation and view themselves as being subjugated to the environment or the supernatural (fate). Often the family relationships are disrupted by desertion

Box 4-1

LEVELS OF FAMILY FUNCTIONING

LEAST ABSTRACT

Level I: Family functions and activities

Level II: Intrafamilial interactions

Level III: Interpersonal relationships

MOST ABSTRACT

Level IV: The family system

Level I deals with family affairs and functions. Included in this level are tangible, pragmatic activities that are either observable or easily identified; more important, these are things that family members are most comfortable in discussing. Four categories of family functioning have been identified in Level I:

1. **Activities of family living.** Families are expected to provide physical safety and economic resources. Included in this category is the ability of family members to obtain such necessities as food, clothing, shelter, and health care.

2. **Ability of the family members to assist one another.** Included in this category is the family's ability to assist one another in developing emotionally and intellectually and at the same time attaining a personal as well as a family identity.

3. **Reproduction, socialization, and release of children.** Included in this category are functioning goals that would allow the family to become closely aligned, thereby allowing the transmission of subcultural roles and values.

4. **Integration between the family, its culture, and society.** Included in this category is the ability of the family to use external environmental resources for support and feedback.

Level II basically deals with communication and various interactions between family members, including what is said, how it is said, patterns of communication over time, the ability of each family member to communicate, and the quality of communication skills. Also included in this level is the transfer of information from family member to family member.

Level III deals with the way family members interact in relationships that occur within the family constellation. The dimensions of closeness and power and the degree of empathy, support, and commitment that exist among family members are important. How the family functions in regard to decision making and problem solving is included in this level.

Level IV deals with the concepts of the family system as well as how the family functions as a system. Level IV is the most abstract level of family functioning. It encompasses the concepts of wholeness, openness or closedness, homeostasis, and rules.

Data from Schneider, R. (1980, June). *Conceptual scheme of family organization and function.* Paper presented at St. Louis University Medical Center conference, St. Louis, Missouri.

of a spouse or by the early emancipation of the children because of severe economic difficulties. These families have been able to survive and adapt by taking in other extended family members' children; for example, a grandmother may provide direct assistance by raising her son's or daughter's children. In these families power is usually authoritarian or not exerted at all.

Middle- and upper-class families in the United States for the most part espouse the Protestant work-ethic values, which dictate the importance of working and planning for the future. These values encompass the belief that although man is somewhat evil, his behavior is changeable by hard work. In the middle- and upper-class family struc-

ture, financial stability and success are viewed as rewards for hard work. Within these classes family relationships center around the nuclear family, socialization occurs with work-related or neighborhood friends, and power may be more egalitarian than in the lower-class family. Power tends to become more male dominated as the economic level of a family rises. Middle- and upper-class families often see themselves as able to control or have mastery over their environment (O'Brien, 1992).

When typical White-American families are compared to Asian-American families, some differences can generally be noted. The typical White-American family defines itself by the present generation, is fiscally independent, has the core relationship as husband-wife, emphasizes happiness of the individual, and is more feeling oriented. In contrast, the Asian family is defined by past, present, and future generations, feels economic obligations to kin, has parent-child as the core relationship, emphasizes the welfare of the family, and is more task oriented (Hsu, 1985). The Asian client's explanatory model of illness is greatly influenced by the family (Smart, 1984), and the discussion of illness is related to a sense of obligation to family (Nilchaikovit, Hill & Holland, 1993).

The nurse must keep in mind that these statements on structure and organization of a family by class are broad generalizations of social class values and in themselves cannot account for cultural differences. For example, many ethnic groups, such as the Newfoundland Inuit family, regardless of socioeconomic status, place great importance on extended family relationships rather than on the individualism valued by White, Protestant, middle-class Canadians. A family with a good income but with a time orientation in the present, such as that commonly found among persons in the lower socioeconomic class, may fail to recognize the importance of saving money and thus may always struggle financially. To understand whether a family system organizes itself around a family unit, such as the extended family, or tends to be a more individualistic system, such as the nuclear family, the nurse must assess the family as a group. The Canadian family is composed of diverse multicultural populations and is defined by three criteria: kinship, function, and location.

Kinship

In the first criterion, kinship, there are three dyads that imply the existence of or location for the individual within the family structure: husband-father, wife-mother, or child-sibling. There are several conventional forms of family structures that are composed of these positions, including the nuclear family and the stem family. The nuclear family, which was discussed earlier, may consist of a husband, a wife, and their nonadult children and is based on all three dyads, with their marital, parental, and sibling elements. Whereas the nuclear family is restricted to

a depth of two generations, the stem family encompasses three generations: grandparents, parents, and children.

Function

The second criterion, function, describes the purpose, goals, and philosophy of the family organization. Family function is defined as the expected action of an individual in a given role. In a description of family organization, the term "function" is used to depict family roles and the assigned tasks for those roles. Every family has unit functions that must be performed to maintain the integrity of the family unit and to meet the needs of the family. If individual family members' needs and societal expectations are to be met, the functioning role of the family must be clearly delineated. In family systems with two or more individuals, the family members have unit functional responsibilities related to their social positions. Depending on the position within the family structure, an individual may function in a variety of roles such as breadwinner, homemaker, companion, health motivator, or sexual partner. It is important for the nurse to remember that the maintenance of the family system is dependent on these various roles. Some cultural groups function in traditional ways in which the family is viewed as a holistic functioning unit. Other cultural groups may function as a disaggregate unit, meaning that the family does not function as a unit but members function independently.

Murray, Meili, and Zentner (1993) have described one approach to examining family functions in relation to the family's physical, affectional, and social properties. Physical functions include providing food, clothing, and shelter; protecting against danger; and providing health care. Affectional functions include meeting emotional needs. Social functions include providing social togetherness, fostering self-esteem, and supporting creativity and initiative. Another approach to examining family functions views the family from a task-oriented perspective (Sussman, 1971). Tasks include socialization of children, strengthening competency of family members in relation to their adjustments within organizations, appropriate use of social organizations, providing an environment that fosters the development of identities and affectional behavior, and creating a satisfying, emotionally healthy environment essential to the family's well-being. Adaptation is essential to the family's ability to carry out functions and tasks and to meet the changing needs of society and other social systems, such as political, health-illness systems.

Location

Family location is also a significant criterion for understanding the family. Martin (1980) and Leininger (1995) discussed the variations that occurred among values of African-American families when families were evaluated in urban versus rural settings. Martin found that when families moved from rural to urban settings, there was an erosion of values emphasizing "mutual aid" and a contrasting increase in individualism, materialism, and secularism. When urban African Americans are compared with their rural counterparts, it appears that urban African Americans may view their counterparts as lacking the toughness and sophistication needed to make headway in a dominant urban culture. Despite the variations that occur with location changes, geographical separation does not mean a severing of kinship ties, according to Martin; rather, geographical separation may serve to strength the emotional bonds between relatives. Today there is a tendency among African Americans, whether urban or rural, toward a migration back home and getting back to their people. For some African Americans there has been an increasing awareness that the urban centers have not met their hopes and aspirations. From the 1940s to the 1970s there was a migration by some African Americans away from the rural South. In the 1980s there was a trend toward migration of some African Americans away from the urban North back to the urban South. For example, the migration of urban northern African Americans has occurred in significant numbers to such cities as Atlanta, Dallas, and Houston (Kunen, 1996).

Religious Groups

According to many sociologists, religion is a social phenomenon (Carroll, Johnson, & Marty, 1979), which implies an interactive relationship with the other social units that constitute a society. However, many persons, particularly those with religious convictions, tend to think of religion in an entirely different way. For some people religion is seen in the context of a person's communion with the supernatural, and religious experiences fall outside ordinary experiences, whereas other people view religion as an expression of an instinctual reaction to cosmic forces (Johnstone, 1988). Another world view of religion depicts religion as an explicit set of messages from a deity. For the most part, all these beliefs tend to deemphasize, ignore, and perhaps even reject the sociological dimensions of religion. Nevertheless, whether it is being considered in general, in regard to a particular religious family such as Christianity or Buddhism, or in regard to a very specific religious group such as Baptists, religion is believed to interact with other social institutions and forces in society and to follow and illustrate sociological principles and laws. In other words, regardless of what religion is or is not, it is a social phenomenon and as such is in a continual reciprocal, interactive relationship with other social phenomena.

Regardless of its definition, be it theological or sociological, many different kinds of groups are based on religion. Generally, religious structures fall into two basic types: the church type and the withdrawal-group type. The church type of structure is broadly based and represents the normative spiritual values of a society that most people adhere to by virtue of their membership in the society, such as Hinduism in India or Catholicism in Spain. For the most part, membership in certain societies dictates the faith that the person should belong to if that person has not made a conscious, deliberate choice to adhere to something else. The church type of structure is generally a comprehensive system that allows for individual variations and in practice does not make extremely rigorous demands on its members. In the United States, the church type of structure is encompassed within numerous major denominations. This denominational structure is in sharp contrast with the church type of structure in other countries, such as India or Spain, where most of the people belong to one faith and one church. In some countries, particularly the United States, individual churches are often closely identified with an ethnic group rather than with a social class, and churches thrive, more or less, as a means of asserting ethnic identity. For example, the Black church, regardless of denominational faith, has become synonymous with the Black life experience. The Amish people, on the other hand, subscribe to one denominational belief; however, the belief is synonymous with the Amish life experience.

The second type of religious structure is the withdrawal group, which expresses the beliefs of those for whom personal commitment and experience are more important than the family and the community functions of religion (Ellwood, 1995). Withdrawal groups meet the needs of those who believe that the faith or lack of faith by the majority is not for them. Persons involved in withdrawal groups define themselves by making a separate choice. These groups include the Amish or Jehovah's Witnesses, which tend to represent a more intense or unbending commitment than that held by the average person adhering to a religion. These groups may be called "sects." Groups that combine separation with syncretism and new ideas and that place emphasis on mystical experience are often referred to as "cults." However, the word "cult" is often used in Western society with caution because it has acquired a negative connotation. In some religious groups such as the Church of the Latter-Day Saints (Mormons), Muslims, Jehovah's Witnesses, Seventh-Day Adventists, Buddhists, or Hindus, as well as that of the Gypsy culture, the extended social organization of the religion is considered more important than membership in the individual family. It is essential to remember that while this view is held by some theological scholars (Ellwood, 1995) many members of these religious groups do not necessarily share this belief. For example, in the Church of the Latter-Day Saints (the Mormon Church), children are taught at a very young age that families are eternal. In this sense, the family is viewed as a stable cohesive group bonded by love and as such is one of the most important units on earth today (Walters, 1994).

As persons from different religions increasingly intermarry, it is becoming more common for parents not to share the same faith. The proportion of Jews who married Gentiles, around 1 in 10 for the first half of the century, according to the American Jewish Committee, doubled in 1960, doubled again by the early 1970s, and in the 1990s has leveled off at just over 50%. Approximately 1 out of 3 American Jews lives in an interfaith household (Wingert, Springen, Stone, et al., 1997). Likewise, the comparable figure for Catholics is 21%, 30% for Mormons, and 40% for Muslims. Thus a new form of religious identification in America is developing and is analogous to a "mixed race." However, although diversity is increasingly acceptable among American religions, observances inevitably involve some sectarianism. Even though raising children in two faiths promotes diversity, it is sometimes confusing for the children who may feel that they are not so good as their all-Jewish or all-Christian cousins. Although attitudes toward intermarriage are becoming more liberal, for some it creates confusion over which holidays to celebrate and which church children should attend. On the other hand, intermarriage is not completely accepted in the United States. There are conservative sects such as Old Colony Mennonites and Missouri Synod Lutherans who are less tolerant of intermarriage and insist on born-again spouses (Wingert, Springen, Stone, et al., 1997).

There are 114 denominations in the United States. Most persons in the United States are Christian, inclusive of 86.2% of the population or 151,225,000 adults) (Bedell, 1997). Of the Christian denominations, the Roman Catholic Church has the largest membership with 60,280,454 reporting, with the Southern Baptist Convention ranking second with 15,663,296 members reporting. The Jewish religion ranks second, with 3,137,000 adult members, or 1.2% of the population. Islam, or the Islamic religion of Muslims, ranks third, with 527,000 adults, or 0.3% of the population, and the Unitarian Universalists ranks fourth with 502,000 adults, or 0.3% of the population (Bedell, 1997).

JEHOVAH'S WITNESSES

Although each group has unique practices, which should be considered by the nurse, two groups with particular significance for the nurse are Jehovah's Witnesses and Seventh-Day Adventists.

The founder of the Watchtower Bible and Tract Society, which is the legal corporation now used by Jehovah's Witnesses, was Charles Taze Russell. The name "Jehovah's Witnesses" was taken in Columbus, Ohio, in 1931 in an attempt to differentiate between the Watchtower Tract Society and the true followers of Russell, who were represented by the Dawn Bible Students and the Layman's Home Missionary Movement. From 1876 to 1879 Russell served as pastor of the Bible class that he organized in Pittsburgh, Pennsylvania, and was also the assistant editor of a small monthly magazine in Rochester, New York. However, he resigned from the editorial position in 1879 when controversy arose over his counterarguments on the "Atonement of Christ." In 1879 he founded the magazine *Herald of the Morning,* which developed into the magazine that is distributed today titled *The Watchtower Announcing Jehovah's Kingdom.* This magazine has grown from a circulation of 6000 to 20.9 million per month and is published in 125 languages. Today there is another Watchtower periodical titled *Awake,* which has a circulation of 18.3 million issues twice a month and is published in 81 languages (Jehovah's Witnesses 1997 Yearbook, 1997).

In 1884 Russell incorporated Zion's Watchtower Tract Society, in Pittsburgh, which published a series of seven books. Russell himself wrote six of these books. The seventh volume, *The Finished Mystery,* caused a split in the group that culminated in a clean division. The larger portion of the group followed Joseph Franklin Rutherford, whereas the smaller portion remained by itself and subsequently became known as the Dawn Bible Students Association. Under Rutherford's leadership the Watchtower Bible Society began to attack the doctrines of organized religion. This group eventually became known as the present-day Jehovah's Witnesses and has branches in 233 countries with 5.9 million members. There are 966,243 Jehovah's Witnesses in the United States (Bedell, 1997). Between 1996 and 1997 the Jehovah's Witnesses were listed as sixth in terms of church-membership increase, with 20,253 new members reported. The United States headquarters are located in Brooklyn, New York (Bedell, 1997).

Modern-day Jehovah's Witnesses still await the Millennium. They regard Christ as a creature who will come to destroy the forces of evil at Armageddon, and they teach that sinners who are not saved will perish, whereas the faithful will enter into the Kingdom of Joy and Happiness. Because they believe in the Second Coming of the Kingdom, they undertake no military services. They also hold the belief that the institutions of government are under the control of Satan. It is this belief that has been the basis for some of the persecution they have undergone over the years. One view of this group is that Jehovah's Witnesses are peaceful but somewhat fanatical and that they know their Bible backward and forward (Smart, 1984). Some theologians believe that this religion appeals to persons of very modest education (Smart, 1984). The Jehovah's Witness faith is based on the doctrines presented in Box 4-2.

Implications for nursing care

There are many implications for nursing care for the nurse who provides culturally appropriate nursing care to a Jehovah's Witness. The paramount concern for the nurse is that Jehovah's Witnesses are opposed to homologous blood transfusions (blood obtained from a blood bank or through donations). However, many but not all Jehovah's Witnesses will submit to certain types of autologous blood transfusions (autotransfusion). Whether autologous blood transfusions will be accepted by a Jehovah's Witness depends on the type of autologous transfusion. Jehovah's Witnesses hold the view that "God's determination is that blood represents life and thus is sacred" (Watchtower, 1989). They believe that it is God's commandment that no human should sustain life by taking blood. Jehovah's Witnesses believe that if blood is taken from a creature and not used for sacrifice, it should be disposed of and covered with dust. This belief clearly rules out autologous transfusions whereby blood is precollected from the client for future use and is stored as either whole blood or as packed cells (Watchtower, 1989). In receiving this type of transfusion, it is believed that stored blood is no longer a part of the person. In refusing this type of autologous transfusion, Jehovah's Witnesses cite God's law: "You should pour it upon the Ground as water" (Deuteronomy 12:24). Yet, there are certain types of autologous transfusions that some Jeho-

---

Box 4-2

BELIEFS OF JEHOVAH'S WITNESSES

1. Jehovah's Witnesses believe that there is one solitary Being from all eternity and that that Being is Jehovah, God, the creator and preserver of the universe in all things that are visible and invisible.

2. Jehovah's Witnesses do not believe in the Holy Trinity of three Gods in one—God the Father, God the Son, and God the Holy Ghost—who are equal in power, substance, and eternity (Watchtower Bible & Tract Society, 1953). Rather, they believe that Satan is the originator of the Trinity doctrine and that this doctrine is just another of Satan's attempts to keep people from learning the truth about Jehovah and his Son, Christ Jesus, which is that there is no Trinity (Watchtower Bible & Tract Society, 1953).

3. Jehovah's Witnesses believe that there is only one God and that he is greater than his Son. They believe that the Son, the firstborn and only begotten, was sent by God but is not God himself and is not equal with God.

4. On the subject of the Virgin Birth, Jehovah's Witnesses believe that Jehovah God took the perfect life of his only begotten Son and transferred it from heaven to the womb of the unmarried virgin, Mary. They believe that Jesus's birth was not an incarnation but that he was emptied of all things heavenly and spiritual. This was a miracle in the sense that Jesus was born a man (and was flesh) instead of a spirit-human hybrid (Martin, 1992).

5. Jehovah's Witnesses believe that the human life that Jesus Christ laid down in sacrifice must be viewed as exactly equal to the life that Adam forfeited for all of his offspring. Thus Jesus's life must be viewed as a perfect human life, no more and no less (Watchtower Bible & Tract Society, 1955).

6. Jehovah's Witnesses believe that immortality is a reward for faithfulness and that it does not come automatically to a human at birth (Watchtower Bible & Tract Society, 1953).

7. On the subject of the Resurrection of Christ, Jehovah's Witnesses believe that Christ was raised from the dead, not as a human creature, but as a Spirit (Watchtower Bible & Tract Society, 1953).

8. Jehovah's Witnesses believe that Christ Jesus will return again, not as a human, but as a glorious spirit. National flags or symbols of the sovereign power of a nation are forbidden by Exodus 20:2-6. Thus those who believe and ascribe salvation only to God may not salute a national emblem without violating Jehovah's commandments against idolatry (Watchtower Bible & Tract Society, 1953).

9. Jehovah's Witnesses believe that the hell mentioned in the Bible is mankind's common grave and that even an honest child can understand it. Thus the doctrine of a burning hell where the wicked are tortured after death cannot be true.

10. Jehovah's Witnesses believe that man is a combination of two things: dust of the ground and breath of life. The combining of these two things produces a living soul, or a creature called man.

11. Jehovah's Witnesses believe that the undefeatable purpose of Jehovah God is to establish a righteous kingdom in these last days and that this purpose has already been fulfilled.

12. Jehovah's Witnesses believe that the Levitical commandments given by God to Moses included the commandment that no one in the House of David should eat blood or he would be cut off from people.

---

vah's Witnesses will accept. One type of autologous transfusion that might be acceptable is blood retrieved through induced hemodilution at the start of surgery (blood that is directed to storage bags outside the client's body). It is essential to remember that some Jehovah's Witnesses believe that if the autotransfusion is halted in any way, the acceptability of the procedure to the client would be questionable. Although this type of autologous transfusion might be acceptable, others such as blood collected from a wound by aspiration, pumped through a filter or a centrifuge to remove debris and clots, and then given back to the client would not be an acceptable

alternative (Watchtower, 1989). In addition, some Jehovah's Witnesses will permit the use of certain blood volume expanders. Many Jehovah's Witnesses carry a card with the types of blood volume expanders permitted. The nurse should ask the client for this card or, if the client is unconscious, examine the client's personal belongings to find this extremely important card. When autologous blood transfusions or blood volume expanders are not plausible alternatives, many physicians look to alternatives to and during major surgery that are acceptable to Jehovah Witnesses, including colloids or colloid replacement fluids, electrocautery, hypotensive anesthesia, or hypothermia. It is important for the nurse to remember that persons who subscribe to this belief are likely to refuse to have any surgical or medical interventions that will require a homologous blood transfusion. Even in the face of ominous danger and with the impending threat of loss of life, a Jehovah's Witness will refuse treatment for self and family members if a homologous transfusion is the only plausible blood replacement option available. There have been many legal battles waged in the courts in regard to minor children and the parents' refusal to allow surgical or medical interventions. The consensus of the court in some countries such as the Supreme Court in the United States has been that a person of adult majority age has the right to refuse treatment but not to withhold treatment from a minor child.

A second concern for the nurse is in regard to the refusal of Jehovah's Witnesses to eat certain foods to which blood has been added, such as certain sausages and lunch meats. The nurse must take extra care to ensure that blood has not been added to foods that are served to Jehovah's Witnesses. Because Jehovah's Witnesses are pacifists and conscientious objectors, the nurse must take extra care to avoid raising such issues during interaction. In general, topics related to politics, government rule, or the like, should be avoided. Because Jehovah's Witnesses do not observe any national holidays or ceremonies, including Christmas, the nurse should avoid any attempts to involve the client in preparations for such celebrations.

SEVENTH-DAY ADVENTISTS

The Seventh-Day Adventist religion sprang from the "Great Second Advent Awakening" that shocked the religious world just before the middle of the nineteenth century. During this period reemphasis on the second advent of Jesus Christ was rampant in England and in Europe. It was not long before many of the Old World views and prophetic interpretations crossed the Atlantic and began to penetrate American theological circles (Martin, 1992). The American Seventh-Day Adventist group began in upper New York (Ellwood, 1995).

The first leader of the Seventh-Day Adventists was William Miller, a Baptist minister from Lower Hampton, New York. The Seventh-Day Adventist religion is based largely on the apocalyptic books of Daniel and Revelation. Many of the early students of the Seventh-Day Adventist religion, following the chronology of Archbishop Ussher, interpreted the 2300 days of Daniel as 2300 years, and thus they concluded that Christ would come back in about the year 1843. In 1818 Miller taught many of his followers that in about 25 years (1843) Jesus Christ would come again. Miller and his associates pinpointed October 22, 1843, as the specific final date on which Jesus Christ would return for his saints, visit judgment on sin, and establish the Kingdom of God on earth. Many theologians disagreed with Miller's contentions because they believed that Miller was teaching in contradiction to the Word of God. According to biblical scripture, "the day and hour knoweth no man, no, not the angels of heaven but God alone" (Matthew 24:36). Because of Miller's early teaching, the first group of Seventh-Day Adventists were called Millerites. However, the mistake of setting an exact date for Christ's Second Coming led to failure for the first Seventh-Day Adventist movement in the United States.

The modern Seventh-Day Adventist movement is based on the prophecy of Ellen G. White. White made an early assertion about Miller's prophecy that supported the prophecy and gave a date that she considered to be correct: October 22, 1844. Despite this failure in prediction, the group has grown and been active in evangelism. Today Seventh-Day Adventists believe Christ will return again very soon and that Christians have an obligation to keep some of the laws of Moses, which includes worship on Saturday, the old Sabbath. Thirteen issues on doctrine that give direction for living and that are upheld by the Seventh-Day Adventist Church are presented in Box 4-3.

There are 790,731 members of the Seventh-day Adventist Church in the United States (Bedell, 1997). The Seventh-day Adventist Church is listed as seventh in the United States between 1996 and 1997 for an increase in membership with 20,253 new members reported. The Worldwide Seventh-Day Adventist Church headquarters are located in Washington, D.C.

Box 4-3

BELIEFS OF SEVENTH-DAY ADVENTISTS

1. **Inspiration and authority of the scriptures.** Seventh-Day Adventists believe that the scriptures of both the Old Testament and the New Testament were inspired by God and constitute the very word of God. They hold the Protestant position that the Bible is the sole root of the faith and practice of Christians.

2. **The nature of Christ.** Christ, called the Second Adam, is pure and holy, and connected with God and beloved by God. Seventh-Day Adventists believe that Christ is God and that he has existed with God for all eternity (Martin, 1985).

3. **The Atonement.** Seventh-Day Adventists do not believe that Christ made partial or incomplete sacrificial atonement on the cross. The all-sufficient sacrifice of Jesus was completed on the cross at Calvary.

4. **The Resurrection.** Seventh-Day Adventists believe that Jesus rose from the grave, ascended literally and bodily into heaven, and serves before God. They believe that there will be a resurrection of both the just and the unjust. For the just, this resurrection will take place at the Second Coming of Christ, whereas the resurrection of the unjust will take place 1000 years later, at the close of the Millennium (Revelation 20:5-10).

5. **The Second Coming.** Seventh-Day Adventists believe that Jesus Christ will assuredly come the second time and that his second advent will be visible, audible, and personal.

6. **The plan of salvation.** Seventh-Day Adventists believe that one must be born again and fully accepted by the Lord. They believe that there is nothing an individual can ever do that will merit the salvation of God. Salvation is by grace (Roman 3:20).

7. **The spiritual nature of man.** Seventh-Day Adventists believe that man rests in the tomb until the resurrection of the just, when the righteous will be called forth by Christ (Revelation 20:4-5). It is at this point that the just will enter into everlasting life in their eternal home in the Kingdom of Glory.

8. **Punishment of the wicked.** Seventh-Day Adventists reject the doctrine of eternal torment because everlasting life is a gift from God (Romans 6:23). The wicked do not possess this and therefore shall not have eternal life (John 3:36).

9. **Sanctuary and investigative judgment.** Seventh-Day Adventists believe that the acceptance of Christ at conversion does not seal a person's destiny; rather, it determines his life's work after conversion.
   Man's record is closed when he comes to the end of his days; he is responsible for his influences during life and is likewise responsible for his evil influences after he is dead.

10. **Scapegoat teaching.** Seventh-Day Adventists repudiate the idea that Satan is the sin bearer.

11. **The Sabbath and the Mark of the Beast.** This doctrine is based on the Bible as interpreted by Seventh-Day Adventists and not according to Ellen White's writings. Seventh-Day Adventists do not believe that keeping the Sabbath is a means of keeping salvation or willing merit before God. They believe that man is saved only by grace.

12. **The question of unclean food.** Seventh-Day Adventists refrain from eating certain foods, not because of the laws of Moses, but because it is a Christian duty to preserve the body in the best of health for the service and glory of God (I Corinthians 3:16).

13. **The "remnant church."** Seventh-Day Adventists believe God has a precious remnant, a multitude of earnest and sincere individuals, in every church. The majority of God's children are scattered throughout the world and may practice their religion on Sunday.

Implications for nursing care

The religious doctrines of Seventh-Day Adventists teach that the body is a temple of God and thus should be kept healthy. Persons who subscribe to this faith may avoid such items as seafood, meat, caffeine, alcohol, drugs, and tobacco in all forms. To provide culturally appropriate nursing care to a Seventh-Day Adventist, the nurse must have a knowledge and understanding of the religious doctrines of the Seventh-Day Adventist Church. A Seventh-Day Adventist may refuse surgical intervention on a Friday evening or Saturday morning or afternoon because the client may interpret such an intervention as being in direct conflict with religious doctrines. This same client may also refuse other medical interventions that might normally take place at these times, such as respiratory or physical therapy.

The religious doctrine in regard to unclean foods may cause some clients to refuse to eat certain foods with shells, such as lobster or crab; scavenger fish, such as catfish; or certain meats. This refusal to eat certain foods high in iodine or protein may cause these clients to have iodine and protein deficiencies; thus it is important for the nurse to teach these clients that iodine and protein substitutes are necessary in the diet. Some specialty shops that have Seventh-Day Adventist clientele stock a variety of protein substitutes for meats. These substitutes are often made from vegetables such as soybeans and may take the place of meats such as ground beef. These substitutes should be encouraged, particularly when they appear to be free of preservatives.

The nurse and the nurse manager should also be aware that a colleague who is a Seventh-Day Adventist may refuse to accept assignments on Friday evenings or Saturday during the day, since the Sabbath begins on Friday at dusk and extends to Saturday at dusk. It is important for the nurse who is a Seventh-Day Adventist to ascertain at the time of employment whether working on Friday evenings or Saturday during the day is a requirement of the job. On the other hand, it is also important for the nurse manager to include staff in making nondiscriminatory policies in this regard. Inclusion of staff in policy making may serve to minimize implementation difficulties.

ETHNIC GROUPS IN RELATION TO FAMILY

On June 30, 1998, there were an estimated 270 million people living in the United States (U.S. Department of Commerce, Bureau of Census, 1998). Of this group 33.8 million (13%) were Black; the American Indian/Eskimo-Aleut populations made up 2.3 million (4%); Asians and Pacific Islanders numbered 10.0 million (4%). An estimated 29.0 million (11%) were of Hispanic origin. About 194.4 million (73%) of the total population classified themselves as non-Hispanic white. Three ethnic groups will be discussed in relation to family. (World Almanac, 1998). It is estimated that by the year 2050 the United States will have 393.9 million people, 49% more than the population today. It is also estimated that the population will be more diverse. The non-Hispanic White share of the population is projected to fall from the current 74% to 53% by 2050. Meanwhile, persons of Hispanic origin will increase from 11% to 24% of the population. Asians and Pacific Islanders will see their population climb from 4% to 9%. Increases are expected to be smaller from American Indian, Eskimo, and Aleut populations from slightly under 1% to more than 1% and for African Americans from 13% to 15% (World Almanac, 1998).

ARAB AMERICANS

According to the 1990 census, there are 3.2 million Arabs in the United States (U.S. Department of Commerce, Bureau of the Census, 1998; 1993a). Arab Americans include people from Egypt, Palestine, Lebanon, Iraq, Jordan, Syria, and other Arabic countries. About 1 million Arab Americans have permanent resident visas in the United States, and another 2 million Arabs are in the United States to study or work (Meleis & LaFever, 1984; U.S. Department of Commerce, Bureau of the Census, 1993b).

For some Arab Americans an affiliation with family is needed if the individual is to cope satisfactorily with stressful events or life crises (Meleis, 1996). On the other hand, family members may be hesitant to seek help actively within the family, waiting instead until help is offered. Visiting between family members is viewed as a social obligation during illness and a variety of other significant events and consequently assumes great importance to the hospitalized client.

Families are expected to be supportive. Particularly in psychiatric care, the extended family of an Arab-American client is often disappointed at the nuclear family's failure to take care of its kin, and the client is angry at being sent to the hospital (Meleis, 1996). Family members may present themselves as overbearing, and the client may seem docile. A family member's overprotectiveness may be better understood when considered in this cultural context. The nurse should understand that family members are often overindulging and may appear to interfere in the client's care.

Meleis (1996) has emphasized that topics of sex and reproduction may have special cultural significance when the client is Arabic. Topics of sex and reproduction are traditionally discussed with female relatives and friends but not with men or strangers. When the nurse wishes to involve the husband in a discussion dealing with sex or reproduction, extreme tact is necessary.

Some Arab-American families are oriented to the present and may believe that planning ahead may be defying God's will. The "efficient, time-conscious" manner in which Americans conduct business varies considerably from what may be construed as a casual Arabic style (Meleis, 1996). With Arab-American clients, as with clients from any other cultural group, the nurse must individualize care rather than provide care based on cultural stereotyping.

NATIVE AMERICANS

According to the 1990 census, there are 2,337,000 American Indians (Native Americans) living in the United States (U.S. Department of Commerce, Bureau of the Census, 1998). Because there are more than 500 different federally recognized tribes of Native American Indians and an additional 200 who do not benefit from federal recognition, it is difficult to predict patterns of residency unless one is dealing with specific tribes (Kramer, 1996). The 1990 census reported large Indian populations in Arizona, Oklahoma, New Mexico, Alaska, California, North Carolina, South Dakota, New York, Montana, Washington, and Minnesota (U.S. Department of Commerce, Bureau of the Census, 1992b). Providing culturally appropriate nursing care is complicated because each nation or tribe of American Indians has its own language and religion, and belief-system practices differ significantly among groups as well as among members of the same tribe (Kramer, 1996).

The American Indian family is composed frequently of extended family members who may encompass several households. Through various religious ceremonies other individuals can become the same as a parent in the family network. In some American Indian tribes, grandparents are viewed as the family leaders, and respect for individuals increases with age. Also in some tribes the family is viewed as important, particularly in periods of crises, when family members are expected to serve as sources of support and security. It is important for the nurse to remember that because some American Indian tribes tend to place great emphasis on the extended family as a unit, the opinions and ideas of the family members should be solicited when one is giving culturally appropriate nursing care. Even though physicians and hospitals may be available to Native Americans, traditional healing ceremonies may still be held in high regard by some families, and it may be important to incorporate old ways to treat illnesses for a treatment plan to be effective.

HMONGS

Hmongs are of Asian descent and are an ethnic-cultural group of people who originally lived in the rural highlands of Laos (Johnson, 1996). Many of the Hmongs living in the United States today were displaced from their homeland because of their alignment with the United States during the Vietnam War (Johnson, 1996). There are 90,082 Hmongs residing in the United States (U.S. Department of Commerce, Bureau of the Census, 1993b). Of this number, 1732 reside in the northeast, 37,166 reside in the Midwest, 1627 reside in the South, and 49,564 reside in the West (U.S. Department of Commerce, Bureau of the Census, 1993a). Of the number of Hmongs residing in this country who immigrated to this country before 1975, 0.4% were foreign born. Of the number of Hmongs residing in this country between 1975 and 1979, 15.3% were foreign born. Of the number of Hmongs residing in the country between 1980 and 1990, 49.5% were foreign born. It is obvious that immigration accounts for the large influx of Hmongs residing in this country today (U.S. Department of Commerce, Bureau of the Census, 1993b).

The median age of Hmongs who make the United States their home is 12.5 years. Hmongs, by median age, are reported to be the youngest ethnic cultural group in the United States (U.S. Department of Commerce, Bureau of the Census, 1993b). Not only are Hmongs one of the youngest cultural groups residing in this country, they also tend to have larger families (6.6 persons) as compared with the rest of Asian Americans (3.8 persons), and the general United States population (3.2 persons) (U.S. Department of Commerce, Bureau of the Census, 1993b). Of the number of Hmongs residing in the United States who are 25 years of age or older, 44.1% of males and 19.0% of females hold a high school degree. Similarly, in this same age group, 7.0% of males and 3.5% of females hold a bachelor's degree or higher. Of the number of Hmongs found in the United States, 96.9% speak Asian or a Pacific Island language at home, 65.0% do not speak English well, and 43.9% are reported to be linguistically isolated (U.S. Department of Commerce, Bureau of the Census, 1993b).

Hmongs are primarily an oral cultural group, a statement implying that some Hmongs have never learned to read Hmong or any other language (Shadick, 1993). In the 1950s French missionaries introduced to the Hmongs a form of written Hmong, which is based on the Roman alphabet (Shadick, 1993). There are two major dialectal variations in the oral Hmong language, which include Hmoo Daw (White Hmong) and Hmoo Ntsua (Blue Hmong) (Dunnigan, 1986). According to Catlin (1985), Hmong is spoken using one of eight tones. For some Hmongs, the oral word holds greater meaning and power than does the written word (Shadick, 1993). Some Hmongs consider the spoken word to be the primary tool and mechanism for passing on traditions, rituals, and information to future generations (Shadick, 1993). It is important for the nurse to remember this when interacting with Hmong clients, and because Hmongs tend to be primarily an oral cultural group, culturally appropriate care is hindered when treatment plans and protocols are given to the client in a written form (even when the client does speak English).

SPECIAL INTEREST GROUPS

Special interest groups are a significant part of the social structure of the United States. Individuals may join a group for many reasons including support and self-help. Support groups provide the opportunity to increase the participant's social network, share solutions to common problems, and reshape perceptions of self and the environment. Examples of support groups include quality-of-life groups, caregiver support groups, and bereavement support groups (McMahon & Presswalla, 1997). Self-help groups are attractive to members because they promote well-being. Self-help groups are usually focused on particular clinical states such as chronic mental illness, a particular social state such as a divorce, or special psychosocial issues such as chemical dependency. Examples include Alcoholics Anonymous (AA), Narcotics Anonymous (NA), and Overeaters Anonymous (OA). Support groups may replace or augment the family or formal health care system and generally aim to link health behaviors with everyday existence. Self-help groups foster self-reliance and are a form of healing (McMahon & Presswalla, 1997). A network of friends, relatives, and neighbors can be crucial to psychological well-being and can help relieve social isolation, promote mental health, facilitate coping, alleviate problems by preventive problem-solving, and assist persons in preparing for stressful events in life (Brown, 1990).

IMPLICATIONS FOR NURSING CARE

When nurses provide care to clients from a sociocultural background other than their own, they must have an awareness of and a sensitivity to the client's sociocultural background, including knowledge of family structure and organization, religious values and beliefs, and how ethnicity and culture relate to role and role assignment within group settings. Any social organization or group can be viewed as the environment in which the client strives for health. The approach to nursing care depends on the situation. The nurse must remember that if even one family member (other than the client), regardless of culture and ethnic heritage, is receptive to nursing care, it is realistic and practical to view the family as an environment. Friedman (1986) contends that nursing care must be directed to the family as a whole as well as to the individual family member. The nurse must therefore view the family as having two separate entities, the first being the family as an environment and the second being the family as the client. Both approaches to client care can be useful when the nurse attempts to provide culturally appropriate nursing care.

If the family is viewed as an environment, the primary focus of nursing care is the health and development of individual family members within a very specific environment. In this context it is important for the nurse to assess the extent to which the family provides the individual basic needs of each person. It is also essential that the nurse remember that individual needs vary depending on developmental level and the current situation. The nurse should be cognizant of the fact that families provide more than just the physical necessities; the ability of the family to help the client meet psychosociological needs is paramount.

When families are viewed as an environment, it is extremely important for the nurse to recognize that other family members may also need intervention. For example, when a child is hospitalized, the parents may feel anxiety and stress; therefore, intervention with them is just as important as intervention with the hospitalized child.

When families are viewed as clients, it is important to assess crucial factors that are germane to family structure and organization. For example, if a hypertensive client is admitted to a hospital unit, it is crucial that the nurse assess several factors related to the family, including the following:

1. The family's current dietary patterns
2. The family's desire, as well as resources, for changing the dietary patterns
3. The family's knowledge about hypertension and its effects on the body
4. The family's capabilities to support a hypertensive family member
5. The family's ability to cope with and manage stress and anxiety

Whether the family is viewed as an environment or as the client, it is essential to incorporate cultural concepts when the nursing plan of care is being developed. The nursing process is used regardless of whether the family is viewed as an environment or as the client. The delineations or differences that occur in the nursing process are the result of cultural variables and beliefs that are germane to a particular ethnic or cultural group. Therefore it is essential that the nurse incorporate cultural beliefs and concerns shared by family members into the plan of care.

Case Study

Susie Chung, a 24-year-old Chinese American, is admitted with right, lower-quadrant abdominal pain. Within a few hours Miss Chung is taken to surgery for an appendectomy. When she returns to the floor, her vital signs remain stable. The nurse notes that even though Miss Chung is rapidly recovering, her immediate and extended family appear to hover about her. The nurse also notes that it is very difficult to administer nursing care because of the number of family members who are keeping a constant vigil.

STUDY QUESTIONS

1. List at least three social organization factors that influence the interactions between members of the same ethnic group or members of varying ethnic groups.
2. List at least two social organization factors that contribute to the development of cultural behavior.
3. Explain the role that religion may play for Susie Chung in regard to sociopsychological adaptation to her illness.
4. List at least three nursing interventions that may serve to minimize the confusion caused by the large number of family members who are keeping constant vigil in Susie Chung's room.
5. List at least two reasons why the family members of Susie Chung have congregated in the hospital room.
6. List at least three factors that would support Susie Chung's family being defined as a behavioral system.

7. List at least two imaginary and two real boundaries that would be found within Susie Chung's family structure.

8. List at least two roles that Susie Chung may take on in a social context within her family structure.

References

Ackerman, N. (1984). *The theory of family systems.* New York: Gardner Press.

Averaswald, E. (1973). Families, change and the ecological perspective. In Ferber, A. (Ed.), *The book of family therapy.* Boston: Houghton Mifflin.

Bailey, E., & Bailey, R. (1995). *Discover Canada.* Oxford, England: Berlitz Publishing Co.

Bateson, G., Jackson, D., Haley, J., & Weakland, J. (1968). Toward a theory of schizophrenia. In Jackson, D.D. (Ed.), *Communication, family and marriage.* Palo Alto, Calif.: Science & Behavior Books.

Bedell, K. (1997). *Yearbook of American and Canadian churches.* Nashville: Abingdon Press.

Beiser, M., Barwick, C., Berry, J., et al. (1988). *After the door has been opened: mental health issues affecting immigration and refugees.* A report of the Canadian Task Force on Mental Health Issues Affecting Immigrants and Refugees. Ottawa: Ministry of Multiculturalism and Citizenship and Health and Welfare.

Berkanovic, E., & Reeder, L.G. (1973). Ethnic, economic and social psychological factors in the source of medical care. *Social Problems, 21,* 246-259.

Berry, J. (1988). Acculturation and psychological adaptation: a conceptual overview. In Berry, J.W., & Annis, R.C. (Eds.), *Ethnic psychology: research and practice with immigrants, refugees, native peoples, ethnic groups and sojourners.* Amsterdam: Swets & Zeitlinger.

Bierck, R. (1997, Dec. 15). Women become the main event. *U.S. News and World Report, 123*(23), 10.

Black, C. (1991). *It will never happen to me.* Denver: MAC.

Bowen, M. (1994). *Family therapy in clinical practice.* Northvale, N.J.: Jason Aronson.

Breitmayer, B., Gallo, A., Knafl, K., & Zoeller, L. (1989, April 3). *Correlates of social competence among children with a chronic illness.* Paper presented at the 13th Annual Midwest Nursing Research Society Conference, Cincinnati, Ohio. (MRNS, Glenview, Ill.)

Brown, S. (1986). Children with an alcoholic parent. In Estes, N., & Heinemann, M. (Eds.), *Alcoholism: development, consequences, and interventions* (ed. 3) (pp. 207-220). St. Louis: Mosby.

Brown, R. (1990). Self-help and therapy groups. In *The Marshall Cavendish encyclopedia of personal relationships: human behavior.* New York: Marshall Cavendish.

Bullough, V.L., & Bullough, B. (1982). *Health care for the other Americans.* East Norwalk, Conn.: Appleton-Century-Crofts.

Campbell, J. (1989, April 3). *Self-care agency in battered women.* Paper presented at the 13th Annual Midwest Nursing Research Society Conference, Cincinnati, Ohio. (MRNS, Glenview, Ill.)

Caplan, G. (1975). The family as a support system. In Caplan, G., & Killilea, M. (Eds.), *Support systems and mutual help: multidisciplinary exploration.* New York: Grune & Stratton.

Carroll, J., Johnson, D., & Marty, M. (1979). *Religion in America: 1950 to present.* New York: Harper & Row.

Casavantes, E. (1976). Pride and prejudice: a Mexican American dilemma. In Hernandez, C.A., Haug, M.J., & Wagner, N.N. (Eds.), *Chicanos: social and psychological perspectives* (ed. 2) (pp. 9-14). St. Louis: Mosby.

Catlin, A.R. (1985). Speech surrogate systems of the Hmong: from singing voices to talking reeds. In Downing, B.T., & Olney, D.P., (Eds.), *The Hmong in the West* (pp. 170-197). Minneapolis: Center for Urban and Regional Affairs, University of Minnesota.

Cloud, J. (1998, Jan. 5). A different fathers' day. *Time, 150*(27), 106.

Coleman, J. (1997). *A long way to go.* New York: Atlantic Monthly Press.

Cose, E. (1997, Nov. 3). Why we can't get along. *Newsweek,* 66.

Danyliw, N. (1997, Dec.15). Got mother's milk? *U.S. News and World Report, 123*(23), 79.

Deuteronomy 12:24 (1984). *New world translation of the holy scriptures* (p. 201). New York: Watchtower Bible and Tract Society of New York, Inc., International Bible Student Association.

Dickerson, D. (1997, Dec. 29). An army-style prep school for minorities. *U.S. News and World Report, 123*(25), 73-74.

Dunnigan, T. (1986). Process of identity maintenance in Hmong society. In Hendricks, G.L., Downing, B.T., & Deinard, A.S. (Eds.), *The Hmong in transition* (pp. 41-53). Staten Island, N.Y.: Center for Migration Studies.

Duvall, E., & Miller, B. (1984). *Marriage and family development* (ed. 6). East Norwalk, Conn.: Appleton-Century-Crofts.

Ellwood, R. (1995). *Many peoples, many faiths* (ed. 5). Englewood Cliffs, N.J.: Prentice Hall.

Fawcett, J. (1975). The family as a living open system: an emerging conceptual framework for nursing. *International Nursing Review, 22,* 113.

Fineman, H.O. (1995, Sept. 18). Mediscare. *Newsweek,* 38-40.

Friedman, M.M. (1986). *Family nursing: theory and assessment.* East Norwalk, Conn.: Appleton-Century-Crofts.

Gary, F. (1991). Sociocultural diversity and mental health nursing. In Gary, F., & Kavanaugh, C. (Eds.), *Psychiatric nursing* (pp. 138-163). Philadelphia: J.B. Lippincott.

Giger, J., Davidhizar, R., Evers, S., & Ingram, C. (1994). Cultural factors influencing mental health and mental illness. In Taylor, C. (Ed.), *Mereness' Essentials of psychiatric nursing* (ed. 14) (pp. 215-238). St. Louis: Mosby.

Giger, J., Davidhizar, R., & Wieczorek, S. (1994). Transcultural nursing: have we gone too far or not far enough? In Strickland, O., & Fishman, D. (Eds.), *Nursing in a diverse society.* New York: Delmar Publications.

Giger, J., Johnson, J., Davidhizar, R., Fishman, D. (1993, March). Strategies for building a supportive faculty. *Nursing and Health Care, 14*(3), 144-159.

Goldsby, R.A. (1977). *Race and races* (ed. 2). New York: MacMillan.

Govaets, K. (1987). Cultural and socioeconomic dimensions in mental health nursing. In Norris, J., Kunes-Connell, N., Stockhard, S., et al. (Eds.), *Mental health–psychiatric nursing: a continuum of care.* New York: John Wiley & Sons.

Gregory, D. (1988). Nursing practice in native communities. In Baumgart, A., & Larson, J. (Eds.), *Canadian nursing faces the future.* Toronto: Mosby.

Grypma, S. (1993, Sept.). Culture shock. *The Canadian Nurse, 89*(8), 33-36.

Guruge, S., & Donner, G. (1996, Sept.). Transcultural nursing in Canada. *The Canadian Nurse, 92*(8), 36-40.

Guttmacher, S., & Elinson, J. (1972). Ethno-religious variation in perception of illness: the use of illness as an explanation for deviant behavior. *Social Science Medicine, 5*(2), 117-125.

Harwood, A. (Ed.). (1981). *Ethnicity and medical care.* Cambridge, Mass.: Harvard University Press.

Headden, S. (1998, Jan. 5). Favor aliens with job skills. *U.S. News and World Report, 123*(25), 83-85.

Henderson, G., & Primeaux, M. (1981). *Transcultural health care.* Reading, Mass.: Addison-Wesley.

Hsu, J. (1985). Asian family interaction patterns and their therapeutic implications. In Pichot, P., Berner, P., Wolf, R., & Thau, K. (Eds.), *Psychiatry: the state of art,* Vol. 8 (pp. 599-606). New York: Plenum Press.

Hyland, S. (1990, Sept.). Helping employees with family care. *Monthly Labour Review,* 22-26.

Information please almanac (1998). Boston: Houghton Mifflin Co.

Jehovah's Witnesses 1997 yearbook (1997). New York: Watchtower Bible and Tract Society.

Johnson, S. (1996). Hmong. In Lipson, J., Dibble, S., and Minarik, P. (Eds.), *Culture and nursing care: a pocket guide.* School of Nursing, University of California, San Francisco: UCSF Nursing Press.

Johnstone, R. (1988). *Religion in society* (ed. 3). Englewood Cliffs, N.J.: Prentice Hall.

Kantrowitz, B. (1997, Nov. 3). Secrets of the ivy league. *Newsweek,* 68.

Kramer, J. (1996). American Indians. In Lipson, J., Dibble, S., & Minarik, P. (Eds.), *Culture and nursing care.* School of Nursing, University of California, San Francisco: UCSF Nursing Press.

Kunen, J. (1996, April 29). The end of integration. *Time,* 39-44.

Leininger, M. (1995). *Transcultural nursing: concepts, theories, research, and practices.* New York: McGraw-Hill.

Lewis, H. (1979). *How's your family?* New York: Brunner/Mazel.

Lewis, J.M., Beavers, W.R., Gossett, J.T., & Phillips, V.A. (1976). *No single thread: psychological health in family systems.* New York: Brunner/Mazel.

Martin, E.P. (1980). *The Black extended family.* Chicago: University of Chicago Press.

Martin, W. (1992). *The kingdom of the cults.* Minneapolis: Bethany House.

Mauksch, H. (1974). A social science basis for conceptualizing family health. *Social Science Medicine, 8,* 521.

McKibbon, J., Généreux, L., & Séguin-Roberge, G. (1996, March).Who cares for the caregivers? *The Canadian Nurse, 92*(3), 38-41.

McMahon, A. (1997). Working with families. In Haber, J., Krainovich-Miller, B., McMahon, A., & Price-Hoskins, P. (Eds.), *Comprehensive psychiatric nursing.* St. Louis: Mosby.

McMahon, A., & Presswalla, J.L. (1997). Working with groups. In Haber, J., Krainovich-Miller, B., McMahon, A., & Price-Hoskins, P. (Eds.), *Comprehensive psychiatric nursing.* St. Louis: Mosby.

McRae, L. (1994). Cultural sensitivity in rehabilitation related to native clients. *Canadian Journal of Rehabilitation, 7*(4), 251-256.

Meleis, A.I. (1996). Arab Americans. In Lipson, J., Dibble, S., & Minarik, P. (Eds.), *Culture and nursing care: a pocket guide.* School of Nursing, University of California, San Francisco: UCSF Nursing Press.

Meleis, A.I., & LaFever, C.W. (1984). The Arab American and psychiatric care. *Perspectives in Psychiatric Care, 22*(2), 42-85.

Minuchin, S. (1974). *Families and family therapy.* Cambridge, Mass.: Harvard University Press.

Misener, T., Sowell, R., Phillips, K., & Harris, C. (1997, July/Aug.). Sexual orientation: a cultural diversity issue for nursing. *Nursing Outlook, 45*(4), 178-182.

Mo, B. (1992, Sept.). Modesty, sexuality, and breast health in Chinese American women. *The Western Journal of Medicine, 157,* 260-264.

Murphy, S. (1986). Family study and nursing research. *Image: Journal of Nursing Scholarship, 18*(4), 170.

Murray, R., & Huelskoetter, M. (1991). *Psychiatric mental health nursing.* Norwalk, Conn.: Appleton & Lange.

Murray, R., Meili, P., & Zentner, J. (1993). The family—basic unit for the developing person. In Murray, R., & Zentner, J. (Eds.), *Nursing concepts for health promotion* (ed. 5). Englewood Cliffs, N.J.: Prentice Hall.

Newman, R. (1998, Jan. 5). A drill for him and a drill for her. *U.S. News and World Report, 123*(25), 33.

Nilchaikovit, T., Hill, J.M., & Holland, J.C. (1993). The effects of culture on illness behavior and medical care: Asian and American differences. *General Hospital Psychiatry, 15*(1), 41-50.

Nolt, S. (1992). *A history of the Amish.* Intercourse, Penna.: Good Books.

O'Brien, S. (1992, Fall). Gender bias in family benefit provision. *Canadian Journal of Community Mental Health, 11*(2), 163-186.

Peitchinis, S. (1989). *Employment standards handbook.* Toronto: McClelland Stewart.

Phipps, S. (1989, April 3). *A phenomenological study of males experience with infertility.* Paper presented at the 13th Annual Midwest Nursing Research Society Conference, Cincinnati, Ohio. (MRNS, Glenview, Ill.)

Prilleltensky, I. (1993, Fall). The immigration experience of Latin American families: research and action on perceived risk and protective factors. *Canadian Journal of Community Health Nursing, 12*(2), 101-116.

Sands, E., & Berry, J. (1993). Acculturation and mental health among Greek-Canadians in Toronto. *Canadian Journal of Community Mental Health, 12*(2), 117-124.

Sartorelli, J. (1994). Gay rights and affirmative action. *Journal of Homosexuality, 27*(3-4), 179-222.

Satir, V. (1983). *Conjoint family therapy* (ed. 3). Palo Alto, Calif.: Science & Behavior Books.

Saunders, L. (1954). *Cultural differences and medical care.* New York: Russell Sage Foundation.

Schneider, R. (1980, June). *Conceptual scheme of family organization and function.* Paper presented at St. Louis University Medical Center Conference, St. Louis, Missouri.

Schneflen, A. (1972). *Body language in social order.* Englewood Cliffs, N.J.: Prentice Hall.

Shadick, K. (1993). Development of a transcultural health education program for the Hmong. *Clinical Nurse Specialist, 7*(2), 48-53.

Shipler, D. (1997). *A country of strangers.* New York: Alfred A. Knopf.

Sleeper, J. (1997). *Liberal racism.* New York: Viking Press.

Smart, N. (1984). *The religious experience of mankind* (ed. 3). New York: Charles Scribner's Sons.

Sniderman, P.M., & Carmines, E.G. (1997). *Reaching beyond race.* Cambridge, Mass.: Harvard University Press.

Spector, R. (1996). *Cultural diversity in health care* (ed. 4). Stamford, Conn.: Appleton & Lange.

Strickland, O., & Giger, J. (1994). Women's health in the decade of the woman. In Strickland, O., & Fishman, D. (Eds.), *Nursing issues and ethics* (pp. 362-399). Albany, N.Y.: Delmar Publishing Company.

Suchman, E.A. (1964). Sociomedical variations among ethnic groups. *American Journal of Sociology, 70,* 319-331.

Sussman, H. (1990, Summer). Are we talking revolution? *Human Resource Development Journal,* 1-3.

Sussman, M.B. (1971, July). Family systems in the 1970s: analysis, politics, and programs. *Annals of American Academy of Political Social Science, 396,* 40-56.

Taylor, C. (Ed.) (1994). *Essentials of psychiatric nursing* (ed. 14). St. Louis: Mosby.

Thompson, M. (1998, Jan. 5). Boys and girls apart. *Time, 150*(27), 104-105.

Thompson, K. (1993, Sept.). Self-governed health. *The Canadian Nurse, 89*(8), 29-32.

U.S. Department of Commerce, Bureau of the Census (1998). *Population profiles of the United States.* Internet Update, June 30, 1998. Washington, D.C.: U.S. Government Printing Office.

U.S. Department of Commerce, Bureau of the Census (1993a). *Current population reports: population profile of the United States, 1993,* Special Studies P23-185. Washington, D.C.: Government Printing Office.

U.S. Department of Commerce, Bureau of the Census (1993b). *We the American Asians.* Washington, D.C.: U.S. Government Printing Office.

U.S. Department of Commerce, Bureau of the Census (1998). *Population projections of the United States by age, sex, race, and Hispanic Origins: 1990 to 2050 (1996).* Washington, D.C.: U.S. Government Printing Office. 1998 Internet update.

Walters, T. (1994, Jan.). Personal communication to J.N. Giger; Salt Lake City, Utah.

Watchtower (1989, March 1). Questions from readers. *Watchtower,* 30-31.

Watchtower Bible & Tract Society. (1953). *Let God be true* (revised ed.). New York: the society.

Watchtower Bible & Tract Society. (1955). *You may survive Armageddon into God's new world.* New York: the society.

Wingert, P., Springen, K., Stone, B., et al. (1997, Dec. 15). A matter of faith. *Newsweek,* 49-53.

Wolfram, W.A., & Clark, H. (Eds.) (1971). *Black-White speech relationships.* Washington, D.C.: Center for Applied Linguistics.

World Almanac (1998). Mahwah, N.J.: World Almanac Books.

York, C. (1991). The labour movement's role in parental leave and child care. In Shibley-Hide, J., & Essex, M. (Eds.), *Parental leave and child care: setting a research and policy agency.* Philadelphia: Temple University Press.

CHAPTER 5

Time

BEHAVIORAL OBJECTIVES

After reading this chapter, the nurse will be able to:

1. Postulate an adequate definition for the term "time" in relation to transcultural nursing care.
2. Understand the significant role that culture plays in the understanding and perception of time.
3. Understand the significant role that the developmental process plays in the understanding and perception of time.
4. Understand the significance of the measurement of time and the relationship to transcultural nursing care.
5. Differentiate the terms "social time" and "clock time."
6. Describe the world view of clock time and social time.
7. Define the three broad areas of the structure of social time: temporal patterns, temporal orientation, and temporal perspectives.

Since the beginning of life on earth, time has been the greatest mystery of all. The mystery of time becomes evident as soon as thought is given to the concept. Our experience with time continuously leads us into puzzles and paradoxes. According to Wessman and Gorman (1977), it is through an awareness and conception of time that the products of the human mind, that is, time itself, seem to possess an existence apart from time's passage, which is perceived as personal and inexorable. We measure time, and time measures us. It is this intimate and personal yet aloof and detached character that constitutes the paradox of human time.

CONCEPT OF TIME

The concept of the passage of time is very familiar to most people regardless of cultural heritage. The days and nights come and go, and with each passing day and night humankind grows older. In the highly mechanized world of today there are numerous clocks and watches that ceaselessly tick away time and determine the schedules by which hundreds of millions of people live. Thus it would seem that the concept of the passage of time should be second nature to humankind and thoroughly understood by all people (Spector, 1996).

However, developing an awareness of the concept of time is not a simple phenomenon but a gradual process (Hymovich & Chamberlin, 1980). Most people, regardless of cultural heritage, remember a time when their perception of the passage of time was altered. Such occasions might have been during times of boredom or of highly emotional and stressful events. During these events time might have seemed to have passed very slowly, or it might have seemed to have passed all too quickly. It must be remembered that a sense of time is not innate but is developed early as a result of everyday experiences that are common to all people. Thus a sense of time results from learning. It becomes a part of human nature before one is conscious of its presence. Even infants perceive the essence of time. Infants are fed on demand or according to a strict timetable and experience the succession of day by night. Thus infants are exposed to regular rhythmic changes that are reflected in rhythmic changes in bodily conditions, including being sated, awake, or asleep. Thus one phenomenon about time is that it is associated with rhythm and change.

Infants grow, develop, and begin to move through crawling. The speed with which crawling occurs determines the time it takes to get from one place to another. Thus even this simple task makes individuals aware that time is associated with speed and velocity, which is the second phenomenon about time. As individuals grow older, speech is learned as they listen to stories that begin with "once upon a time." It is through these storytelling sessions that children learn that things did happen before they were born; thus time is associated with history and goes backward as well as forward with the succession of events. As the growth and development of the child continues, an awareness of punctuality is developed. Children may be punished for being slow or late, and regardless of their reaction to it, the punishment contributes to the formation of character and the development of the understanding of time. Thus the third phenomenon about time is that it is associated with social behavior (Sideleau, 1992).

The child begins to become conscious of time and asks questions such as, "Where was I before I was born?" "What did God do before He created the world?" "What will happen to me after I die?" Such questions lead to an understanding that time is associated with philosophy and religion. Children are taught to read time on a clock, and as they grow to adulthood, they learn that the clock is ubiquitous and that life is governed by the clock. Thus there is an erroneous identification of time with the clock. Through questioning, individuals begin to contemplate existence on earth and to develop an understanding that time is associated with something external over which there is no control and that appears absolute (Elton, 1975; Sideleau, 1992).

Developing an understanding of the definition of time by looking at the developmental process is clearly too simple. The development of the awareness of time is directly influenced by earlier ideas and prejudices that are mostly unconscious. However, because it is the nature of humankind to have a questioning frame of mind, ideas and prejudices may become conscious.

Other considerations concerning time include the question of whether time is concrete or abstract. Time is perceived as real in the sense of being concrete and having direct effects, or it is regarded as not real in the sense of being abstract. The mathematical and physical sciences adopt the view that time is an abstract dimension with only a locational or reference function (McGrath & Kelly, 1986). On the other hand, the biological sciences adopt the view that time is an essential ingredient in many life and behavioral processes such as gestation, healing, and metamorphosis. This difference in conceptualization of time may be related to an obvious difference between the physical and biological sciences and how each treats the concept of entropy. For the physical sciences entropy, or randomness, continuously increases over time, whereas the biological sciences see organization, structure, and information residing within the organism and in the organism's relation to its environment as increasing over time.

MEASUREMENT OF TIME

Time has two distinct, though related, meanings. The first meaning is that of duration, which is an interval of time. The second meaning is that of specified instances, or points in time. These two meanings are related because a point in time is identified as being the end of a time interval that starts at an arbitrary or fixed reference point, such as the founding of Rome or the birth of Christ. Thus, if one asks the question, "What is the time?" and the answer given is, "It is 10:00 A.M.," this answer refers to a point in time. At the same time, the answer refers to a time interval, since it indicates the time from a certain reference point, which in this case is midnight the previous night (Elton, 1975; Sideleau, 1992). The two meanings are quite different and must not be confused with each other. Measuring devices are meant to determine intervals of time, and clocks and watches are designed to read direct points in time. Clocks and watches therefore have to be standardized against a standard clock. The purpose of a standard clock is to measure accurately the time interval up to the present time. This phenomenon goes back to one universal standard clock against which all standard clocks are calibrated.

The purpose of a universal standard clock is to define operational time in terms of both time interval and point in time (Landes, 1983). The purpose of measuring devices is to define time; however, people need to have intuitive ideas about time to specify the properties of the instrument. Measuring devices of a phenomenon such as time are more accurate than measuring devices of some other phenomena. For example, if person wanted to measure the weight of another person, this weight could be defined operationally as a point or reading on a scale. Thus a good scale would give accurate weight, just as any good clock would give accurate time. On the other hand, if an individual wanted to define a person's intelligence quotient (IQ) as the score obtained on an intelligence test but there was no general agreement about what constituted intelligence and what constituted a good intelligence test, the scores would not be so relevant or so meaningful as the weight or time measures.

Throughout the history of humankind there have been two obvious standards of time: the day and the year. The day is a remarkably easy period of time to recognize because of the experience of daylight and darkness, which result from the earth's spinning on its axis. The year is also easy to recognize because of the passage of the seasons, which are caused by the tilting of the earth's axis. Thus a day is the period of time for one complete revolution of the earth about its axis, whereas a year is the time taken for the earth to move one complete revolution around the sun, which takes just under 365.25 days. Therefore it is completely natural that we choose to mark the passage of time by first marking the days and then marking the years. Time measurement during the day has been divided into hours, and the hours in turn have been divided by 60 to give minutes. The minutes have been divided by 60 to give seconds.

Very early in the history of civilization the middle of each day was determined as the point when the sun was at its highest point during the day. This point was defined as noon, and clocks were made to read 12 when it occurred. Thus, if it is noon in one place, it is midnight at the opposite side of the earth and different times at other places on the earth. To understand how time varies, the earth must be viewed as a circle that passes through both the North Pole and the South Pole.

Traditionally in science, Greenwich, the observatory in London, has been taken to have 0 degrees of longitude; the longitude of all other places on earth are given as so many degrees east or west of Greenwich. Therefore, one half of the earth's surface has a longitude of up to 180 degrees east of Greenwich, whereas the other half has a longitude of up to 180 degrees west of Greenwich. The times of all places east of Greenwich are ahead of that of Greenwich, and the times of all places west of Greenwich lag behind that of Greenwich. For example, if a person started from Greenwich and traveled eastward to a longitude of 45 degrees, the time would be 3 hours ahead of Greenwich time. The converse is that if a person started at Greenwich and traveled westward to a longitude of 180 degrees, the time would be 12 hours behind that of Greenwich. In simpler terms, if it were 2 A.M. on Sunday morning at Greenwich, it would be 2 P.M. on Sunday at a longitude 180 degrees east of Greenwich and 2 P.M. on Saturday at a longitude 180 degrees west of Greenwich (Elton, 1975).

This phenomenon of time presents some interesting effects on persons who travel great distances. For example, it is possible for an international traveler to have two birthdays (birthday anniversaries); that is, if a person crosses the international date line traveling eastward at 2 A.M. Sunday morning, at which point it suddenly becomes 2 A.M. Saturday, that person has Saturday all over again and thus is able to celebrate the birthday again. If this same international traveler who is about to celebrate a birthday on Saturday leaves from the point of origin at 2 A.M. on Saturday but crosses the international date line westward, the traveler suddenly finds that it is 2 A.M. Sunday morning and apparently has missed almost the entire day of Saturday and the birthday (Elton, 1975).

Clocks

According to historians and philosophers the earliest clocks were undoubtedly sundials of various kinds, which were probably followed by devices that used the regular flow of a substance such as water, oil, or sand, or the steady combustion of oil or candles. The earliest clocks have been dated back to 1600 B.C. in Egypt and were used throughout classical times and the Middle Ages.

The thirteenth century saw the invention of a rhythmic motion clock, which was a saw-toothed crown wheel. However, the most important development in clock construction occurred with the introduction of the pendulum, which was first discovered by Galileo in 1581. Galileo discovered that a swinging pendulum would readily tick away a unit of time by a specific number of swings and that even if the swings gradually died the unit of time would remain relatively unaffected. Thus for the first time in history, time was measured more accurately.

Tropical years

An important distinction that has been made by scientists is the difference between a calendar year and a tropical year. According to scientists, a calendar year consists of 365 days, whereas a tropical year consists of 365.242199 solar days (the word "tropical" in this instance has nothing to do with a hot climate). The difference between these two numbers (tropical year and calendar year) is the reason for the necessity of leap years. Time that is based on the length of a tropical year is called "ephemeris time." One tropical year is defined in terms of having 31,556,925.9747 seconds. Today atomic clocks have replaced the old, outdated pendulum and weight- and gravity-driven clocks. Atomic clocks are so accurate that in due course scientists speculate that the difference between atomic time and ephemeris time will become very apparent. In fact, atomic clocks are said to be 10 million times more accurate than any other clock on earth and are never more than 1 billionth of a second off. Atomic clocks are considered to be so accurate that the exact second of an event can be obtained at the time of the event.

Solar time

Solar time is perhaps the earliest way that time was measured (Dossey, 1982). Solar time takes into consideration a focal point, 12:00 noon, which is precisely the point at which the sun passes directly overhead (vertically above the meridian). The time between successive crossings of the sun directly over the same meridian is called a solar day. However, this measurement of time is not without its problems. When days are measured in this way, they turn out to be not exactly constant. A solar day varies slightly in length throughout the year because of the orbiting of the earth around the sun.

The concept of solar time has many implications for nurses who work at extreme southern or northern points of the earth, for example, at the North or South Pole. A nurse working in the northern most part of Canada may find Indians operating on "Indian time" because the sun remains up during most of the summer and down during much of the winter. Activities requiring daylight can therefore be done anytime during a 24-hour period. Staying up much of the night and sleeping in the daytime is consistent with an orientation to do what feels right at the present time. On the other hand, "White man's time" is more future oriented and adheres to clocks and schedules rather than to the sun (Wuest, 1992, England, 1986; Young & Hayne, 1988). Generally White men who have not grown up in the northernmost part of Canada but have relocated to this area tend to work during familiar working hours and to sleep during familiar sleeping hours. However, this pattern may not necessarily correlate with the same time orientation for others who are native to the northernmost part of Canada.

Calendar

Inventing a simple yet efficient calendar has presented difficulties since the invention of the first calendar. Scientists believe that these difficulties lie in the fact that the three obvious periods are due to the rotation of the earth about the sun. These three revolutional periods are not simply related one to the other. In fact, they have obvious differences. For example, 1 tropical year equals 365.224 solar days, and 1 month is considered to be the observed time between one full moon and the next, or 29.5306 solar days.

Throughout history we have measured time by counting the months and the calendar years and combining the two. However, this combination of months and years has proved to be most confusing. Even if we ignored the moon, there would still be the problem of the solar year not being a whole number of days, though this problem has conceivably been dealt with by the system of leap years. With so many different civilizations contributing to the development of the calendar, it is no wonder that we are left with a complicated system that children and even adults, regardless of ethnic or cultural heritage, find difficult to remember or understand. Many of the significant events linked with the calendar can be traced to specific persons in history such as Julius Caesar, who decreed that months should alternately have 30 and 31 days with the exception of February (which at that time was the last month of the Roman calendar). Historians believe that all would have been well with the calendar if Julius Caesar had not decided to call the fifth month Julius in his honor. The problem began when Augustus followed Julius Caesar and also wanted a month. He promptly chose the month that followed Julius and named it "Augustus." However, he very soon realized that his month was shorter than Caesar's month and promptly took a day from February, added it to his month, and readjusted the rest of the year. The result was that there were 3 long months in succession, that is June, July, and August. Even today, because of the vanity of Emperor Augustus, children continue to chant "Thirty days hath September."

According to the earlier decree by Julius Caesar, September would have been an alternate month with 31 days if August had been given 30 days as originally planned (Elton, 1975). Although there have been attempts over the last 50 years to standardize the calendar by international agreement through the League of Nations and the United Nations, these attempts have uniformly failed. For example, the day that is considered the beginning of the New Year in the United States is January 1, but the beginning of the New Year differs in many countries.

SOCIAL TIME VERSUS CLOCK TIME

The word "time" immediately presents an image of a clock or calendar. However, the term "social time" is not equivalent with clock time. Social time refers to patterns and orientations that relate to social processes and to the conceptualization and ordering of social life. For centuries, many of the great thinkers of the universe have recognized and argued that social time must be distinguished from clock time. As early as 1910, Henri Bergson insisted that the homogeneous time of newtonian physics was not the time that revealed the essence of humankind. On the other hand, Phillip Bock (1964), an anthropologist, showed that an Indian wake could be meaningfully analyzed in terms of "gathering time," "prayer time," "singing time," "intermission time," and "meal time." None of these times has a particular relationship to clock time. They all simply imply the passage of the mourner from one time to another by consensual feelings rather than by the clock.

According to some sociologists, certain kinds of psychological disorders may be viewed in terms of the individual living wholly in the present, the implication being that the past and the future are completely severed from the consciousness. The difference therefore between social time and clock time is that the former is a more inclusive concept whereas the latter may or may not be. Hoppe and Heller (1974) conducted a study on Mexican Americans and proposed that Mexican Americans have a present-time orientation that may possibly account for the tendency to be late for appointments. It is believed that present-time orientation, particularly in high-risk settings such as mental health facilities, may result in a crisis approach rather than a preventive one. For example, a client who has an immediate need at home may be late for appointments at the clinic or hospital, or may miss them altogether. The nurse should also keep in mind that clients with a present-time orientation may be reluctant to leave an appointment simply because the time is up.

This same lack of correlation between social time and clock time can be seen in mystical beliefs. According to mystical thought, magic can be employed to negate the temporal order that infers causality. For example, an Indian warrior who is wounded by an arrow may attend to his pain by hanging the arrow up where it is cool or by applying ointment to the arrow. What the Indian warrior is attempting to do is to reverse the clock time, that is, wrench the present back into the past to alter the course of events. For people who have mystical beliefs, temporal intervals are not simple, homogeneous series; rather, they contain an inherent quality and meaning or an essence and efficacy of their own (Cassirer, 1955). Therefore the objectivity represented by clock time is unknown to a person with mystical beliefs.

Many sociologists believe that people who lack or minimize clock time also lack regularity or temporal measurement. The natural and social phenomena may dictate regularity and measurement. Ariotti (1995) provides several examples of natural events that have been used to time human activities: (1) The arrival of the cranes in ancient Greece marked the time for planting. (2) The return of the swallow marked the time for the end of pruning. (3) The South African bushmen note the rising of Sirius and Canopus and are able to depict the progress of winter across the night sky by the movement of these celestial bodies across the night sky.

Archeologists have been able to piece together the history of humankind by measuring the passage of time, using the method of geologists. This measure of time is based on rates of deposits to and erosion of natural early elements. An example of this kind of measurement is tree-ring chronology (Weyer, 1961).

WORLD VIEW OF SOCIAL TIME VERSUS CLOCK TIME

People throughout the world view social time and clock time differently (Giger & Davidhizar, 1995; Davidhizar, Dowd, & Giger, 1997). For example, Sorokin (1964) noted that the division of time by weeks reflects social conditions rather than mechanical newtonian divisions. Most societies have some kind of week, but the weeks vary in length from 3 to 16 or more days. In most cases weeks are a reflection of the cycle of market activities. The Khasi people have an 8-day week because they hold market every eighth day. The Khasi people have named the days of the week after the places where the principal markets occur (Sorokin, 1964).

Some cultural groups exhibit a social time that not only is different from clock time, but is actually scornful of clock time. For example, there are peasants in Algeria who live with a total indifference to the passage of clock time and who despise haste in human affairs. These peasants have no notion of exact appointment times; they lack exact times for eating meals; and they have labeled the clock as the "devil's mill" (Thompson, 1967). Some Amish keep "slow time." When those around them adjust their time to go from "day light savings time" to "standard time," the Amish set clocks one-half hour ahead (Randall-David, 1989; Gingerich, 1972; Wenger, 1991; Nolt, 1992). This has important implications for the nurse in trying to emphasize the importance of keeping medical appointments.

Despite the way people in various cultures view clock time as opposed to social time, the nurse must remember that clock time should not be regarded as unimportant or irrelevant. Although for some people in some cultural groups there is no necessary correlation of clock time and social time, clock time does not take on paramount importance in a social context such as the modern Western world, where the watch or the clock can become something of a tyrant. In Jonathan Swift's *Gulliver's Travels,* Gulliver never did anything without looking at his watch, which he called his "oracle." He said that his watch pointed out the time for every action of his life. Because of Gulliver's obsession with his watch, the Lilliputians concluded that the watch was Gulliver's god.

Aside from literature, many actual examples of human obsessive behavior in regard to clock time can be found. Lebhar (1958) wrote that he was exactly 43 years old and had probably only 227,760 hours to live, and he proceeded to detail how he would maximize the use of those remaining hours of his life. He concluded that if he reduced his sleep time from 8 hours to 6 hours, the 2 hours a day saved from sleeping would amount to 18,980 hours over a period of 26 years. If this savings were converted into 18-hour days, which is the equivalent of about 2 years and 11 months, he could virtually lengthen his remaining years by 2 years and 11 months. This example illustrates how human life can be turned into a lengthy succession of minutes and hours, with the individual's existence reduced to a compulsive and frantic effort to avoid waste.

Gilles and Faulkner (1978) conducted a study of the role of time in television news work. They found that time is a major factor in the production of unscheduled "hard" news. The definition for "hard" news refers to events such as fires, homicides, and accidents, which have a certain urgency to them. They summarized the findings of their research in three propositions. In the first proposition they concluded that the news value of an event is directly proportional to the time invested in covering it. An event may turn out to be relatively minor in the sense of not involving the trauma or shock value that was anticipated, but this factor was not considered when a film crew invested time in the event, and the story is likely to be used in the evening news program anyway. They found in the second proposition that what is considered news by the news crew depends on when it happens and how long it lasts. Although viewers tend to believe that what they see on the evening news is a compilation of the universal news events for that particular day, what is telecast each evening is actually a compilation of news events that the news crew was able to learn about, get a story line on, capture on film, and then process and edit the film. The researchers found in the third proposition that bias in the news reflects occupational assumptions and temporal constraints more than it does the political or social views of the news crew. More important than political and social biases are the assumptions that the news crew makes about what will make good news on television and the severe time constraints on those persons assigned to locate film and write about events in time for the evening news program. The researchers concluded that because of deadline pressures, it is inevitable that events are reduced to surface actions and that the visuals seen each evening are of only the most dramatic events.

In today's modern technological society clock time is of paramount importance. However, we must remember that even in a modern society the clock may be a relatively peripheral part of social life. Not all people in a modern technological society function under the inevitable tyranny of the clock. In a survey of a representative sample of the French population, approximately 21% of the respondents indicated a belief that there was no urgency about being punctual and also stated that they had not experienced the feeling of wasting time (Stoetzel, 1953). It is the perception of some people in some cultural groups that there is little correlation between being punctual and wasting time (Hein, 1980). Hein further postulated that assumptions and definitions in regard to time are determined by culture and cultural variables and are reflected in interactions with others, personal views concerning punctuality, use or waste of time, and value and respect for time or a lack thereof. Waiting is a cultural counterpart to time because a particular behavior, person, or event is anticipated within a particular time frame. Waiting may have a meaning similar to that of time for some African-American clients. The nurse may schedule an appointment for an African-American client and wait for the client to arrive for the appointment. However, the client may not arrive for several hours, or perhaps even a few days, because of other important issues that in the client's mind took precedence over the appointment. Although the nurse viewed this time as waiting and therefore wasting time, the client for whom the appointment was made was not wasting time (Randall-David, 1989).

In some cultures, for example, among some persons of Asian origin, time is viewed as flexible and so there is no need to hurry or be punctual except in extremely important cases. Asians may spend hours getting to know people and view predetermined abrupt endings as rude (Stauffer, 1995). Nonetheless, the nurse should emphasize the importance of keeping scheduled appointments. Hispanics or Latinos as well often have difficulty with scheduled appointments. In fact, Hispanics or Latinos are sometimes attributed by others as being on "Latin time." However, this is sometimes explained by Hispanics as the result of consideration for others who were not ready to leave for the appointment (Ruiz, 1981; Ruiz & Padella, 1977; Hoppe & Heller, 1974).

In the American nursing profession, many nurses have related professionalism and success in their career to a sense of precision about clock time. For example, in many health care facilities, a medication error is considered to occur when a medication is not given within 30 minutes of the prescribed time, even when the medication is given daily and is not a time-released medication. Thus the nurse must complete a medication error form for not giving a routine daily medication such as a vitamin or laxative, which is neither time released nor urgent.

Most agencies relate medication errors to disciplinary action and dismissal. In some facilities the nurse is expected to complete all morning or evening care in a precise time frame even though many clients may not operate in the same time sphere as the facility schedule for client care. For example, a client may become upset when the night nurse refuses to help the client to shower at 3 A.M. because showering is a stated day-shift activity. In this case the client may be used to starting the day at 3 A.M. and unwilling to wait until 7 A.M. to do so. Another example is early morning vital signs, which may be taken by the night nurse to facilitate a timely assessment of the client's condition for the physician who makes early morning rounds. The client may be annoyed at being awakened for such a brief procedure and then instructed by the nurse to return to sleep.

According to Zerubavel's (1979) analysis of the temporal order of the hospital, any unit of clock time is equal to any other unit whether one is talking about minutes, hours, days, or weeks. However, Zerubavel concluded that different days mean quite different things to different people. Because people perceive days differently, it is important to remember that some days are more or less desirable for some people. For example, some health care personnel may perceive the fact of working two weekends in succession as unfair. Similarly, evening or night duty is usually considered less desirable than day duty. Thus it is important for hospital administrators to understand the necessity for fairness in scheduling. Some hospitals have a policy that all personnel are expected to work their share of the less desirable times. In other hospitals the staff are paid differentials for working what is perceived as the less desirable times, that is, evenings, nights, weekends, and holidays.

STRUCTURE OF SOCIAL TIME

The structure of social time is a complex phenomenon. To understand the structure of social time, three broad areas of social time must be analyzed: temporal pattern, temporal orientation, and temporal perspective.

Temporal pattern

Hawley (1986) identified the temporal pattern of social time as one of the most important aspects of ecological organization. He concluded that there are five basic elements in the temporal pattern of any social phenomenon: periodicity, tempo, timing, duration, and sequence.

Periodicity Periodicity refers to the various rhythms of social life and is characterized by activities related to both the needs and the activities of people. For example, every community has a functional routine that is supposedly peculiar to that community, such as the search for food, shelter, and mates, which occurs more or less with regular periodicity. People also have transcendental needs that are pursued with regular periodicity. For example, people may attend church weekly in pursuit of satisfying transcendental needs. Even physical functions of the body occur in a periodic manner. There are cyclical variations in physiological functions of the body, such as body temperature, blood pressure, and pulse.

Nelkin (1970) studied the behavior patterns of migrant workers and found several daily, weekly, and seasonal rhythms that were germane to their existence. Nelkin concluded that these migrant workers seemed to alternate between compact and diffuse time. Migrant time was seen to be very present oriented, irrational, and highly personal. Nelkin concluded that migrant time was in sharp contrast to the typical time perception, which was future oriented, rational, and impersonal. Findings from the study indicate that social time for the migrants differed because it was a series of disconnected periods rather than a continuous and predictable process, which in part accounted for maladaptive behaviors such as excessive drinking, gambling, volatile social relationships, and apathy.

Periodicity is also considered important at the managerial level. An important aspect of managerial life concerns the periodicity of meetings. For example, it is inappropriate for managers of a volunteer organization to plan frequent meetings for the membership. It is believed that a volunteer organization can engage in systematic self-destruction and ensure itself of a high turnover of membership if the body seeks to gather its members too often. These organizations must justify their demands on the members' time and at the same time create the novelty necessary to maintain the interest of the membership. In contrast to this are nonvoluntary groups, such as those that are part of a job assignment. For example, in nursing administration, regular meetings are necessary as part of the required management structure and are not usually planned with the intent of being novel and interesting. Because the management structure requires regular meetings, the meetings are planned regardless of specific agenda items.

Periodicities are also noted at the individual level. It is believed that when people are able to control their own work patterns (periodicity), satisfaction and productivity are maximized (Strauss, 1963). Some individuals spontaneously choose to alternate bouts of intense work with periods of idleness.

It is important for the manager to realize that productivity is cyclic and that equal periods of productivity cannot always be maintained. For example, after a period in which a nursing care unit experiences high client acuity necessitating an extremely heavy work load for staff, employees will need to recover with a period of less intense pressure. It is unwise to follow a period of high acuity with another assignment that requires major time on the task. However, some work environments by their very nature cannot provide for individual periodicity. For example, industrial workers often must work at a continuous rhythmic pace, such as that seen on an automobile assembly line.

To understand periodicity, the nurse must remember that it is an important aspect of human life and the first aspect of the temporal pattern. Periodicity therefore refers to the recurrence of a social phenomenon with some kind of regularity that can be measured by clock time or by comparison of the social phenomenon with other social phenomena.

Tempo Tempo is the second aspect of the temporal pattern and refers to rate (Morgenstern, 1960). Tempo may refer to the frequency of activities in some unit of social time or to the rate of change of some phenomenon. An example of this is the industrialization of the United States, which differs from that of Russia and China because of different rates (Gioscia, 1970). In a study done by the Southern Illinois University Foundation (Veterans World Project, 1972) it was suggested that one major problem among Vietnam veterans resulted from the rapidity with which they were brought home. The study concluded that the sudden transition from combat back to the United States by way of jet flights required a psychological adjustment that was often quite traumatic for these veterans.

Tempo also includes perceived rapidity of time and experience and the rapidity of various modes of social life, such as urban versus rural and work versus leisure. For example, the tempo of life in a large city such as Chicago or New York is much different from the tempo of life in a smal rural Midwestern town. Thus a person who relocates may have difficulty adjusting to the different tempo.

Tempo has several important consequences at the individual level because control of the tempo of one's work seems to be important for a healthful self-concept (Kohn, 1977). The tempo of change in social order appears to be related to emotional health; thus the more rapid the change, the greater is the stress of the individual. This thought became the theme of Alvin Toffler (1970), who coined the term "future shock"—the psychological disruptions that result from experiencing too much change in too short a time. An example of this is noted with Japanese people, who traditionally have had to change their culture and society at a very rapid pace. The very rapid tempo of the deliberate transformation of the Meiji era in Japan produced considerable stress for the Japanese people. Some historians have concluded that the 1878 revolution of Japan did save Japan from Western domination, but the generations that followed experienced the brunt of the hectic rate of change and suffered extraordinary mental agonies as a result of these forced changes (Pyle, 1969).

Timing Timing is the third element in the temporal pattern and is referred to as "synchronization." Timing involves the adjustment of various social units and processes with each other. The necessity for synchronization has led to the emphasis on clock time in modern society. Timing can be a crucial factor in the initiation of planned social changes and is of obvious importance in numerous social contexts, such as industrial processes, military campaigns, and political campaigns. A presidential candidate who supports a particular view that is not popular or timely may lose an election but win at a later time when the view becomes popular or another view emerges. For example, Richard Nixon ran for president of the United States in 1960 and lost. Eight years later he ran for president again at the height of the Vietnam War, and because the issue of the war was a timely one, he campaigned on this issue and won. Success is related to being at the right place at the right time with popular ideas.

Another example of the importance of timing is provided by research data on institutionalized disturbed children. These children, because of their psychological limitations, can be permitted to engage in activities such as competitive sports for only limited amounts of time. The restrictions on time are necessary because the process of the game and the psychological processes can mesh for only limited periods of time before the two processes begin to conflict and lead to destructive behavior (Doob, 1970).

Some researchers have concluded that one of the most serious problems of the modern American family is the difficulty of synchronizing family life because of the diverse activities in which each member is engaged. Another difficulty that has emerged over the years lies in the efforts of rural immigrants to adjust to the stringent demands of industrial life. Some researchers have suggested that habitual functioning of these rural immigrants must be synchronized with the industrial process and that such synchronization disallows the individual's self-actualization.

Duration Duration is the fourth element of the temporal pattern and has been the concern of psychologists more than it has been the concern of sociologists. The psychological concern of duration is related to the duration of which the individual is conscious, or to what has been referred to as the "spacious present." According to the classic early work of James (1890), one of the early writers in the field of social psychology, longer or shorter periods are conceived symbolically by adding to or dividing the vaguely bound unit that is the spacious present.

Duration has significance beyond the psychological level, however. Some noted sociologists have set forth a number of laws that relate to duration and behavior in organizations (Parkinson, 1970). Parkinson developed the laws of triviality and delay. The law of triviality states that the amount of time spent on any item in the agenda of an organizational meeting is inversely proportional to the money involved with that item. People may quibble far more about an item costing $50 than about an item costing $10,000. For example, in professional staff meetings at a state psychiatric hospital, an inordinate amount of time was spent discussing the purchase of a 75-cent plastic receptacle for holding clients' personal items such as toothbrushes and soap. A year later, when some plastic lids were missing, several meetings were devoted to developing a strategic nursing procedure for safeguarding these "valuable plastic receptacles." The policy developed to safeguard these receptacles mandated that the staff send a written requisition to the director of nursing, who in turn was required to write a written justification for replacement of the receptacle or the lid. The law of delay asserts that delay is the deadliest form of denial. In addition, duration is perceived as a useful variable.

Researchers continue to investigate the effects of various phenomena such as perceived importance of time, anxiety, and boredom on the perception of time. For example, researchers have concluded that morale may be improved among workers if time is subjectively made to pass more quickly and if there are several methods whereby the apparent length of a period of time can be manipulated (Meade, 1960).

Sequence Sequence is the fifth element of the temporal pattern and is derived from the fact that there are activities requiring order. An obvious evidence of the utility of sequence is the measuring of values. For example, work before play is an ordering of activities that reflects a valuing hierarchy. In a classic 1946 study, Friedman measured values relating to physical activities, theoretic-scientific interests, and esthetic interests and found that subjects made similar choices on both time and money scales. Friedman concluded that when cost and time are equalized, similar preferential orderings are made for various activities.

In modern American society time is indeed money. It is conceivable, however, that the sequential ordering of activities may reflect necessity rather than values as an industrial process. It is also possible that conflict may arise over whether the sequence actually does represent necessity rather than values. Generally, this kind of conflict is more common in organizational settings in which disputes arise over the necessity of sequential orderings that are demanded by bureaucratic rules.

Finally, sequential ordering may reflect habit. Rituals of primitive societies are ordered in accordance with custom. Modern rituals also fall in this category, even though some are more appropriately viewed as reflections of values. For example, the ritual of a man removing his hat before entering a room or elevator is a habitual sequence. However, the ritual of the same man removing his hat before the national anthem is played is a sequence demanded by values.

Temporal orientation

Temporal orientation refers to the ordering of past, present, and future and to the fact that individuals and groups may be differentiated according to whether behavior is primarily related to the past, present, or future. Psychologists and sociologists, however, have raised objections to this particular ordering. One objection is that past, present, and future are perceived to make up an organic whole that cannot be separated (Cassirer, 1955; Sideleau, 1992). A second objection involves variations in the ordering of past, present, and future among various groups. For example, the argument is made that an actor's orientation to a situation always contains an "expectancy aspect," which implies that all orientations are to a future state of a situation as well as to the present. However, this may be true only in a limited sense, because actors generally do not anticipate their demise in the situation. It is also untrue that orientation to the future is a universal and inherent aspect of all social action.

Future orientation refers to the fact that the future is a dominant factor in present behavior, and as such this kind of orientation is by no means universal. For example, the Navajo Indians' view of time does not include the expectancy aspect. In years past, efforts to get the Navajo Indians to engage in range control and soil conservation programs were extremely frustrating for government employees because the Navajos simply do not have a view of temporality that would lead them to act on the basis of an expected future (Hall & William, 1960). For the Navajo people the only real time, like the only real space, is that which is here and now (Iverson, 1992). For some Navajo Indians there is little reality of the future; thus the promise of future benefits is not worth thinking about (Hall & William, 1960). It is important for the nurse to remember that the way in which a society, group, or individual orders past, present, or future will be consequential for behavior.

Kluckhohn and Strodtbeck (1961) have argued that the knowledge of rank ordering of these three modes can tell much about a social unit and the direction of change for that unit. Some Americans have typically placed a dominant emphasis on the future, which does not imply that they ignore either the past or the present. Although there are some undesirable connotations for the label "old fashioned," few Americans express total contentment with the present state of affairs. According to Kluckhohn and Strodtbeck, American values change easily as long as the change does not contradict what is perceived as the American way of life. There is a direct relationship between the extended future orientation and the amount of change. However, the change perceived is not expected to be the kind that threatens the existing order.

Generally speaking, resistance to change should be expected where there is a past orientation. Thus it should be expected that serious problems would arise in efforts to industrialize a society where a future orientation was lacking. For example, in a classic 1953 study, Ritzenthaler found that among the Chippewa Indians, who traditionally lack any concern for the future, there were serious problems when attempts were made to industrialize their work. Ritzenthaler also noted that the Chippewa Indians quit work as soon as they had sufficient money for immediate needs.

Temporal orientations are not immutable; they can change, and along with change come various behavioral changes. Therefore a shift of orientation to the present may have significant consequences in several contexts (Ketchum, 1951). For example, in a crowd situation the orientation may be drawn to the present, wherein some of the typical behaviors of crowds may manifest themselves as overreacting behaviors, such as struggling at a department store sale, racing to the exit doors in a fire, or panic in an airplane during turbulence. Similarly, in a marriage or relationship where the partners perceive the relationship to be of uncertain duration, they may begin to act in accordance with feelings rather than stable values. For example, one of the partners may transfer joint banking accounts and charge card accounts to individual status. In other words, when situations are structured so that people function in a present orientation that lacks future and past orientations, a variety of self-destructive and self-limiting behaviors may result.

Whenever a change is anticipated, orientation to the change may be resisted by individuals or groups, and serious consequences generally follow. The intermingling of traditional orientation, which is somewhat past oriented, with the pressures manifested by modernization, which may be somewhat present or future oriented, may cause societal agony. For example, many problems arose in a factory in Cantal, Guatemala, because the management refused to be sensitive to market variations or to the problem of obsolete equipment (Nash, 1967). Worse situations occurred in Iran, which is a past-oriented society. In past-oriented societies the past is of primary importance and the future of minimal significance. In Iran businessmen invested considerable sums of money in factories without any real plan on how to use these factories (Hall & William, 1960).

Temporal orientation is an important variable in societal behavior and is also significant at the societal level. Some psychological studies indicate that temporal orientation may be directly related to various kinds of emotional disorders, such as alcoholism, and to certain kinds of deviant behaviors, such as juvenile delinquency.

Temporal perspective

Temporal perspective refers to the image of past, present, and future that prevails in a society, a social group, or individuals. The rank ordering of past, present, and future is of significance, yet it is insignificant in gaining an adequate understanding of social time. For example, if a particular group is future oriented, that is, it ranks the future highest in its hierarchy of values, its behavior will depend largely on the way it perceives the future. If people in a society perceive that they may be extinct in the future, efforts may be made to ensure survival. The converse of this is that if people in a society perceive that they do not have a future (for example, they will be eradicated in a nuclear holocaust), they may adopt a present orientation, desiring to live life now to its fullest. An excellent example of this is found with the dying client's perception of time. For the dying client, living in the present is very important; however, the nurse should recognize other realms of time perception. The nurse should ascertain precisely how the client views the past, present, and future because these views may assist the nurse in helping the client cope with death and the challenges faced in the process (Maguire, 1984). An image of the future functions to direct present behavior in accordance with specific values, and some sociologists view a society as being magnetically pulled toward a future fulfillment of their own image of the future as well as being pushed from behind by their past (Polick, 1973).

A future orientation to illness, disease, and health care is essential to preventive medicine. Actions are taken in the present to safeguard the future, particularly regarding certain disease conditions, such as using condoms to prevent AIDS, practicing safe sex, adhering to a diet to prevent elevated cholesterol or blood glucose levels, not driving while under the influence of alcohol, and using seat belts.

TIME AND HUMAN INTERACTION

Up to this point an effort has been made to create an awareness that social time arises out of interaction. Regardless of the cultural heritage of an individual or group, there is no kind of time that is natural to humans. Instead, time is a result of the structuring and functioning of social order. When a particular temporality emerges, it tends to persist and to influence subsequent interaction. Various cultural groups construct systems of time that have diverse meanings and therefore diverse consequences on social interactions. The most fundamental differences in the meaning of time occur when cultural groups measure time predominantly by either social events or the clock.

Cultural groups that measure time predominantly by social events construct time according to the activities of the group. Conversely, cultural groups that measure time by the clock schedule activities according to the clock. In this regard, time is perceived basically as qualitative for those who measure time by social life and activities and as quantitative for those who measure time by the clock. When measured by social activities, time has significance only in terms of the activities that are occurring. When time is measured by the clock, it has significance only in terms of money, which is perceived to be a scarce commodity, and all activities that take place do so in the shadow of the clock.

There are few cultural groups or societies that could be characterized as bound exclusively by the clock or as wholly independent of any constraints of temporality. How a group perceives time, nevertheless, has implications for interactions. For example, the Balinese people have a detemporalizing concept of time (Geertz, 1973). For these people social time includes a calendar with a complex system of peri-odicities. According to Geertz, this is called a "premutational calendar" because it contains 10 different cycles of days ranging in length from 1 to 10 days. Although this is a complex system, it nevertheless serves various religious and practical purposes; it identifies nearly all the holidays and temple celebrations and at the same time guides the individual in daily activities. According to Geeretz, the structure of this complex system allows and disallows certain activities on certain days. For example, certain days are good or bad for building a house, starting a business enterprise, moving from one location to another, going on a trip, and harvesting and planting crops.

In contrast to the belief of the Balinese people is the belief held by some Americans that time is money and therefore a scarce commodity. Thus human interactions are controlled in accordance with some notion of the appropriate amount of time for a particular situation. For example, some Americans distinguish the amount of time that can rightfully be consumed by strangers from that which can be given to friends and relatives. Weigert (1981) concluded that interaction time is a measure of the meaning of the relationship between two persons. In the event that two casual acquaintances meet somewhere, it is unlikely that they will take more than a few minutes to express recognition or perhaps exchange a pleasantry or two; therefore, the interaction time for such a meeting is limited. The converse of this is that if two good friends meet and one of the friends attempts to limit the interaction, the other friend may feel rejected. Therefore the violator is expected to account for the behavior, and if this accounting is not forthcoming, the friendship may be severely strained. A single logical conclusion is that interaction can be evaluated in terms of time consumption.

In the United States methods to save time or to use time more effectively are in high demand. Numerous books, articles, workshops, tapes, and seminars imply that most Americans value time but at the same time do not think they use it wisely. Many busy professionals feel torn between wise use of time and taking time for interpersonal relationships with fellow workers or friends. For example, a dilemma may arise when a person is busy and a coworker drops in and asks, "Do you have a minute?" If time is considered money, a minute is costly. Because this worker values time, a reply of "yes," may be viewed as costly and thus unjustifiable. On the other hand, "no" may be perceived by the other person as a lack of sensitivity, coldness, and a lack of interest. Therefore much of the advice given by time-efficiency experts can do much to depersonalize human interactions. A person who follows the advice of these experts to the letter may have far more hours in which to accomplish tasks but at the same time may have fewer friends and fewer intimate relationships.

Drucker (1966) called the executive a captive because everyone can move in on an executive's time, and, generally speaking, everybody does. An executive's time is often preempted by matters that are important to other people; therefore, the executive has little or no time for self. A nurse manager who is responsive to others may find there is little time to do paperwork in the office and thus may take a lot of paperwork home. A nurse manager's personal priorities are often modified when employees present "more urgent" problems.

CULTURAL PERCEPTIONS OF TIME

Appreciating cultural differences regarding time is important for the nurse in relating to both peers and clients. When people of different cultures interact, as is frequently the case in health care settings, there is a great potential for misunderstanding. If nurses are to avoid misreading issues that involve time perceptions, they must have an understanding of how other persons in different cultures view time (Tripp-Reimer & Lively, 1993).

Campinha-Bacote (1997) compared time orientation among certain groups in relation to future-time and present-time orientation:

Dominant American	Future over present
African Black	Present over future
Puerto Rican American	Present over future
Mexican American	Present
Chinese American	Past over Present
Native American	Present

Individuals with future-oriented perceptions

Most middle-class Americans, regardless of ethnic or cultural heritage, tend to be future oriented (Tripp-

Reimer & Lively, 1993). For example, some middle-class Americans tend to defer gratification of personal pleasure until some future objective has been met, such as advanced education. Thus they will delay starting families, purchasing homes, buying an expensive car, or investing money until they have prepared for a profession through advanced education, and so on. Another noted difference among members of the dominant American culture is that these individuals tend to structure time rigidly. For these people, adhering to a time-structured schedule is a way of life, regardless of whether the schedule involves work or leisure. For the nurse who works with future-oriented individuals, it is important to talk about events in relation to the future and to adhere to the schedule for planned events in a timely and precise manner.

Individuals with present-oriented perceptions

Present-oriented individuals do not necessarily adhere strictly to a time-structured schedule. The present takes precedence over the future and the past with these individuals. More specifically, whatever is occurring at a precise moment may be more important than a future appointment. It is important for the nurse to avoid labeling such individuals as lazy, disrespectful, or lacking interest. Hoppe and Heller (1974) concluded that present-time orientation may be a reason why some Hispanic clients are late for appointments. Carter (1979) noted that it is important to gain an awareness of differences in values for African Americans from low socioeconomic groups and proposed that instead of labeling tardiness as a blatant disregard for time, problems related to health, economics, and transportation should be considered with these individuals. Another explanation of individuals with present-time orientation is that they tend to react to time in a linear fashion. Because they perceive time as being on a straight plane, they believe that a present moment spent on a particular task or with a particular individual cannot be regained: "We will never have this moment again," or "We must do it now because we'll pass this way only once." This idea is in contrast to the thoughts held by persons with circular-time orientation, who say,

"I'll get back with you," or "We can do it later." The implication of these latter statements is that both persons will be around and the essence of the moment can be relived. In relation to health care, present-oriented individuals are not likely to be involved in preventive care; however, they will seek out emergency care in acute care facilities (Grypma, 1993: Guruge & Donner, 1996). Grypma (1993) notes that after setting up a prenatal class for some American Indian women residing on a reservation, although these individuals had preregistered for the class and confirmed their appointment, they did not keep the appointment. The reason given by these women for not attending the class was a sudden weather shift and the low tide, which provided optimal conditions for picking abalone at islands nearby. For these women, the present-oriented need for food took precedence over plannng for the future event of having a baby (Thompson & McDonald, 1989).

A common belief shared by some African Americans and Mexican Americans is that time is flexible and events will begin when they arrive. For African-Americans this belief has been translated through the years as a perception of time wherein lateness of 30 minutes to an hour is acceptable. Mbiti (1970) traced this perception of time back to West Africa, where the concept of time was elastic and encompassed events that had already taken place, as well as those that would occur immediately.

Many American Indians and Inuits believe that only what is needed for the day should be used and nature will continue to provide for future needs (McRae, 1994). Atcheson (1987) noted that health, and therefore life, is a spiritual experience for Indians and the gifts of the Great Spirit should never be abused. Some American Indians and Inuits believe that the person who gives the most to others should be respected. This is also in keeping with the notion of being present oriented. Many American Indians and Inuits have been taught to live in the present and not be concerned with the future. Therefore they share what they have today (McRae, 1994; Hagey & Buller, 1983; Young, Ingram, & Swartz, 1990).

It is important for the nurse to remember that time perception may also be related to socioeconomic status. For example, although some African Americans and Mexican Americans can be characterized as present-oriented individuals, others have been assimilated into the dominant culture and are very time conscious and take pride in punctuality. These African-Americans and Mexican Americans are more likely to be future oriented and therefore are more likely to save and plan for important events. They are also likely to be well educated and to hold professional positions. This may not always be the case, since some individuals may not be well educated or hold professional positions yet may value time and have future hopes for themselves and their children. According to Pouissant and Atkinson (1970), these individuals are more likely to encourage their children to seek higher education and to begin saving for the future.

Time perception may also be related to religious orientation. Some Native Americans, Mexican Americans, and African Americans hold strong religious beliefs, and their concept of time is therefore very future oriented. These individuals, who may come from all socioeconomic and educational levels, have in common the belief that life on earth, with all of its pain and suffering, is bearable only because of the chance for future happiness after death. Such individuals, according to Smith (1976), may plan future activities related to their deaths; for example, they may plan their funeral, including their eulogy; purchase a grave plot; make a will; and otherwise prepare to die. Such individuals may also threaten heirs with disinheritance and talk about what the heirs will do with their hard-earned money.

Levine and Wolff (1985), with the assistance of colleagues Laurie West and Harry Reis, compared the time sense of male and female students in Niterói, Brazil, with similar students at California State University at Fresno. A total of 91 Brazilian students and 107 students from California were surveyed. The universities selected in Brazil and California were similar in academic quality and size, and the cities in which they were located were secondary metropolitan centers with populations of approximately 350,000. The researchers asked students about their perception of time in several situations, including what they considered late or early for a hypothetical lunch appointment with a friend. According to the data, the average Brazilian student defined lateness for the hypothetical lunch as 33 minutes after the scheduled lunchtime, whereas the Fresno students defined lateness for the hypothetical lunch as 19 minutes after the scheduled lunchtime. The Brazilian students allowed an average of 54 minutes before they considered someone early for an appointment, whereas the Fresno students drew the line for earliness at 24 minutes. When the Brazilian students were asked to give typical reasons for lateness, they were less likely to attribute it to a lack of caring than their North American counterparts were. Instead, the Brazilian students pointed to unforeseen circumstances that an individual could not control without prior knowledge. In addition, the Brazilian students appeared less inclined to feel personally responsible for their own lateness. The question that comes to mind for the nurse is, "Are Brazilians more flexible in their concepts of time and punctuality?" Another question for the nurse to consider is, "If Brazilians are more flexible in their concepts of time and punctuality, how does this relate to the stereotypical picture of the fatalistic and irresponsible temperament associated with Latins?" This example illustrates the need for nurses to guard against formulating stereotyped images of persons from other cultures. Instead, the nurse must have an understanding of cultural variables that differ among cultures, such as the variation in viewing time.

Levine and Wolff (1985) found similar differences in how students from North America and Brazil characterize people who are late for appointments. In the survey, the Brazilian students indicated that a person who is consistently late is probably a person who is more successful than one who is consistently on time. These students seemed to accept the premise that someone of great stature is expected to arrive late; therefore a lack of punctuality is a badge of success. In contrast, according to the North American students, persons who arrive late for scheduled appointments, rush in late to meetings, turn in assignments late, or fail to notify others when they find that they are going to be late are generally unorganized, have trouble with priorities, are inconsiderate, and thus will fail to advance professionally and will be less successful. Popular literature in the United States on creating a successful business and professional image espouses the need for continued punctuality.

PHYSIOCHEMICAL INFLUENCES IN RELATION TO TIME

Research on biological rhythms has found that internal body rhythms fluctuate within a 24-hour period. Biological capacities for some individuals are on a low ebb in the daytime, whereas for others, they are at a high level during the day (Biological Rhythms, 1970; Yogman, Lester, & Hoffman, 1983; Ziac, 1984). Research has shown that the time of day in which medication is given influences its effectiveness and its side effects; drugs may be more potent when biological capacities are at a low ebb. However, it is important for the nurse to remember that although drugs might be more potent with low biological capacities, the treatment may be less therapeutic. Health care professionals often fail to take into account the client's biological rhythms when scheduling surgical procedures and diagnostic tests. For example, surgical interventions should be avoided when a client's biological capacities are low. Persons who are at a low ebb of biological functioning may be at greater risk for an exaggerated response to anesthesia or may be less able to respond to blood loss (Bremner, Vitiello, & Prinz, 1983; Sideleau, 1992). Evidence also exists that diagnostic tests and treatments may be tolerated better by certain clients when they are timed according to biological rhythms. Hormones and other homeostatic physiological mechanisms fluctuate in the body in a rhythmic way. The timing of the collection of blood and urine samples is important and influences the interpretation of the information obtained.

Physiochemical levels also are related to age. Children have a higher metabolic rate, which tends to make time appear to move more slowly for children. On the other hand, older individuals have a slower metabolic rate, which results in time appearing to move more quickly.

Body rhythms may influence waking at a preselected time. Waking, however, is also a conditioned response. Body systems, including the nervous and endocrine systems, are the result not only of internal biological rhythms, but also of psychological phenomena, such as the time or date of previous traumatic events.

Psychological phenomena can greatly affect the client's time perception. For example, according to Sideleau (1992), persons with psychiatric problems can manifest several types of time impairments, including the following:

1. Perception as related to rate and flow of time; that is, a sense that time passes too quickly or too slowly.
2. Failure to recognize finite division of time, which is manifested by confusion related to the inability to distinguish night from day.
3. Attention or inattention to time; that is, adhering too rigidly to schedules or the complete disregard for the value of time constraints or schedules.

It is important for the nurse to carefully discern whether the client's time perception is attributable to cultural phenomena or to some biochemical or psychological manifestation. For example, drug abusers tend to have an altered sense of time. If a hallucinogenic or excitatory drug is being used, the individual may experience temporal contraction and spatial expansion. For these persons, the distortion in time is so profound that they often arrive early for appointments (Sideleau, 1992). In stark contrast, individuals who are influenced by the effects of tranquilizers experience time expansion and space contraction. These individuals are more likely to arrive late for an appointment. Although all these phenomena can be experienced by clients who have a biochemical imbalance or a psychological disorder, the nurse must carefully determine if the faulty perception is caused by the disorder or by a cultural phenomenon (Giger, Davidhizar, Evers, & Ingram, 1994; Giger, Davidhizar, Johnson, & Poole, 1997).

IMPLICATIONS FOR NURSING CARE

The nurse who gains an understanding of time as a cultural variable with a significant effect on clients and ultimately on client care must also gain an understanding of how time is managed to give quality client care. A general attitude shared by health care professionals is that time is irreplaceable and irreversible and that to waste time is to waste life. Moreover, there is no such thing as a lack of time; regardless of the way individuals spend time, it goes at the same pace (Salmond, 1986). That is, each individual has 168 hours to live per week, no more and no less. As health care needs have changed over the years, so have the demands that are placed on nurses. Nurses are constantly being challenged to work in a more time-efficient manner, causing high levels of stress. Some nurses maintain that they are losing control and lack personal satisfaction and thus are becoming burned out. However, it is important for the nurse to remember that one way to remain in control and to have personal satisfaction as opposed to burnout is to adopt an efficient system of time management. Getting organized and precisely articulating priorities is related to job satisfaction (Feldman, Monicken, & Crowley, 1983; MacStavic, 1978; McNiff, 1984). Nurses have long known the importance of working smarter rather than longer or harder (Barros, 1983).

Conflicts between nurses and physicians are sometimes complicated by differences in time perception. Nurses tend to operate on an hourly time sense with adherence to rigid schedules to complete client care assignments. Physicians tend to measure time with the client not in actual time spent with the client, which often is quite brief, but in the duration of the illness or its treatment. Physicians are less likely to schedule time strictly and often appear not to appreciate the nurse's sense of time (Sheard, 1980; Young & Hayne, 1988).

For the nurse, time management issues involve how to manage both personal time and time at work to meet professional goals. In addition, as cost-containment issues are gaining increased attention in nursing, time management concerns also necessitate precise assessment of client care needs to plan the hours of nursing time required to meet these needs and to manage the time of staff who are supervised in the delivery of care (Vestal, 1987). In the 1970s the concern with cost effectiveness of client care and the realization that census may not be an adequate determinant of the demand for care prompted the development of client classification systems. These classification systems were used initially in general hospitals to determine needs for nursing resources by grouping clients into categories that reflected the magnitude of nursing care time. By 1979 over 1000 hospitals reported using some method of classifying levels of care and the time required (Schroder, Washington, Deering, & Coyne, 1986). In 1983 the development of client classification systems received a significant impetus when the Joint Commission on Accreditation for Hospitals and American Hospital Association Standards recommended client classification systems in all hospitals. As psychiatric hospitals began to seek accreditation under the American Hospital Association Standards, increasing attention was given to client classification systems in psychiatric hospital settings.

Appropriate grouping of clients in a hospital (such as having a unit for colostomy clients) can contribute to effective use of staff time. In addition, grouping client activities into a logical sequence (such as changing the client's bed after the colostomy irrigation is finished) can save the nurse time.

Organization of supplies and tasks is important when activities are grouped together. Organizing items prevents multiple interruptions during a procedure to collect things that were forgotten. A nurse who must leave a procedure to get items that are needed but were forgotten not only wastes time but appears incompetent.

Nursing efforts to reduce hospitalization time are a serious concern today as health care costs spiral (Midgley & Osterhage, 1973). Yet another dimension of time management for nurses in the 1990s involves appropriately timed data collection to determine client needs and to collect data about the nursing process (Felton, 1970; Polit & Hungler, 1990). If assessment of client and nursing needs is inadequately timed, inaccurate solutions may be planned. The nurse who is aware of the importance of time must also consider the time constraints of data collection. Although a 24-page nursing assessment may provide optimal client data, if the time taken to collect these data would result in other client care being neglected, time constraints will by necessity influence the length of the assessment. Time constraints also influence data collection for research purposes in a health care setting. If financial restraints prohibit additional staff for research purposes, a decision must be made about the priority of the research versus the priority of other nursing staff duties (Monette, Sullivan, & Dejong, 1986).

As change agents, nurses are also concerned with time in relation to change. According to organiza-

tional change theory, if change merely involves knowledge, change can be achieved in a short time with little difficulty. If attitudes are involved, somewhat longer periods of time are needed. If the behavior of an individual is involved, a moderate amount of time is required, and moderate difficulty may be encountered. If the behavior of a group is involved, a large amount of time may be required and a high level of difficulty may be encountered (Hersey & Blanchard, 1982).

Lest the nurse stereotype all persons in the United States as valuing timeliness, it must be emphasized that time and punctuality vary considerably from place to place and region to region. Each region and even each city has its own rhythm and rules. Words such as "now" and "later" can convey vastly different meanings. "Now" and "later" may also be interpreted differently by persons from different ethnic or cultural groups. For some African Americans, "now" may not really imply 'immediately'; rather, "now" may mean 'soon,' so that it could be hours before an action is taken. For the same African American, "later" may not really imply 'within a few hours' but 'when you get around to it' (Mbiti, 1990). In contrast, for some future-oriented Americans, "now" means 'immediately,' and thus action is expected at once. For these same persons, "later" means 'within a few hours.'

For Americans who travel abroad, major differences encountered, surpassed only by language problems, are the contrasting paces of life and the punctuality differences of people from other countries. These differences can also be noted in the United States when one travels from region to region. For example, in the South, regardless of whether the area is rural or urban, the general pace of life is slow and laid back, and punctuality is not of paramount importance; thus people from this region may be stereotyped as "country." In contrast, in a large metropolitan area such as New York, the pace of life is associated with more rapid activity, such as walking fast, talking fast, and making decisions quickly. Time differences are also seen in various agencies and among various health professionals. For example, the nurse may find that a more rapid pace is required in a particular hospital setting. The pace may also vary in different clinical disciplines.

Duties may differ, and the pace may be more accelerated in high-risk areas such as the intensive care unit, coronary care unit, emergency room, operating room, and psychiatric unit. On the other hand, these areas also experience "slow time" or "down time" when the census is low.

When caring for clients who may have present-oriented time perceptions, such as some Black Americans, some Americans from Puerto Rico, some American Indians, some Mexican Americans, and some Chinese Americans, the nurse must remember that it is necessary to avoid adhering to time as a fixed resource (an example would be rigid schedules for nursing care procedures such as baths, medications, and meals). In this case the nurse may find that the standards of the institution regarding time and the time orientation of the client may be in conflict with each other. Again, it is important for the nurse to remember that such persons may perceive time as flexible and that what is happening now is more important than what is going to happen in the future. Therefore the nurse must be able to adapt

client care within a range in time rather than fixed hours. It is important for the nurse to be cognizant of the fact that time is perceived differently by some individuals from diverse ethnic, cultural, age, and socio-economic groups (Gaglione, 1988). Accepting that there are different ways of perceiving time is the first step to increasing tolerance for time related cultural behaviors. The nurse should appreciate the breadth of factors that affect perception of time. For example, Carter, Green, Green, and Dufour (1994) noted that homeless individuals are very present-time oriented. This can significantly affect follow-up care and compliance with treatment recommendations. On the other hand, certain illnesses may affect time perception. Individuals with schizophrenia tend to be present oriented and have a limited ability to focus on the future. This can significantly affect adjustment to the hospital and community living situations (Suto & Frank, 1994). Chronic illness may affect perception of time for the future. For some persons, hope is important for an orientation to the future (Alberto, 1990).

Case Study

Miss Susie Jones is a 37-year-old Black-American client who has been coming to the hospital's outpatient clinic because she is a brittle diabetic. Miss Jones's diabetes was diagnosed 6 months previously; however, the diabetes remains uncontrolled by insulin. The client was put on a regimen of 40 units of lente insulin with 5 units of regular insulin at 7 A.M. and at 4 P.M. When Miss Jones comes to the clinic today, she relates to the nurse that she had an episode of "blacking out," or an "insulin reaction," because she forgot to eat after taking her morning insulin. This morning, as frequently in the past, Miss Jones is at least 1 hour late for her scheduled appointment. The following questions relate to variable time and its significance in relation to Susie Jones.

STUDY QUESTIONS

1. List at least two things in relation to the perception of time and culture that may be contributing factors in Susie Jones's tardiness for appointments.
2. List at least two things that the nurse could suggest to Susie Jones that would assist her in being on time for future clinic appointments.
3. List at least two factors about time that contribute to Susie Jones's noncompliance with the medical regimen.

4. Identify ways that the nurse could assist Susie Jones in developing an understanding about time and its relationship to important medications such as insulin.
5. Identify a contributing factor to the insulin reaction that was described to the nurse by Susie Jones.

References

Alberto, J. (1990). *A test of a model of the relationships between time orientation, perception of threat, hope, and self-care behaviors of persons with chronic obstructive pulmonary disease.* Doctoral dissertation, Indiana University School of Nursing, Bloomington, Indiana.

Ariotti, P.E. (1995). The concept of time in Western antiquity. In Fraser, J.T., & Lawrence, N. (Eds.), *The study of time* (vol. 3) (pp. 69-80). New York: Springer-Verlag.

Atcheson, J. (1987). *Traditional health beliefs and compliance in Native American tuberculosis patients.* Unpublished master's thesis, McMaster University, Hamilton, Ontario.

Barros, A. (1983, August). Time management: learn to work smarter, not longer. *Medical Laboratory Observer,* 107-111.

Biological rhythms in psychiatry and medicine. (1970). Chevy Chase, Md.: U.S. Department of Health, Education, and Welfare, National Institute of Mental Health.

Bock, P. (1964). Social structure and language structure. *Southwestern Journal of Anthropology, 20,* 393-403.

Bremner, W.J., Vitiello, M.V., & Prinz, P.N. (1983). Loss of circadian rhythmicity in blood testosterone levels with aging in normal man. *Journal of Clinical Endocrinology and Metabolism, 56*(6), 1278-1281.

Campinha-Bacote, J. (1997). Understanding the influence of culture. In Haber, J., Krainovich-Miller, B., McMahon, A., & Hoskins, P. (Eds.), *Comprehensive psychiatric nursing* (ed. 5) (pp. 76-90). St. Louis: Mosby.

Carter, J. (1979). Frequent mistakes made with Black clients in psychotherapy. *Journal of the National Medical Association, 71*(10), 56-64.

Carter, K., Green, R., Green, L., & Dufour, L. (1994). Health needs of homeless clients accessing nursing care at a free clinic. *Journal of Community Health Nursing, 11*(3), 139-147.

Cassirer, E. (1955). *An essay on man.* New York: Bantam Books.

Davidhizar, R., Dowd, S., & Giger, J. (1997). Model for cultural diversity in the radiology department. *Radiology Technology, 68*(3), 233-240.

Doob, L. (1970). *Patterning of time.* New Haven, Conn.: Yale University Press.

Drucker, P. (1966). *The effective executive.* New York: Harper & Row.

Elton, L. (1975). *Time and man.* New York: Pergamon Press.

England, J. (1986). Cross-cultural health care. *Canada's Mental Health, 34*(4), 13-15.

Feldman, E., Monicken, L., & Crowley, M. (1983). The systems approach to prioritizing. *Nursing Administration Quarterly, 7*(2), 57-62.

Felton, J.S. (1970). Communicating in writing. I and II. Occupational Health Nursing, 18(5), 13-19; 18(6), 13-25.

Friedman, B. (1946). *Foundations of the measurement of values.* New York: Columbia University Press.

Gaglione, B. (1988). *Cognitive orientations of three healthy retired American men.* Doctoral dissertation, New Brunswick, N.J.: Rutgers—The State University of New Jersey.

Geertz, C. (1973). *The interpretation of cultures.* New York: Basic Books.

Giger, J., Davidhizar, R., Evers, S., & Ingram, C. (1994). Cultural factors influencing mental health. In Taylor, C. (Ed.), *Essentials of psychiatric nursing,* (ed. 14) (pp. 215-238). St. Louis: Mosby.

Giger, J., Davidhizar, R., Johnson, J., & Poole, V. (1997). The changing face of America. *Health Traveler, 4*(4), 11-17.

Gilles, R., & Faulkner, R. (1978). Time and television news work: task temporalization in the assembly of unscheduled events. *Sociological Quarterly, 19,* 89-102.

Gingerich, O. (1972). *The Amish of Canada.* Waterloo, Ontario: Conrad Press.

Gioscia, V. (1970). On social time. In Yaker, H., Osmond, H., & Cheek, F. (Eds.), *The future of time* (pp. 73-141). New York: Doubleday.

Grypma, S. (1993). Culture shock. *The Canadian Nurse, 89*(9), 33-37.

Guruge, S. & Donner, G. (1996). Transcultural nursing in Canada. *The Canadian Nurse, 92*(9), 34-39.

Hagey, R., & Buller, E. (1983). Drumming and dancing: a new rhythm in nursing care. *The Canadian Nurse, 79*(4), 28-31.

Hall, E., & William, F. (1960). Intercultural communication: a guide to men of action. *Human Organization, 19,* 7-9.

Hawley, A. (1986). *Human ecology.* New York: Ronald Press.

Hein, E.C. (1980). *Communication in nursing practice* (ed. 2). Boston: Little, Brown & Co.

Hersey, & Blanchard, K. (1982) *Management of organizational behaviors.* Englewood Cliffs, N.J.: Prentice Hall.

Hoppe, S. & Heller, P. (1974). Alienation, familism, and the utilization of health services by Mexican American. *Journal of Health and Social Behavior, 15,* 304.

Hymovich, D.P., & Chamberlin, R.W. (1980). *Child and family development.* New York: McGraw-Hill.

Iverson, P. (1992). *The Navajos.* New York: Chelsea House Publishers.

James, W. (1890). *Principles of psychology* (vol. 1). New York: Dover Publications.

Ketchum, J.D. (1951). Time, values, and social organization. *Canadian Journal of Psychology, 5,* 97-109.

Kluckhohn, F., & Strodtbeck, F. (1961). *Variations in value orientation.* Evanston, Ill.: Row, Peterson.

Kohn, M. (1977). *Class and conformity* (ed. 2). Chicago: Dorsey Press.

Landes, D. (1983). *Revolution in time.* Cambridge, Mass.: Belknap Press of Harvard University Press.

Lebhar, G. (1958). *The use of time* (ed. 3). New York: Chain Store.

Levine, R., & Wolff, E. (1985, March). Social time: the heartbeat of culture. *Psychology Today,* 29-35.

MacStavic, R.E. (1978). Setting priorities in health planning: what does it mean? *Inquiry, 45*(1), 20-24.

Maguire, D.C. (1984). *Death by choice* (ed. 2). New York: Schocken Books.

Mbiti, S.S. (1970). *African religions and philosophies* (ed. 2). New York: Anchor Press.

McGrath, J., & Kelly, J. (1986). *Time and human interaction* (ed. 2). New York: Guilford Press.

McNiff, M. (1984, June). Getting organized—at last. *RN, 47,* 23-24.

McRae, L. (1994). Cultural sensitivity in rehabilitation related to native clients. *Canadian Journal of Rehabilitation, 7*(4), 251-256.

Meade, R. (1960). Time on their hands. *Personnel Journal, 39,* 130-132.

Midgley, J.W., & Osterhage, R.A. (1973). Effect of nursing instruction and length of hopitalization on postoperative complications in cholecystectomy patients. *Nursing Resident, 22*(1), 69-72.

Monette, F.C., Sullivan, T., & Dejong, C. (1986). *Applied social research.* New York: Holt, Rinehart, & Winston.

Morgenstern, I. (1960). *The dimensional structure of time.* New York: Philosophical Library.

Nash, M. (1967). *Machine age Maya.* Chicago: University of Chicago Press.

Nelkin, D. (1970). Unpredictability and life style in a migrant camp. *Social Problems, 17,* 472-487.

Nojima, Y., Oda, A., Nishii, H., et al. (1987). Perception of time among Japanese inpatients. *Western Journal of Medicine, 9*(3), 288-300.

Nolt, S. (1992). *A history of the Amish.* Intercourse, Pa.: Herald Press.

Parkinson, C. (1970). *The law of delay.* London: John Murray.

Polick, F. (1973). *The image of the future* (vols. 1-2). New York: Oceana Publications.

Polit, D. & Hungler, B.P. (1990). *Nursing research: principles and methods.* Philadelphia: J.B. Lippincott.

Pouissant, A., & Atkinson, C. (1970). Black youth and motivation. *Black Scholar, 1,* 43-51.

Pyle, K. (1969). *The new generation of Meiji Japan.* Stanford, Calif.: Stanford University Press.

Randall-David, E. (1989). *Strategies for working with culturally diverse communities and clients* [Brochure]. Washington, D.C.: U.S. Department of Health and Human Services.

Ritzenhaler, R. (1953). The impact of small industry on an Indian community. *American Anthropologist, 55,* 143-148.

Ruiz, R. (1981). Cultural and historical perspectives in counseling Hispanics. In Sue, D. (Ed.), *Counseling the culturally different: theory and practice* (pp. 186-215). New York: Wiley.

Ruiz, R.A., & Padella, A.M. (1977). Counseling Latinos. *The Personnel and Guidance Journal, 55,* 401-408.

Salmond, S. (1986). Time management: the time is now. *Orthopedic Nursing, 5*(3), 25-32.

Schilder, E. (1981). On the structure of time with implications for nursing. *Nursing Papers, 13*(3), 17-26.

Schroder, P.J., Washington, W.P., Deering, C.D., & Coyne, L. (1986). Testing validity and reliability in a psychiatric patient classification system. *Nursing Management, 17*(1), 49-54.

Sheard, T. (1980). The structure of conflict in nurse-physician relations. *Supervisor Nurse, 11*(8), 14-16.

Sideleau, B. (1992). Space and time. In Haber, J., Leach-McMahon, A., Price-Hoskins, P., & Sideleau, B., (Eds.), *Comprehensive psychiatric nursing* (ed. 4). St. Louis: Mosby.

Smith, J.A. (1976). The role of the Black clergy as allied health care professionals in working with Black patients. In Luckraft, J.D. (Ed.), *Black awareness: implications for Black care* (pp. 12-15). New York: American Journal of Nursing Company.

Sorokin, P. (1964). *Sociocultural causality, space, time.* New York: Russell & Russell.

Spector, R. (1996). *Cultural diversity in health care* (ed. 4). Stamford, Conn.: Appleton & Lange.

Stauffer, R. (1995). Personal communication. Harrisburg, Virginia.

Stoetzel, J. (1953). The contribution of public opinion research techniques to social anthropology. *International Social Science Bulletin, 5,* 494-503.

Strauss, G. (1963). Group dynamics and intergroup relations. In Lewis, Jr., A.O., (Ed.), *Of men and machines* (pp. 321-327). New York: E.P. Dutton.

Suto, M., & Frank, G. (1994). Future time perspective and daily occupations of persons with chronic schizophrenia in a board and care home. *American Journal of Occupational Therapy, 48*(1), 7-18.

Thompson, E. (1967). Time, work-discipline, and industrial capitalism. *Past and Present, 38,* 58-59.

Thompson, P., & McDonald, J. (1989). Multicultural health education: responding to the challenge. *Health Promoting, 28*(2), 8-11.

Toffler, A. (1970). *Future shock.* New York: Random House.

Tripp-Reimer, T. (1984). Cultural assessment. In Bellack, J., & Bamford, P. (Eds.), *Nursing assessment: a multidimensional approach.* Monterey, Calif.: Wadsworth.

Tripp-Reimer, T., & Lively, S.H. (1993). Cultural considerations in mental health—psychiatric nursing. In Beck, C.K., Rawlins, R.P., & Williams, R.S. (Eds.), *Mental health-psychiatric nursing* (ed. 3) (pp. 166-177). St. Louis: Mosby.

Vestal, K. (1987). Management concepts for the new nurse. Philadelphia: J.B. Lippincott.

Veterans World Project. (1972). *Wasted men: the reality of the Vietnam veteran.* Edwardsville, Ill.: Southern Illinois University Foundation.

Weigert, A. (1981). *Sociology of everyday life.* New York: Longman.

Wenger, A. (1991). The culture care theory and the older order Amish. In Leininger, M. (Ed.), *Cultural care diversity and universality: a theory of nursing.* New York: National Leauge for Nursing.

Wessman, A., & Gorman, B. (1977). The emergence of human awareness and concepts of time. In Gorman, B.S., & Wessman, A.E. (Eds.), *Personal experience of time* (p. 3). New York: Plenum Press.

Weyer, E. (1961). *Primitive peoples today.* New York: Doubleday.

Wuest, J. (1992). Joining together: students and faculty learn about transcultural nursing. *Journal of Nursing Education, 31*(2), 90-92.

Yogman, M.W., Lester, B.M., & Hoffman, J. (1983). Behavioral rhythmicity and circadian rhythmicity during mother, father, stranger, infant social interaction. *Pediatric Research, 17*(11), 872-876.

Young, L., & Hayne, A. (1988). *Nursing administration: from concepts to practice.* Philadelphia: W.B. Saunders.

Young, D.E., Ingram, G., & Swartz, L. (1988). Cree healer attempts to improve the conpetitive position of native medicine. *Arctic Med Res, 47*(supp. 1), 313-316.

Young, D.E., Ingram, C., & Swartz, L. (1990). *Cry of the eagle: encounters with a Cree healer.* Toronto: University of Toronto Press.

Zerubavel, E. (1979). *Patterns of time in hospital life.* Chicago: University of Chicago Press.

Ziac, D.C. (1984). Menstrual synchrony in university women. *American Journal of Physical Anthropology, 63*(2), 237.

Environmental Control

Environmental control refers to the ability of an individual or persons from a particular cultural group to plan activities that control nature. Environmental control also refers to the individual's perception of ability to direct factors in the environment. This definition in itself implies that the concept of environment is broader than just the place where an individual resides or where treatment occurs. In the most practical sense, the term "environment" encompasses relevant systems and processes that affect individuals (Sideleau, 1992).

Systems are organized structures that may influence and be influenced by individuals. Processes may be viewed as organized, purposeful patterns of operations. Processes generally include the dynamics and interactions between families, groups, and the community at large. On the basis of these definitions, it is evident that the environment and humans have a reciprocal relationship in the sense that humans and the environment are constantly exchanging matter and energy. When this exchange has purpose and is goal directed, the interaction and exchange processes are considered functional and useful. However, when the exchange has no purpose

and lacks goal direction, a dyssynchronous relationship occurs (Haber & Giuffra, 1992).

In the broadest sense, health may be viewed as a balance between the individual and the environment. Health practices such as eating nutritiously, subscribing to preventive health services available in the community, and installing hazard- and pollution-control devices are all believed to have a positive effect on the individual, who in turn can positively affect the environment (Spector, 1996).

Complex systems of health beliefs and practices exist across and within cultural groups. In addition, variations, whether extreme or modest, to cultural beliefs and practices are found across ethnic and social class boundaries and even within family groups. Today the most widely accepted approach to health care is the biomedical model. This model emphasizes biological concerns, which are considered by those who support this model as more "real" and significant in contrast to psychological and sociological issues (Kleinman, Eisenberg, & Good, 1978).

Today in modern Western society, health care practitioners remain primarily interested in abnormalities in the structure and function of body systems and in the treatment of disease. According to Kleinman, Eisenberg, and Good (1978), the biomedical approach is culture specific, culture bound, and value laden. The biomedical model represents only one end of a continuum. At the opposite end of the continuum is the traditional model, which espouses popular beliefs and practices that diverge from medical science (Chrisman, 1977). Persons who subscribe to beliefs encompassed in the traditional model have varying health beliefs and practices, including folk beliefs and traditional beliefs that are also shaped by culture (Spector, 1996).

DISTINCTION BETWEEN ILLNESS AND DISEASE

During the last decade, scientists and anthropologists began to make a distinction between the terms "illness" and "disease." The individual experiences that relate to illnesses do not necessarily correlate with the biomedical interpretation of disease. Illness can be defined as an individual's perception of being sick. On the other hand, disease is diagnosed when the condition is a deviation from clearly established norms based on Western biomedical science (Fabrega, 1971). Illness can and does occur in the absence of disease; approximately 50% of visits made by individuals to physicians are for complaints without a definite basis. According to Kleinman, Eisenberg, and Good (1978), illness is culturally shaped in the sense that it is individually perceived. In other words, how one experiences and copes with disease is based on the individual's explanation of sickness. Disease is described in detail in medical-surgical nursing textbooks. However, nurses need to remember to incorporate both personal and cultural reactions of the client to illness, disease, and discomfort to give culturally appropriate nursing care.

Just as culture influences health-related behavior, it also has a profound effect on expectations and perceptions of sickness that shape the labeling of sickness and on how, when, and to whom communication of health problems occurs (Campinha-Bacote, 1997). The astute nurse must keep in mind the fact that perceptions of health and illness are shaped by cultural factors. As a direct result of cultural shaping, individuals vary in health care behav-

iors, health status, and health-seeking attitudes (Grypma, 1993, Thompson, 1993; McRae, 1994; Guruge & Donner, 1996).

The term "health care behavior" is defined as the social and biological activities of an individual that are based on maintaining an acceptable health status or manipulating and altering an unacceptable condition (Bauwens & Anderson, 1988). The term "health status," on the other hand, is defined as the success with which an individual adapts to the internal and external environment (Bauwens & Anderson, 1988). Thus health care behavior influences health status, which in turn influences health care behavior. Because health care behavior and health care status are reciprocal in nature, they both can be affected by sociocultural forces such as economics, politics, environmental influences, and the health care delivery system itself (Elling, 1977).

CULTURAL HEALTH PRACTICES VERSUS MEDICAL HEALTH PRACTICES

Cultural health practices are categorized as efficacious, neutral, dysfunctional (Pillsbury, 1982), or uncertain.

Efficacious cultural health practices

According to Western medical standards, efficacious cultural health practices are those practices that are viewed as beneficial to health status, though they can differ vastly from modern scientific practices. Because efficacious health practices can facilitate effective nursing care, nurses need to actively encourage the use of these practices among and across cultural groups. Nurses must keep in mind that a treatment strategy that is consistent with the client's beliefs may have a better chance of being successful. For example, persons from cultural groups who subscribe to the theory of hot and cold, such as some Mexican Americans, may actually benefit from this particular belief. Individuals who subscribe to this theory may avoid hot foods in the presence of stomach ailments such as ulcers, a practice that is consistent with the bland diet used in a medical regimen for the treatment of ulcers. Thus scientific health care practices may be blended with efficacious cultural health practices.

Neutral cultural health practices

Neutral cultural health practices have no effect on the health status of an individual. Although some health care practitioners may consider neutral health practices irrelevant, the nurse must remember that such practices may be extremely important because they may be linked to beliefs that are closely integrated with an individual's behavior (Pillsbury, 1982). Greene (1981) cited several examples of neutral practices, including "the ritual disposal of the placenta and cord," interpretation of signs in the cord, avoidance of sexual activity during various stages of pregnancy, certain hygiene practices, and avoidance of exposure to luminous rays of the moon during a lunar eclipse. Many Southeast Asian women believe that sitting in a door frame or on a step while they are pregnant will complicate labor and delivery. In waiting and examination rooms, these women will avoid areas near doors. These women may also think that overeating or inactivity during pregnancy will cause a difficult delivery. For many of these women, it is believed that sleeping late or during the day will have the same effect. Hill tribeswomen (Hmong and Mien) avoid contact with scissors and knives because they fear sharp instruments may cause cleft lip or abortion. There is a general belief among these women that reaching overhead for something or working too hard may cause miscarriage or birth defects (Lew, 1989; Mattson, 1995). Although these practices require no planned nursing interventions, the astute nurse must recognize their significance and respect the client's right to subscribe to and practice such beliefs.

Dysfunctional cultural health practices

Dysfunctional cultural health practices are harmful. An example of a dysfunctional health care practice found in the United States is the excessive use of such items as overrefined flour and sugar. The nurse must be aware of practices that are dysfunctional and should work to establish educational training programs that will help individuals identify dysfunctional health practices and develop beneficial practices. A dysfunctional health care practice was noted among women of various racial, ethnic, and cultural groups in British Columbia in Canada (Hislop,

Deschamps, Band, et al., 1992). Findings from this study noted that implementation of a population-based cervical cytology screening program in British Columbia that began in 1955 decreased the mortality from invasive squamous cervical cancer by over 70%. However, the mortality from cervical cancer, despite the implementation of this innovative program, remained high among the Canadian Native population (Inuits, Indians, the Metís). In fact, the mortality was four times higher among Canadian Native women than that of their non-Native counterparts (Threlfall, 1986). Although approximately 85% of the women in the general population complied with screening recommendations, the compliance by Native women was approximately 30% less. Whether this underparticipation by Native woman resulted from beliefs and attitudes or lack of availability of resources was not determined.

Uncertain cultural health practices

In 1972 Williams and Jelliffe developed a cultural assessment system that included a category of cultural health practices with unknown effects. Classified as uncertain, these practices included such things as swaddling a newborn infant to maintain body temperature and using an abdominal binder for mother and infant to prevent umbilical hernias.

The nurse must remember that in most instances health practices do not fit perfectly into one category or another. According to Greene (1981), health practices are subjectively evaluated as more or less beneficial or harmful when they are compared with the alternative practices available to the user.

VALUES AND THEIR RELATIONSHIP TO HEALTH CARE PRACTICES

Values may be viewed as individualized sets of rules by which people live and are governed. They serve as the cornerstone for beliefs, attitudes, and behaviors. Cultural values are often acquired unconsciously as an individual assimilates the culture throughout the process of growth and maturation. It is important for the nurse to recognize that because cultural values are believed to exist almost solely on an unconscious level, they are the most difficult to alter. Cultural values therefore have a pervasive and profound influence on the individual (Giger, Davidhizar, Johnson, & Poole, 1997).

Value orientations

Kluckhohn and Strodtbeck (1961) defined value orientations as "complex but definitely patterned principles . . . which give order and direction to the ever-flowing stream of human acts and thoughts as they relate to the solution of common human problems." Kluckhohn and Strodtbeck also proposed that it is entirely possible for an individual to hold a value orientation different from the rest of the same cultural group. However, they concluded that despite differences in value orientation within a cultural group, dominant value orientations can be identified for most persons of a particular cultural group.

Kluckhohn and Strodtbeck (1961) compared the way people in different cultural groups organize their thinking about such things as time, personal activity, interpersonal relationships, and the relationship to nature and the supernatural. They developed an orientation framework that includes temporal, activity, relational, people-to-nature, and innate human nature orientations.

Temporal orientation

Temporal orientation refers to the method by which persons from particular cultural groups divide time. Time is generally divided into three frames of reference: past, present, and future. According to Kluckhohn and Strodtbeck (1961) and Haber and Giuffra (1992), most cultures combine all three orientations, but one is more likely to dominate than another.

Activity orientation

Activity orientation refers to whether a cultural group is perceived as a "doing"-oriented culture, which is oriented toward achievement, or as a "being"-oriented culture, which values "being" and views people as an important link between generations. In other words, the "doing"-oriented culture values accomplishments, whereas the "being"-oriented culture values inherent existence.

Relational orientation

Relational orientation from a cultural perspective distinguishes interpersonal patterns. More specifi-

cally, relational orientation refers to the way in which persons in a culture set goals for individual members. Relational orientations are found in three modes: lineal, individualistic, and collateral.

Lineal mode When the lineal mode is dominant within a particular cultural group, the goals and welfare of the group are viewed as major concerns. Other major concerns are the continuity of the group and the orderly succession of the group over time. Cultures that are perceived as subscribing to the lineal mode view kinship bonds as the basis for maintaining lineage.

Individualistic mode Cultures in which the dominant mode is individualistic value individual goals over group goals. Thus each individual is responsible for personal behaviors and ultimately is held accountable for personal accomplishments.

Collateral mode When the collateral mode is dominant in a cultural group, the goals and welfare of lateral groups such as siblings or peers are of paramount importance. Examples are found in Russia and in Israel, where the goals of individuals are subordinate to those that affect the entire lateral group.

People-to-nature orientation

People-to-nature orientation implies that people either dominate nature, live in harmony with nature, or are subjugated to nature. The conceptual framework of people dominating nature is based on the view that humans dominate nature and further indicates that humankind can master or control natural events. When people live in harmony with nature, there is an integration among them, nature, and the universe. When the view that humans are subjugated to nature is held, a philosophy of fatalism is adopted; that is, fate is considered inevitable and individuals perceive themselves as having no control over nature or their future—they consider themselves powerless to guide personal destiny. An example is the belief held by some Appalachian people that, "If I'm going to get cancer, I'm going to get it," so that taking preventive measures to avoid cancer would be of no benefit. This fatalistic attitude, however, is not completely consistent because most Appalachians will go to a physician or hospital if they believe they are extremely ill.

Innate human nature orientation

The innate human nature orientation distinguishes an individual's human nature as being good, evil, or neutral. Some cultural groups view human beings as having a basic nature that is either changeable or unchangeable. For example, an individual may be viewed as evil and unchangeable, evil but changeable, or neutral (subject to both good and negative influences).

LOCUS-OF-CONTROL CONSTRUCT AS A HEALTH CARE VALUE

The locus-of-control construct, which originated in social learning theory, is defined as follows:

When a reinforcement is perceived as following some action but not being entirely contingent upon (personal) action then in our culture it is typically perceived as a result of luck, chance, and fate, as under the control of powerful others, or unpredictable because of the great complexity of the forces surrounding [the individual]. When the event is interpreted in this way by an individual, we have labeled this belief in external control. If a person perceives that the event is contingent upon his own behavior or his own permanent characteristics, we have termed this a belief in internal control (Rotter, 1966).

The above definition presupposes that individuals who believe that a contingent relationship exists between actions and outcomes have internal feelings of control and thus act to influence future behaviors and situations. Individuals who believe that efforts and rewards are uncorrelated, and who thus have external feelings of control, view the future as the result of luck, chance, or fate and are less likely to take action to change the future. The locus-of-control construct can be applied to a variety of phenomena, including the weather, preventive health, curative health actions, and feelings of well-being. For example, individuals who believe that a contingent relationship exists between compliance to preventive and treatment regimens and health have an internal locus-of-control and are likely to respond positively to affect the future and thus promote good health. On the other hand, individuals who believe that compliance behaviors and health are unrelated have an external locus-of-control and have little motivation to develop behaviors that could affect the future and enhance good health. Rotter (1975) concluded

that the locus-of-control does not in itself represent a behavior trait and can be modified by interaction with others.

The astute nurse should recognize that persons who subscribe to an external locus-of-control tend to be more fatalistic about nature, health, illness, death, and disease. For example, some Hispanics, Appalachians, and Puerto Ricans are reported to have an external locus-of-control. Some American Indians, Chinese Americans, and Japanese Americans or Japanese Canadians are said to be more or less in harmony with nature; therefore their cultural beliefs fall outside the locus-of-control construct. However, northern European Americans and African Americans are reported to fall within both the internal and the external locus-of-control construct (Kluckhohn & Strodtbeck, 1961). The nurse can help the client modify behaviors that fall within the realm of the external locus-of-control construct by showing the effects of certain behaviors on illnesses, health, and disease and thus promote the development of an internal locus-of-control.

FOLK MEDICINE

Folk medicine, or what is commonly referred to as "Third World beliefs and practices," is often called "strange or weird" by nurses and other health professionals who are unfamiliar with folk medicine beliefs (Snow, 1981; Giger, Davidhizar & Turner, 1992). In reality, whether or not something is considered "strange or weird" depends on familiarity with the beliefs. In most instances folk medicine practices will not be considered "strange or weird" once health care providers become familiar with them.

The astute nurse must distinguish between practices that are familiar and practices that are desirable, since becoming familiar with something does not imply acceptance. In this situation, tolerance becomes a two-way process: people who subscribe to folk medicine practices need not feel compelled to abandon these beliefs and practices when they become familiar with modern medicine, and health care practitioners should not feel compelled to abandon modern medical practices when they become familiar with folk medicine practices.

An individual's world view largely determines beliefs about disease and the appropriate treatment interventions. For example, a belief in magic may lead to the assumption that a disease is a result of human behavior and that a cure can be achieved by magical techniques. A religious belief may lead to the assumption that the disease is a result of supernatural forces and that a cure can be achieved by appealing to supernatural forces. The scientific view may lead to the assumption that the disease is a result of the cause-and-effect relationship of natural phenomena and that a cure is achieved by scientific medicine (Henderson & Primeaux, 1981).

Folk medicine beliefs as a system

The folk medicine system classifies illnesses or diseases as natural or unnatural. This division of illnesses or diseases into natural and unnatural phenomena is common among Haitians, persons from Trinidad, Mexicans and Mexican Canadians, African Canadians, and some Southern White Americans (Snow, 1981).

Distinction between natural and unnatural events

The simplest way to distinguish between natural and unnatural illnesses is to state that, according to this belief system, natural events have to do with the world as God made it and as God intended it to be. Thus natural laws allow a measure of predictability for daily life. Unnatural events, on the other hand, imply the exact opposite because they upset the harmony of nature. Unnatural events can therefore be viewed as events that interrupt the plan intended by God and at their very worst represent the forces of evil and the machinations of the devil. Unnatural events are frightening because they have no predictability. They are outside the world of nature, and so when they do occur, they are beyond the control of ordinary mortals.

Germane to the tendency to view phenomena in terms of opposition, such as good versus evil and natural versus unnatural, is the belief held by some folk medicine systems that everything has an exact opposite. For example, some African Canadians who subscribe to a folk medicine system believe that for every birth there must be a death, for every marriage there must be a divorce, and for every person with good health there must be someone with bad health. This belief is so encompassing that such individuals believe that every illness has a cure, every poison has an antidote, every herb has a healing purpose, and so forth (Snow, 1981). This belief contributes to the lack of acceptance by persons in some cultural groups to the chronicity of such diseases as AIDS, herpes, or syphilis.

Today, herbal medicine is enjoying a "rebirth" (French, 1996). Eisenberg, Kessler, Foster, et al. (1993) noted that 34% of all United States citizens use herbal products in some way. In 1990 United States citizens spent $13.7 billion dollars on "unconventional" therapy, with 75% of this cost being "out-of-pocket." Canadians are also participating in this resurgence with an increased use of herbal medicines (Abarts, 1995).

Distinction between natural and unnatural illnesses

Illnesses are generally classified as natural or unnatural, which affects the type of cure or practitioner sought. All illnesses can be viewed as representing disharmony and conflict in some particular area of life and thus tend to fall into two general categories: natural illnesses as environmental hazards and unnatural illnesses as divine punishment.

Natural illness as environmental hazards Natural illnesses in the folk medicine belief system are those that occur because of dangerous agents, such as cold air or impurities in the air, food, and water. Natural illnesses are based on the fact that everything in nature is connected and that events can be both interpreted and directed by an understanding of these relationships. Sympathetic magic, the basis for popular folk medicine beliefs and practices, can be divided into two categories: contagious and imitative magic. At the root of contagious magic is the premise that the parts do represent the whole. Many witchcraft practices are based on contagious magic, including such practices as an evildoer obtaining a lock of the victim's hair or shavings from other victim's skin to do harm. Imitative magic, on the other hand, is based on the premise that like will follow like. For example, a knife under the bed will cut labor pains. To assist the client in preventing natural illnesses, the nurse must comprehend the direct connections between the body and natural phenomena such as the phases of the moon, the position of the planets, and the changing of the seasons. Because in this belief system good health is contingent on these phenomena, it is imperative that one be able to read these signs if the body is to remain in harmony with nature.

Unnatural illnesses as divine punishment Unnatural illnesses are beleved to occur because a person may become so grave a sinner that the Lord withdraws His favor. In fact, illnesses may be attributed to punishment for failure to abide by the proper behavior rules given to man by God (Gregory, 1988). The cause of unnatural illnesses, for those who subscribe to these beliefs, is based on the continual battle between the forces of good and evil as personified in God and the devil. Evil influences may be blamed for any unnatural illness, which may range from nightmares to tuberculosis or cancer (Boston, 1993). An example of a person subscribing to this belief would be a diabetic African-Canadian woman who consistently refuses to inject herself with insulin because she believes her illness is the direct result of punishment by the devil for her sinful youth. However, unnatural illnesses are also believed to occur as a result of witchcraft. Witchcraft is based on the belief that there are individuals who have the ability to mobilize unusual powers for good and evil.

Comparison of the folk medicine system and other medical systems

To develop an understanding of folk medicine as a system, the system itself must be examined along with the ecological model, the Western medical system, alternative therapies, and religious systems. Every medical system is based on the philosophy of survival of the human organism. According to the classic work of Thomas Weaver (1970), both folk practices and Western medical practices are social systems with interdependent parts or variables that include beliefs, attitudes, practices, and roles associated with the concepts of health and disease and with the patterns of diagnoses and treatment.

All medical systems have an adaptive nature. As such, the term "medical system" can be defined as the pattern of cultural tradition and social institutions that evolves from deliberate behavior to improve health status regardless of the outcome of a particular behavior (Dunn, 1975).

To achieve good health, an individual must develop an idea of what constitutes disease, with its counterpart conditions of pain and suffering. Once a philosophy of health is adopted by an individual, various health roles are delineated. These health roles require specific health care practitioners who are duly initiated into the rights of practice. Practitioner status may be granted by medical societies or, in the case of folk medicine practices, by supernatural forces. The body is an integral part of each individual; therefore, all medical systems use body parts or excreta for diagnostic purposes. In addition, folk medicine practices, in most cases, prescribe medicine to rub into the skin, to irrigate the body, or to anoint the sick.

Ecological model The ecological model is closely related to the folk medicine system. Kay (1979) defined ecology as having three foci: (1) biological, or the branch of biology that deals with the relationship between organisms and the environment; (2) social, or the relationship between people and institutions and the interdependence between the two; and (3) cultural, or the relationship between culture and the environment, which also includes culture and societies in the environment. Ecological dimensions of health care can assist the nurse in providing plausible explanations as to why certain individuals contract specific diseases and why other individuals do not. Over the past decade, health care practitioners have become increasingly concerned with the ecological dimensions of race and ethnic minority group health problems such as AIDS, sickle cell anemia, and other such diseases.

Western medical system In contrast to the folk medicine system, which attempts to explain illness in terms of balances between an individual and the physical, social, and spiritual worlds, is the Western medical system of diagnoses and scientific explanations for illness. Western medical practices focus on preventive and curative medicine, whereas folk medicine practices focus on personal rather than scientific behavior. In the folk medicine system, it may make all the sense in the world to burn incense and to avoid certain individuals, cold air, and the "evil eye." According to Kay (1979), one person's religion is another person's magic, witchcraft, or superstition. However, it is very difficult for health care professionals to see these entities as directly relevant to medical practice or to recognize that for some cultural groups religion is the equivalent of a science.

Although many differences in focus can be seen when a comparison between Western and folk medicine health practice is made, some of these differences may not be that significant. For example, Western medical relationships are generally dyads, such as physician-client, physician-nurse, and nurse-client relationships, whereas folk medicine networks are generally multiperson health care networks that may consist of parents, other relatives, and nonrelatives as health care givers. However, today multiperson health care networks are no longer dismissed by Western health care practitioners as being irrelevant and thus dysfunctional. In fact, multiperson networks are slowly being incorporated into the Western medical system of health care.

Ethnic diets are an important aspect of human ecology because health care providers are beginning to incorporate into practice the use of ethnic diets and to understand their significance. A person, regardless of ethnic group, must consume enough food to meet nutritional requirements for energy, fat, protein, vitamins, and minerals to keep the body functioning. Rittenbaugh (1978) noted that very little is known regarding the range of human variability both among and within human populations, particularly regarding common parameters such as nutritional requirements, physiological response to malnutrition, and digestive capabilities. It is perhaps this lack of knowledge that has in the past resulted in Western-oriented health care providers prescribing diets unacceptable to persons from diverse and multicultural backgrounds. In fact, some individuals from diverse cultural backgrounds may have physical incompatibility with certain Western foods. Therefore factors regarding ethnic diets and other such folk practices must be considered by the nurse when developing care plans for culturally specific nursing care.

Alternative therapies In 1990, 34% of Americans, approximately 61 million people, used one or more nonmedical forms of therapy to treat illness. Most of these individuals used these alternative therapies without informing their health practitioner (Eisenberg, Kessler, Foster, et al., 1993). In contrast, Dr. William LaValley, founder of the Nova Scotia Medical Society's Complementary Medicine Section, estimates that 25% of the Canadian population seeks health care from alternative practitioners (University of Calgary—Complementary Medicine Seminar, 1995). Other presenters at the University of Calgary—Complementary Medicine Seminar (1995) reported that 18% of patients seen at the Calgary HIV/AIDS clinic and 27% of those seen at the University of Calgary gastroenterology clinic had tried alternative therapies. Some 44% of physicians from Alberta indicated that they made referrals to practitioners of alternative therapies, though only 10% considered themselves informed on the subject (Petersen, 1996). Although Western medicine tends to focus on illness care, alternative therapy addresses the whole patient (Peterson, 1996). In alternative therapy, symptoms are seen as the tip of the iceberg and the body's means for communicating to the mind that something needs to be changed, removed, or added to one's life (Petersen, 1996). In alternative therapy, the mind and the body are seen as a whole. Acupuncture, holistic healing, therapeutic touch, aromatic therapy, and meditation, guided imagery, and a variety of other techniques prevail as feasible alternative therapies (Barnum, 1994). Practitioners of alternative therapies include homeopaths, naturopaths, massage therapists, and reflexologists (Cronsberry, 1996). According to Dossey (1993), scientists working in the new field of psychoneuroimmunology have demonstrated the existence of intimate links between parts of the brain concerned with thought and emotion and the neurological and immune system. Based on these discoveries, Dossey (1993) concluded that there is no doubt that thought can become biology. Although the scientific value of alternative, or complementary therapies, is yet to be proved, there is a psychological component that allows the client to have a sense of control. For this reason, nurses should be well informed about nontraditional methods (Cronsberry, 1996).

Religious systems Some religious groups have elaborate rules concerning health care behaviors, including such things as the giving and receiving of health care. Religious experiences are based on cultural beliefs and may include such things as blessings from spiritual leaders, apparitions of dead relatives, and even miracle cures. Healing power based on religion may also be found in animate as well as inanimate objects. Religion can and does dictate social, moral, and dietary practices that are designed to assist an individual in maintaining a healthy balance and in addition plays a vital role in illness prevention. Examples of religious health care practices include illness prevention through such acts as the burning of candles, rituals of redemption, and prayer. Religious practices such as the "blessing of the throats" on St. Blaise Day are performed to prevent illnesses such as sore throats and choking. Baptism may be seen as a ritual of cleansing and dedication as well as a prevention against evil. In addition to being related to dedication to God's will and a preparation for death, anointing the sick is related by some religious and cultural groups to recovery and may be performed in the hope of a miracle. Circumcision is also a religious practice in that it may be viewed as having redemptive values that may prevent illness and harm (Morgenstern, 1966; Spector, 1996).

It is important for the nurse to learn to distinguish between a shaman and a priest. A shaman derives power from the supernatural, whereas a priest learns a codified body of rituals from other priests and from biblical laws. In traditional folk medicine systems, some of the most significant religious rituals are those that meditate between events in the "here and now" and events in the hereafter or "out there" in the "nether" world (Morley & Wallis, 1978).

Another example of a religious system is the Amish. For the Amish, religion and custom are inseparable and blend into a way of life (Randall-David, 1989). Religious considerations determine hours of work, occupation, means, destination of travel, and choice of friends and mates. The Amish value the importance of working with the elements of nature rather than mastery over these elements.

Closeness to soil, animals, plants, and weather is valued. Salvation is viewed as obedience to the community (Wenger, 1991). The Amish have the belief that the human body was created by God and should not be tampered with. Some Amish believe that although medication may help, it is God who heals (Randall-David, 1989).

Many Amish have been increasingly influenced by special health food interests, vitamins, and food supplement industries (Wenger, 1988). Folk medical practices and opposition to health care seems to be dominant in some family systems (Hostetler, 1980). Egeland (1967) hypothesized that there is a relationship between the concept of family culture and health behavior. Clusters of family cultures serve as basic socializers of health (Egeland, 1967). *Friendshaft*, a concept that crosses distinct church lines, produces distinct patterns of behavior and personality in the Amish community related to choice of type of physician. It also influences choice of curative diet therapy, folk remedies, and family coding of preference of treatment in reference to presumed cause of symptoms (Brewer & Bonalumi, 1995; Wenger, 1995).

IMPLICATIONS FOR NURSING CARE

The nurse must keep in mind that regardless of whether a client believes in internal or external locus-of-control or whether the client uses a folk medicine system, religious system, or ecological system, there is still safety in harmony and balance, and there may be danger in anything that is done to the extreme. In other words, it is bad for the body to eat too much, drink too much, stay out too late, and so on. In a classic 1972 study in Harlem, it was reported that 90% of African-American adolescents surveyed believed that good health was largely a matter of looking after oneself. These adolescents concluded that the results of excess may not be immediately visible but sooner or later will affect the individual because the body has become weakened (Brunswick & Josephson, 1972).

There seemingly is a gender and age differential that is associated with strengths and weaknesses among individuals. Generally speaking, strength is correlated with a person's ability to withstand illness, whereas weakness is correlated with a person's heightened susceptibility. For example, strength has been related to the male of our species. In Canada, females are generally regarded as weaker than their male counterparts, and this gender weakness is generally perceived as women being more prone to illness primarily because of functional blood loss and anatomical differences. Certain age groups have also been related to individual strength and weakness. Infants and unborn fetuses are considered the weakest of all and are perceived to be at the mercy of the mother's behavior, including prenatal behavior. During pregnancy, harmony and moderation are the keys to a healthy baby; thus the pregnancy period carries the greatest taboos among most cultural groups. For example, some Mexican Americans, Amish, Hutterites, and both White and African Americans subscribe to the doctrine of maternal moderation in pregnancy (Bauer, 1969). It is even believed that the mother's emotional state during pregnancy may affect the baby, particularly in the case of pity, fear, mockery, or hate. For example, some southern African Americans believe that feelings of hate for a particular individual may cause the baby to resemble that person or that a child could be subjected to seizures if the mother saw someone having a seizure and felt pity. Some African Americans, persons from the southern United States, and Mexican Americans also believe that when a pregnant woman makes fun of someone with a physical affliction, the baby may be born with the same affliction, thus punishing the mother for lack of charity (Snow, 1981).

Because some cultural groups believe in a direct connection between the body and the forces of nature, it is important for the nurse to recognize the relevance of natural phenomena such as phases of the moon, positions of the planets, and seasons of the year.

In the rural South in the United States, there is a dependence on natural signs to regulate behavior. Some of these people rely on the *Old Farmer's Almanac* to guide such events as planting crops, setting hens' eggs, destroying weeds, weaning babies, and fishing. The *Almanac* is consulted for many health needs, such as the best time to extract teeth or to have teeth filled (according to the *Almanac,* the best

time to have teeth extracted is during the moon's increase, and the best time to have teeth filled is during the moon's decrease). The *Almanac* may also be used to determine the optimal time to undergo surgical procedures. The nurse must remember that the *Almanac* is not only used by rural Southern people, but also in Northern urban areas many African-American pharmacists give *Almanacs* as gifts to their customers for the New Year. Interestingly, the first *Old Farmer's Almanac* is reported to have been written by a physician in 1897.

It is also important for the nurse to remember that many people from diverse cultural groups use the zodiacal signs to manipulate health regimens but do not mention this to health professionals for fear of being ridiculed. Use of zodiacal signs illustrates how external forces are brought to bear on the individual; these signs are the basis for a lively practice of self-medication, dietary regulation, and behavior modifications. The nurse should remember that some of these practices are harmful, some are neutral, and some are beneficial. For example, it would be extremely detrimental for a client in need of a lifesaving surgical procedure to wait for a full moon to have the procedure done. It is important for the nurse to devise training programs that will teach clients to manipulate behaviors and interpret zodiacal signs in a way that will maintain health and prevent illness and disease.

The nurse should also appreciate that dreams may have a role in health. Many Haitians believe that dreams are important events that allow the individual to communicate with inhabitants of the supernatural world. When dead relatives appear in a dream, they bring messages from the other world, upon which the Haitian individual is likely to rely on (Randall-David, 1989; Holcomb, Parson, Giger & Davidhizar, 1996).

In a study of the folk medicine system, it may become obvious that this system reflects a view of the world as a dangerous place, where the individual must be constantly on guard against nature, other persons, and possible punishment from God. This world view teaches the individual that it is best to look out for oneself and that mistrust is wiser than trust. For example, Hispanics or Latinos may believe that illness has its roots in physical imbalances or supernatural forces that include God's will, magical powers, evil spirits, powerful human forces, or emotional upsets. For some Hispanics or Latinos, treatment comes primarily through a variety of healers which include the *curandero* (uses prayer, artifacts); *yerbero* (herbalist); *espiritista* (practitioner of *espiritismo,* a religious cult concerned with communication with spirits and the purification of the soul through moral behavior); *santero* (practitioner of *Santería* a religious cult concerned with teaching people how to control or placate the supernatural) (Randall-David, 1989; Richardson, 1982; Wanderer and Rivera, 1986; Ruiz, 1985; Weclew, 1975). It may be necessary to involve spiritual healers and priests in crisis intervention therapy to treat the client.

The presence of an alternative medical (folk medicine) system that is different from and possibly in direct conflict with the Western medical system can serve to complicate matters. It not only becomes a matter of offering health care in the place of no health care, or offering superior health care in lieu of inferior health care, but the nurse must remember that persons from diverse cultural backgrounds have deeply ingrained beliefs about how to attain and maintain health. These beliefs, which may be linked to the natural and supernatural worlds, may adversely affect the physician-client and nurse-client relationships and thus influence the individual's decision to follow or not follow prescribed treatment regimens. For exmple, in certain cultures, the occurrence of cancer may be attributed to insufficient use of herbal medicine, an insult to an ancestor, or the result of a perceived punishment. Thus, standard Western medical approaches may not always appear relevant to certain clients in multicultural populations (Boston, 1993).

The nurse might correctly assume that when a low-income African American, southern White American, Pureto Rican, or Mexican American arrives for professional care, every home remedy known to the client has already been tried. It is important for the nurse to determine what the client has been doing to combat the illness. If the home remedy is harmless, it is best left in the treatment plan with the nurse's own suggestions added. However, harmful practices must be eliminated. One of the best ways for the nurse to eliminate harmful practices is to inquire whether the practice has worked. If the client assumes that it has not worked, the nurse can simply suggest that something else be tried. If the client perceives that a harmful practice is beneficial, the nurse must provide education that will illuminate the dangers of this harmful practice.

Nurses have recently begun to explore the relationship of person and environment in nursing research. An exploratory study by Pyles (1989) related Etzioni's compliance theory to satisfaction by nursing employees in a school of nursing. Data from the study indicated that a normative power structure in the school and the resultant moral-involvement profile in the faculty were compatible for an organization such as a university, which displays cultural goals. In a more clinical study, Gould (1989) studied 112 elderly residents in three metropolitan nursing homes. The data indicated that life satisfaction is an indicator of well-being, which is useful as a measure of quality of care because of its linkage to health. The data additionally indicated that bonding develops between institutionalized elderly persons and their caregivers, which precludes the drive for self-determination. Thus the data provided an explanation of why lower-income elderly persons demonstrated high levels of life satisfaction despite low levels of perceived influence over the institutional environment.

Case Study

Martha Brown is a 27-year-old woman who lives in northern Kentucky in a small cabin in the hills that has no indoor plumbing. She lives with her husband and six small children. The public health nurse makes a home visit after three of the children have been diagnosed by the school nurse as having lice. While the nurse is explaining the use of Rid (lice treatment) to the mother, she notes that

---

Case Study—cont'd

Mrs. Brown has a persistent cough that she states she has had for 2 years. The nurse notes that the cough is productive, that Mrs. Brown looks emaciated, and that her color is extremely ashen. She tires easily. Although health insurance is a benefit of her husband's job in a nearby mine, Mrs. Brown's children were born at home, and she has never had a complete physical. When asked why she has not gone to a nearby free health clinic, Mrs. Brown replies, "Sickness is God's will, and He will cure me if He wants to. Anyway, my family comes first, and I don't have the time. Besides, doctors can't be trusted. My Aunt Jane went to one once, and she died the next week."

STUDY QUESTIONS

1. Based on the fact that Mrs. Brown is Appalachian and taking into consideration the fact that every individual is unique, decide whether Mrs. Brown is more likely to be "being" oriented or "doing" oriented in regard to activity orientation.
2. Decide what the relational orientation is for Mrs. Brown based on her reply to the public health nurse about why she has not sought treatment.
3. Based on Mrs. Brown's reply to the public health nurse and on the fact that she is Hispanic, what people-to-nature orientation is she likely to have?
4. Decide, on the basis of Mrs. Brown's comment and the fact that she is Hispanic, what view of human nature she is likely to hold.
5. List at least three reasons why Mrs. Brown might be apprehensive about seeking medical help.

References

Abarts (1995, February). University of Calgary hosts complementary medicine society. *Holistic and Complementary Medical Society of Alberta Newsletter, 1*(1), 1.

Barnum, B.S. (1994). *Nursing theory* (ed. 4). Philadelphia: J.B. Lippincott Co.

Baskett, T.F. (1977). Grand multiparity—a continuing threat: a 6-year review. *Canadian Medical Association Journal, 116*(9), 1001-1004.

Bauer, W.W. (1969). *Potions, remedies, and old wive's tales.* New York: Doubleday.

Bauwens, E., & Anderson, S. (1988). Social and cultural influences on health care. In Stanhope, M., & Lancaster, J. (Eds.), *Community health nursing: process and practice for promoting health* (ed. 2) (pp. 89-108). St. Louis: Mosby.

Boston, P. (1993). Culture and cancer: the relevance of cultural orientation within cancer education programmes. *European Journal of Cancer Care, 2,* 72-76.

Brewer, J.A., & Bonalumi, N.M. (1995, December). Cultural diversity in the emergency department. *The Journal of Emergency Nursing, 2*(6), 494-497.

Brunswick, A.F., & Josephson, E. (1972, October). Adolescent health in Harlem. *American Journal of Public Health, 72*(suppl), 7-47.

Campinha-Bacote, J. (1997). Understanding the influence of culture. In Haber, J., Krainovich-Miller, B., McMahon, A., & Price-Hoskins, P. (Eds.), *Comprehensive psychiatric nursing* (ed. 5). St. Louis: Mosby.

Chrisman, N.J. (1977). The health seeking process. *Culture and Medicine in Psychiatry, 1,* 351-377.

Cronsberry, T. (1996, April). Alternative cancer therapies. *The Canadian Nurse, 92*(4), 35-38.

Davidhizar, R.E., & Giger, J. (1998). *Canadian Transcultural Nursing.* St. Louis: Mosby.

Dossey, L. (1993). *Healing words.* San Francisco: Harper.

Dunn, F.L. (1975). Transcultural Asian medicine and cosmopolitan medicine as adaptive systems. In Leslie, E. (Ed.), *Asian medical systems: a comparative study* (p. 135). Berkeley: University of California Press.

Egeland, J. (1967). Belief and behavior as related to illness: a community case study of the old order Amish (Doctoral dissertation, Yale University). *Dissertation Abstracts International, X,* Ann Arbor, Mich.: University Microfilms International.

Eisenberg, D., Kessler, R., Foster, C., et al.: (1993). Unconventional medicine in the United States: prevalence, costs, and patterns of use. *New England Journal of Medicine, 328*(4), 246-252.

Elling, R.H. (1977). *Socio-cultural influences on health care.* New York: Springer Publishing.

Fabrega, H. (1971). Medical anthropology. In Siegel, B.J. (Ed.), *Biennial review of anthropology.* Stanford, Calif.: Stanford University Press.

French, M. (1996, July). The power of plants. *Advances for Nurse Practitioners,* 16-18.

Giger, J., Davidhizar, R., & Turner, G. (1992). Black American folk medicine. *The ABNF Journal,* 42-46.

Giger, J., Davidhizar, R., Johnson, J., & Poole, V. (1997). The changing face of America. *Health Traveler, 4*(4), 11-17.

Godel, J., Pabst, H., Hodges, P., & Johnson, K. (1992, Sept.-Oct.). Iron status and pregnancy in a northern Canadian population: relationship to diet and iron supplementation. *Canadian Journal of Public Health, 83*(5), 339-343.

Gould, M. (1989, November 14). *The relationship of perceived social-environmental factors and functional health status to life satisfaction in the elderly.* Paper presented at the Sigma Theta Tau International Conference, Indianapolis, Ind.

Greene, L. (1981). *Social and biological predictors of nutritional status, growth, and development.* New York: Academic Press.

Gregory, D. (1988). Nursing practice in native communities. In Baumgart, A., & Larson, J. (Eds.), *Canadian nursing faces the future.* Toronto: Mosby.

Grypma, S. (1993, September). Culture shock. *The Canadian Nurse, 89*(8), 33-37.

Guruge, S., & Donner, G. (1996, September). Transcultural nursing in Canada. *The Canadian Nurse, 92*(8), 36-40.

Haber, J., & Giuffra, M. (1992). Sociocultural issues. In Haber, J., Hoskins, P., Leach, A., & Sideleau, B. (Eds.), *Comprehensive psychiatric nursing* (ed. 4) (pp. 244-246). St. Louis: Mosby.

Henderson, G., & Primeaux, M. (1981). *Transcultural health care.* Reading, Mass.: Addison-Wesley.

Hislop, T.G., Deschamps, M., Band, P.R., et al. (1992). Participation in the British Columbia Cervical Cytology Screening Programme by Native Indian women. *Canadian Journal of Public Health, 83*(5), 344-345.

Holcomb, L.O., Parsons, L.C., Giger, J.N., & Davidhizar, R. (1996). Haitian American: implications for nursing care. *Journal of Community Health Nursing, 13*(4), 249-260.

Hostetler, J. (1980). *Amish society* (ed. 3). Baltimore: The Johns Hopkins University Press.

Kay, M. (1979). Clinical anthropology. In Bauwens, E.E. (Ed.), *The anthropology of health* (pp. 3-11). St. Louis: Mosby.

Kleinman, A., Eisenberg, L., & Good, B. (1978). Culture, illness and care. *Annals of Internal Medicine, 88,* 251-258.

Kluckhohn, K., & Strodtbeck, F. (1961). *Variations in value orientations.* New York: Row, Peterson.

Lew, L. (1989). *Southeast Asian Health Project: application for mother, children and infants demonstration grant.* Unpublished manuscript (grant proposal). Ottawa.

Mattson, S. (1995, May). Culturally sensitive perinatal care for southeast Asians. *Journal of Obstetric and Gynecological Neonatal Nursing, 24*(4), 335-341.

McRae, L. (1994). Cultural sensitivity in rehabilitation related to native clients. *Canadian Journal of Rehabilitation, 7*(4), 251-256.

Morgenstern, J. (1966). *Rites of birth, marriage, death, and kindred occasions among the Semites.* Chicago: Quadrangle. (1973, New York: Ktav Publishing House.)

Morley, P., & Wallis, R. (1978). *Culture and caring.* London: Peter Owen.

Peterson, B. (1996, January). The mind-body connection. *The Canadian Nurse, 92*(1), 29-31.

Pillsbury, B. (1982). Doing the month: confinement and convalescence of Chinese women after childbirth. In Kay, M. (Ed.), *Anthropology of human birth.* Philadelphia: F.A. Davis.

Pyles, C. (1989, November 13). *Power compatibility profile in a school of nursing.* Paper presented at the Sigma Theta Tau International Conference, Indianapolis, Ind.

Randall-David, E. (1989). *Strategies for working with culturally diverse communities and clients* [Brochure]. Washington, D.C.: U.S. Department of Health and Human Services.

Richardson, L. (1982). Caring through understanding: Part 2. Folk medicine in the Hispanic population. *Imprint, 29*(2), 21.

Rittenbaugh, C. (1978). Human foodways: a window on evolution. In Bauwens, E.E. (Ed.), *The anthropology of health.* St. Louis: Mosby.

Rotter, J.B. (1966). Generalized expectancies for internal versus external control of reinforcement. *Psychological Monographs, 80*(1), 1-28.

Rotter, J.B. (1975). Some problems and misconceptions related to the construct of internal versus external control of reinforcement. *Journal of Consulting and Clinical Psychology, 43,* 56-67.

Ruiz, P. (1985). Cultural barriers to effective medical care among Hispanic-American patients. *Annual Review of Medicine, 36*(63).

Scott, K. (1991, November). Northern nurses and burn out. *The Canadian Nurse, 87*(10), 18-21.

Sideleau, B. (1992) Space and time. In Haber, J., McMahon, A., Price-Hoskins, P., & Sideleau, B. (Eds.), *Comprehensive psychiatric nursing* (ed. 4). St. Louis: Mosby.

Snow, L.F. (1981). Folk medical beliefs and their implications for the care of patients: a review based on studies among black Americans. In Henderson, G., & Primeaux, M. (Eds.), *Transcultural health care.* Reading, Mass.: Addison-Wesley.

Spector, R. (1996). *Cultural diversity in health care* (ed. 4). Stamford, Conn.: Appleton & Lange.

Thompson, K. (1993, September). Self-governed health. *The Canadian Nurse, 89*(8), 29-32.

Threlfall, W.J. (1986). Cancer patterns in British Columbia Native Indians. *Medical Journal, 28,* 508-510.

University of Calgary—Complimentary Medicine Seminar. (1995). University of Calgary, Alberta.

Wanderer, J., & Rivera, G. (1986). Black magic beliefs and white magic practice: the common structures of intimacy, tradition and power. *Social Science Journal, 23*(4), 419.

Weaver, T. (1970). Use of hypothetical situations in a study of Spanish-American illness referral systems. *Human Organisms, 29,* 141.

Weclew, R.V. (1975). The nature, prevalence, and level of awareness of *curanderismo* and some of its implications for community mental health. *Community Mental Health Journal, 11*(2), 145-154.

Wenger, A. (1988). *The phenomenon of care in a high context culture: the old order Amish.* (Doctoral dissertation. Detroit, Mich.: Wayne State University.

Wenger, A. (1991). The culture care theory and the older order Amish. In Leininger, M. (Ed.), *Cultural care diversity and universality: a theory of nursing.* New York: National League for Nursing.

Wenger, A. (1995). Cultural context, health, and health care decision making. *The Journal of Transcultural Nursing, 7*(1), 3-14.

Williams, C., & Jelliffe, D. (1972). *Mother and child health: delivering the services.* London: Oxford University Press.

CHAPTER 7   Biological Variations

BEHAVIORAL OBJECTIVES

After reading this chapter, the nurse will be able to:

1. Articulate biological differences among individuals in various racial groups.
2. Relate the importance of knowledge of biological differences that may exist among individuals in various racial groups to the provision of health care by the nurse.
3. Describe nursing implications that may arise when providing care for individuals in different cultural and racial groups.
4. Describe nutritional preferences and deficiencies that may exist among persons in different cultural groups.
5. Explain how psychological characteristics may vary from one culture to another.
6. Explain how susceptibility to disease may differ among individuals in different racial groups.

It is a well-known fact that people differ culturally. Cultural differences are evident in communication, spatial relationships and needs, social organizations (family, kinships, and tribes), time orientation, and ability or desire to control the environment. Less recognized and understood are the biological differences that exist among people in various racial groups. It is becoming more evident to nurses that a body of scientific knowledge does exist about biological cultural differences. References to and information about biocultural differences are mushrooming in the literature and have resulted in a field of study known as "biocultural ecology" (Bennett, Osborne, & Miller, 1975), which has as its major focus the study of human adaptation and homeostasis. The purpose of biocultural ecology is to transcend the fragmentation inherent in the separation of culture, human biology, and ecology and the environment. Biocultural ecology is an examination of diverse human populations by means of this three-way interaction system and focuses on spe-cific, localized individuals and populations within a given environment. Data relative to all the variables significant to people within a racial group are essential for complete understanding of the people. Not only are no two persons alike, but also no two cultural or racial groups are alike, and all phenomena relative to both individuals and cultural or racial groups must be understood.

Although the significance of biocultural ecology concepts has existed in other disciplines, such as sociology and medical anthropology, the nursing literature has only recently documented the importance of this field for nurses. A focus on transcultural issues that began in the mid-1960s with the impetus of nurses such as Madeleine Leininger (1970) has helped nurses to develop cultural insights and a deeper appreciation for human life and values from a cultural perspective. However, despite the introduction of transcultural nursing concepts, the nursing literature remains scanty on biological variations existing among people in various racial

129

groups. The strongest argument for including concepts on biological variations in nursing education and subsequently nursing practice is that scientific facts about biological variations can aid the nurse in giving culturally appropriate health care. Nurses who care for people transculturally need to be cognizant of certain basic biological differences to give nonharmful and competent care.

Most nurses in the United States have been educated in a system of nursing practice based on biological baselines of the dominant White race. Because studies on biological baseline data in growth and development, nutrition, and other biological phenomena have been conducted using White subjects, standardized norms available to the nurse do not reflect biological variations existing among different racial groups. That people in various racial groups differ tremendously is evidenced externally and is related to biogenetic variations that have occurred internally. Therefore, values uniracially normed are inappropriate when applied across racial groups. In the United States, White-standardized values for factors related to growth and development, nutrition, and susceptibility to disease are often applied to African Americans, Orientals, and American Indians. Therefore significant deviations from the norm that may be labeled "nonnormal" might be more appropriately labeled "non-White" (Overfield, 1977, 1995). In fact, biological variations among racial groups are so diverse that multiple dimensions are encompassed.

DIMENSIONS OF BIOLOGICAL VARIATIONS

A direct relationship exists between race and body structure, skin color, other visible physical characteristics, enzymatic and genetic variations, electrocardiographic patterns, susceptibility to disease, nutritional preferences and deficiencies, and psychological characteristics. Differences among people in various racial groups in each of these areas are discussed in the following sections.

Body structure

One category of difference between racial groups is body structure, which includes both body size

and body shape. Newborn body proportions differ among racial groups. Although research on this topic remains scanty, it has been postulated that newborn body proportions appear to be genetically programmed to conform to the pelvic shape of the mother (Overfield, 1977, 1995).

Body structure as well as bone density also differs among adults. For example, the prevalence of osteoporosis and the incidence of vertebral fractures are both reported to be substantially lower in African-American women than in White American women (Cummings, Kelsey, Nevitt, & O'Dowd, 1985; Gilsanz, Roe, Mora, et al., 1991; Melton & Riggs, 1987; Pollitzer & Anderson, 1990). This finding is generally attributed to racial differences in adult bone mass (Pollitzer & Anderson, 1990).

Among adults, bone density is greater in African Americans than in White Americans of either sex (Reid, Cullen, Schooler, et al., 1990). However, differences in adult bone density are not necessarily confined to these two racial groups. In fact, the bone density of adult Polynesians is reported to be greater than that of age-matched Whites (Reid et al., 1990). In contrast, Asian Americans generally have lower values for bone density compared with other racial groups (Reid et al., 1990).

Biological markers that account for the variations in adult bone mass among racial groups are unknown. In addition, the time of life at which these differences are manifested is uncertain. According to Li, Specker, Ho, and Tsang (1989), prepubertal African-American children tend to have higher values for bone density than their White counterparts have. Some researchers (Garn, Nagy, & Sandusky, 1972; Li, Specker, Ho, & Tsang, 1989) have speculated that such findings indicate that racial differences in skeletal mass develop early in childhood and persist throughout life.

In regard to body structure and size, the face is perhaps one of the most fascinating areas of the body because it has many parts that combine to make the whole. The face tends to be the one prominent area that can visibly categorize people by race. For example, eyelids vary from racial group to racial group. In some racial groups the eyelids droop over the cartilage plate above the eye, and in other racial groups the eyelids do not droop. The epicanthic fold, another variation of the eyelids, is found predominantly in persons with Oriental characteristics but may be present in other racial groups.

Ears are another fascinating part of the face because they have a variety of shapes. Earlobes can be free and floppy, or attached close to the face as if the intent were to make sure the lobe stayed in place. Earlobes that are free and floppy are very handy for attaching earrings. When earlobes are attached, they are the least defined, and the wearing of objects such as earrings may be difficult.

Noses come in all sizes and shapes; however, nose size and shape correlate directly with one's racial ancestry. It has been postulated that small noses were an evolutionary result of living in cold climates, such as the classic Oriental nose. On the other hand, noses with high bridges were a result of living in climates that were dry, such as the classic Iranian and American Indian noses. People who lived in moist, hot climates developed broad, flat noses, such as those found on Africans and African Americans (Overfield, 1977, 1995).

Teeth offer another important variation in body size and shape. Tooth size, which is important because the teeth help shape the size of the lower face, varies among racial groups. For example, Australian aborigines have the largest teeth in the world, as well as four extra molars. Oriental Americans and African Americans have very large teeth, whereas White Americans have very small teeth. People with very large teeth tend to have their jaws projecting beyond the upper part of the face. This projection tends to be a normal variation and not an orthodontic problem. There is also a tendency among some racial groups for fewer teeth. For example, some racial groups do not have a third molar or maxillary lateral incisors. Peg teeth are sometimes a step in the evolutionary process that facilitates the presence or absence of a particular type of tooth (Overfield, 1977, 1995).

As teeth vary among racial groups, so do tongues. The most common variances are scrotal tongues, which occur in 5% of the population in some racial groups; geographic tongues, which occur in 3% of the population in some racial groups; and fissured tongues, which occur in 5% to 40% of the population in some racial groups (Witcop et al., 1963).

The mandibular or palatine torus is also of concern to the nurse when inspecting the mouth. The torus is a bony protuberance, and the palatine torus occurs on the midline of the palate, whereas the mandibular torus occurs as a lump on the inner side of the mandible near the second molar. Tori are fairly common, with palatine tori occurring in up to 25% of the population in most racial groups studied. Mandibular tori occur in 7% of Whites, 2% of African Americans, and 40% of Orientals (Jarvis, 1972).

Another variation in body size and structure is attributable to muscle size and mass. In certain racial groups specific muscles are absent altogether. The peroneus tertius muscle, which is found in the foot, and the palmaris longus muscle, which is found in the wrist, are absent in individuals in some racial groups. However, muscle absence in general does not appear to be more prevalent in any particular racial group, nor does absence of a particular muscle correspond with absence of another muscle.

Numerous studies have been conducted regarding inheritability of stature (Overfield, 1995). In general, the conclusions are that people by virtue of race vary in height as a result of race and that in the United States African Americans and White Americans are the tallest, American Indians are either similar in height or a few inches shorter than Mexican Americans, and Asian Americans are the shortest. Individuals of higher socioeconomic status in all ethnic groups are taller (Overfield, 1995). In regard to physical growth and developmental rates, African Americans are generally advanced, whereas Orientals are generally retarded when these groups are compared with White norms.

Body weight

It is well-known fact that weight differs in individuals both by race and by gender. African Americans and Whites are less similar in weight than they are in height. This is believed to be attributable to the fact that African Americans have heavier bone and muscle mass than Whites have (Greaves, Puhl, Baranowski, et al., 1989; Kuh, Power, & Rodgers, 1991; Laor, Seidman, & Danon, 1991; Ortiz, Russell, Daley, et al., 1992). On the average, African-American men weigh less than their White counterparts (166.1 compared to 170.6 pounds) (Najjar, 1987). In stark contrast, African-American women are consistently heavier at every age group than their White American counterparts (149.6 compared to 137.0 pounds). In addition, African-American women average about 20 pounds heavier than their White American counterparts from 35 to 65 years of age (Haffner, Stern, Hazuda, et al., 1986; Greaves, Puhl, Baranowski, et al., 1989). Similarly, Mexican-American Whites, on the average, weigh more than non-Hispanic Whites as result of truncal fat (Haffner, Stern, Hazuda, et al., 1986; Greaves, Puhl, Baranowski, et al., 1989). Although race does appear to have an influence on body weight, perhaps one of the best predictors of obesity is socioeconomic status (Overfield, 1995). This is evident by the fact that on the average obesity is more pronounced in the low class, less pronounced in the middle class as compared to their low-class counterparts, and even less pronounced in the upper class as compared to their middle-class counterparts (Garn, Sullivan, & Hawthorne, 1989).

Skin color

When working with people from diverse cultural backgrounds, the nurse should have an understanding of how different races evolved in relation to the environment. Biological differences noted in skin color may be attributable to the biological adjustments a person's ancestors made in the environment in which they lived. For example, it has been scientifically postulated that the original skin color of humans on earth was black (Overfield, 1977; Overfield, 1995). Further postulations state that white skin was the result of mutation and environmental pressures exerted on persons living in cold, cloudy northern Europe. The mutation is believed to have occurred because light skin was better able to synthesize vitamin D, particularly on cloudy days. It is believed that black skin became a neutral trait in climates where protection from the sun and heat of the tropics was not a factor (Overfield, 1977, 1995).

Skin color is probably the most significant biological variation in terms of nursing care. Nursing care delivery is based on accurate client assessment, and the darker the client's skin, the more difficult it becomes to assess changes in color. When caring for clients with highly pigmented skin, the nurse must first establish the baseline skin color, and daylight is the best light source for doing so. If possible, dark-skinned clients should always be given a bed by a window to provide access to sunlight. When daylight is not available to assess skin color, a lamp with at least a 60-watt bulb should be used. To establish the baseline skin color, the nurse must observe those skin surfaces that have the least amount of pigmentation, which include the volar surfaces of the forearms, the palms of the hands, the soles of the feet, the abdomen, and the buttocks. When observing these areas, the nurse should look for an underlying red tone, which is typical of all skin, regardless of how dark its color. Absence of this red tone in a client may be indicative of pallor. Additional areas that are important to assess in dark-skinned clients include the mouth, the conjunctivae, and the nail beds. Generally speaking, the darkness of the oral mucosa correlates with the client's skin color. The darker the skin, the darker the mucosa; nevertheless, the mucosa is lighter than the skin.

The nurse must be aware that oral hyperpigmentation can occur on the tongue and the mucosa and is a condition that can alter the value of the oral mucosa as a site for observation. The occurrence of oral hyperpigmentation is directly related to the darkness of a person's skin. Oral hyperpigmentation appears in 50% to 90% of African Americans, compared with 10% to 50% of Whites. Another important consideration for the nurse is the appearance of a hard palate because it takes on a yellow discoloration, particularly in the presence of jaundice. The hard palate is frequently affected by hyperpigmentation in a manner similar to that of the oral mucosa and the tongue. The nurse should also assess the lips because they may be helpful in assessing skin-color changes (such as jaundice or cyanosis). It is important for the nurse to remember, however, that the lips of some Black people have a natural bluish hue (Rouch, 1977). Thus it is important for the nurse to have established the baseline color of the lips if they are to be of value in detecting cyanosis (Branch & Paxton, 1976).

It is also important for the nurse to establish the normal color of the conjunctivae when working with persons from transcultural populations. The conjunctivae will reflect the color changes of cyanosis or pallor and is a good site for observing petechiae. Another excellent source for determining the presence of jaundice is the sclera. The nurse should first establish a baseline color for the sclerae because the sclerae of dark-skinned persons often have a yellow coloration caused by subconjunctival fatty deposits. A common finding of persons with highly pigmented skin is the presence of melanin deposits or "freckles" on the sclerae.

The final area of assessment should be the nail beds, which are useful when attempting to detect cyanosis or pallor. In dark-skinned persons it is difficult to assess the nail beds because they may be highly pigmented, thick, or lined or contain melanin deposits. Regardless of color, for baseline assessment, it is important for the nurse to notice how quickly the color returns to the nail bed after pressure has been released from the free edge of the nail (Rouch, 1977). A slower return of color to the nail bed may be indicative of cyanosis or pallor. It is also difficult to detect rashes, inflammations, and ecchymosis in dark-skinned persons. It may be necessary to palpate rashes in dark-skinned persons because rashes may not be readily visible to the eye. When palpating the skin for rashes, the nurse should notice induration and warmth of the area.

Other visible physical characteristics

In addition to looking for changes in pallor and cyanosis, the nurse should note other aberrations in the skin. For example, mongolian spots may be present on the skin of African American, Asian-American, Native-American, or Mexican-American newborns. Mongolian spots are bluish discolorations that vary tremendously in size and color and are often mistaken for bruises. Another aberration that is more common in African Americans than in other racial groups is keloids. These ropelike scars represent an exaggeration of the wound-healing process and may

occur as a result of any type of trauma, such as surgical incisions, ear piercing, or insertion of an intravenous catheter.

Enzymatic and genetic variations

The basic genetic makeup of an individual is determined from the moment of conception. At the moment of conception, among other things, the upper limits of achievement are set; the "map," so to speak, is drawn. In other words, a person can be only what he or she is genetically determined to be. More specifically, growth and development cannot go beyond what the genes make possible. An individual will not grow 1 inch taller than genetic structure allows regardless of the amount of exercise or vitamins consumed. By the same token, an individual will be no more intelligent than genetic structure allows, despite the amount of tutoring or special schooling the individual receives (Burt, 1966; Lorton & Lorton, 1984).

In medical terms, a person's race represents his or her genetic makeup. Although race may be irrelevant in some situations, knowing the racial predisposition to a certain disease is often helpful in evaluating clients and diagnosing their illness as well as in assessing risks (Divan, 1989). The genetic and enzymatic predisposition to certain diseases is discussed in this chapter under Susceptibility to Disease (p. 139); lactose intolerance and glucose-6-phosphate dehydrogenase (G-6-PD) deficiency are discussed under Nutritional Deficiencies (p. 155).

Genes are the working subunits of chemical information that carry a complete set of instructions for making the needed protein for a cell (Lewis, 1997). It is essential to remember that genes contain a particular set of instructions by way of coding for a particular protein (Collins, 1997). These coded instructions are known as deoxyribonucleic acid (DNA). DNA is composed of two long, paired strands that are spiraled into what is known as a "double helix" (Collins, 1997). Although there are only four different chemical bases in DNA, (1) adenine, (2) thymine, (3) cytosine, and (4) guanine, the order in which these bases occur determines specifically what information is available in a matter similar to the way in which the specific letters in the alphabet combine to form particular words and connect to form sentences (Collins, 1997). DNA itself resides in a core, or what is known as the nucleus of each of the cells in the body. In fact, every human cell, with one notable exception in the form of mature red blood cells, which have no nucleus, has the same DNA. All somatic cells have 46 molecules of double-stranded DNA. Likewise, each molecule consists of 50 to 250 million bases which are housed in a chromosome (Collins, 1997).

There are several levels of genetic investigation including molecular genetics and cytogenetics. *Molecular genetics* is the study of genes at a biochemical or cellular level (Lewis, 1997). A gene and its effects are often separable, and, as such, geneticists are able to distinguish the gene responsible for a trait or illness from the actual expression of a particular trait or illness (Lewis, 1997). For example, the genes themselves compose what is termed the *genotypes,* whereas the actual expression of these genes is called the *phenotype.* In contrast to molecular genetics, *cytogenetics* is the study of genes that involves matching phenotypes to chromosomal variants. As the twentieth century progressed, cytogenetics rapidly matured as geneticists built upon the mapping of all four chromosomes of the fruit fly. By 1950, the arduous task of mapping genes on the 22 pairs of autosomes was begun (Lewis, 1997). Today this process of sequencing a genetic map is known as the "Human Genome Project" (Collins, 1997). The purpose of the Human Genome Project is to identify the three billion code letters of a representative human genome by the year 2005 (Collins, 1997). At the same time, geneticists will identify the exact location of all genes on the sequencing map. Work relative to the 15-year international Human Genome Project was officially inaugurated in the United States on October 1, 1990. The U.S. project is currently jointly funded by the National Institute of Health through the National Center for Human Genome Research and the Department of Energy (Collins, 1997).

Another area of genetic study is termed *population genetics*. Population genetics is the study of allele frequencies in populations (Lewis, 1997). Population genetics is extremely important because human beings tend to marry or mate with people primarily like themselves, that is, the same racial, ethnic, and cultural groups. Because of this there is a tendency for a frequency of certain alleles in that given population. For example, although 1 out of 800 women in the general United States population are affected by the BRCA1 breast cancer gene, this figure climbs dramatically to 1 out every 100 women among Ashkenazi Jews (Lewis, 1997).

Today the relative role that genetics plays in understanding the etiology of disease is becoming evident. It is important to remember that all diseases, except for trauma, have a genetic linkage. The earliest introduction to the concept of genetic inheritance comes from the nineteenth-century work of Gregor Mendel. Mendel's work involved the identification and breeding of a variety of pea plants (Overfield, 1995). From his work, Mendel noted that these pea plants had two different expressions of an inherited trait. For example, Mendel noted that when short plants were bred with short plants they were "true breeding," that is, giving rise to the production of only short plants. However, when tall plants were bred with short plants or another tall plant, the next generation resulted in offsprings of only tall plants. This phenomenon indicates that a gene can and does exist in alternative forms. In genetics, these alternative forms are called *alleles* (Lewis, 1997).

Ordinarily a gene is a stable entity, but over the course of time a gene can suffer a change in sequence (Lewis, 1997). This change is termed a *mutation.* The new form of the gene is inherited in a stable manner as in the case of the previous form when the mutation occurs (Lewis, 1997). When a mutation occurs, the organisms carrying the altered gene is called a *mutant,* whereas the organism that carries the normal, or unaltered, gene is called the *wild type.* The term "wild type" is used to describe either the *genotype* or the *phenotype.*

To understand how copies of a gene are transmitted, it is essential to understand that the life cycle of an organism passes through a diploid phase and essentially has two copies of each gene. At conception, one of two copies is passed from the parent to a gamete (a germ cell, egg or sperm). At this point, the gamete contains one copy of each gene of the organism, and this is called the *haploid* set. Consequently the alternative types of gametes produced by the parents unite to form what is called the *zygote* (the fertilized egg) (Lewis, 1997).

With a mutation, new alleles arise. Generally, when a mutation occurs, the particular frequency is represented by only one copy among all the copies of that particular gene in the population (Thompson, McInnes, & Willard, 1991). The probability that a new mutation will survive from one generation to the next is largely dependent on both chance and by natural selection. From one generation to the next, depending on chance, allele frequencies fluctuate (Thompson, McInnes, & Willard, 1991). This entire phenomenon is termed *genetic drift*.

When an individual has two identical alleles for a gene, this individual is said to be *homozygous* for that gene. Similarly, an individual with two different alleles is *heterozygous*. In other word, a person inherits essentially one allele from each parent. These alleles can be the same or different. Therefore, at any locus on a chromosome pair there is a gene composed of two alleles. For example, the blood types A, B, and O are the alleles for the ABO blood type locus (Overfield, 1995). If there is only one allele at a particular locus, then the gene is said to be *monomorphic*. In contrast, when there are multiple alleles at a particular gene locus, the gene is said to be *polymorphic* (Overfield, 1995). An excellent example of this concept is found in the enzyme deficiency glucose-6-phosphate dehydrogenase (G-6-PD) deficiency, which is said to be caused by the most polymorphic genes known, having more than 320 alleles (Luzzatto, 1986).

In Mendel's classic work, he noted that each of the genes identified had two alleles, which is suggestive of two obvious expressions. A gene may have many alleles (variants) as a result of changes in any of the hundreds or thousands of DNA base pairs that make up a gene. However, because the concept of DNA and DNA sequencing had not yet been identified, Mendel was able to detect a gene variant only if the phenotype was altered. For example, if a green pea produced a yellow pea, this phenomenon would be a phenotypic alteration (Lewis, 1997). As Mendel continued his work, he noted that in some instances one gene could mask the expression of another. In this case, the gene that masks the expression of the other is considered to be completely *dominant,* whereas the mask allele is considered to be *recessive.* An excellent example of this concept was noted when Mendel crossed a "true-breeding" tall plant with a short plant. In this case, the tall plant (or the tall allele) was completely dominant to the short plant (short allele), and thus all the plants in the next generation were tall (Lewis, 1997; Overfield, 1995). An inherited trait is said therefore to be either dominant or recessive. Whether this trait is dominant or recessive depends on the particular nature of the phenotype. Often the heterozygote, on a biochemical level, is actually intermediate, or a mixture of the homozygous dominant and homozygous recessive, though the heterozygote and the homozygous-dominant genotypes are indistinguishable (Lewis, 1997; Overfield, 1995). For example, in the case of Tay-Sachs, a genetically inherited disease commonly found among Jews, the heterozygote (with one dominant and one recessive allele) actually produces half the normal amount of the enzyme that the gene encodes, yet this amount appears to be sufficient for normal function, and so that person remains as healthy as a person with two dominant alleles. A phenotypic (disease itself) expression of the gene would occur only if a person inherited two recessive alleles.

How a person inherits a particular gene depends on two basic characteristics which include (1) the dominant or recessive nature of the allele and (2) the type of chromosome that the gene in question is part of (Lewis, 1997). If a person has dominant alleles, that is, has only one copy of the gene, this dominant allele can affect the phenotype. In contrast, a person who has a recessive allele must have two copies of the gene if the phenotype is to be expressed. For example, the cancer-predisposing alleles BRCA1, BRCA2, and the newly discovered BRCA3 are dominant. Therefore an individual would need to inherit one copy of the gene from one parent to have an odds ratio of 1 in 2 chances of developing the disease. The second mode of inheritance depends on the chromosome location that the particular gene is a part of. For example, human beings have

46 chromosomes including two that determine sex—X and Y (sex chromosomes). The presence or absence of a single gene on the Y chromosome is responsible for determining sex. The remaining chromosomes are termed "non-sex chromosomes," or "autosomes." Specially, a female has 44 autosomes and two X chromosomes. In contrast, a male has 44 autosomes and one X and one Y chromosome. In other words, there are actually 23 pairs of chromosomes consisting of 22 pairs of autosomes, and one pair of X and Y chromosomes (Harper, 1993, Lewis, 1997). Because there is a difference in sex chromosome constitution, it is believed that genes on the sex chromosomes follow different, sex-linked, patterns of inheritances in the two sexes. In case of X-linked dominant inheritance, it is essential to remember that male-to-male transmission never occurs because men cannot pass their X chromosomes to their sons. In addition, all daughters of an affected male with an X-linked gene will actually receive the gene either in a recessive or a dominant form (Harper, 1993). For example, if the father passes an X-linked recessive gene onto his daughter, the daughter will be a carrier. However, if the father passes an X-linked dominant gene to his daughter, the daughter will be affected (Harper, 1993). Thus modes of inheritance of a particular trait can depend on the recessive and dominant characteristics of the allele or on whether the gene is located on the sex chromosome or an autosomal chromosome (Saito et al., 1992).

To understand the significance of genetics, it is essential to develop an awareness of the relative role of single mendelian traits in humans. Single mendelian traits in humans are associated with disorders or traits linked to a single gene. For example, the most prevalent mendelian disorders are believed to be cystic fibrosis, Tay-Sachs disease, and Duchenne muscular dystrophy (Lewis, 1997). Yet, although these mendelian traits are considered to be prevalent, they are extremely rare in occurrence, affecting 1 in 10,0000 or fewer births (Lewis, 1997). Today, about 2500 mendelian disorders are known, and some 2500 other identifiable conditions are suspected to be mendelian related because of their recurrence patterns in large families (Lewis, 1997).

Some disease cannot be explained by the single-gene mendelian-trait theory. Although every individual has two alleles for any autosomal gene (one allele for each chromosome), a gene can exist in a given population in more than two allelic forms (Lewis, 1997). This different allele combination often leads to variations in phenotype (Harper, 1993; Lewis, 1997). In addition, there is a difference in the dominance relationship of an allele. For example, as previously indicated, in the case of complete dominance, one allele is expressed, and the other is not. However, in some instances, some genes demonstrate what is termed "incomplete dominance." Incomplete dominance occurs when the heterozygous phenotype is intermediate between that of either homozygote (Harper, 1993; Lewis, 1997). For example, in the case of familial hypercholesterolemia (FH), an individual with two disease-causing alleles actually lacks the liver receptors that take up cholesterol from the bloodstream (Lewis, 1997). In this case, the phenotype will actually parallel the number of receptors. Individuals with one mutant allele die in young adulthood, and those with two of the wild type (the most common expression of a particular gene in a given population) do not develop this inherited form of heart disease (Lewis, 1997).

Understanding genetics and its transcultural and racial implications is of paramount importance. Understanding race and the genetic implications is also important. There are scientists who recognize only Black, White, and Orientals/American Indians as racial groups (Overfield, 1995; Polednak, 1989; Brues, 1977). Orientals/American Indians are often placed by these scientists in one major group because of some genetic similarities (Overfield, 1995; Brues, 1977). Race is an important term because races of people are not static. What is implied by this is that all races have evolved over time as a direct response to environmental stimuli. Thus the characteristics that define a race will not necessarily define any specific individual from that particular race of people (Overfield, 1995). For example, the Yupik Eskimos are said to have a 75% gene frequency of M in the MN blood system, 61% in the O, 25% in the A, and 16% in the B within the ABO blood groups (Overfield, 1995). These same individuals are believed to have no prevalence for Rh-negative blood (Overfield, 1995). A health care professional working with this group of people might assume incorrectly therefore that the most common array of traits for the Yupiks would be blood types M and O and that these individuals would be invariably Rh positive. Although some Yupiks might actually display this array of traits, it must be remembered that because of genetic heterogeneity, some individual Yupiks might differ (Overfield, 1995).

It has been reported that among some races, the incidence of dizygote twinning is highest in African Americans, occurring in 4% of births. Dizygote twinning occurs in approximately 2% of births in Whites and in 0.5% of births in Asians (Bulmer, 1970; Giger, Davidhizar, & Wieczorek, 1993).

Some research interpretations (Jensen, 1969, 1974, 1977) have indicated that the small but persistent differences between the average intelligence quotients (IQs) of African-American children and those of White children reflect a genetic difference. Jensen (1969) claimed to have controlled for variables, including income and education. He reported that he found a difference in IQ that he believed to be indicative of a genetic difference. Others have refuted Jensen's claim (Kamlin, 1974). In 1977 Jensen conducted a study of children between 5 and 16 years of age in the rural South in which analysis of the data indicated that the IQs of African-American children, but not those of White children, drop substantially as they grow older. Jensen believed that this contrast between African Americans and Whites possibly meant that the decrement in IQ was genetically determined. This has not been supported by research by others.

Drug interactions and metabolism Reactions to drugs vary with race. Some evidence indicates that drugs are metabolized by different races in different ways and at different rates (Echizen, Horai, & Ishizaki, 1989). For example, Zhou, Koshakji, Silberstein, et al. (1989) demonstrated that Chinese subjects are more sensitive to the cardiovascular effects of propranolol than White subjects are. In the body there are three classes of reactions to foreign chemicals or drugs: hydrolysis, conjugation, and oxidation (Kalow, 1982, 1986, 1989). The following are examples of reactions to specific drugs.

Isoniazid is a drug commonly used to treat tuberculosis. People metabolize this drug in one of two ways: they will inactivate it either very slowly or very rapidly. Those persons who inactivate this drug very slowly are at risk for developing peripheral neuropathy during therapy (Vessell, 1972). Rapid inactivation of this drug occurs in 40% of Whites, 60% of African Americans, 60% to 90% of American Indians and Eskimos, and 85% to 90% of Orientals (Vessell, 1972). Pyridoxine is given with isoniazid, and the doses are spaced at larger intervals for slower reaction during treatment for tuberculosis. Primaquine is metabolized by oxidation and is used in the treatment of malaria. When this drug is given to individuals who lack the enzymes necessary for glucose metabolism of the red blood cells, hemolysis of the red blood cells occurs. Approximately 100 million people in the world are affected by this particular enzyme deficiency and thus are unable to ingest primaquine. Approximately 35% of African Americans have this particular enzyme deficiency.

Succinylcholine is a muscle relaxant used during surgery. It is inactivated by hydrolysis by the enzyme pseudocholinesterase. In most individuals it is rapidly inactivated, but some individuals have the atypical form of the enzyme and suffer prolonged muscle paralysis and an inability to breathe after administration of the drug. African Americans, Orientals, and American Indians are at risk for having pseudocholinesterase deficiency; Whites have a slightly higher risk than these groups. Some Jews and Alaskan Eskimos have a considerably greater risk: 1 out of 135 Alaskans is unable to metabolize the drug succinylcholine normally (Kalow, 1982, 1986, 1989; Vessell, 1972).

Alcohol is metabolized differently depending on race. There are two enzymes involved in the metabolism of alcohol: alcohol dehydrogenase (ADH) and acetaldehyde dehydrogenase (ALDH). Alcohol metabolism is a two-step process: alcohol dehydrogenase (ADH) converts alcohol to acetaldehyde, and acetaldehyde dehydrogenase (ALDH) converts acetaldehyde (a toxic substance) to acetic acid (a nontoxic substance). Both of these enzymes have more than one variant. Alcohol dehydrogenase (ADH) has a high-activity type, which converts alcohol to acetaldehyde rapidly, and a low-activity variant, which converts it slowly (Kalow, 1986; Kalow, 1972). ALDH has four variants (ALDH-1 through 4). Acetaldehyde dehydrogenase–1 (ALDH-1) is considered "normal"; other types are less efficient in their ability to metabolize acetaldehyde (Goedde, 1983, 1986).

In Whites, with "normal" levels of both ADH and ALDH-1, alcohol is metabolized fairly efficiently. In contrast, American Indians and Asians have an excessive level of high-activity ADH and a low level of ALDH-1. Consequently, alcohol is metabolized to acetaldehyde rapidly by persons in these groups. However, the metabolism to acetic acid is delayed. Because acetaldehyde is toxic and acetic acid is not, the net result is unpleasant effects such as facial flushing and palpitations (Keltner, 1994; Kudzma, 1992). Data from some studies indicate that American Indians and Orientals experience noticeable facial flushing and other vasomotor symptoms after ingesting alcohol, compared with their White and African-American counterparts, who experience less severe reactions. Facial flushing, after ingestion of alcohol, occurs in 45% to 85% of Asians versus 3% to 29% of Whites (Chan, 1986).

Caffeine, a component of many drugs as well as coffee, tea, and colas, appears to be metabolized and excreted faster by Whites than by Asians (Grant et al., 1983). It is thought that the differences noted in caffeine metabolism are directly correlated with liver-enzyme differences (Kudzma, 1992).

Another category of drugs that is metabolized differently depending on race is antihypertensives. Several studies suggest that there are notable differences between African Americans and their White counterparts in the metabolism of antihypertensive drugs (Freis, 1986; Moser & Lunn, 1982; Zhou et al., 1989). Fries (1986) noted that African Americans tend to need higher doses of beta-adrenergic receptor blocking agents such as propranolol (Inderal). In contrast, Moser and Lunn (1982) found that angiotensin-converting enzyme inhibitors (captopril) tend to be less effective as a single therapy for African Americans compared with Whites with the same treatment regimen. Zhou, Koshkji, Silberstein, et al. (1989) noted that even when body surface area and body weight were taken into account Chinese men tend to

need only about half as much propranolol compared with White American males.

Psychotropic drugs are also metabolized differently depending on race. When blood plasma levels of alprazolam (Xanax) were studied in 42 healthy men (14 American-born Asians, 14 foreign-born Asians, and 14 Whites), it was noted that the Asian clients needed smaller doses to achieve the same blood plasma levels as their White counterparts (Lin, Lau, Smith, et al., 1988). Body heights and weights were not a factor in the study results. Nonetheless, in both Asian groups (American-born and foreign-born), the drug remained in the blood longer (Lin, Lau, Smith, et al., 1988). It is important for the nurse to remember that certain psychotropic drugs can cause higher blood levels in certain individuals by virtue of race (such as Asian Americans). It is essential to modify the dosage of these drugs based not only on body surface area and weight, but also by racial consideration.

Lawson (1986) noted that third-world clients are routinely given smaller doses of neuroleptics because some racial groups metabolize drugs more slowly and therefore experience a greater drug effect. For neuroleptic medications, these same variations by race are found in the United States.

In a prospective study of tardive dyskinesia, Glazer, Morgenstern, and Doucette (1993) found that among psychiatric outpatients treated with neuroleptic medications, race was a probable factor for this iatrogenic movement disorder. The data indicated that non-White clients, 97% of whom were African American, were about twice as likely to develop tardive dyskinesia as their White counterparts. To ensure the accuracy of the results, the researchers controlled for other demographic and clinical risk factors.

In a follow-up study, Glazer, Morgenstern, and Doucette (1994) found that, compared with Whites, non-Whites were more likely to be younger, less skilled, unmarried, and more likely to have a diagnosis of schizophrenia. Non-Whites were also more likely to receive higher doses of neuroleptics principally because they were frequently given more high-potency depot medications. Despite the control for known tardive dyskinesia factors, the estimated rate of tardive dyskinesia was nearly twice as high for non-Whites as for Whites. According to Glazer et al. (1994), none of the other demographic, clinical, psychosocial, or general health variables measured in the study appeared to explain the association between race and the propensity for tardive dyskinesia. Despite these findings, the correlation between race as a biological marker for tardive dyskinesia remains unclear (Glazer et al., 1994). Habits such as drinking and smoking are known to speed drug metabolism and thus the fact that some White and African Americans drink significantly more alcohol than some Asian Americans is an important consideration.

Lefley (1990) contends that African-American clients are significantly misdiagnosed as psychotic. Because they are viewed as more violent, they receive more medication and spend more time in seclusion than Whites, Hispanics, or Asians (Lefley, 1990). The higher dose of medication prescribed for African Americans may result more from staff perception than a decision based on serum levels and careful observation (Keltner & Folks, 1992).

Gender is another cultural consideration that may have profound effect on the metabolism of drugs. Yonkers, Kando, Cole, and Blumenthal (1992) suggest that women have the potential for higher blood plasma levels of psychotropic drugs especially when used with oral contraceptives. In addition, they note that women have greater efficacy of antipsychotic agents and a greater likelihood of adverse reactions such as hypothyroidism and, in older women, tardive dyskinesia. Although plausible explanations for these differences have been offered, women have traditionally been excluded from clinical trials measuring the efficacy and metabolism of certain drugs.

Electrocardiographic patterns

A common finding in African Americans, particularly in African-American men, is the occurrence of inverted T waves in the precordial leads of the electrocardiogram. This aberration is a normal variant in the African-American population but would indicate a pathological condition if found in other racial groups, such as Whites.

Susceptibility to disease

Another category of differences between racial groups is susceptibility to disease. The increased or decreased incidence of a particular disease may be genetically determined.

Tuberculosis Historically, some American Indians have had a tuberculosis incidence that is 7 to 15 times that of non-Indians, whereas African Americans have had a tuberculosis incidence three times higher than that of White Americans (Williams, 1975). Urban American Jews have been the most resistant to tuberculosis (Overfield, 1977). The increased susceptibility of African Americans to tuberculosis may be a result of their tendency toward overgrowth of connective tissue components concerned with protection against infection because tuberculosis is a granulomatous infection (Polednak, 1971).

At the turn of the twentieth century, tuberculosis was the leading cause of death in the United States. Tuberculosis remained the leading cause of death until the introduction of antituberculosis drug therapy in the1940s and early 1950s (Phipps, 1993). The case rates for tuberculosis steadily declined from 83,304 reported cases in 1953, to 22,225 reported cases in 1984 (Centers for Disease Control and Prevention [CDC], 1991). Since 1986, there has been a resurgence in the number of reported cases of tuberculosis in the United States (CDC, 1991). The percentage of reported cases of tuberculosis has steadily increased from 3.0% in 1986 to 6.0% in 1996. Between 1985 and 1990, the highest reported case rates occurred in Miami, Atlanta, San Francisco, Tampa, Newark, and New York City (CDC, 1992a). It is postulated that these cities have higher case rates than other cities have because their states also report the highest number of human immunodeficiency virus (HIV)–positive persons, particularly among intravenous (IV) drug abusers. In addition, these states have a larger influx of immigrants from countries in which tuberculosis is endemic (Phipps, 1993). Many persons with HIV infection have organisms that are resistant to most of the chemotherapeutic agents used to treat this type of tuberculosis. When an individual has drug-resistant tuberculosis, he or she may pass the resistant organisms to others. In such cases, effective treatment of this type of tuberculosis becomes nearly impossible (Phipps, 1993).

The number of reported cases of tuberculosis among certain racial groups has changed dramatically over the last several years. For example, in 1988, the incidence of tuberculosis was seven times higher among African Americans than among non-Hispanic Whites, nine times higher among Asians and Pacific Islanders, and four times higher among American Indians and Hispanics (CDC, 1989a). Ethnic minorities now account for more than two thirds of all the reported cases of tuberculosis in the United States, partly as a result of the increased incidence of tuberculosis among ethnic minorities affected with the HIV (CDC, 1998). It is also interesting to note that, of the cases of tuberculosis reported for children, ethnic minorities account for nearly 83% of the number of cases (U.S. Department of Health and Human Services Healthy People 2000, 1990).

In 1972, the National High Blood Pressure Education Program (NHBPEP), in concert with the National Heart, Lung, and Blood Institute (NHLBL) of the National Institutes of Health, was implemented (Joint National Committee, 1997). Up to now, this program has succeeded in its original mission of increasing awareness, prevention, and treatment of hypertension. The trends in awareness, treatment, and control of hypertension among United States adults from 1976 to 1994 (Burt, Cutler, & Higgins, 1995). Data from NHANES III (1991-1994) indicate a level of adult public awareness of hypertension that was 68.4% of the total population. Similarly, knowledge of the adult United States population regarding treatment of hypertension has increased from 31% (NHANES II, 1976-1980) to 53.6%, Likewise, knowledge of adults in the general United States population regarding control of hypertension in that population increased from 10% (NHANES II, 1976-1980) to 27.4% (NHANES III, 1991-1994) (Burt, Cutler, & Higgins, 1995).

It is important to remember that susceptibility to disease may also be environmental or a combination of both genetic and environmental factors. The evidence indicates that tuberculosis can occur in response to both socioenvironmental and psychological stress factors. In a classic study of clients in Seattle, Holmes et al. (1957) found that environmental factors appeared to be relevant in relation to the onset of tuberculosis. In this classic study, data in the life experiences of each client were plotted for a 12-year period preceding hospitalization. Analysis of the data revealed that in the majority of clients there was a gradual increase in experiences that were perceived by the individual as significant and stressful. The combination of stressful life experiences and personal perception resulted in a psychological crisis situation that was evidenced in the 2-year period preceding hospitalization. Further analysis of the data done by Holmes et al. indicated that clients who are poorly equipped to deal with social relationships, especially when a lot of tension is present, may be at risk for tuberculosis.

Blood groups, Rh factor, and disease Blood groups also differentiate people in certain racial groups. A prevalence for type O blood has been found among Native Americans, with some incidence of type A blood and virtually no incidence of type B blood. Almost equal incidences of types A, B, and O blood are found in Japanese and Chinese people, with the AB blood type found in only about 10% of the Japanese and Chinese population. African Americans and Whites have been found to have equal incidences of A, B, and O blood types. The predominant blood types of African Americans and Whites are A and O, with fewer incidences of AB and B types (Overfield, 1995; Jick et al., 1969).

Statistically, persons with type O blood are at a greater risk for duodenal ulcers, whereas persons with type A blood are more likely to develop cancer of the stomach. In addition, there is some evidence that women with type O blood have a diminished chance of getting thromboembolitic disease, particularly when taking birth control pills, in comparison with women with other ABO blood types (Jick et al., 1969).

The Rh-negative factor in blood is most common in Whites, much rarer in other racial groups, and apparently absent in Eskimos (Lewis, 1942). Because there are at least 27 different antigens in the Rh system, this system is complex and difficult to understand. Of clinical significance is the D antigen because it is more immunogenic than any other Rh antigen and is usually the antigen involved in hemolytic disease of the newborn. When antigen D is present, the term "Rh positive" is used. Approximately 85% of persons in the world have Rh-positive blood. The term "Rh negative" is used when antigen D is absent. Persons with the Rh-negative factor who are exposed to Rh-positive blood form Rh antibodies. After continued exposure to Rh-positive blood, the Rh antibody will bind to corresponding antigens on the surface of red blood cells, which contain the Rh antigen. Ordinarily Rh antibodies do not fix complement. As a result, there is no immediate hemolysis, such as that occurring with ABO incompatibility. Rather, Rh-antigen red blood cells are broken down rapidly by macrophages in the spleen, resulting in a conversion of hemoglobin to bilirubin, which causes jaundice. Thus the multigravida woman with the Rh-negative factor who has a Rh-positive mate and has either delivered or aborted a Rh-positive infant will be more likely to have babies who are susceptible to jaundice. This condition can be prevented in subsequent pregnancies if the Rh-negative woman is given RhoGAM immediately after aborting or delivering an Rh-positive infant.

Diabetes Other conditions that appear to have biocultural or racial prevalence include diabetes mellitus, hypertension, sickle cell anemia, and systemic lupus erythematosus (SLE). Reportedly there is a high incidence of diabetes mellitus in certain American Indian tribes, including the Seminole, Pima, and Papago. However, diabetes is believed to be quite rare among Alaskan Eskimos (Westfall, 1971). Diabetes mellitus is a major health problem in the United States, with an incidence of over 8 million diagnosed cases, which accounts for more than 3% of the total population in the United States (American Diabetic Association, 1998; Centers for Disease Control and Prevention [CDC], 1998). The incidence of diabetes mellitus is so widespread that it is postulated that, for every person with diagnosed diabetes, there is another person who remains undiagnosed (Carter Center of Emory University, 1985). In fact, it is estimated that there are more than 7.2 million people in the United States with undiagnosed diabetes (Horton, 1992). Diabetes is so prevalent in the United States population that it was the seventh leading cause of death in the United States in 1998 (CDC, 1998; National Centers for Health Statistics, 1998). Diabetes was reported as the under-

lying cause for more than 40,000 deaths and a contributory factor in approximately 160,000 other deaths (CDC, 1998; National Centers for Health Statistics, 1998). By race, diabetes is ranked as the seventh leading cause of death in the United States among Whites, Blacks, Chinese, and Filipinos. In contrast, diabetes is ranked as the fourth leading cause of death among American Indians (CDC, Diabetes Surveillance Report, 1998). Women in the general United States population have a higher mortality associated with diabetes than their male counterparts have. In fact, diabetes is ranked as the fourth leading cause of death among Black, American Indian, Hawaiian, and Filipino women (CDC, Diabetes Surveillance Report, 1998).

It is important to note that the prevalence of diabetes varies according to race and gender. The prevalence of diabetes increases with age and at all ages is highest among African-American women. In 1988, the prevalence rate of diabetes for African-American women (50.9 per 1000) was twice as high compared with their White counterparts (23.4 per 1000) (Horton, 1992).

There are three types of diabetes: insulin-dependent diabetes mellitus (IDDM), non-insulin-dependent diabetes mellitus (NIDDM), and gestational diabetes mellitus (GDM). IDDM has a peak incidence between 10 and 14 years of age, apparently affects boys at a somewhat higher frequency than girls, has a higher incidence in Whites, and accounts for 10% to 20% of cases (Krolewski & Warram, 1985). NIDDM dramatically increases with age, has a higher frequency in women, has a higher incidence in non-White persons (particularly Hispanics and American Indians), and accounts for 80% to 90% of cases (Carter Center of Emory University, 1985). GDM has been reported in 20% of all pregnant women and increases with maternal age but is not affected by race or culture (Rifkin, 1984).

Hypertension The incidence of hypertension has been reported to be significantly higher in African Americans than in White Americans. The onset by age is earlier in African Americans, and the hypertension is more severe and associated with a higher mortality in African Americans. Studies that demonstrated obvious differences in blood pressure between African Americans and their White counterparts date back to 1932 (Adams, 1932). Since that time other studies have also clearly indicated that there is a remarkable difference in blood pressure levels between African Americans and individuals of other races (Lerner & Kannel, 1986; Stokes, Kannel, Wolf, et al., 1987).

For many years, it has been postulated that 35% of African Americans more than 40 years of age are hypertensive (Tipton, 1974). In a study with a random sample of adults 18 to 79 years of age, 9% of non-Blacks and 22% of African Americans were found to be hypertensive according to standards set by the World Health Organization, wherein hypertension is indicated when a diastolic blood pressure of 95 mm Hg or greater is evidenced (Boyle, 1970). In another study done by the Chicago Health Association, the analysis of the data confirmed previous findings of a higher prevalence rate for hypertension among African Americans in all age groups than for White Americans. Further analysis of the data indicated an equal prevalence of hypertension among both sexes in the Black race and an increased incidence with advancing age (Merck, Sharp, & Dohme, 1974). However, contrasting opinions indicate that hypertension may occur slightly more often in men than in women (Joint National Committee, 1997).

Data from the 30-year follow-up study to the classic Framingham study indicate that hypertension may be an independent risk factor for coronary heart disease for both men and women between 35 and 64 years of age (Stokes, Kannel, Wolf, et al., 1987). Other data indicate that the prevalence of hypertension may be highest among Black, non-Hispanic women (National Center for Health Statistics, 1991). In the Maryland Statewide Household Survey of 6425 adults 18 years of age and older, 28.2% of the African-American population showed a prevalence of mild to moderate hypertension (a systolic blood pressure greater than 160 mm Hg and a diastolic blood pressure greater than 95 mm Hg) compared with 20.1% of their White counterparts (Saunders, 1985; State of Maryland Demonstration, 1977-1983).

Because the traditional terms "mild hypertension" and "moderate hypertension" failed to convey the major influence of high blood pressure as a risk factor for cardiovascular disease (CVD), the Joint Na-

tional Committee on Detection, Evaluation, and Treatment of High Blood Pressure (1997) has attempted to clarify terminology. According to the committee's report, 50 million Americans have elevated blood pressure, which by current definition implies a systolic blood pressure 140 mm Hg or greater and a diastolic blood pressure 90 mm Hg or greater, or both (Joint National Committee, 1997). The Committee concluded that the prevalence of hypertension increases with age, is greater in African Americans than in Whites, is greater in both races in less educated individuals than in more educated individuals, and is especially prevalent and devastating in lower socioeconomic groups (Joint National Committee, 1997). In addition, the data indicate that, in young adulthood and early middle age, high blood pressure prevalence is greater in men than in women. However, after middle age the reverse is true (Joint National Committee, 1997; Roccella & Lenfant, 1989).

The prevalence for hypertension is also greater by geographical region. For example, both African Americans and Whites residing in the southeastern United States have a greater propensity for hypertension and a greater stroke death rate as a direct result of the condition than African Americans and Whites residing in other areas of the country have (Roccella & Lenfant, 1989). The new classifications for hypertension as proposed by the Joint Committee on Detection, Evaluation, and Treatment of Hypertension (1997)* are as follows:

Category	Systolic (mm Hg)		Diastolic (mm Hg)
Optimal	<120	and	<80
Normal	<130	and	<85
High-normal	130-139	or	85-89
Hypertension (based on the average of two or more readings)			
Stage 1	140-159	or	90-99
Stage 2	160-179	or	100-109
Stage 3	≥180	or	≤110

As indicated previously a diagnosis of hypertension is confirmed when there is a consistent systolic

*Excerpted from the *Sixth Report of the National Committee on Detection, Evaluation, and Treatment of High Blood Pressure* (1997). Bethesda, Md.: National Institutes of Health—National Heart, Lung, and Blood Institute.

blood pressure level of 140 torrs or above and a consistent diastolic blood pressure level of 90 torrs or above (based on the average of two or more readings). Reportedly, as a result of this definition, hypertension is of concern for approximately 50 to 60 million Americans (Joint National Committee, 1997; Walsh, 1993). It is essential to remember that hypertension should never be diagnosed on the basis of a single measurement except when the systolic blood pressure is 210 mm Hg or greater and the diastolic blood pressure is 120 mm Hg, with average levels of diastolic blood pressure of 90 mm Hg or greater and systolic blood pressure levels of 140 mm Hg or greater (Joint National Committee, 1997).

Many individuals who are hypertensive remain symptom free for a long time; thus researchers at the National Heart, Lung, and Blood Institute have estimated that more than 50% of persons with hypertension do not know that they are hypertensive. Hypertension continues to be the major cause of heart failure, kidney failure, aneurysm formation, and congestive heart failure. Primary hypertension is evidenced in 90% of reported cases, whereas only about 10% of reported cases are classified as secondary. The diagnosis for primary hypertension may be supported when the following risk factors are present:

1. Positive family history
2. Increased sensitivity to the renin-angiotensin system
3. Obesity
4. Hypercholesterolemia
5. Hyperglycemia
6. Smoking
7. Abnormal sodium and water retention

The diagnosis for secondary hypertension is made when the following causes are present (Walsh, 1993):

1. Coarctation of the aorta
2. Pheochromocytoma (a catecholamine-secreting tumor)
3. Cushing's disease
4. Chronic glomerulonephritis
5. Toxemia from pregnancy
6. Thyrotoxicosis
7. Effects of certain drugs such as contraceptives
8. Collagen disease

Primary hypertension affects more African Americans than White Americans. Researchers at the National Health Examination Survey indicated that in persons 24 to 34 years of age, 3.6% of non-Black men and 12.5% of African-American men have primary hypertension as well as 2.3% of non-Black women and 8.6% of African-American women. According to this study, these figures appear to rise steadily with age and are at all age levels conspicuously higher in African Americans. Thus the overall ratio of African Americans to non-Blacks for incidence of primary hypertension is estimated to be 2:1. In addition, primary hypertension is believed to be more severe for African Americans regardless of age level. The death rate for primary hypertension at all age levels up to 85 years of age is higher in African Americans than in non-Blacks. It was reported that men between 24 and 44 years of age have a mortality from primary hypertension of 14.8% for African Americans and 1% for non-Blacks. In this same age group female mortality from primary hypertension was reported to be 12.3% for African Americans and 0.8% for non-Blacks (Merck, Sharp, & Dohme, 1974). These data indicate that African Americans succumb to primary hypertension almost 15 times more often than non-Blacks do. Furthermore, the death rate for hypertension is probably an underestimation. The nurse must be aware of significant risk factors for hypertension to assist in early detection and continued maintenance and treatment, which can aid in reducing the mortality.

Data are available to indicate that African Americans have a higher propensity for hypertension (Lerner & Kannel, 1986; Stokes, Kannel, Wolf, et al., 1987; CDC, 1992b; Joint National Committee, 1997; National Center for Health Statistics, 1998). In fact, the prevalence of hypertension among persons 20 years of age and older was down from 48.1 per 1000 in 1960-1962 to 34.9 from 1988-1994 in African-American males as compared to 39.3 from 1960-1962 and 24.3 from 1988-1994 in their White counterparts (National Center for Health Statistics, 1998). African-American women do not fare any better than their male counterparts. The prevalence rate for African-American women 20 years of age from 1988-1994 was 30.6, down from 50.5 from

1960-1962 as compared to a prevalence of 20.4 from 1988-1994, which is a decrease from 34.9 for 1960-1962 (National Center for Health Statistics, 1998). It remains controversial as to whether there are genetic markers such as skin color that can be related to hypertension prevalence among African Americans and other persons with dark skin color (Braithwaite & Taylor, 1992; CDC, 1998). However, in a classic study of African Americans residing in Charleston, South Carolina, it was noted that these subjects showed significant association between blood pressure and skin darkness among both men and women (Boyle, 1970). The effect for this study was independent of age but was minimized by consideration of socioeconomic status.

A later but totally different study was done with African Americans in the population from the same geographical location. Contrary to the earlier study, the data indicated that skin color was not significantly associated with a 15-year incidence of hypertension noted in African-American women over 35 years of age in this geographical location (Keil, 1981). In this study, skin color was measured by a photoelectric reflectometer on the medial aspect of the upper arm. In addition, the effect for the study was independent of socioeconomic status. Both these studies differ remarkably from a study reported by Braithwaite and Taylor (1992) that was conducted in Detroit on African-American men. According to Braithwaite and Taylor (1992), the data from this study indicate that there is a significant relationship between high blood pressure and skin color as measured by subjective coding of skin color of the forehead, between the eyes.

In a recent study, Klag, Whelton, Coresh, et al. (1991) found that there was an association between skin color and systolic and diastolic blood pressures higher in darker-skinned persons than that in lighter-skinned persons. In the study, 457 African Americans were surveyed in three United States cities by use of a reflectometer to note the intensity of skin color and the correlation with blood pressure. The findings from the study indicate that both systolic and diastolic blood pressures may be higher in darker persons than in lighter ones and increased by 2 mm Hg for every 1-SD (standard deviation) in-

crease in skin darkness. However, the data indicated that the association was dependent on socioeconomic status, whether measured by education or on another index consisting of education, occupation, and ethnicity. Significant findings were present only in persons on the lower level of either index (Klag et al., 1991). Using multiple linear regression, the researchers found that both systolic and diastolic blood pressures remained significantly associated with darker skin in the lower socioeconomic status, independent of age–body mass index, and concentration of blood glucose. The researchers concluded that the findings may be attributed to two factors:

1. Either the inability of such groups to deal with psychosocial stress associated with darker skin or
2. the findings may be consistent with an interaction between the environmental factors associated with low socioeconomic status and a susceptible gene that has a higher prevalence in persons with darker skin (Klag et al., 1991).

Regardless of the race of the client, to obtain blood pressure measurements with values that are representative of the client's usual levels, it is important that the individual be seated with the arm bared, supported, and at heart level. The client should not have smoked or ingested caffeine within 30 minutes before the measurement is taken (Joint National Committee, 1997). If the measurement must be repeated, it should not be taken for at least 5 minutes after the first reading. To ensure an accurate measurement, the appropriate cuff size must be used. In addition, it is also essential that the bladder of the cuff should nearly (or at least 80%) or completely encircle the arm (Joint National Committee, 1997).

Sickle cell anemia The most common genetic disorder in the United States is sickle cell anemia, which occurs predominantly in African Americans. It has been projected that 50,000 African Americans have sickle cell anemia (Wyngaarden & Smith, 1985). Sickle cell anemia or the trait also occurs in people from Asia Minor, India, the Mediterranean, and the Caribbean area but to a lesser extent than what has been reported in African Americans. Sickle cell anemia is characterized by chronic hemolytic anemia and is a homozygous recessive disorder. In sickle cell anemia the basic disorder lies within the globin of the hemoglobin (Hb), where a single amino acid (valine) is substituted for another (glutamic acid) in the sixth position of the beta chain. It is believed that this single amino acid substitution profoundly alters the properties of the Hb molecule; Hb S is formed instead of normal Hb A as a result of the intermolecular rearrangement. The normal oxygen-carrying capacity of the blood is found in Hb A. As a result of deoxygenation, however, there is a change in solubility of protein, which causes the Hb molecules to lump together, causing the cell membrane to contract, with the resultant "sickle cell shape."

The affected cells have a shortened life span of 7 to 20 days, which is profoundly different from the life span of normal cells, which is 105 to 120 days. Hb SA is the heterozygous state and is often an asymptomatic condition referred to as sickle cell trait.

Sickle cell anemia is believed to have occurred for many years in Africa along the Nile river valley as an adaptive disease. In Africa this disorder was believed to produce resistance from malaria transmission by the *Anopheles* mosquito (Williams, 1975). In Africa sickle cell anemia or the trait affects approximately 10% of the Black population, and the death rate before 21 years of age has been 100% in those affected with the disease. Before full recognition of the clinical significance of sickle cell anemia in the United States, the death rate was almost of the same magnitude as that in Africa. Today in the United States, as a result of improved and comprehensive care, as well as early recognition of the crisis of the disease, persons with sickle cell anemia may live through their third and fourth decades of life.

A differential diagnosis for sickle cell anemia should be made for all African-American persons who (1) have chronic anemia of undetermined origin, (2) demonstrate an increased susceptibility to infections, or (3) have unexplained attacks of joint, bone, or abdominal pain. Making the diagnosis of sickle cell anemia is done in the laboratory through a technique called "hemoglobin electrophoresis." Hemoglobin electrophoresis provides a definitive diagnosis. In addition to hemoglobin electrophoresis, a complete history including a physical examination and laboratory data base should be done. The labo-

ratory data base should include a complete blood cell count (CBC) with a differential and reticulocyte count, electrolytes, blood urea nitrogen (BUN), glucose, direct bilirubin, and urinalysis (Satcher & Pope, 1974). In addition, radiographs of the chest, abdomen, and bones are indicated if there is evidence of pain or fever. However, a bone scan is preferable.

For persons with sickle cell anemia the indications for prompt admission to a hospital include the following (Leffall, 1974):
1. Vaso-occlusive pain crisis that does not respond to analgesics within 4 hours of administration
2. Aplastic crisis
3. Splenic sequestration, a life-threatening condition that requires immediate admission to the intensive care unit for continuous observation and therapy
4. Hyperhemolytic crisis, which can occur if the hemoglobin and hematocrit levels continue to drop
5. Infections indicated by a temperature greater than 101° F or a white blood cell count greater than 15,000 (However, viral ear, nose, and throat infections may not indicate admission for pediatric clients.)
6. Thromboembolic phenomena in the lungs, cerebrum, and long bones
7. Pregnancy, which indicates an increased risk

A common problem associated with sickle cell anemia is drug use and abuse. At the Martin Luther King, Jr., Hospital, a team of health professionals working through the National Sickle Cell Center was involved in the care of clients with sickle cell anemia. Their work revealed three kinds of problems (Satcher et al., 1973):
1. Clients with sickle cell anemia were typically stereotyped as drug abusers by many health professionals.
2. The delay in seeking medical care during a sickle cell crisis was caused by the client's desire to tolerate pain and avoid drug dependence.
3. Drug abuse in clients with sickle cell anemia was found in those clients with severe and disabling conditions. These clients required drugs so frequently that they often became mentally and physically dependent.

The nurse must be able to identify early signs of sickle cell crisis and teach the client to recognize these symptoms when they occur. The nurse should impress on the client the significance of early recognition and treatment of crisis symptoms. Ongoing surveillance of signs and symptoms of sickle cell crisis can promote appropriate treatment and perhaps prevent early death (Platt, Brambilla, Rosse, et al., 1994).

Systemic lupus erythematosus Systemic lupus erythematosus (SLE) is a chronic disease of unknown cause that affects organs and systems individually or in a variety of combinations. The disease affects women 8 to 10 times more often than it does men. The age distribution for the disease spans from 2 to 97 years. SLE was named after the classic butterfly rash, which is erosive and thus "likened to the damage caused by a hungry wolf" (Rodnan & Schumacher, 1983). This disease was once believed to be relatively rare and always fatal. However, with the advent of better techniques for recognition, the disease has come to be thought of as fairly common, and its course can be controlled by corticosteroids. Even today, however, some clients do die as a result of lesions that affect major organs or as a result of secondary infections. Although the cause of the disease is still unknown, three major causative factors are being investigated. The first factor is an aberration of the immune system that causes immune complexes containing antibodies to be deposited in tissue, which in turn causes tissue damage. The second factor is a viral infection that is caused by or results from some immunological abnormality. The third factor is the combination of the above factors to produce the disease. In addition, some drugs are known to induce lupuslike syndromes, including procainamide (Pronestyl), isonicotinic acid hydrazide (INH, isoniazid), and penicillin (Rodnan & Schumacher, 1983).

As previously indicated, SLE was believed to be a very rare disease. However, because of sophisticated detection procedures, researchers now postulate that this is not so—its incidence has been estimated to be 2.6 per 100,000 population. Although it occurs more frequently in African Americans than in non-Blacks, it is reported to be extremely rare among the Asian population.

The nurse who understands that signs and symptoms of arthritis may be indicative of SLE, especially when combined with weakness, fatigue, and weight loss, can assist in early detection. In addition, the nurse should look for symptoms of sensitivity to sunlight, including development of a rash or symptoms of fever or arthritis as a result of exposure to sunlight. The butterfly lesions of SLE generally appear over the cheeks and bridge of the nose. These lesions are often bright red and may extend beyond the hairline, thus causing alopecia (loss of hair), particularly above the ears. Lesions may also be noted on the neck and may spread slowly to the mucous membranes and other tissues of the body. These lesions generally do not ulcerate; however, they do cause degeneration and atrophy of tissues. Other clinical findings may also be present, depending on the organs involved, including glomerulonephritis, pleuritis, pericarditis, peritonitis, neuritis, and anemia. The most severe manifestations of SLE are renal and neurological in nature.

Laboratory tests used to diagnose SLE may need to be specific to the organs involved, such as proteinuria, abnormal cerebrospinal fluid, or radiographic evidence of pleural reactions. Before the advent of the LE-cell preparation, or what is commonly referred to as the "LE-cell test," the diagnosis was made by the presentation of the butterfly rash and systemic complications, and the prognosis for the client was generally fatal. However, as a result of the LE-cell test and other sensitive tests, including the antinuclear antibody (ANA) or the antinuclear factor (ANF) test, clients with more varied symptoms have been confirmed earlier. Thus through early detection appropriate treatment has been initiated. Client teaching by the nurse should include instructions on the need for appropriate exercise, appropriate balance of rest and activity, and the necessity of avoiding direct exposure to sunlight. As indicated earlier, SLE is a disease with prevalence among some racial groups, and the nurse who recognizes the biocultural significance of the disease is more apt to give culturally appropriate nursing care.

AIDS According to the *Surgeon General's Report* (1987), one fact that is emerging with clarity is the increasing incidence of acquired immunodeficiency syndrome (AIDS) among African Americans and Hispanics. In the United States 1 of every 8 Americans is African American, but among Americans with AIDS, 1 of every 4 is African American. These numbers reflect the fact that 24% of the total AIDS cases reported thus far involve African-American persons. In the United States 1 of every 12 Americans is Hispanic, but 1 of every 7 Americans with AIDS is Hispanic (National AIDS Clearinghouse, 1998).

From June 1981 through December 1997, there were 641,086 reported cases of AIDS in the United States (CDC, 1998). Estimates are that the total number of HIV and AIDS cases in the United States number between 650,000 and 900,000 people (National AIDS Clearinghouse, 1998). Of the number of reported cases of AIDS, 264,652 were White males; 170,141 were Black males; 93,584 were Hispanic males; 4037 were Asian/Pacific Islander males; 1477 were American Indian/Alaska Native males; and 641 males reported no race. Similarly, of the number of reported AIDS cases among women in the United States, 22,463 were White of European descent; 55,191 were Black; 19,894 were Hispanic; 508 were Asian/Pacific Islander; 279 were American Indian/Alaska Native; and 133 cases involved women of unknown races (National AIDS Clearinghouse, 1998).

While women represented just 17% of the total of AIDS cases, this figure nearly doubles to 28% of all HIV cases. Proportionately, heterosexual women and in particular heterosexual African-American women continued to be the fastest growing segment of the population to be diagnosed with AIDS. In addition, proportionately by population size, African-Americans continue to be infected by AIDS at a disproportionately high rate (CDC, 1998). In fact, over the past decade AIDS has moved ahead of cardiovascular disease to become the leading cause of death among African Americans 25 to 44 years of age (National AIDS Clearinghouse, 1998).

Of the number of pediatric cases reported in the United States that involve children under 13 years of age, 1426 were White; 4697 were Black; 1876 were Hispanic; 44 were Asian; 27 were Native American; and 16 reported cases were persons of unknown races (National AIDS Clearinghouse, 1998). Although these numbers are alarming, they do not accurately reflect the full scope of this widespread problem in the United States. It is estimated that the data available on reported cases of AIDS indicate that the prevalence of AIDS in the United States is so widespread that 1 out of every 300 Americans has AIDS, representing 0.3% of the total population (National AIDS Clearinghouse, 1998). Yet, in 1998, only 25 states had initiated an integrated name-based reporting system for HIV and AIDS. These states include:

Alabama	Massachusetts	South Carolina
Arizona	Mississippi	South Dakota
Arkansas	Nevada	Tennessee
Colorado	New Jersey	Utah
Idaho	North Carolina	Virginia
Indiana	North Dakota	West Virginia
Louisiana	Ohio	Wisconsin
Michigan	Oklahoma	Wyoming
Minnesota		

Since the reporting of these data, three other states have initiated an integrated name-based reporting system for HIV and AIDS, and they are Florida, Mexico, and Nebraska (CDC, 1998). From June 1981 through December 1997, 390,692 people have succumbed to AIDS or AIDS-related conditions in the United States. Of the total number of deaths in 1996 alone, 14,500 were White; 16,000 were Black; 6900 were Hispanic; 280 were Asian/Pacific Islander; and 100 were American Indian/Alaska Native (CDC, 1998).

Nutritional preferences and deficiencies

Another category of differences among cultural groups is nutritional preferences and deficiencies.

Nutritional preferences Nutritional preferences include habits and patterns. When it comes to food choices, people are creatures of habit (Zifferblatt, Wilbur, & Pinsky, 1980). The term "habit" connotes inflexibility, though people do change their habits for many reasons. The term "food patterns" is more descriptive of food choices. Many factors are associated with the formation of food patterns and preferences. Food patterns are developed during childhood as a result of family life-style and ethnic or cultural, social, religious, geographical, economic, and psychological components. All of these variables influence an individual's attitudes, feelings, and beliefs about certain foods. However, the paramount factors that seem to determine food choices are cultural and ethnic in nature. Adults in a particular culture set the tone for cultural food patterns, which establish the foundation for a child's lifelong eating customs regarding the timing of meals, the number of meals per day, foods acceptable for specific meals, methods of preparation, dislikes and likes, and table manners. Over time, children develop a sense of stability and security in regard to certain food patterns and attitudes.

Schwerin, Stanton, and Smith (1982) indicated that people exhibit distinct patterns of consuming foods in different combinations or forms and that for the most part these patterns have remained constant over the past decade. For example, many southern Americans would routinely choose grits as a food but would not routinely choose lentils. However, American diets are becoming more homogeneous because of many factors, including transportation, advertising, mobility, economic status, methods of production, and appreciation of other people's cultural heritage (Katz, Hediger, & Valleroy, 1974; Pangborn, 1975; Riggs, 1980; Saldana & Brown, 1984).

Some people, based on their culture, have not been traditionally known to make food choices solely on the basis of nutritional and health values of food. For example, one of the most nutritious vegetables is broccoli; however, broccoli ranks twenty-first among vegetables consumed in the United States. On the other hand, the tomato, which is the most commonly eaten vegetable in the United States, ranks sixteenth as a source of vitamins and minerals (Farb & Armelagos, 1980).

When people relocate, they carry established food habits to the new location, but these habits are retained only if the foods are available in the new location and are affordable. Foods in various cultures have different prestige or status. For example, beef and certain seafoods, such as lobster, are regarded as high-status foods among people in the United States. Hindus from India consider cows to be sacred and therefore do not eat beef. In seafaring countries

seafoods have no status value because they are common. Foods obtain their status rating from various factors, including religious beliefs, availability, cost, cultural values, and traditions, or because a highly respected individual has endorsed them. Even today, in many cultures men and their opinions regarding food preferences are more highly regarded than women and their opinions. In fact, in certain cultures men are so highly regarded that they are served meals first, before women and children. As a result of this practice, women and children may receive insufficient quantities and fewer varieties of foods.

Food also has symbolic meaning, in some cultures, that has nothing to do with nutritional value. In these cultures eating becomes associated with sentiments and assumptions about oneself and the world (Chang, 1974; Farb & Armelagos, 1980). Food becomes symbolic to people not only because of religious connotations, but also because it can be used as a reward. For example, a mother who gives a child candy or ice cream as a reward for good behavior may be reinforcing that food as a good food. On the other hand, a mother who serves a particular food (such as broccoli or cabbage) and says she is doing so because of bad behavior may be reinforcing that food as a bad food or punishment.

Food patterns and nutrition among African Americans. Food patterns among African Americans are not significantly different from those of non–African Americans living in the same geographical area. However, distinct differences do exist for African Americans living and raised in the North as compared with those living and raised in the South. African Americans, as a cultural group, are in the low socioeconomic groups, which may precipitate nutritional problems. As a result of nutritional deficiencies African Americans tend to have medical problems that are somewhat different from those of White Americans. As mentioned earlier, hypertension is a medical problem that is twice as great in African Americans as in White Americans. Another medical problem, particularly in women, that has been linked to food patterns and selections is obesity. Soul foods, which are generally cooked for long periods and well seasoned, may also contribute to many of the medical problems that African Americans encounter. Taking their roots from southern African Americans who saw their preparation as economical, soul foods include:

Name of food	Region	Type of food	Description
Poke salad	Southern U.S.	The cooked young shoots of pokeweed	Prepared with spicy seasoning and fatback
Collard greens	Southern U.S.	Garden raised	Prepared with spicy seasoning and fatback
Fatback	Southern U.S.	Pork fat	Prepared from loin of pig
Chicken wings	Southern U.S.	Chicken	Prepared by frying with spicy seasoning
Chitterlings	Southern U.S.	Meat	Intestines of young pigs that are boiled or fried
Hog maws	Southern U.S.	Meat	Stomach of pig
Grits	Southern U.S.	Grain	Hulled and coarsely ground corn that is boiled and simmered
Hoppin' John	Southern U.S.	Combination	Black-eyed peas and rice
Dandelion	Southern U.S.	Wild greens	Prepared with spicy seasoning and fatback greens
Ribs	Southern U.S.	Pork meat	Prepared with spicy seasoning and slow heat

A cultural pattern that has been established among African-American pregnant women is the consumption of nonfood items (pica), which supposedly originated because of nutritional needs. Another common practice among children under 3 years of age, pregnant women, and some men is the eating of earthy substances such as dirt or clay. This practice is known as geophagy and is practiced mainly in the lower socioeconomic groups. For many years in African society the biological need for calcium, iron, and other minerals, especially by pregnant and lactating women, was partially met by eating clays that were high in nutrients. An analysis of some clays has revealed significant amounts of calcium, magnesium, potassium, copper, zinc, and iron, which are the same substances that have been prescribed for pregnant and lactating women in modern societies (Farb & Armelagos, 1980). Africans who were brought to the United States as slaves continued to eat clay, which is still bought in some areas of the South and shipped to relatives in the North. However, geophagy leads to iron deficiency, mainly because clay inhibits the absorption of iron, potassium, and zinc (Halsted, 1968). It is believed that geophagy is both a cause and a consequence of anemia. In areas where clay is not readily available, laundry starch is sometimes substituted, though it can irritate the stomach and is almost completely lacking in valuable minerals.

There are many clinical implications for the nurse in meeting the nutritional needs of African Americans, who normally have lower hemoglobin and hematocrit levels than non–African Americans have (Dalman, Bar, & Allen, 1978; Garn, Ryan, & Abraham, 1980). Although these lower hemoglobin and hematocrit levels are believed to be partially caused by genetics, some studies suggest that nutritional factors may also be responsible (Jackson et al., 1983).

Another clinical implication for the nurse who cares for African Americans is that of lactose intolerance. Many African Americans are lactose intolerant but can tolerate milk products such as buttermilk, yogurt, fermented cheese, and small quantities of milk. In addition certain nutrients known to be low in the African-American diet include iron, calcium, and vitamin A.

Another clinical implication for African Americans is the high incidence of hypertension, which may necessitate a low-sodium diet. Because African Americans habitually use large amounts of salt and other spicy seasonings, special attention must be given to the importance of seasoning foods to make them acceptable and at the same time limiting the use of salt.

Food patterns and nutrition among Puerto Ricans. Many Puerto Ricans, like persons from other Latin American cultures, subscribe to the theory of "hot" and "cold." The major difference for Puerto Ricans is that they classify diseases as hot and cold and foods and medications as hot, cold, and cool. Both Indian and Spanish influences are reflected in Puerto Rican native dishes. Foods enjoyed by Puerto Ricans include the following:

Name of food	Type of food	Description
Acerola	Fruit	Barbados cherry (*Malpighia* and *Bunchosia* species)
Arroz blanco	Grain	Enriched white rice
Bacalao	Meat	Salted codfish
San cocho	Combination	Soup prepared with meat and viandas
Safrito	Seasoning	Specially treated tomato sauce
Viandas	Vegetable	Starchy tropical vegetable dish that includes plantains, green bananas, and sweet potatoes

The common fare of Puerto Ricans is rice, cooked grainy and dried, and red or white beans stewed with bacon or olive oil, garlic, and onions. Another common fare is *safrito,* which is a tasty mixture of tomatoes, green peppers, sweet chili peppers, onions, garlic, oregano, and fresh coriander cooked in lard or vegetable oil and used as a relish to season foods. Other foods eaten regularly in Puerto Rico include a variety of foods such as *viandas* (starchy vegetable dish, including plantains, sweet potatoes, and green bananas), cassava, breadfruit, acerola, mango, avocado, corn, okra, chayotes, and tubers. The acerola, which is also called the West Indian, or Barbados, cherry, is the highest known source of vitamin C. The acerola contains 1000 mg (1 g) of vitamin C per 100 g portion. Many of the food items that are common in the United States are very expensive because they have to be imported. Chicken, pork, and beef, which are normally fried, are usually limited in the diet because of their cost. Eggs are generally used as the main dish and may be served as omelets. Milk is a very popular food item in Puerto Rico but is seldom drunk as a beverage. The intake of milk is believed to be low in native Puerto Rico because of its cost. A popular beverage is *cafe con leche,* which is a combination of coffee with 2 to 5 ounces of milk. This beverage constitutes the largest portion of milk that is consumed. For the most part, foods are cooked for very long periods, or they are fried. Lard and salt pork are commonly used to flavor many dishes. One food item that has an exaggerated reputation for being nutritious and is often given to children and lactating women is malt beer.

There are many clinical implications for the nurse in meeting the nutritional needs of Puerto Ricans. Pregnant Puerto Rican women have a high incidence of megaloblastic anemia and therefore should be instructed to increase their intake of foods high in folic acid (Parker & Bowering, 1976). For the client who needs to control carbohydrate intake, the nurse should instruct the client about the necessity of counting *viandas* as bread exchanges. The nurse must also be aware that the diet of Puerto Ricans who have moved to mainland cities may lack variety because of the inability of some Puerto Ricans to afford the native island foods that they were accustomed to getting previously. Therefore the nurse and the client should look for acceptable food items that are comparable in health value.

Food patterns and nutrition among Cubans. A major portion of the Cuban diet includes cut-up vegetables, stews, and casseroles that have been flavored with sage, parsley, bay leaves, thyme, cinnamon, curry powder, capers, onions, cloves, garlic, and saffron. An integral part of Cuban food preparation is saffron, which is so heavily used in the Cuban diet that some dishes are considered anemic looking and unpalatable unless they have a deep golden saffron hue. Chicken, fish, or meat soup is served at least once a day, before each major meal. Salad is also served every day, along with fried foods, especially fish, poultry, and eggs. Most Cuban people eat rice and beans of many different varieties. Although fruits and vegetables are plentiful, most Cuban refugees do not consume fruits and vegetables on a regular basis (Gorden, 1982). The typical breakfast of Cuban people consists of coffee and bread. Some Cuban adults drink a lot of strong coffee and rum. Foods enjoyed by Cubans include the following:

Name of food	Type of food	Description
Guava	Fruit	Small yellow or red sweet tropical fruit
Plantains	Fruit	Banana-like fruit that tastes like sweet potatoes and is boiled or fried

There are many clinical implications for the nurse in meeting the nutritional needs of Cuban people. The nurse should be aware that in most Cuban diets calcium intake is normally low; therefore, the nurse should instruct the client to incorporate some cheese and milk into the diet. In addition, the nurse should advise the client to replace fried foods with other methods of food preparation, such as boiling or broiling. In addition, the client should be advised that long cooking periods for some foods such as pork are beneficial.

Food patterns and nutrition among Native Americans. A problem for Native Americans living on reservations that is as prevalent today as it was in the past is food scarcity and a lack of food variety. For Native Americans fresh fruits, vegetables, and meats are very expensive, if they are available at all. Traditional foods may vary among tribes; however, the basic Native American diet consists of corn, beans, and squash. A status food for most tribes is corn. Chili pepper is widely used among tribes because it adds spice to the diet and is considered to be a good source of vitamin C. On some reservations and particularly among some tribes, diets are considered to be very poor, supplying less than two thirds of the recommended daily allowances for one or more nutrients (Miller, 1981). The diets tend to be inadequate in calories, calcium, iron, iodine, riboflavin, and vitamins A and C (Owens et al., 1981).

Poor nutrition has been directly related to several leading causes of death among Native Americans, including heart disease and cirrhosis of the liver. Diabetes is three times more common among some Native American tribes than in the general United States population (Miller 1981). Native Americans have the highest reported prevalence of NIDDM (type II diabetes mellitus). In the Pima tribe hyperinsulinemia reflects a resistance to insulin action (Nagulesparan, Savage, & Knowler, 1982). Among some Native American tribes there is a prevalence for low hemoglobin values and mild thyroid deficiencies (Interdepartmental Commission on National Defense and Division of Indian Public Health [ICND & DIPH], 1964). Foods enjoyed by Native Americans include the following (of which these are only a few):

Name of food	Type of food	Description
Acorns (from some oak trees)	Nut	Leached-out nut paste
Amaranth	Vegetable, cereal	Leaves, seeds
American lotus	Vegetable	Kernels, tuber
Arrowhead (*Sagittaria*)	Vegetable	Tuber
Arrowroot (*Maranta*)	Vegetable	Tuber
Basswood	Cooked vegetable	Buds, flowers
Cattail	Vegetable, salad	Shoots, spikes, pollen
Chickory	Cooked salad	Young leaves
Dandelion	Salad	Leaves
Ginseng (American ginseng)	Vegetable	Roots
Groundnut	Vegetable	Tuber
Jack-in-the-pulpit	Vegetable	Long-term roasted corn
Jerusalem artichoke	Vegetable	Tuber
Jícama	Vegetable	Tuber
Nettle (collected with gloves)	Vegetable	Cooked shoots
Pawpaw	Pie, pudding	Fruit
Pigweed	Vegetable	Tops of leaves
Pine nuts (piñons)	Nuts	Nuts in pinecones of neoza pine, stone pine, and piñon
Pokeweed	Vegetable	Boiled sprouts, boiled roots
Prickly pear (Spanish *tuna*)	Fruit	Red fruit of cactus
Rose	Salad, jelly	Fruit high in vitamin C
Smartweed (knotweed)	Salad	Leaves
Sorrel	Salad	Leaves
Sumac (smooth sumac)	Beverage	Steeped berries
Violet	Vegetable	Leaves, entire plant
Water cress	Salad	Leaves
Wild ginger	Vegetable	Root
Yucca	Salad, vegetable	Flowers, pods

There are many clinical implications for the nurse in meeting the nutritional needs of Native Americans. The nurse must recognize that the diets of most Native American tribes tend to be inadequate in protein, calcium, and vitamins C and A, which may result from unavailability or economics. Another problem found among Native

American tribes is the prevalence of lactose deficiency. The nurse should advise the client to consume foods, other than milk, that are high in calcium and riboflavin.

Food patterns and nutrition among the Japanese. Most Japanese dishes are ideally suited for American life because they are economical and nutritious. Japanese people take great pride in the visual effect of foods that they prepare. In the Japanese culture the arrangement of food, color contrasts, and even shape are considered to be as important as the cooking and seasoning of a particular food. In addition, the rules for picking up chopsticks, holding bowls and teacups, and eating soups are traditions that are well established and regularly observed. These traditional rules of etiquette are as important to the Japanese people as the preparation of the food.

Most of the foods are cooked on a *hibachi* (a small earthen grill) by broiling, steaming, and stir frying. It is thought by the Japanese that stir frying preserves vitamins because the food is cooked only briefly. Meat, which is very expensive in Japan, is stretched with vegetables. Fish is used in some fascinating ways, such as being served raw. Soybean products, which are considered to be an important source of protein, and *tofu* are common fare of the Japanese people. In the Japanese culture salads are rarely served with meals, and bread is often replaced by rice or noodles. The Japanese people have a tendency to use extraordinary flavors when cooking, such as wheat germ powder, which is called *aji-no-moto.* Another important seasoning in Japanese cooking is soy sauce. The common beverages included in the Japanese diet among adults are unsweetened green tea (which is the national beverage), beer, and *sake* (rice wine). Milk is often included in the children's diet in the Japanese culture but is rarely used by adults. Foods enjoyed by the Japanese people include the following:

Name of food	Type of food	Description
Aji-no-moto	Grain—wheat germ	Wheat germ
Sake	Beverage	Rice wine
Sashimi	Meat	Raw fish
Shoyu	Seasoning	Soy sauce
Tempura	Combination	Deep-fried seafoods and vegetables
Tofu (Chinese *dòfu*)	Vegetable	Soybean curds

There are many clinical implications for the nurse in meeting the nutritional needs of the Japanese people. A common clinical problem found among the Japanese people is lactose intolerance. In working with a Japanese client, the nurse should advise the client to consume sources of calcium other than milk, such as *tofu.* The nurse should also advise the client to use enriched rice and to avoid washing the grains before cooking to preserve the nutrient value. When working with a Japanese client on a sodium-restricted diet, the nurse should teach the client to measure the amount of soy sauce used and to avoid eating the many types of pickles that are ordinarily eaten. Another important clinical implication the nurse should remember is the high incidence of stomach cancer among Japanese people, which has been associated with their high intake of raw fish (Qureshi, 1981). Eating raw fish is believed to carry the risk of infestation with fish tapeworms (Goldman, 1985) and has been associated with outbreaks of gastroenteritis (Morse, Guzewich, & Hanrahan, 1986).

Food patterns and nutrition among Koreans. Just as in other Oriental cultures, the main staple of the Korean diet is rice, which is mixed with other grains. Korean people generally mix rice with barley, millet, and red beans because it is believed that a diet consisting of only white rice causes health problems. Most Korean people eat three meals daily, which are of equal proportions. Before cooking, foods are cut into small pieces to facilitate the use of chopsticks. Soups containing seaweed, meat, or fish are always served. One of the most popular condiments in Korea is ginseng; Korean people believe that ginseng has roots resembling the human fetus, is a panacea for curing illnesses regardless of age or sex and is a supposed aphrodisiac.

Korea is surrounded on three sides by water; thus fish products are plentiful and account for 85% of the nation's animal protein intake. Almost every conceivable kind of fish is served, whether raw, freshly steamed, or salted and dried. One of the most expensive food items in Korea is eggs because they are scarce. The preferred meat of Koreans is beef, which is prepared by marination of it with lots of sugar to provide a crispy coating.

Kimchi involves one of the most nutritious preservative processes available in Korea and does not require refrigeration. *Kimchi* is prepared with chopped vegetables that are highly seasoned, salted, and fermented underground or in a special earthenware container. *Kimchi* can also be prepared from naturally grown vegetables such as cabbage, turnips, cucumbers, and other seasonable vegetables that are soaked in salt water overnight and seasoned the next day with garlic, scallions, ginger, and hot pepper. *Kimchi* is fermented without disturbance for at least 1 month and is best after 2 or 3 months.

Many vegetables are grown in Korea; thus Koreans serve both fresh vegetables and *kimchi* routinely. Vegetables are never overcooked and are seasoned with red and black pepper, garlic, sesame seed oil, and soy sauce. Because Korea is surrounded by water on three sides, seaweed is plentiful and is a food item that is highly prized for its nutritive value. In the Korean culture seaweed is a must for the expectant mother. Another common fare in Korea is noodles made from rice flour. A Korean diet includes many products made from soybeans, such as soy sauce, soybean paste, bean sprouts, bean curds, and soybean milk. The dairy products of Korea include bean curd and soybean milk. Because Korea is a densely populated country, there is no room for a dairy industry; thus milk is very expensive and scarce and is served only to children. Because milk is so scarce, babies are often weaned from the breast as late as 2 years of age.

Fresh fruits are readily available in Korea and include apples, peaches, strawberries, pears, watermelons, blackberries, pomegranates, currants, and cherries. Fruit is generally served with each meal. Pastries such as cakes and pies are usually not served with meals; however, they can be found in many small specialty shops.

The national beverage of Korea is made from ginseng; Korea has never been a tea-drinking nation. Another beverage that usually accompanies a Korean meal is barley water, which is served cold in the summer and warm in the winter. Barley water is prepared with grains that stick to the pan after the rice for the meal has been removed. A cup or two of water is added to this rice, and the liquid is allowed to simmer slowly while the meal is being eaten; it is then served after the meal. Foods enjoyed by the Korean people include the following:

Name of food	Type of food	Description
Barley water	Beverage	Prepared from leftover rice grains
Ginseng	Condiment	Spice
Kimchi	Combination	Vegetables that are highly seasoned, salted, and fermented underground for 1 to 3 months

There are many clinical implications for the nurse in meeting the nutritional needs of Korean people. Up to now, the medicinal properties of ginseng have been poorly researched (Barna, 1985). However, it is believed that the long-term abuse of ginseng may be a contributing factor of hypertension. Other, less frequently seen adverse reactions from the long-term abuse of ginseng include nervousness, sleeplessness, skin eruptions, morning diarrhea, edema (Siegel, 1979), and irregularities in blood glucose levels (Ginseng, 1980). The nurse who works with Korean-American clients must remember that in the United States rice is not commonly mixed with other grains, as is practiced in Korea. To increase the nutritional value of rice, the client should use whole-grain or enriched rice.

Because Korean people are accustomed to the taste of seaweed, which is expensive, the nurse should encourage the client to substitute seaweed with stronger-tasting greens such as turnip greens, kale, and mustard greens. Lactose intolerance is a common problem among adults in Korea. Thus the nurse should encourage the client to substitute other dairy products for fresh milk, such as cottage cheese, yogurt, and aged cheese, as well as the nondairy product *tofu*. For a diabetic Korean client, a sugar substitute may be dissolved in hot water and poured over meat that is broiled until the crispy texture has been achieved (Maras & Adolphi, 1985). Although *kimchi* is a zesty accompaniment to plain, broiled foods, it is not readily available in the United States; therefore, a Mexican *salsa* ('sauce') may be used as a substitute (Maras & Adolphi, 1985).

Food patterns and nutrition among Middle Easterners. The Middle East is composed of nine separate countries around the eastern Mediterranean Sea: Greece, Turkey, Lebanon, Syria, Iraq, Iran, Israel, Jordan, and

Egypt. These countries are bound together by foods and certain attitudes about foods. The common staples of Middle Easterner people are lamb and goat. Because of the climate and the lack of suitable pasture land, beef is uncommon in the Middle Eastern countries. In most Middle Eastern countries, *dolma,* a very popular meat dish, is often served. *Dolma* is made of ground meat mixed with rice, herbs, and spices and then wrapped in leaves or stuffed in vegetables. Because many of these countries are contiguous to the eastern Mediterranean seaboard, all varieties of saltwater and freshwater fish, shellfish, and roe are served. In some of the Mediterranean countries bound by religious tradition, some foods are restricted. For example, many Muslims avoid eating pork and wild birds; the main dish of the Muslim people is vegetables and legumes.

For most Middle Easterner people, bread is the staple of life; for every mouthful of food, most Middle Easterners eat a mouthful of bread (Valassi, 1962). A meal without bread is unthinkable for most Middle Easterner people. Bread is generally homemade, fresh, and warm, and the more compact dark bread is preferred to refined white bread. *Pilaf* is a festive dish that is served throughout the Middle East. Other common fares of Middle Eastern countries include beans and lentils, which rank directly behind bread and rice.

In the Middle East boiled beans are served cold with olive oil dressing and lemon juice. In addition, a variety of vegetables, both cooked and raw, are served. Seasonings commonly used by Middle Easterners in food preparation include onions, fresh tomato paste, olive oil, and parsley. There are more than 120 ways of preparing eggplant, which is a favorite of most Middle Easterners.

Baklava is one of the most popular and best-known sweets in the Middle East. However, sweets are generally served only on holidays or during social calls. Unlike Americans, Middle Easterners seldom serve sweets as dessert. Instead, a bowl of fresh fruit consisting of cucumbers, guavas, mangos, citrus fruits, dates, figs, pomegranates, or bananas is the usual dessert. Cooking fats used in Middle Eastern cooking include olive and sesame oil, butter, and gee, which is a clarified butter made from goat's, sheep's, or camel's milk. Middle Easterners use animal fat to cook foods when the dish is to be eaten hot and oils when the dish is to be eaten cold. Meals are not considered tasteful and well prepared unless a large quantity of fat is used. The popular spices in the Middle East include mint, oregano, and cinnamon. The most popular herb is garlic. The exception to this is found in Iran, where garlic is considered vulgar. Olives in many shapes and colors are popular.

Milk is not commonly served to adults; however, it is given to children. Yogurt is considered to be a supreme health food that cures many ills, confers long life and good looks, prolongs youth, and fortifies the soul. Yogurt is served in many foods; for example, it is mixed with diced cucumbers and is used as a topping for rice, fried vegetables, and desserts. Thin yogurt that has been diluted with water is considered safer, less perishable, and more thirst quenching than milk. A specialty cheese served by Greek people is *feta,* a white cheese made from sheep's or goat's milk.

Wine is a forbidden drink in the Muslim faith, Islam. Other than Christians and Jews, many Near Easterners do not drink alcoholic beverages of any kind. Every meal ends with coffee or tea; however, coffee takes precedence most of the time. The exception to this is found in Iran, where the favorite drink is tea served hot and sweet. Foods enjoyed by Middle Easterner people include the following:

Name of food	Culture	Type of food	Description
Baklava	Greek	Dessert	Layered pastry made with honey
Bulgur	Middle Eastern	Grain	Granular wheat product with netlike flavor
Dolmades (*dholmadhes*)	Greek	Combination	Grape leaves stuffed with beef
Feta	Greek	Dairy product	Soft, salty, white cheese made from sheep's or goat's milk
Kibbeh	Middle East	Meat	Fresh, raw lamb, ground and seasoned, similar to meat loaf
Moussaka	Greek	Combination	Meat and eggplant casserole
Phyllo	Greek	Grain	Paper-thin pastry for meat, vegetable, cheese, and egg dishes and pastries

There are many clinical implications for the nurse in working with people from the Middle East. Because fresh milk is not normally consumed by adults from most Middle Eastern countries, the protein and calcium content of the diet must be increased. The nurse should encourage the Middle Eastern client to substitute yogurt for fresh milk because yogurt is a favorite of most Middle Easterners. White cheese, cottage cheese, and aged sharp cheese can also be substituted for fresh milk. For the client on a carbohydrate-restricted diet, the nurse must remember that bread should be restricted or eliminated from the diet because it is high in carbohydrates. The elimination of bread from the diet of persons in cultures where bread is a main staple is difficult. However, the nurse must stress to the client the importance of reducing carbohydrate intake. Because fat is used in large quantities to add taste to meals, the amount of fat in the diet could pose problems for clients on low-calorie, diabetic, or low-fat diets. For clients using sodium-restricted diets, feta cheese and olives should be eliminated from the diet.

Nutritional deficiencies Racially related nutritional deficiencies include lactose intolerance and glucose-6-phosphate dehydrogenase (G-6-PD) deficiency. Lactose intolerance, or intolerance to milk, is a relatively common condition that is considered normal in many ethnic groups. It is found in over 66% of Mexican Americans and is very common in African Americans, some American Indian tribes, Orientals, and Ashkenazic Jews (Bayless, 1975; Burns & Neubort, 1984; Kisch, 1953). In fact, it has been reported to be found in approximately 90% of adult African Blacks and 79% of African Americans, American Indians, and Orientals. Although lactose intolerance is very common among these racial groups, it is reported to be much less common among Whites of northern European descent, with only 5% to 15% of this population having the disorder. Yet the statistical significance reported among Whites of northern European descent indicates that this condition is more than a rare phenomenon.

The cause of lactose intolerance is an insufficient amount of lactase, the enzyme responsible for converting the nonabsorbable milk sugar, lactose, into the absorbable sugars glucose and galactose. With lactase deficiency, any undigested lactose will remain in the small intestine, where, because of its osmotic capacity, it draws water. When the lactose reaches the colon, it begins to combine acetic acid and hydrogen gas, which results in the symptoms of lactose intolerance: cramping, flatulence, abdominal bloating, and diarrhea. These symptoms are dose related, meaning that they occur only if the person ingests more food containing lactose than the person's supply of available lactase can metabolize. Foods containing large amounts of lactose include milk, yogurt, and milk chocolate. Of these food items, nonfat dry milk contains the most lactose. Foods containing moderate amounts of lactose include cream, cottage cheese, and most cheeses. Even unlikely foods such as dried soup, cookies made from prepared mixes, cold cuts, and bread and butter contain small amounts of lactose (When Patients, 1976).

The nurse must be cognizant of foods that can cause lactose intolerance symptoms, particularly when working with persons who are extremely lactose intolerant. For the majority of clients, treatment of this condition is usually a matter of restricting lactose-containing foods rather than eliminating them altogether. An adult who is advised to restrict milk and milk products but otherwise eat a well-balanced diet should not need any nutritional supplements. However, for pregnant or lactating women, nutritional supplements (such as calcium tablets) may be necessary. Lactose intolerance does not generally develop until after childhood; children who are lactose deficient should be encouraged to eat aged cheeses because the aging process changes lactase to lactic acid. In addition, some physicians may recommend a soybean-based milk substitute as well as vitamins and calcium supplements. Even for the adult lactose-deficient client, the astute nurse can suggest alternatives to milk products, such as cheese aged over 60 days. The nurse should be aware that telling the client to drink milk may not necessarily be good advice for many adults in the world and should give special consideration to the pregnant or lactating woman because most racial groups, except for Whites, cannot tolerate milk in adulthood (Bayless, 1975).

G-6-PD deficiency is another enzyme deficiency disorder that is more prevalent in certain racial or ethnic groups. Although it is more prevalent in certain groups, these groups may have different forms of the deficiency. Williams (1975) reported that the type A variety, which moves rapidly on starch-gel electrophoresis, is found in 35% of African Americans who have the deficiency. The slow-moving type B variety is found in 65% of Blacks who have the deficiency and in nearly all non-Blacks who have the deficiency. However, all forms affect males more than females because the genetic inheritance is carried on the X chromosome. The Canton/Chinese disorder of G-6-PD has been found among the Chinese and the people of Southeast Asia. The incidence of the Cantonese Chinese form ranges from 2% to 5% (Williams, 1975). Still another form of G-6-PD deficiency is the Mediterranean variety, which is the most clinically severe type. This form of G-6-PD deficiency affects up to 50% of male Greeks, Sardinians, and Sephardic Jews.

G-6-PD is an enzyme constituent of the red blood cells and is involved in the hexose monophosphate pathway, which accounts for 10% of glucose metabolism of the red blood cells. Under normal circumstances the proportion of glucose metabolized through this pathway may increase greatly if the cells are subjected to oxidants causing metabolic stress. The result is the formation of increased methemoglobin and degradation of hemoglobin. In addition, certain medications tend to overwhelm the protective mechanism, especially when older red blood cells are involved, because of a decline in G-6-PD activity with the aging of these cells. Red blood cells with a genetically determined deficiency of G-6-PD are unable to withstand lesser oxidative stresses, and as a result, a hemolytic process ensues that precipitates a significant anemia.

In the presence of certain conditions, G-6-PD–deficient red blood cells hemolyze, resulting in hemolytic anemia. Conditions that precipitate hemolytic anemia in susceptible persons include the administration of certain drugs such as quinine, aspirin, phenacetin, chloramphenicol, probenecid, sulfonamides, and thiazide diuretics. The presence of infection and the ingestion of fava beans (also called broad beans, or horse beans) are also linked to the precipitous onset of hemolytic anemia. The fava bean is a dietary staple in some of the Mediterranean countries such as Greece and those of northern Africa. Favism, a condition induced by ingestion of the fava bean, is one of the most severe forms of G-6-PD hemolysis. G-6-PD deficiency has also been related to an adaptive process that prevents malaria. The discerning nurse should assist the client in identifying substances that are likely to precipitate hemolytic episodes. In addition, the client should be taught to exercise caution to prevent serious infections. G-6-PD deficiency is a condition that remains asymptomatic until an exposure occurs. The nurse must understand that hemolytic episodes are the result of culturally related nutritional habits and geographical and environmental location.

Psychological characteristics

Gaitz and Scott (1974) have indicated that although cultural factors may influence mental health scores in research studies such scores are not indicative of whether one cultural group has more or fewer incidences of mental illness than another. There are many different definitions of mental health, one of which postulates that a person is mentally healthy when there is a balance in the person's internal life and adaptation to reality. Thus it can be determined that normal behavior is relative to a specific culture and that different psychological characteristics are promoted by each culture. Other variables that influence mental health include family relationships, childbearing practices, language, attitudes toward illness, and social and economic status.

Some cultural groups have a low socioeconomic status, which consequently affects mental health. For example, some Mexican Americans have a low socioeconomic status in terms of substandard housing, education, physical health, political influence, communication, and social exclusion. The concept of social exclusion must be considered as a contributing factor in the failure of any particular cultural group to assimilate the culture of the wider society. Broad exposure to other life-styles, cultures, environments, and ideas facilitates an understanding and flexibility on the part of an individual when dealing with other people or when solving problems. Feelings of insecurity may also be related to cultural background. For example, psychological adjustment may be difficult for a Native American who has lived on a reservation and goes to a college where there are few other Native Americans. The difficulty in adjustment may be attributable to the fact that this person has lived in an isolated environment in which there is a failure to become assimilated into the mainstream of society. Therefore, health care providers must consider both ethnicity and economic factors when assessing mental health status.

There has been no consistent attack on problems of mental illness around the world. While no continent or island area has been immune from mental illness, the study of mental illness in relation to culture has been restricted and often localized. There may have been a hesitancy to study cultures and mental illness because of possible implications of racism (Griffith & Griffith, 1986). Some authorities cite that psychiatrists have also not seriously discussed the possibility that racism may be a manifestation of an individual psychological disorder (Poussaint, 1975). In any case, research on mental illness on a broad world perspective has been seriously lacking.

Although research, for the most part, is lacking, some interesting cultural data and implications are available in the studies that have been reported. Not only do mental illnesses seem to vary among cultures, but treatment does also. In Japan, psychiatric institutions are small; in the United States, they are large. Societies also have differing demands on individuals emerging from the treatment milieu. Not only do hospitals and treatment milieus differ around the world, but also the paths into illness show a different pattern in each culture. Variations in class identity or in the pace of acculturation of class segments may produce differences in deviant types. Similarly, personalities seem to vary among persons from different geographical regions. There is some evidence that the cultural backgrounds and forms of illness vary apart from the question of how these illnesses are treated. For example, stresses placed on a traditional Chinese family are different from those placed on Hindus and Malays (Opler, 1959).

Lawson (1986) reported findings suggesting that racial and ethnic differences exist in the clinical presentations of psychiatric disorders. Significant racial differences have been noted among proposed biological markers for various psychiatric disorders, such as serum creatinine phosphokinase, platelet serotonin, and HLA-A2 determinations. Racial and ethnic differences in response to psychotropic medication, such as higher blood levels of the drugs found among Asians, affect dosage requirements and potential side effects. All these developments underline the importance of considering ethnic and racial factors in caring for psychiatric clients.

In the United States the incidence of mental illness has been found to vary among certain racial groups. For example, posttraumatic stress disorder (PTSD) had been studied among Vietnam veterans. Because of racism in the military and racial and social upheaval in the United States during the Vietnam War years, as well as limited opportunities for African Americans in the postwar period, African-American veterans of the Vietnam War often have harbored conflicting feelings about their wartime experiences. African-American veterans have been found to suffer PTSD at a higher rate than White veterans have. Diagnosis and treatment of PTSD in African Americans is complicated by a tendency to misdiagnose African-American clients, by the varied manifestations of PTSD, by clients' frequent alcohol and drug abuse, and by medical, legal, personality, and vocational problems (Allen, 1986).

Also, in the United States there is evidence that schizophrenia has been consistently overdiagnosed and affective disorders underdiagnosed, particularly in African Americans and low socioeconomic groups (Gurland, 1976; Taylor & Abrams, 1978; World Health Organization, 1976). General causes of such misdiagnoses include overreliance on the classic thought disorder symptoms pathognomonic of schizophrenia and, for affective disorders, lack of clearly defined boundaries between normal and abnormal mood, as well as failure to realize that clients with affective illness can manifest cognitive thought processes. In addition, according to Jones and Gray (1986), misdiagnoses among African Americans result from such factors as cultural differences in language and mannerisms, difficulties in relating between African-American clients and White therapists and staff, and the myth that African Americans rarely suffer from affective disorders. The effects of cultural and racial differences on baseline behaviors and symptoms have thus far received little consistent attention. Research is needed to investigate more closely how the general diagnostic problems in psychiatry affect certain racial groups. Research is also needed on how cultural and racial differences may affect diagnosis. Finally, baseline behaviors and symptoms for racial groups must be established.

Meinhardt and Vega (1987) have reported that most studies of use of mental health services by ethnic groups have used parity as a measure of whether members of ethnic groups are receiving a fair share of services. The level of services is assumed to be adequate if the percentage of ethnic group members in the treatment population is the same as the group's percentage in the general population. However, service planning based on achieving parity fails to consider that some groups may have higher levels of need than others. Equitable care among ethnic and racial groups based on need is another issue that mental health professionals are addressing (López, 1981).

A better understanding of the differences among various cultures in the area of mental health and treatment for mental illness will enable culturally appropriate mental health care. Griffith and Griffith (1986) have pointed out that mental health professionals should give more consideration to the fact that cultural issues such as racism can cause psychological injury. It is evident from the increasing quantities of literature on culture and mental health that there is a growing awareness among health professionals that care for clients with mental problems must be culturally appropriate and that cultural factors do affect mental health. Although rice and tea may not be the most potent tools of modern psychiatry, they may play an important role in making psychiatric care acceptable to the acutely disturbed Asian or Pacific American psychiatric client (Lu, 1987). It is important for the nurse to study what is available about the population groups being served and consider the important differences that may be required in the care provided. Not only must nurses appreciate that caring for clients from different cultural groups may require different care methods, but they must also assist other mental health workers in being sensitive to differing care needs.

Domestic violence

Between 1979 and 1987, approximately 5.6 million violent crimes were committed against women (Strickland & Giger, 1994). In fact, it is estimated that some 2 million women are "battered" in the United States each year (Hamberger, Saunders, & Hovey, 1992; Newman, 1993). This number may be grossly underestimated because it is derived from the use of the Conflict Tactics Scale (CTS). The CTS relies quite heavily on self-reports of abusive incidents or behaviors (Horton, 1992). It is estimated that "woman battering" is underreported by as much as 40% (Newman, 1993; Shipley & Sylvester, 1982).

By definition, the term "battering" implies that an individual is either physically or emotionally abused (Campbell, 1989; Flitcraft, 1991; Newman, 1993). Although there are reported cases of "male battering" perpetrated by women, the victims of abuse are women in more than 90% of all reported domestic violence cases (Flitcraft, 1991; Newman, 1993). Although battered women syndrome has been heavily documented in the literature (Campbell, 1989; Chez, 1988; Flitcraft, 1991; Newman, 1993), it has not received the adequate attention it has needed as a social concern until recently. Battered women syndrome has moved to the forefront of social concerns with the murders of Nicole Brown Simpson (wife of famed running back O.J. Simpson) and her friend Ronald Goldman. Simpson, who pled "no-contest" to "wife-beating" in 1989, was later acquitted of the murder of his ex-wife (Brown Simpson) and her friend (Goldman). However, in the civil trial bought by the estate of Nicole Brown Simpson and the father of Ronald Goldman, Simpson was found liable for the murders of Brown Simpson and her friend Ron Goldman. The plaintiffs were awarded an astounding 33 million dollars. At this writing, Simpson has appealed this verdict. Nonetheless, because of Simpson's celebrity status, more adequate attention has now been focused on battered women syndrome.

In the majority of cases involving "woman battering," the assailants were usually an intimate who was either a family member, spouse, or a boy friend. The phenomenon of battered women syndrome has become so widespread that it is believed to be the leading cause of injury among women in the United States (Chez, 1988). Battering accounts for one in every five visits to the hospital emergency room by women in this country (Stark & Flitcraft, 1982).

The incidence of battering may have a direct relationship to other violent crimes committed against women, such as rape and homicide. Homicide is the eleventh leading cause of death in the United States (National Center for Health Statistics, 1998). In fact, it is estimated that one of every six homicides in this country involves a family member (U.S. Department of Health and Human Services, 1991). Of the number of murders committed in the United States, about half are committed by a spouse. According to Mercy and Saltzman (1989), women are 1.3 times-more likely to be victims of partner homicides than their male counterparts.

Between 1973 and 1987, approximately 155,000, or 1 in every 600, women were raped. Like the number of actual domestic violence cases, this number is greatly underestimated because 53% of women fail to report a rape (Strickland & Giger, 1994). The incidence of rape varies with race and ethnicity. Women who are raped are likely to be African-American women who have been raped by African-American men. Of the number of rapes, 65% occur at night (between the hours of 8 PM and 4 AM), 43% occur near the victim's home, and 15% occur at a friend's house. Although a greater number of women report "stranger rape," the incidence of acquaintance rape (date rape) and domestic violence rape is greatly underreported.

Case Study

Sarah Jennings is a 21-year-old African-American, married woman and the mother of a 12-month-old daughter. Mrs. Jennings was diagnosed at age 11 as having sickle cell anemia. For the last 3 years, she has remained largely asymptomatic. She is admitted to the hospital in sickle cell crisis. Her admitting complaints include severe joint pains in both the upper and lower extremities, a temperature of 101.8° F, and shortness of breath. On physical examination, the nurse notes that Mrs. Jennings has coarse rales in the base of both lungs and that her lips are cyanotic and dry. Her nail beds are also cyanotic, and when they are blanched, capillary refill is slow. Initial laboratory examination reveals a hemoglobin of 8 g/dL. While taking the nursing history, it is revealed that Mrs. Jennings has also had problems drinking milk and eating certain dairy products for most of her adult life.

STUDY QUESTIONS

1. List at least two contributing factors for Mrs. Jennings's sickle cell anemia that relate to biological variations by race and ethnic heritage.
2. List at least one other racial group with a predisposition for sickle cell crisis.
3. List the basic causes of sickle cell anemia.
4. List at least two other conditions that Mrs. Jennings could be at risk for developing because of her race and ethnic heritage.
5. Describe at least two differences noted when the nurse is assessing the skin color of dark-skinned individuals.

References

Adams, J.M. (1932). Some racial differences in blood pressures and morbidity in groups of white and colored workmen. *American Journal of Medical Science, 184,* 342-350.

Allen, I. (1986). Posttraumatic stress disorder among Black Vietnam veterans. *Hospital and Community Psychiatry, 37*(1), 55-60.

American Diabetic Association (1998). *Vital statistics.* Alexandria, Va.: the Association.

Barna, P. (1985). Food or drug? The case of ginseng. *Lancet, 2,* 548.

Bayless, T. (1975). Lactose and milk intolerance: clinical implications. *New England Journal of Medicine, 292*(5), 1156-1159.

Bennett, K.A., Osborne, R.H., & Miller, R.J. (1975). *Biocultural ecology: Annual review of anthropology.* Palo Alto, Calif.: Annual Reviews.

Boyle, E. (1970). Biological patterns in hypertension by race, sex, body weight, and skin color. *Journal of the American Medical Association, 213,* 1637-1643.

Braithwaite, R., & Taylor, S. (1992). *Health issues in the Black community.* San Francisco: Josey-Bass.

Branch, M., & Paxton, P. (1976). *Providing safe nursing care for ethnic people of color.* East Norwalk, Conn.: Appleton-Century-Crofts.

Brues, A.M. (1977). *People and race.* New York: Macmillan Publishing Co. (Reprinted 1990. Waveland Press, Inc., Prospect Heights, Ill.)

Bulmer, M. (1970). *The biology of twinning in man.* New York: Oxford University Press.

Burns, E., & Neubort, S. (1984). Sodium content of koshered meat [letter]. *Journal of the American Medical Association, 252(21),* 2960.

Burt, C. (1966). The genetic determination of difference in intelligence: a study of monozygote twins reared together and apart. *British Journal of Psychology, 57,* 137-153.

Burt, V.L., Cutler, J.A., Higgins, M., et al. (1995). Trends in the prevalence, awareness, treatment, and control of hypertension in the adult U.S. population. *Hypertension 26*(1), 60-69.

Burt, V.L., Whelton, P., Roccella, E.J., et al. (1995). Prevalence of hypertension in the U.S. adult population. *Hypertension, 25*(3), 305-313.

Campbell, J. (1989). A test of two exploratory models of women's response to battering. *Nursing Research, 38*(1), 18-24.

Carter Center of Emory University (1985). Closing the gap: the problem of diabetes mellitus in the United States. *Diabetes Care, 8,* 391-401.

Centers for Disease Control and Prevention (1998, June). HIV/AIDS surveillance report: U.S. HIV and AIDS cases reported through December 1997. 9(2). Atlanta, Ga.: U.S. Department of Health and Human Services.

Centers for Disease Control and Prevention (1998, June). Diabetes surveillance report, 1997. Atlanta, Ga.: U.S. Department of Health and Human Services.

Centers for Disease Control and Prevention (1989a). A strategic plan for the elimination of tuberculosis in the United States. *Morbidity and Mortality Weekly Report, 38*(suppl. 3), 1-27.

Centers for Disease Control and Prevention (1991). Nosocomial transmission of multi-drug resistant tuberculosis among HIV-infected persons—Florida and New York, 1988-1991. *Morbidity and Mortality Weekly Report, 40*(34), 585-591.

Centers for Disease Control and Prevention (1992a). CDC surveillance summaries, Dec. 1991; tuberculosis morbidity in the United States: final data, 1990. *Morbidity and Mortality Weekly Report, 40*(SS3), 23-28.

Centers for Disease Control and Prevention (1992b). Recommendations of the Advisory Council for the reduction of hypertension among minority populations. *Morbidity and Mortality Weekly Report, 40,* 1-7.

Chan, A.W. (1986). Racial differences in alcohol sensitivity *Alcohol & Alcoholism, 21*(1), 93-104.

Chang, B. (1974). Some dietary beliefs in Chinese folk culture. *Journal of the American Diet Association, 65*(4), 436.

Chez, R. (1988). Woman battering. *American Journal of Obstetrics and Gynecology, 156,* 1-4.

Collins, F. (1997, January). Sequencing the human genome. *Hospital Practice, 32*(1), 35-55.

Cummings, S., Kelsey, J., Nevitt, N., & O'Dowd, K. (1985). Epidemiology of osteoporosis and osteoporotic fractures. *Epidemiology Review, 7,* 178-208.

Dalman, P.R., Bar, G.D., & Allen, C.M. (1978). Hemoglobin concentration in White, Black and Oriental children: is there a need for separate criteria in screening for anemia? *American Journal of Clinical Nutrition, 31*(3), 377.

Divan, D. (1989). Letter to the editor. *New England Journal of Medicine, 321*(4), 259.

Echizen, H., Horai, Y., & Ishizaki, T. (1989). Letter to the editor. *New England Journal of Medicine, 321*(4), 258.

Farb, P., & Armelagos, G. (1980). *Consuming passions: the anthropology of eating.* Boston: Houghton Mifflin.

Flitcraft, A. (1991). Domestic abuse: diagnosing, treating, and understanding its victims. *Clinical Nurse Practitioner, 9*(2), 3-5.

Freis, E. (1986). Antihypertensive agents. In Kalow, W., Goedde, H.W., & Agarwal, D. (Eds.), *Ethnic differences in reactions to drugs and xenobiotics.* New York: Liss.

Gaitz, C., & Scott, J. (1974). Mental health of Mexican Americans: do ethnic factors make a difference? *Geriatrics, 1*(11), 110-113.

Garn, S., Nagy, A., & Sandusky, S. (1972). Differential sex dimorphism in bone diameters of subjects of European and African ancestry. *American Journal of Anthropology, 37,* 127-130.

Garn, S., Ryan, A., & Abraham, S. (1980). The Black-White difference in hemoglobin levels after age, sex, and income matching. *Ecology of Food Nutrition, 10*(2), 69.

Garn, S., Sullivan, T., & Hawthorne, V. (1989). Educational level, fatness, and fatness differences between husbands and wives. *American Journal of Clinical Nutrition, 50,* 535.

Giger, J., Davidhizar, R., & Wieczorek, S. (1993). Culture and ethnicity. In Bobak, I., & Jensen, M. (Eds.), *Maternity and gynecologic care* (ed. 5) (pp. 43-67). St. Louis: Mosby.

Gilsanz, V., Roe, T., Mora, S., et al. (1991, Dec. 5). Changes in vertebral bone density in black girls and white girls during childhood and puberty. *New England Journal of Medicine, 325*(23), 1597-1600.

Ginseng. (1980). *Medical Letter Drugs Therapy, 22*(17), 72.

Glazer, W.M, Morgenstern, H., & Doucette, J.T. (1993). Predicting the long-term risk of tardive dyskinesia in outpatients maintained on neuroleptic medications. *Journal of Clinical Psychiatry, 54*(4), 133-139.

Glazer, W.M., Morgenstern, H., & Doucette, J.T. (1994). Race and tardive dyskinesia among outpatients at a CMHC. *Hospital and Community Psychiatry, 45*(1), 38-45.

Goedde, H.W. (1983). Population genetic studies on aldehyde dehydrogenase isoenzyme deficiency and alcohol sensitivity. *American Journal of Human Genetics, 35,* 769.

Goedde, H.W. (1986). Ethnic differences in reactions to drugs and other xenobiotics: outlook of a geneticist. In Kalow, W., Goedde, H.W., & Agarwal, D. (Eds.), *Ethnic differences in reactions to drugs and xenobiotics* (pp. 9-20). New York: Liss.

Goldman, D.R. (1985). Hold the sushi [Letter]. *Journal of the American Medical Association, 253*(17), 2495.

Gorden, A.M. (1982). Nutritional status of Cuban refugees: a field study on the health and nutrition of refugees processed at Opa-Locka, Florida. *American Journal of Clinical Nutrition, 35*(3), 582.

Grant, D., Tang, B.K., & Kalow, W. (1983). Variability in caffeine metabolism. *Clinical Pharmacology Therapy, 33,* 591-602.

Greaves, K., Puhl, J., Baranowski, T., et al. (1989). Ethnic differences in anthropometrics characteristics and their parents. *Human Biology, 61*(3), 459.

Griffith, E., & Griffith, E. (1986). Racism, psychological injury, and compensatory damages. *Hospital and Community Psychiatry, 37*(1), 71-75.

Gurland, B. (1976). Aims, organization, and initial studies of the cross-national project. *International Journal of Aging and Human Development, 7,* 283-293.

Haffner, S.M., Stern, M.P., Hazuda, H.P, et al. (1986). Upper body and centralized adiposity in Mexican Americans and non-Hispanic Whites: relationship to body mass index and other behavioral and demographic variables. *International Journal of Obesity, 10,* 493.

Halsted, J.A. (1968). Geophagia in man: its nature and nutritional effects. *American Journal of Clinical Nutrition, 21*(12), 1384.

Hamberger, L., Saunders, D., & Hovey, M. (1992, May-June). Prevalence of domestic violence in community practice and rate of physician inquiry. *Family Medicine, 24*(4), 283-287.

Harper, P. (1993). *Practical genetic counseling* (ed. 4). Oxford, England: Butterworth-Heinemann.

Healthy People 2000. National Health Promotion and Disease Prevention Objectives. (DHHS Publication No. PHS 91-50212). U.S. Department of Health and Human Services. U.S. Government Printing Office. Washington, D.C.

Holmes, T.H., et al. (1957). Psychosocial and psychophysiological studies of tuberculosis. *Psychosomatic Medicine, 19,* 134-143.

Horton, J. (Ed.) (1992). *The women's health data book: a profile of women's health in the United States* (pp. 60-62). Washington, D.C.: The Jacob's Institute of Women's Health.

Interdepartmental Commission on National Defense and Division of Indian Public Health (ICND & DIPH) (1964). *Fort Belknap Indian Reservation: nutrition survey.* Washington, D.C.: U.S. Public Health Service.

Jackson, R.T., Sauberlich, H.S., Skala, J.H., et al. (1983). Comparison of hemoglobin values in black and white male U.S. military personnel. *Journal of Nutrition, 113*(1), 165.

Jarvis, A. (1972). Minor orofacial abnormalities in an Eskimo population. *Oral Surgery, 33,* 417-427.

Jensen, A.R. (1969). How much can we boost IQ and scholastic achievement? *Harvard Education Review, 29,* 1.

Jensen, A.R. (1974). Cumulative deficits: a testable hypothesis? *Developmental Psychology, 10,* 996.

Jensen, A.R. (1977). Cumulative deficit in IQ of blacks in the rural South. *Developmental Psychology, 13,* 184.

Jick, H., Slone, D., Westerhom, B., et al. (1969). Venous thromboembolic disease and ABO blood type. *Lancet, 1,* 539-542.

Joint National Committee. (1997). *The report of the Joint National Committee on Detection, Evaluation and Treatment of High Blood Pressure.* Washington, D.C.: National Institutes of Health, National Heart, Lung, and Blood Institute.

Jones, B., & Gray, B. (1986). Problems in diagnosing schizophrenia and affective disorders among blacks. *Hospital and Community Psychiatry, 37*(1), 61-65.

Kalow, W. (1972). Pharmacogenetics of drugs used in anesthesia. *Human Genetics, 60,* 415-427.

Kalow, W. (1982). The metabolism of xenobiotics in different populations. *Canadian Journal of Physiological Pharmacology, 60,* 1-19.

Kalow, W. (1986). Outlook of a pharmacologist. In Kalow, W., Goedde, H., & Agarwal, D. (Eds.), *Ethnic differences in reactions to drugs and xenobiotics.* New York: Liss.

Kalow, W. (1989). Race and therapeutic drug response. *New England Journal of Medicine, 320* (9), 588-589.

Kamlin, L.J. (1974). *The science and politics of IQ.* New York: John Wiley & Sons.

Katz, S.H., Hediger, M.L., & Valleroy, L.A. (1974). Traditional maize processing techniques in the New World. *Science, 184,* 765.

Keil, J. (1981). Skin color and education effects on blood pressure. *American Journal of Public Health, 71,* 532-534.

Keltner, N. (1994, Oct.). Personal communication to J.N. Giger.

Keltner, N., & Folks, G. (1992). Psychopharmacology update: culture as a variable in drug therapy. *Perspectives in Psychiatric Nursing, 28*(1), 33-35.

Kisch, B. (1953). Salt poor diet and Jewish dietary laws. *Journal of the American Medical Association, 153*(16), 1472.

Klag, M., Whelton, P., Coresh, J., et al. (1991, Feb. 6). The association of skin color with blood pressure in U.S. blacks with low socioeconomic status. *Journal of the American Medical Association, 265*(5), 599-602.

Krolewski, A., & Warram, G. (1985). Epidemiology of diabetes mellitus. In Joslin, E.P. (Ed.), *Joslin's diabetes mellitus* (ed. 12). Philadelphia: Lea & Febiger.

Kudzma, E. (1992, Dec.). Drug responses: all bodies are not created equal. *American Journal of Nursing, 92,* 48-50.

Kuh, D.L., Power, C., & Rodgers, B. (1991). Secular trends in social class and sex differences in adult height. *International Journal of Epidemiology, 20*(4), 1001-1009.

Laor, A., Seidman, D., & Danon, Y.L. (1991). Changes in body height among selected ethnic groups. *Journal of Epidemiology and Community Health, 45*(2), 169-170.

Lawson, W. (1986). Racial and ethnic factors in psychiatric research. *Hospital and Community Psychiatry, 37*(1), 50-54.

Leffall, L.D. (1974). Cancer mortality among blacks. *CA: a Cancer Journal for Clinicians, 24,* 42-46.

Lefley, H. (1990). Culture and chronic mental illness. *Hospital and Community Psychiatry, 41,* 277.

Leininger, M. (1970). *Nursing and anthropology: two worlds to blend.* New York: John Wiley & Sons.

Lerner, D., & Kannel, W. (1986). Patterns of coronary heart disease morbidity and mortality in the sexes: a 26-year follow-up of the Framingham population. *American Heart Journal, 11,* 383-390.

Lewis, J.H. (1942). *The biology of the Negro* (Chicago University Monographs in Medicine). Chicago: University of Chicago Press.

Lewis, R., (1997). *Human genetics: concepts and applications* (ed. 2). Dubuque, Iowa: William C. Brown Publishers.

Li, J., Specker, B., Ho, B., & Tsang, R. (1989). Bone mineral content in black and white children 1 to 6 years of age: early appearance of race and sex differences. *American Journal of Disorders in Children, 143,* 1346-1349.

Lin, K.M., Lau, J.K., Smith, R., et al. (1988). Comparison of alprazolam plasma levels in normal Asians and Caucasian male volunteers. *Psychopharmacology, 96,* 365-369.

López, S. (1981). Mexican Americans' usage of mental health facilities: underutilization reconsidered. In Baron, A. (Ed.), *Explorations in Chicano psychology.* New York: Praeger.

Lorton, J., & Lorton, E. (1984). *Human development through the life span.* Belmont, Calif.: Brooks/Cole.

Lu, F. (1987). Culturally relevant inpatient care for minority and ethnic patients. *Hospital and Community Psychiatry, 38*(11), 1126-1127.

Luzzato, L. (1986). Glucose-6-phosphate dehydrogenase and other genetic factors interacting with drugs. *Progress in Clinical and Biological Research, 214,* 385.

Maras, M.L., & Adolphi, C.L. (1985). Ethnic tailoring improves dietary compliance. *Diabetes Education, 11*(4), 47.

Meinhardt, K., & Vega, W. (1987). A method of estimating underutilization of mental health services by ethnic groups. *Hospital and Community Psychiatry, 38*(11), 1186-1190.

Melton, L., & Riggs, B. (1987). Epidemiology of age-related fractures. In Avioli, L. (Ed.), *The osteoporotic syndrome: detection, prevention, and treatment* (ed. 2) (pp. 1-30). Orlando, Fla.: Grune & Stratton.

Merck, Sharp, & Dohme (1974). *Hypertension handbook for clinicians.* Westpoint, Pa.: Merck, Sharp, & Dohme.

Mercy, J., & Saltzman, L. (1989). Fatal violence among spouses in the United States, 1976-1985. *American Journal of Public Health, 79,* 595-599.

Miller, M.B. (1981). Supplementing and adding variety to the diets of Indians on a reservation in Minnesota. *Journal of the American Dietetic Association, 78*(6), 626.

Morse, D.L., Guzewich, J.J., & Hanrahan, J.P. (1986). Widespread outbreaks of clam- and oyster-associated gastroenteritis. *New England Journal of Medicine, 314*(11), 678.

Moser, M., & Lunn, J. (1982). Responses to captopril and hydrochlorothiazide in black patients with hypertension. *Clinical Pharmacology Therapy, 32,* 307-312.

Nagulesparan, M., Savage, P.J., & Knowler, W.C. (1982). Increased in vivo insulin resistance in nondiabetic Pima Indians compared with Caucasians. *Diabetes, 31*(11), 952.

Najjar, M. (1987). Anthropometrics reference data and prevalence of overweight, United States 1976-1980. *Vital and Health Statistics Series II,* No. 238.

National AIDS Clearinghouse. (1998, Aug.). National AIDS Hot Line. Operator ID 586.

National Center for Health Statistics (1998). *Health, United States, 1998* (DHHS Publication No. PHS 91-1232). Hyattsville, Md.: Public Health Service.

Newman, K. (1993, June). Giving up: shelter experience of battered women. *Public Health Nursing, 10*(2), 108-113.

Opler, M. (Ed.) (1959). *Culture and health.* New York: Macmillan.

Ortiz, O., Russell, M., Daley, T.L., et al. (1992). Differences in skeletal muscle and bone mineral mass between Black and White females and their relevance to estimates of body composition. *American Journal of Clinical Nutrition, 55*(1), 8-13.

Overfield, T. (1977). Biological variations. *Nursing Clinics of North America, 12*(1), 19-27.

Overfield, T. (1995). *Biologic variations in health and illness: race, age and sex differences* (ed. 2). New York: CRC Press.

Owens, G.M., Garry, P.J., Seymore, R.D., et al. (1981). Nutrition studies with White Mountain Apache pre-school children in 1976 and 1969. *American Journal of Clinical Nutrition, 34*(2), 266.

Pangborn, R.M. (1975). Cross-cultural aspects of flavor preferences. *Food Technology, 29*(6), 34.

Parker, S.L., & Bowering, J. (1976). Folacin in diets of Puerto Ricans and black women in relation to food practices. *Journal of Nutrition Education, 8*(2), 73.

Phipps, W. (1993). The patient with pulmonary problems. In Long, B.C., Phipps, W.J., & Cassmeyer, V. (Eds.), *Medical surgical nursing: concepts and clinical practice.* St. Louis: Mosby.

Platt, O., Brambilla, D., Rosse, W., et al. (1994, June 9). Mortality in sickle cell disease: life expectancy and risk factors for early death. *New England Journal of Medicine, 330*(23), 1639-1644.

Polednak, A.P. (1971). Connective tissue responses in Negroes in relation to disease. *American Journal of Physical Anthropology, 41,* 49-57.

Pollitzer, W., & Anderson, J. (1990). Ethnic and genetic differences in bone mass: a review with a hereditary vs environmental perspective. *American Journal of Clinical Nutrition, 52,* 181.

Poussaint, A.F. (1975). Interracial relations. In Freedman, A.M., Kaplan, H.I., & Sandock, B.J. (Eds.), *Comprehensive textbook of psychiatry* (ed. 2, vol 2). Baltimore: Williams & Wilkins.

Qureshi, B.A. (1981). Nutrition and multi-ethnic groups. *Royal Social Health Journal, 101*(5), 187.

Reid, I.R., Cullen, S., Schooler, B.A., et al. (1990). Calcitropic hormone levels in Polynesians: evidence against their role in interracial differences in bone mass. *Journal of Endocrinology Metabolism, 70*(5), 1452-1466.

Rifkin, H. (Ed.). (1984). *The physician's guide to type II diabetes (NIDDM): diagnosis and treatment.* New York: The American Diabetes Association.

Riggs, S. (1980). Tastes of America. *Regionality Institutions, 87*(12), 76.

Roccella, E.J., & Lenfant, C. (1989). Regional and racial differences among stroke victims in the United States. *Clinical Cardiology, 12*(IV), 1213-1220.

Rodnan, G.P., & Schumacher, H.R. (1983). *Primer on the rheumatic diseases* (ed. 8). Atlanta, Ga.: Arthritis Foundation.

Rouch, L. (1977). Color changes in dark skin. *Nursing '77, 7*(1), 48-51.

Saito, S., Okui, K., Tokino, T. et al.: (1992). Isolation and mapping of 68 RFLP markers on human chromosome 6. *American Journal of Human Genetics* *50*(1):65-70.

Saldana, G., & Brown, H.E. (1984). Nutritional composition of corn and flour tortillas. *Journal of Food Science, 49*(4), 202.

Satcher, D., & Pope, L. (1974). *Emergency evaluation and management of persons with sickle cell disease.* Bethesda, Md.: National Institutes of Health.

Satcher, D., et al. (1973). *Sickle cell counseling: a committee's study and recommendations.* New York: National Foundation-March of Dimes.

Saunders, E. (1985). Special techniques for management of hypertension in blacks. In Hall, W.D., Saunders, E., & Shulman, N.B. (Eds.), *Hypertension in blacks: epidemiology, pathophysiology, and treatment* (pp. 209-236). St. Louis: Mosby.

Schwerin, H.S., Stanton, J.L., & Smith, J.L. (1982). Food, eating habits, and health: a further examination of the relationships between food eating patterns and nutritional health. *American Clinical Nutrition, 35* (suppl. 5), 1319.

Shipley, S., & Sylvester, D. (1982). Professional attitude toward violence in close relationships. *Journal of Emergency Room Nursing, 8*(2), 88-91.

Siegel, R.K. (1979). Ginseng abuse syndrome: problems with the panacea. *Journal of the American Medical Association, 24*(15), 614.

Stark, E., & Flitcraft, A. (1982). Medical therapy as repression: the case of the battered woman. *Health Medicine, 1,* 29-32.

State of Maryland Demonstration of Statewide Coordination for the Control of High Blood Pressure (1977-1983, October). NHLBL Contract No. 1-HV-2986.

Stokes, J., Kannel, W., Wolf, P., et al. (1987). The relative importance of selected risk factors for various manifestations of cardiovascular disease among men and women from 35 to 64 years old: 30 years of follow-up in the Framingham study. *Circulation, 75*(6): 65-73.

Strickland, O., & Giger, J. (1994). Women's health in the decade of the woman. In Strickland, O., & Fishman, D. (Eds.), *Nursing issues in the 1990s* (pp. 362-400). Albany, N.Y.: Delmar.

Surgeon General. (1987, April). Speech to the media and the nation on AIDS.

Taylor, M.A., & Abrams, B. (1978). The prevalence of schizophrenia: a reassessment using modern diagnostic criteria. *American Journal of Psychiatry, 135,* 945-948.

Tipton, D. (1974, May). Physiological assessment of black people. In Care of black patients (X428.1). A group of papers presented at a conference on care of the black patient, sponsored by Continuing Education in Nursing, University of California, San Francisco.

U.S. Department of Health and Human Services, Healthy people 2000 (1991). *National health promotion and disease prevention objectives* (DHHS Publication No. PHS 91-50212). Washington, D.C.: Government Printing Office.

Valassi, K.V. (1962). Food habits of Greek Americans. *American Journal of Nursing, 11*(3), 240.

Vessell, E.S. (1972). Therapy-pharmacogenetics. *New England Journal of Medicine, 287*(18), 904-909.

Walsh, E. (1993). The patient with peripheral vascular problems. In Long, B.C., Phipps, W.J., & Cassmeyer, V. (Eds.), *Medical surgical nursing: concepts and clinical practice* (pp. 705-742). St. Louis: Mosby.

Westfall, D. (1971, Nov.). Diabetes mellitus among the Florida Seminoles. *HSMHA Health Reports, 86,* 1037-1041.

When patients can't drink milk. (1976, Aug.). *Nursing Update,* pp. 10-12.

Williams, R.A. (Ed.). (1975). *Textbook of black-related disease.* New York: McGraw-Hill.

Witcop, E., et al. (1963). Oral and genetic studies of Chileans, 1960: 1. Oral anomalies. *American Journal of Physical Anthropology, 21,* 15-24.

World Health Organization. (1976). *Schizophrenia: a multinational study.* Geneva: World Health Organization Press.

Wyngaarden, J.B., & Smith, L.H. (Eds.) (1985). *Cecil textbook of medicine.* Philadelphia: W.B. Saunders.

Yonkers, K.A., Kando, J.C., Cole, J.O., & Blumenthal, S. (1992). Gender differences in pharmacokinetics and pharmacodynamics of psychotropic medication. *American Journal of Psychiatry, 149*(5), 587-595.

Zhou, H.H., Koshakji, R.P., Silberstein, D.J., et al. (1989). Racial differences in drug response: altered sensitivity to and clearance of propranolol in men of Chinese descent as compared with American Whites. *New England Journal of Medicine, 320,* 565-570.

Zifferblatt, S.M., Wilbur, C.S., & Pinsky, J.L. (1980). Understanding food habits. *Journal of American Diet Association, 76*(1), 9.

Application of Assessment and Intervention Techniques to Specific Cultural Groups

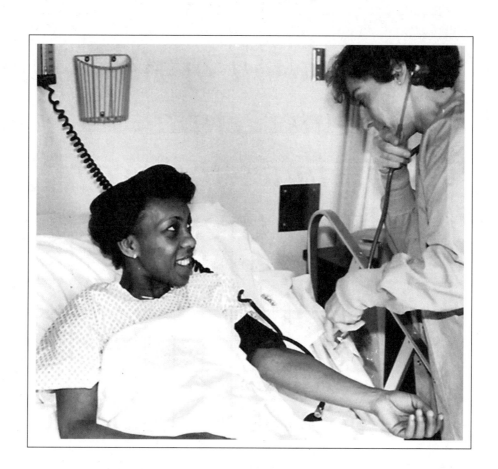

CHAPTER 8 African Americans

Brenda Cherry and Joyce Newman Giger

BEHAVIORAL OBJECTIVES

After reading this chapter, the nurse will be able to:

1. Identify ways in which the African-American culture influences African-American individuals and health-seeking behaviors.
2. Recognize the need for an in-depth understanding of variables that are common within and across cultural groups to provide culturally appropriate nursing care when working with African Americans.
3. Recognize physical and biological variances that exist within and across African-American groups to provide culturally appropriate nursing care.
4. Develop a sensitivity and an understanding for communication differences evidenced within and across African-American groups to avoid stereotyping and to provide culturally appropriate nursing care.
5. Develop a sensitivity and an understanding for psychological phenomena that influence the functioning of an African American when providing nursing care.

In a time when people are seeking to become more culturally aware, it is important to note distinctions in terminology regarding cultural groups. This is certainly true of African Americans. Some African-American individuals and groups are encouraging the use of the term "Black Americans," whereas others are encouraging the use of the term "African Americans." The term "African Americans" is used to refer to a cultural heritage that is a combination of African and American. On the other hand, the term "Black Americans" is believed to place more focus on biological racial identity than on cultural heritage. The term "African Americans" is used in this book except in instances where its descriptive characteristic is inappropriate, for example, Black skin, Black race, non-Black, Black English, and Black dialect. We have chosen this term because it is now commonly used in the literature. As a note: the hyphen is used only when the compound adjective appears before a noun.

OVERVIEW OF AFRICAN AMERICANS

According to the United States Census Bureau, there are approximately 34,333,000 African Americans residing in the United States, who represent approximately 12.7% of the American population (U.S. Department of Commerce, Bureau of the Census, Internet release, 1998). Of the number of African Americans residing in this country, 53.0% live in the South, 19% live in the Midwest, 19% live in the Northeast, and 9.0% live in the West (U.S. Department of Commerce, Bureau of the Census, 1993b).

Although African Americans live throughout the United States, the states with the greatest number of African Americans are New York (2,859,000), California (2,209,000), Texas (2,022,000), Florida (1,760,000), and Georgia (1,747,000).

The cities with the largest number of African Americans are metropolitan New York (2,103,000), Chicago (1,080,000), Detroit (778,000), Philadelphia (632,000), and Los Angeles (488,000) (U.S. Department of Commerce, Bureau of the Census, 1993b). In 1991, African Americans represented more than 50% of the total population in five United States cities: Detroit (778,000), Washington, D.C. (400,000), New Orleans (308,000), Baltimore (436,000), and Memphis (335,000) (U.S. Department of Commerce, Bureau of the Census, 1993b).

The median age of African Americans residing in the United States is 29.9 years, compared with 33 years for the rest of the general population (U.S. Department of Commerce, Bureau of the Census, Internet release, 1998). This number is up from 25 years of age in 1980. African-American men have a lower mean age than African-American women. In 1990, only 8.4% of African Americans were 65 years of age or older, compared with 14% of their White counterparts and 13% of the rest of the general population. The number of African Americans 65 years of age or older was 2.5 million in 1990 (up from 2.1 million in 1980). It is interesting to note, however, that African-American women dominated the older age groups (62%), compared with their male counterparts (38%). It is believed that the disproportionately low number of African-American males 65 years of age or older is a result of the higher mortality for African-American males (U.S. Department of Commerce, Bureau of the Census, 1993b).

In 1990, 66.2% of African-American males 25 years of age or older held a high school diploma, compared with 78.5% of their White male counterparts. Similarly, 63.8% of African-American women 25 years of age or older held a high school diploma, compared with 77.4% of their White counterparts. In 1990, 11.0% of African-American males 25 years of age or older held a bachelor's degree or higher, compared with 25.3% of White males. Among African-American women, 11.7% held a bachelor's

or higher degree, compared with 18.4% of White women (U.S. Department of Commerce, Bureau of the Census, 1993b). In 1989, 62.7% of African Americans participated in the work force, compared with 65.4% of Whites. In addition, African Americans are less likely to participate in the work force than other racial and ethnic groups.

From the sixteenth to the nineteenth centuries, more than 10 million Africans were brought to the United States and bonded into slavery (Ploski & Williams, 1989). By historical accounts, nearly 600,000 slaves arrived in the United States in the sixteenth century, 2,000,000 in the seventeenth century, 5,000,000 in the eighteenth century, and 3,000,000 in the nineteenth century (Ploski & Williams, 1989). Because of these historical accounts, the perception held by most Americans is that African Americans may be the only cultural and ethnic group who reside in the United States today who did not immigrate to this country voluntarily. Although this perception has merit, in reality, the history of the arrival of Africans in the United States has become somewhat distorted throughout the years. In actuality, many Europeans (meaning those persons of English, German, and Scotch-Irish ancestry) voluntarily immigrated to the American colonies as laborers and became "indentured servants" (Ploski & Williams, 1989). Many of these people were paupers or debtors who used indentured servitude to gain a better way of life.

The first 20 African Americans to land at Jamestown in 1619 (preceding the *Mayflower*) were accepted into the community as "indentured servants." Although it is true that these 20 African Americans did not have freedom of choice in the decision to come to the colonies because they were systematically captured against their will, they nonetheless, over the same course of time (7 years), enjoyed the same liberties and privileges of the "free working class," including the right to own property (Ploski & Williams, 1989).

Two of the most notable African Americans who arrived in this country as "indentured servants" were Anthony Johnson, who became a "freeman" as early as 1622, and Richard Johnson. Anthony Johnson prospered so well that by 1651, he himself was able to acquire five "indentured servants." Likewise, Richard Johnson, having been given 100 acres of land of his own, acquired two indentured servants by 1654, two of whom were White (Ploski & Williams, 1989). However, it is appropriate to note that both of these men were the exception, not the rule. In fact, a fissure was cracking open, and African-American servitude and White servitude were beginning to be viewed differently. By 1640, African Americans had ceased to be viewed as servants and were assigned the status of chattel (meaning one who remained a fixed item of personal property for the duration of life).

In 1661, the Virginia House of Burgesses formally recognized the institution of African-American slavery (Ploski & Williams, 1989). Of the 13 original colonies, only Pennsylvania protested the system of slavery. By 1667, Virginia had written into its statutes that even purifying the African-American soul through baptism could not alter the condition of the African-American regarding bondage or freedom. Thus, color became the real "cutting edge" that separated the African, now American, from the rest of the colonists (Ploski & Williams, 1992).

Even today, the cultural roots of African Americans are entrenched in the African-American life experience. According to Bloch (1983), it is the African-American life experience that has established what has become known as the African-American view of the external world. The African-American life experience has shaped the internal attitudes and belief systems of African Americans, and it continues to influence interactions of African Americans with persons from other cultural groups.

Some of the health problems noted particularly in African Americans are believed to be the result of varying genetic pools and hereditary immunity. However, many of these problems have been found to be more closely associated with economic status than with race. Three intervening and reinforcing variables include poverty, discrimination, and social and psychological barriers. These variables are regarded as being so profound in their effect on African Americans that they tend to keep these individuals from using the health care services that are available. These variables may also explain why morbidity and mortality rates are higher among African

Americans than for the rest of the general population. Although underrepresented in the general population, African Americans remain overrepresented among the health statistics for life-threatening illness.

The life expectancy for African Americans continues to lag behind that for Whites. The life expectancy for African Americans is 71.0 years, compared with 76.4 years for Whites (U.S. Department of Commerce, Bureau of the Census, 1993a). African-Americans continue to have a higher infant mortality (11.2 per 1000 live births in 1993), compared with White Americans (9.4 per 1000 live births in 1993) (National Center for Health Statistics, Healthy People 2000 Review, 1993). Although the average life expectancy for African Americans at birth edged upward to the low 70s, it is important to note that the life expectancy for African-American male babies born between 1986 and 1988 actually shrank (NCHS, Healthy People 2000 Review, 1993). A portion of the shrinkage is attributable to infant mortality, which is twice as high for African-American babies, compared with White babies. Yet another portion of the shrinkage is attributable to disparities in health concerns, especially chronic illnesses, that contribute significantly to premature deaths before 65 years of age among African-American males. In fact, in 1987, the rate of deaths for African-American males was 55% higher for heart disease, 26% higher for cancer, 180% higher for stroke, and 100% higher for lung disease than for the rest of the general U.S. population (NCHS, Healthy People 2000 Review, 1993). Perhaps the greatest disparity was the rate of deaths or the potential for life lost for African-American males attributable to homicides, which was 630% higher, compared with White males (NCHS, Healthy People 2000 Review, 1993). In health status disparities, African-American women do not fare much better than their male counterparts. When the life expectancy of White women is compared with the life expectancy of African-American women, the data indicate that African-American women have a shorter life expectancy compared with their White counterparts (73.4 years versus 78.9 years) (NCHS, Healthy People 2000 Review, 1993).

COMMUNICATION

Communication is the matrix for thought and relationship between all people regardless of cultural heritage (Murray & Huelskoetter, 1991). Verbal and nonverbal communication is learned in cultural settings. Difficulties arise if a person does not communicate in the way or manner prescribed by the culture because the individual cannot conform to social expectation. Communication, therefore, is basic to culturally appropriate nursing care.

Dialect

Dialect refers to the variations within a language. African Americans speak English; however, there are widespread differences in the way English is spoken between African Americans and other ethnic and cultural groups. Different linguistic norms evolve among groups of people who are socially or geographically separated. Social stratification alters the nature and frequency of intercommunication between groups. When social separation by factors such as ethnic origin or class is responsible for the origin and perpetuation of a particular dialect, the dialect is referred to as a stratified dialect. When differences in dialect emerge as a result of geographical separation of people, the dialect is called a "regional, or geographical, dialect."

Origins of African-American dialect in the United States Accurate and reliable data concerning the different dialects spoken by most African Americans are unavailable to the public or to educators (Turner, 1948). The study of pidgin and Creole language has facilitated an intelligent study of Black English and of the notable differences between Black English and Standard English (Hymes, 1970). Research into the languages of Brazilians of African descent, as well as Haitians, Jamaicans, and the present-day African-American inhabitants off the seacoasts of South Carolina and Georgia, indicates a correlation of structural features of several of the languages spoken in parts of West Africa as well as a similarity to the English spoken by Whites in the United States (Hymes, 1970).

The first Africans brought to the United States as slaves were systematically separated during transportation, and this separation continued after arrival. As a result, the various African languages combined with the languages of other cultural groups in the New World, such as the Dutch, the French, and the English. This combination of the different African languages with other different languages fostered a need for a "common language" for all African Americans, which ultimately led to the restructuring of grammar of all language, including English. This process is referred to as "pidginization" and "creolization." Pidgin English is not a language but a dialect. Pidgin tends to be simple in grammar and limited in vocabulary. Typically, in communities where pidgin is spoken, its use is limited to trade purposes, task-oriented activities, and communication between cultural or ethnic groups (Hymes, 1970). When a pidgin dialect undergoes internal expansion and extension of use, the results are creolization. It is from a pidgin dialect that a Creole language was born. In the United States several Creole dialects developed that still exist, particularly in the rural South in such places as New Orleans, Louisiana; Hattiesburg and Vicksburg, Mississippi; and Mobile, Alabama. Furthermore, the migration of African-Americans from the South saw the development of pidginization and creolization in some northern cities such as New York, Chicago, and Detroit. Evidences of past migration and its effect on dialect and Black English remain obvious even today.

Language usage The dialect that is spoken by many African Americans is sufficiently different from Standard English in pronunciation, grammar, and syntax so as to be classified as "Black English." The use of Standard English versus Black English varies among African Americans and in some instances may be related to educational level and socioeconomic status, though this is not always the case. The use of Standard English by African Americans is important in terms of social and economic mobility. However, the use of Black English has served as a unifying factor for African Americans in maintaining their cultural and ethnic identity. It is not uncommon for some African Americans to speak Standard English when serving in a professional capacity or when socializing with Whites and then revert to Black English when interacting in all African-American settings. Some African Americans who have not mastered Standard English may feel insecure in certain situations where they are required and expected to use Standard English. When confronted with such situations, they may become very quiet, with the result that they may be labeled hostile or submissive.

Pronunciation of Black English

There is a tendency for users of what is often referred to as "Black dialect" to pronounce certain syllables and consonants somewhat differently. For example, *th,* as in *the, these,* or *them,* may be pronounced as *d,* as in *de, des,* and *dem* (Dillard, 1972; Wolfram & Clark, 1971). In Black English there is also a tendency to drop the final *r* or *g* from words; thus *father* and *mother* becomes *fatha* and *motha.* The words *laughing, talking,* and *going* are pronounced *laughin, talkin,* and *goin.* Speakers of Black English may also place more emphasis on one syllable as opposed to another; for example, *brother* may be pronounced *bro-tha.* In addition, the final *th* of words is pronounced as *f* in Black English; thus *bath, birth, mouth,* and *with* are pronounced *baf, birf, mouf,* and *wif.*

Copula deletion of the verb "to be" is a common omission in some environments; for example, the speaker of Black English might say, "He walking" or "She at work" in contrast to the Standard English, "He is walking" or "She is at work." Black English speakers may also use the unconjugated form of the verb "to be" where Standard English speakers would use the conjugated form. An example of this would be, "He be working" in contrast to the Standard English, "He is working."

In Standard English every verb is in sequence and must be marked as either present or past tense. However, in Black English only past tense verbs need to be marked. For example, in Black English the *s* marking the present tense may be omitted, thus "He go" or "She love." Attempts to correct this can result in phrases such as "I goes" and "We loves." Speakers of Black English may also omit the possessive suffix. For example, in Black English one might say, "Richard dog bit me" or "Mary dress," in contrast to the Standard English, "Richard's dog bit me" or "Mary's dress" (Dillard, 1972).

Speakers of Black English also have some words that are classified as slang. These words are different from slang words used in other dialects and may or may not convey the same meaning. For instance, African Americans may use the word *chilly* or *chillin* to infer sophistication, whereas a White individual may use the word *cool* or (formerly) *groovy* to convey the same meaning. Some African Americans may use the verb "to fix" to denote planned actions, for example, "I'm fixin to go home," whereas the user of Standard English would say, "I am getting ready to go home."

The speech of some African Americans is very colorful and dynamic. For these persons, communication also involves body movement (kinesics). Some African Americans tend to use a wide range of body movement, such as facial gestures, hand and arm movements, expressive stances, handshakes, and hand signals, along with verbal interaction. This repertoire of body movements can also be seen in sports and in dance, which is the highest communicative form of body language.

Some African Americans will use sounds that are not words to add expression to their conversation or to music, such as *oo-wee* or *uh huh,* which have analogies in some of the West African languages as expressed in the surviving Gullah dialect (Sea Islands, South Carolina) but not in English.

The term *signifying* describes an approach wherein one attempts to chide or correct someone indirectly. For example, one might correct someone who is not dressed properly by saying, "You sure are dressed up today."

Most African Americans use Black English in a systematic way that can be predictably understood by others; thus Black English cannot and should not be regarded as substandard or ungrammatical. It is estimated that approximately 80% of African Americans use Black English at least some of the time (Dillard, 1972).

Implications for nursing care

The nurse must develop a sensitivity to communication variances as a prerequisite for accurate nursing assessment and intervention in multicultural situations. In all nursing environments the potential for misunderstanding the client is accentuated when the nurse and the client are from different ethnic groups. Perhaps the most significant and obvious barrier occurs when two persons speak different languages. However, the nurse must be cognizant of the fact that barriers to communication exist even when individuals speak the same language. The nurse may have difficulty explaining things to a client in simple, jargon-free language to facilitate the client's understanding. The nurse must develop a familiarity with the language of the client because this is the best way to gain insight into the culture. Every language and dialect is special and has a unique way of looking at the world and at experiences (Kluckhohn, 1972). Every language also has a set of unconscious assumptions about the world and life. According to Kluckhohn (1972), people see and hear what the grammatical system of their language makes them sensitive to perceive.

The nurse who works with African-American clients may find that although the language is the same the perception of what message is being sent and received by the nurse and the client may be different. Therefore it is of the highest priority for the nurse who is working with African Americans, particularly those who speak Black English, to understand as much of the context of the dialect as possible.

The nurse must bear in mind that Black English cannot be viewed as an unacceptable form of English. Thus it is important for the nurse to avoid labeling and stereotyping the client. The nurse should avoid chiding and correcting the speech of African Americans because this behavior can result in the client's becoming quiet, passive, and, in some cases, aggressive or hostile. On the other hand, although the nurse should attempt to use words common to the client's vocabulary, mimicking the client's language can be interpreted as dehumanizing. For example, if a nurse were to say *dem* for *them,* or *dese* for *these,* the client may perceive this as ridicule.

When working with persons who speak Black English, the nurse must keep in mind that the client may use slang to convey certain messages. However, slang terms often have different meanings between individuals and especially between cultural groups. For example, an African-American client's response to questioning about a diagnostic test, "It was a real bad experience," may actually mean that it was

a unique and yet positive experience. The nurse working with this client will need to clarify the exact meaning of the word *bad*. In Black English the word *bad* is often used for the exact opposite, in other words, 'good'. In another example, an African-American client who states that the medication has been taken "behind the meal" may mean the medication has been taken 'after eating'. A nurse may interpret *behind* to mean 'before' rather than 'after' because the dictionary definition states that *behind* means 'still to come'. The nurse must be cautious about interpreting particular words each time an African American uses certain terms.

It is essential that the nurse identify and clarify what is happening psychologically and physiologically to the African-American client. When possible, the nurse should substitute words commonly understood by the African-American client for more sophisticated medical terms. When this is done, the nurse will find that the African-American client is more receptive to instructions and more cooperative. Stokes (1977) offers a list of terms commonly used by nurses and equivalent words used by some African-Americans:

Conditions (medical/Black English)	Functions (medical/Black English)
Diabetes/sugar	Constipation/locked bowels
Pain/miseries	Diarrhea/running off, grip
Syphilis/bad blood, pox	Menstruation/red flag, the curse
Anemia/low blood, tired blood	Urinate, urine/pass water, tinkle, peepee
Vomiting/throw up	

The nurse must remember that some African Americans place a great deal of importance on nonverbal elements of communication and that the verbal pattern of some African-American clients may differ significantly from that of a non-African-American nurse. It is also important for the nurse to remember that words used by some African-American clients may be the same as those used by the nurse but have different, idiosyncratic meanings. When working with African-American clients, the nurse must also remember that eye contact, nodding, and smiling are not necessarily essential or direct correlates that the African-American client is paying attention (Sue, 1981).

SPACE

According to Hall (1966), the degree to which people are sensorially involved with each other, along with how they use time, determines not only at what point they feel crowded or have a perception that their personal space is collapsing inwardly, but the methods for alleviating crowding as well. For example, Puerto Ricans and African Americans are reported to have a much higher involvement ratio than other cultural groups such as German Americans or Scandinavian Americans. It is believed that highly involved people, such as African Americans, require a higher density than less involved people. However, highly involved people may at the same time require more protection or screening from outsiders than people with a lower level of involvement do.

To understand the variable of space, it is essential to understand time and the way it is handled because the variable of time influences the structuring of space. According to Hall (1966), there are two contrasting ways in which people handle time, monochronic and polychronic, and each affects the way in which an individual perceives space. People with low involvement are generally monochronic because such individuals tend to compartmentalize time; for example, they may schedule one thing at a time and tend to become disoriented if they have to deal with too many things at once. On the other hand, polychronic individuals tend to keep several operations going at once, almost like jugglers, and these individuals tend to be very involved with each other.

Implications for nursing care

The nurse who works with Latin Americans, Africans, African Americans, or Indonesians may feel somewhat uncomfortable because these cultures generally dictate a much closer personal space when personal and social spaces are involved (Sue, 1981). Because some African Americans are perceived as polychronic individuals, it is important for the nurse to remember that polychronic individuals tend to collect activities.

When polychronic individuals interact with monochronic individuals, some difficulties may be experienced because of the different ways in which these individuals relate to space and to each other. An example of a difficulty encountered between monochronic and polychronic individuals is when monochronic individuals become upset or angry because of the constant interruptions of polychronic individuals.

Some monochronic individuals believe that there must be order to get things done. On the other hand, polychronic individuals, such as some African Americans, do not believe that order is necessary to get things done. The nurse who works with African Americans must keep in mind that, to reduce polychronic effects, it is necessary to reduce multiple-activity involvements on the part of the client. The nurse can accomplish this by separating activities with as much screening and scrutiny as necessary (Hall, 1966). One goal of nursing intervention should be to help the client structure activities in a ranked order that will produce maximal benefits for the client.

SOCIAL ORGANIZATION

Social organization refers to how a cultural group organizes itself around particular units (such as family, racial or ethnic group, and community or social group). Most African Americans have been socialized in predominantly African-American environments. Historically, because of legalized segregation, African Americans were separated or isolated from the mainstream of society. Consequently, African Americans are the only cultural group in the United States that has not been assimilated into the mainstream society. Even today, African Americans maintain separate and in most cases unequal lifestyles, compared with other Americans. Evidence of the failure to assimilate on the part of African Americans is seen in the existence of predominantly African-American neighborhoods, churches, colleges and universities, and public elementary and high schools.

Historical review of slavery and discrimination

Patterns of discrimination have existed in the United States since the inception of slavery. With the inception of slavery came the foundations of attitudes and beliefs that were and continued to be the pillars that support the institution of racism. Racism, discriminatory practices, and segregation combined have produced insularity or separatist feelings and attitudes on the part of some African Americans. As a result, African Americans are often accused of having more separate and more insular patterns of communication, which have restricted some African Americans from participating in the wider White society. Thus some African Americans prefer to maintain themselves within their own group. Accordingly, this insularity has promoted the retention of culturally seeded beliefs that differ from the beliefs held by the dominant culture. Leininger (1978) noted that every cultural group has unique beliefs that influence their attitudes regarding health. These beliefs tend to determine the type of behavior and health care practices that a particular cultural group views as appropriate or inappropriate. In other words, the attitudes and beliefs regarding health and illness vary in the United States between African Americans and Whites and even among African Americans themselves.

Attitudes, beliefs, values, and morals are the basic structural units of any culture. Culture is an outward manifestation of a way of life; it is dynamic, fluid, and ever evolving. The family is the basic social unit of most cultures and is the means by which culture is passed down from one generation to the next. The inception of slavery in the United States precipitated the beginning of the destruction of the transplanted African culture. In Africa, Africans had been accustomed to a strictly regulated family life with rigidly enforced moral codes. The family unit was closely knit, well organized, connected with kin and community, and highly functional for the economic, social, psychological, and spiritual well-being of the people (Jones, 1966). The family was the center of African civilization.

The destruction of the African family began with the capture of slaves for transplantation to the New World, which began in 1619. As slaves were captured, the young, healthy men and women and children were forcibly removed from their families and tribes. This separation continued as these slaves journeyed to the New World because they were placed on ships without regard for family unity, tribe, or kinship. On the arrival of the slaves in the United States, this systematic separation of individuals from families continued.

The cruelest form of emasculation of the Black Africans, now Americans, was the breeding of slaves for sale. Infants and children were taken from their mothers and sold as chattel. Marriage between slaves was not legally sanctioned and was generally left to the discretion of the owners. Some slave owners assigned mates when slaves reached breeding age. Others would not permit their slaves to marry a slave from another plantation. Most slave owners sold husbands, wives, and children without consideration for family ties. The children who were produced of the slave union belonged to the slave owner, not to the parents. The African-American family in the United States during slavery lacked autonomy because the family members were someone else's property. The parents were unable to provide security or protection for their children. Husbands were unable to protect their wives. In a documentary of the lives of 75 African-American women, Angelou (1989) describes the heartbreaking tenderness of African-American women and the majestic strength they needed to survive the subjugation and horror of the slavery experience.

In contrast to the above view of the destruction of the African-American family during slavery, Gutman (1976) contends that the African-American family was not disaggregated because of slavery. In fact, Gutman (1976) presents compelling evidence to suggest not only that some African-American families remained intact during slavery, but also many slave marriages were officially documented as the names of their offspring were. Gutman (1976) cautions, however, that no more misleading inference could be drawn from these data than to argue that the data alone show that slaves lived in stable families.

Changing roles of the African-American family

Under the system of slavery in the United States, the role of the African-American man as husband and father was obliterated. The African-American man was not the head of the household, nor was he the provider or the protector of his family. Instead, he was someone else's property. Under the system of slavery, the African-American man remained powerless to defend his wife and children from harm, particularly when they were beaten or sexually assaulted by the White overseer or owner or by any White person. The African-American male slave was often referred to as "boy" until he reached a certain age, at which point he became "uncle." The only crucial function for the African-American man within the African-American family was siring children.

In the United States under the system of slavery, the African-American woman became the dominant force in the family. She was forced to work side by side with her male counterpart during the day and additionally had the responsibility of caring for family members at night. The African-American woman was forced to bear children for sale and to care for other children, including those of the slave owner. Some African-American women during slavery were also forced to satisfy the sexual desires of any White man, and any children born out of this union were considered slaves. If the African-American woman had a husband, he was merely her sexual companion and was referred to as her "boy" by the slave owner and by White society in general. The inception of slavery, the division of the African family and subsequently the African-American family, and the subordinate role of the African-American man played a significant part in the establishment of the female-dominated African-American household that exists even today in the United States.

Even after slavery was abolished in the United States, the destructive forces against the African-American family persisted. Today, the residual effects of slavery are still evident in some parts of the country. After slavery was abolished and during the emancipation period and the years that followed, the African-American man was either denied jobs or given tasks that were demeaning and dehumanizing. From the time of the abolition of slavery until the mid-1960s, African-Americans in some parts of the country were attacked, lynched, and murdered. Sexual attacks on African-American women also continued. Such actions further served to drive some African-American men away from their families. Thus there was further weakening of the family and subsequently of the African-American male role (Bullough & Bullough, 1982).

Despite the discriminatory practices and the continued hostile attacks against African Americans, some African-American families nevertheless were able to establish themselves. As these African-American families were increasingly able to develop a secure economic status, they began to establish schools, churches, and other social organizations.

Characteristics of the African-American family

In the United States there are basically two types of family structures: the male-headed (patriarchal) family structure and the female-headed (matriarchal) family structure. The number of African-American female-headed households doubled between 1950 and 1991. Today, such families constitute 46% of African-American families. In addition, between 1950 and 1991 the number of African-American female-headed householders who had never been married quadrupled, from 9% in 1950 to 41% in 1991 (U.S. Department of Commerce, Bureau of the Census, 1992). The fact that approximately half of the African-American families in the United States are female-headed is attributable in part to factors related to and carried over from slavery. For example, the African-American family has not been able to overcome deficits related to education and income. According to the U.S. Department of Commerce, Bureau of the Census (1993a), the average income for African-American men, compared with men in other cultural groups with similar skills and educational levels, is significantly lower. African-American males, in particular, have not made significant strides in gaining entry into the work force since the 1980 census. The annual labor participation for African-American males was 69.5 in 1991, compared with 70.6 in 1980. In addition, the annual salary for African-American males remains disproportionately low, compared with their White counterparts. The annual salary for African-American males 25 years of age or older with less than a high school education was $16,832, compared with $19,560 for their White counterparts. Similarly, for African-American males 25 years of age or older with a high school diploma, the annual salary was $20,271, compared with $26,526 for their White counterparts. For African-American males 25 years of age and older with 4 years or more of college, the annual salary was $32,145, compared with $41,661 for their White counterparts (U.S. Department of Commerce, Bureau of the Census, 1992).

Implications for nursing care

Even today, the African-American family is often oriented around women; in other words, it is matrifocal. This has implications for the nurse because within the African-American family structure the wife or mother is often charged with the responsibility for protecting the health of the family members. The African-American woman is expected to assist each family member in maintaining good health and in determining treatment if a family member is ill. This responsibility has both positive and negative effects because African-American clients often enter the health care delivery system at the advice of the matriarch of the family. The nurse must recognize the importance of the African-American woman in disseminating information and in assisting the client in making decisions. Although the African-American family may be matrifocal, it is nevertheless essential to include the African-American man in the decision-making process.

Some African-American families are composed of large networks and tend to be very supportive during times of crisis and illness. Large-network groups can have both positive and negative effects on wellness, illness, and recovery behaviors. Jackson, Neighbors, and Gurin (1986) found that network size was positively related to distress: the more informal helpers there were, the higher the distress score on the instrument used in the survey. One conclusion of the study is that network size is not a good measure of perceived social support. According to the findings from the study, the more serious the problem, the more people within the network are consulted for help. But the more people consulted does not necessarily reduce the severity of the problem; rather, an individual with an acute illness may spend so much time seeking assistance within the network that necessary and timely treatment is delayed. The nurse should include all the members of the network in planning and implementing health care because

some members of the network may provide advice or care that could be detrimental to the client. For example, an African-American client who is admitted with an electrolyte imbalance and is brought laxatives from home by a relative may have additional electrolyte problems when the laxatives are taken without consulting members of the health care team. In this case the nurse must emphasize the importance of the nurse's role in providing health care. Once the family develops a feeling of trust, the nurse is more likely to be consulted should perceived health needs arise, for example, when the client needs a laxative.

TIME

Time is a concept that is universal and continuous. All emotional and perceptual experiences are interrelated with the concept of time. The perception of time is individual and is determined by cultural experience (Hall, 1976). In the United States, time has become the most important organizing principle of the dominant culture (Hall, 1976). The majority of individuals of the dominant culture are time conscious and very future oriented; they make it a common practice to "plan ahead" and "save for a rainy day." Time has become very important and comparable to money in the American society. Doing things efficiently and faster has become the American way.

It is impossible to characterize African Americans and their perceptions of time as one way or the other because African Americans, just as individuals from other cultural groups, vary according to social and cultural factors. Some African Americans who have become assimilated into the dominant culture are very time conscious and take pride in punctuality. These individuals are likely to be future oriented and believe that saving and planning are important. They are likely to be well educated and to hold professional positions, though this is not always the case, because some African Americans who are not well educated and do not hold professional jobs still value time and have hopes for the future (they are likely to encourage their children to seek higher education and to save for the future) (Poussaint & Atkinson, 1970).

On the other hand, some African Americans react to the present situation and are not future oriented; it is their belief that planning for the future is hopeless because of their previous experiences and encounters with racism and discrimination. They believe that their future will be the same as their present and their past (Poussaint & Atkinson, 1970). These individuals are likely to be jobless or have low-paying jobs. Educational levels may vary from junior high school to college degrees among persons who share this belief. Such individuals are unlikely to value time; thus they do not value the concept of punctuality and may not keep appointments or may arrive much later than the scheduled time. It is the belief of some African Americans that time is flexible and that events will begin when they arrive. This belief has been translated down through the years to imply an acceptable lateness among some African-Americans of 30 minutes to 1 hour. This perception of time can be traced back to West Africa, where the concept of time was elastic and encompassed events that had already taken place as well as those that would occur immediately (Mbiti, 1970).

Finally, some African Americans have a future-oriented concept of time because of their strong religious beliefs. These individuals may be from all socioeconomic and educational levels. It is their belief that life on earth, with all its pain and suffering, is bearable because there will be happiness and lack of pain after death. African Americans who hold this belief plan their funerals and even purchase their grave plots long before their deaths (Smith, 1976).

Implications for nursing care

Because some African Americans perceive time as flexible and elastic, it is essential for the nurse to include the client and family in the planning and implementation of nursing care. When planning nursing care with the client and family, the nurse should emphasize events that have flexibility where time is concerned, such as morning care and bathing. On the other hand, the nurse must also emphasize events that have no flexibility where time is concerned and where delay in doing something, such as taking time-released medications or medications for certain conditions, would have serious implications

for the client's well-being. For example, a client with high blood pressure must be made to understand that the medication must be taken as and when prescribed, not as and when desired. A medication missed today cannot be made up by taking double the amount tomorrow. As another example, an insulin-dependent diabetic client cannot delay the time between meals.

Some African Americans are perceived as individuals with present-time orientations. Such persons may have a more flexible adherence to schedules and may believe that immediate concerns are more relevant than future concerns. Because appointment schedules may lack meaning, the nurse must emphasize the importance of adhering to the appointment schedule. If the nurse knows a particular client has a pattern of arriving late, the nurse may advise that client to arrive for scheduled appointments at least half an hour early. For the nurse who works with clients who are focused on the present, it is essential to avoid crisis-oriented nursing and promote preventive nursing (Sue, 1981).

ENVIRONMENTAL CONTROL
Health care benefits

In the United States the system of health care beliefs and practices is extremely complex and diverse among cultural groups. Variations in health care beliefs and practices cross ethnic and social boundaries. These variations are evidenced even within families. Culture influences individual expectations and perceptions regarding health, illness, disease, and symptoms related to disease. Accordingly, culture, cultural beliefs, and cultural values influence how one copes when confronted with illness, disease, or stress (Anderson & Bauwens, 1981).

In the United States a distinction between "illness" and "disease" has been made by anthropologists and sociologists (Staples, 1976). Illness has been defined as an individual's perception of being sick, which is not necessarily related to the biomedical definition of disease. Disease has been defined as a condition that deviates from the norm. Thus illness may exist in the absence of disease and vice versa (Staples, 1976). Norms used to determine a disease condition, using Western standards, have for the most part been taken from studies conducted on White subjects. Thus, when these norms are applied to other cultural groups, such as African Americans, the norm values may be meaningless and may lead to erroneous conclusions. For example, to receive a 2 for color on the Apgar scoring system for newborns, the infant must be completely pink. Another example of a Western norm expectation is that an inverted T wave may be an ominous, pathological finding. However, in the case of African Americans, and particularly African-American men, such a finding should be the expectation, rather than being perceived as ominous and pathological. Also, growth as related to body size and physique is often normed by White Western standards. Thus African Americans, who mature at an earlier age and typically have larger physiques than those of their White counterparts, may be perceived as being either overweight or oversized when White Western norms are applied.

Health care beliefs and the African-American family

African Americans in the United States are a highly heterogeneous group; thus, it is impossible to make a collective statement about their health care beliefs and practices. Many health care beliefs that are exhibited by African Americans in the United States are derived from their African ancestry (Smith, 1976). For example, in West Africa, where most African Americans originated, man was perceived as a monistic being, that is, a being from which the body and soul could not be separated (Smith, 1976). Man was also perceived as a holistic individual with many complex dimensions. Religion was interwoven into health care beliefs and practices. (West Africans continue even today to believe that illness is a natural occurrence resulting from disharmony and conflict in some area of the individual's life.) Because life was centered around the entire family, illness was perceived as a collective event and subsequently a disruption of the entire family system. The traditional West African healers always involved the individual's entire family in the healing process, even when the disorder was believed to be somatic. Thus the traditional West African healer based treatment on the premise of wholeness, the necessity for rein-

corporation of the client into the family system, and involvement of the entire family system in the care and treatment of the individual (Smith, 1976).

Perception of illness In the United States some African Americans perceive illness as a natural occurrence resulting from disharmony and conflict in some aspect of an individual's life. This belief is a cultural value that has been passed down through the generations to African Americans as a result of West African influences and tends to involve three general areas: (1) environmental hazards, (2) divine punishment, and (3) impaired social relationships (Snow, 1977). An example of an environmental hazard would be injuries as the result of being struck by lightning or being bitten by a snake. Divine punishment would include illnesses or diseases that the individual would attribute to sin. Impaired social relationships may be caused by such factors as a spouse leaving or parents disowning a child (Snow, 1977).

Another belief held by some African Americans is that everything has an opposite. For every birth, there must be a death; for every marriage, there must be a divorce; for every occurrence of illness, someone must be cured (Snow, 1978). Some African Americans may not be able to distinguish between physical and mental illness and spiritual problems and as a result may present themselves for treatment with a variety or combination of somatic, psychological, and spiritual complaints (Smith, 1976). For example, a client may present real symptoms of an ulcer but may relate the symptoms to past sins or grief over a financial loss. The client desires assistance not only for the somatic disorder, but also for the psychological and spiritual complaints.

African Americans who share mainstream attitudes about pain may respond to pain stoically out of a desire to be a perfect client. This means that they tend not to "bother" the nurse by calling for attention or for pain medication. For such clients the nurse must make it clear that the client has a right to relief from pain. On the other hand, some African-American clients exhibit a different form of stoicism. Hard experience has convinced them that trouble and pain are God's will. In this case the nurse needs to help the client understand that pain retards healing and is medically undesirable (LoBiondo-Wood, Zimmerman, & Gaston-Johansson, 1989).

Folk medicine

Folk medicine is germane to many cultural and ethnic groups. Individuals from all aspects of society may use folk medicine either alone or with a scientifically based medical system. The importance of folk medicine and the level of practice vary among the different ethnic and cultural groups, depending on education and socioeconomic status (Bullough & Bullough, 1982). In contrast to the scientifically based health care system in the United States, folk medicine is characterized by a belief in supernatural forces. From this perspective health and illness are characterized as natural and unnatural.

According to Snow (1983), it matters whether an African-American person comes from a rural background when it is necessary to select health care providers. Some African Americans who were reared in the rural South may have grown up being treated by folk practitioners and may not have encountered a physician until they reached adulthood. Therefore these people are more likely to turn to a neighborhood folk practitioner when they become ill. According to White (1977), folk medicine is still used within the African-American community because of humiliation encountered in the mainstream health care system, lack of money, and lack of trust in health care workers. Today, some African Americans go to physicians in order to get prescribed medications, not because they believe the physician is superior in knowledge or training (Murray & Huelskoetter, 1991).

Witchcraft, voodoo, and magic are an integral aspect of folk medicine (McKenzie & Chrisman, 1977). Natural events are those that are in harmony with nature and provide individuals who believe in and practice folk medicine with a certain degree of predictability in the events of daily living. Unnatural events, on the other hand, represent disharmony with nature, and so the events of day-to-day living cannot be predicted (Snow, 1983). Another aspect of the folk medicine system is a belief in opposing forces, or the belief that everything has an opposite. For example, for every birth, there must be a death.

Also incorporated into the system of folk medicine is the belief that health is a gift from God, whereas illness is a punishment from God or a retribution for sin and evil (Snow, 1983). This concept is evidenced by the belief held by some African Americans that if a child is born with a physical handicap, it is a punishment from God for the past wrongdoings of the parents. In this way, sins of the father and mother are passed on for retribution by the children (Snow, 1983). Such beliefs are not limited to African Americans but are also found among other cultural groups in the United States; for example, some Mexican Americans believe that illness is a punishment for some sin or misdeed (Snow, 1983).

Practice of African-American folk medicine There are still some African Americans in the rural South and in the urban northern ghettos who practice folk medicine based on spirituality, including witchcraft, voodoo, and magic (McKenzie & Chrisman, 1977). Some of these individuals may also use the orthodox medical system. Historically, such cities as New Orleans and Baton Rouge, Louisiana, were very much voodoo oriented, and such beliefs were held not only by African Americans, but also by members of other cultural groups. Even today, the African-American folk medicine system is practiced by the high-ranking voodoo queen in some Louisiana cities. The Louisiana Voodoo Society is a carryover from a combination of Haitian and French cultural influences (Mitchel, 1978). Voodoo and witchcraft are not restricted to Louisiana but are also practiced in such places as the Georgia sea islands, which are just off the coast of Savannah. Interestingly enough, some of the inhabitants of the Georgia sea islands remain pure-blooded descendants of West African ancestry. Even today, some inhabitants of the Georgia sea islands have refused to intermarry with members of other cultural groups, thus maintaining the tradition of "pure-blooded" lineage (Wolfram & Clark, 1971). Pure-blooded descendants of West Africans are also found off the coast of South Carolina. Very few of these people still speak Gullah (English with an admixture of various African languages) and tend to isolate themselves when possible from the mainstream of society (Wolfram & Clark, 1971).

African-American folk medicine system defined
In the system of African-American folk medicine, illness is perceived as either a natural or an unnatural occurrence. A natural illness may occur because of exposure to the elements of nature without protection (such as a cold, the flu, or pneumonia). Natural illnesses occur when dangerous elements in the environment enter the body through impurities in food, water, and air. However the words *natural* and *unnatural* are connoted to mean more or less than the dictionary definitions of these words. For example, cancer, which is linked to such environmental hazards as smog, cigarette smoke, toxic waste, and other chemical irritants, would be considered a natural illness in a professional medical system. However, those persons who share beliefs in African-American folk medicine might view cancer as an unnatural illness, perceiving it as a punishment from God or a spell cast by an evil person doing the work of the devil (Snow, 1974). Such persons may not readily acknowledge the fact that cancer, for example, may be caused by environmental factors such as cigarette smoking; thus they may continue smoking even after being diagnosed with cancer. Unnatural illnesses are perceived as either a punishment from God or the work of the devil. This perception is in contrast to the dictionary definition of illness as an unhealthy condition of the body or mind (Webster's, 1984).

Types of folk practitioners Jordan (1975) identified distinct types of folk practitioners. The first type is the "old lady" or "granny" who acts as a local consultant. This individual is knowledgeable about many different home remedies made from certain spices, herbs, and roots that can be used to treat common illnesses. Another duty of this individual is to give advice and make appropriate referrals to another type of practitioner when an illness or a particular medical condition extends beyond her practice (Jordan, 1975). The second type of practitioner is the "spiritualist," the most prevalent and diverse type of folk practitioner. This individual attempts to combine rituals, spiritual beliefs, and herbal medicines to effect a cure for certain illnesses or ailments. The third type of practitioner is the voodoo priest or priestess. In some West Indies islands, the voodoo

practitioner can be a man, whereas in some rural southern areas of the United States, the voodoo practitioner must be a woman and may inherit this title only by birthright and a perceived special gift (Snow, 1974).

In contrast to the type of voodoo priest or priestess found in some West Indies islands and in some rural or urban southern United States areas is the type of voodoo priest or priestess found in some larger urban areas such as Chicago; Queens or Jamaica, New York; or Los Angeles. In these cities the voodoo folk practitioner may be either male or female, does not have to inherit the right to practice by virtue of bloodline, and does not have to possess significantly powerful gifts (Snow, 1974). Historically, the voodoo priestess found in cities such as New Orleans must possess certain physical characteristics; that is, she must be African American, and more specifically, she must be of mixed ancestry, either an octoroon (a person of one-eighth Black ancestry) or a quadroon (a person of one-fourth Black ancestry) if her powers are to be superior (Snow, 1974).

Even today, some southern and northern African Americans still turn to one of these three types of practitioners when seeking medical advice. Educational level or socioeconomic status does not appear to alter or affect how some African Americans perceive folk practitioners. Similar views are shared by some members of other cultural groups. In the summer of 1988, newspaper articles throughout the United States carried the story that the first lady of the United States refused to make any moves or to allow her husband, the president of one of the most powerful countries in the world, to make decisions unless an astrologer was consulted.

Witchcraft: an alternative form of folk medicine
The practice of witchcraft is quite widespread and is not limited to the boundaries of the United States. Various degrees of witchcraft are practiced in countries throughout the world. In addition, the practice of witchcraft is not limited to any one particular cultural group. Persons who believe in witchcraft believe that it can be used not only to cure illness or disease but also to cause illness or disease. For example, strokes, dementia, and some gastrointestinal disorders may be perceived by some persons who

believe in witchcraft to be the direct result or influence of witchcraft (Henderson & Primeaux, 1981).

The practice of witchcraft is based on the belief that there are some individuals who possess the ability to mobilize the forces of good and evil. These abilities are based on the principles of sympathetic magic, which underlie many of the beliefs of folk medicine practice. The basic premise of sympathetic magic is that everything in the universe is connected. There is a direct connection between the body and the forces of nature. Interpretation and direction of events are accomplished by understanding these connections. Sympathetic magic is categorized into contagious and imitative magic. The basic premise of contagious magic is the perception that physically connected objects can never be separated; therefore, any actions against the parts constitute an action against the whole (Henderson & Primeaux, 1981). Individuals who practice witchcraft may use a piece of clothing or nail clippings from someone to cast an "evil" spell or to protect the individual. The basic premise of imitative magic is that like follows like, or that one will imitate what one desires to achieve. For example, a knife placed under the bed will cut pain; an evil charm put on when the moon is waxing will increase the moon.

A recurring theme in the practice of witchcraft is that of animals being in the body. Lizards, toads, snakes, and spiders are believed to be the most common types of intruders. These animals are dead and pulverized and are generally believed to enter the body by means of food or drink. It is not uncommon for persons who believe in witchcraft to refuse to eat or drink food prepared by someone they believe may have put a hex on them. Individuals who believe that such a spell has been cast on them may present themselves at health care facilities with symptoms described as "reptiles crawling over the body or snakes wiggling in their stomach." Some of these individuals may also share the belief that the physician is powerless to help them once they have been "hexed" (Jordan, 1979).

Perceptions concerning folk medicine and other alternative medical solutions The prevalence of the belief in and the use of folk medicine remedies and other alternative forms of health care is not fully understood (Jacques, 1976). It is impossible to generalize or postulate how widespread the use of folk medicine remedies is among African Americans. However, evidence does exist that there are some African Americans in all areas of the United States who believe in and practice folk medicine as well as other alternative forms of health care such as witchcraft, voodoo, and spiritualism (Snow, 1983). There is also evidence to support the notion that different levels of folk medicine are practiced (Jacques, 1976). The boundaries of folk healers for some African Americans may also vary. For example, the "granny" folk healer may possess the skills and knowledge to cure only simple illnesses or ailments. In contrast, a "witch doctor" is believed to possess supernatural powers that allow the "casting out of such things as animal demons" (Jordan, 1979). In addition, African-American folk medicine practitioners may have titles different from those of folk practitioners found in other cultural groups in the United States, such as "conjure doctor," "underworld man," "father divine," the "root doctor," and the "root worker" (Jacques, 1976).

Origins of African-American folk medicine African-American folk medicine practices in the United States can be traced back to regions of West Africa (Smith, 1976). There are also influences on African-American folk medicine that originated in other countries such as Haiti, Jamaica, and Trinidad (Smith, 1976). Because of slavery, there was a blending of various African tribes, particularly in slave cities and states such as New Orleans, Louisiana, and Savannah, Georgia, with other cultural groups such as the French, the Creoles, and the Indians. Various folk medicine practices found among some African Americans in the North and the South have been handed down from generation to generation. Even today, the consistent use of some form of African-American folk medicine continues, and such continuity indicates that these practices have withstood the test of time and are presumed to be valid, though no empirical data exist that would indicate the validity or reliability of such practices.

Rationale for the use of African-American folk medicine Some African Americans choose to use folk medicine because of tradition, whereas others have made this choice based on previous discriminatory practices and unfair treatments that have existed throughout some regions of the United States. In this regard, the delivery of health care services were not exempt from "Jim Crow" laws, which were legally sanctioned until the mid-1960s throughout the South. However, the northern regions of the United States also were not exempt from such discriminatory practices in regard to health care. This is evident in the passage of the Hill-Burton Act in 1946, which was not abolished until 1966 with the passage of the Federal Medicare Act (Bullough & Bullough, 1982).

The Hill-Burton Act, also known as the Hospital Construction Survey Act, provided federal grants for hospitals, both private and public, that admittedly did not service African Americans. Under this law, hospitals, whether private or public, were allowed to discriminantly service populations based on race. In addition, these same hospitals were allowed to continue these discriminatory practices in regard to hiring and staffing patterns. From such practices were born the all-African-American hospitals, which were found not only in the South but also in the North. Inclusions and exclusions for purposes of rendering health care services to those persons in need were left to the proprietors of the hospital. Thus patterns of admission and service to African Americans varied throughout the country without regard to regional locale. In some northern and western states, admission to and service by some hospitals remained theoretically open to all races on equal terms, whereas in other states the courts upheld the rights of hospital proprietors to segregate as they saw fit.

This discriminatory practice was dramatically emphasized by the deaths of two famous African Americans: Bessie Smith, in 1937, and Charles Drew, in 1950. Bessie Smith was a legendary "blues" singer who was critically injured in an automobile accident while traveling from Jackson, Mississippi, to Memphis, Tennessee. White attendants at the scene of the accident surmised correctly that Smith had a severed right arm and therefore needed immediate medical attention. The attendants took Smith to a hospital designated as "all White," and the administrators at the hospital refused to treat her despite the severity of her injuries. The ambulance attendants were forced to take Smith to Memphis, where she could be treated. On arrival, Smith was in profound shock, having lost a great quantity of blood. It has been said that despite Bessie Smith's obvious fame and the great admiration shown her by millions of fans, both African American and White, the fact that she was African American ultimately caused her death (Albertson, 1982).

Charles Drew, a surgeon, discovered blood plasma and developed the procedure for blood plasma transfusion. Even today, people throughout the world, regardless of race, benefit from his discovery. However, despite his profoundly important contribution to the medical field, the discovery of blood plasma was of no benefit to Drew when he, like Smith, was involved in an automobile accident and similarly was refused treatment in an "all-White" hospital. Although Drew was responsible for the technique of blood plasma transfusion, it was not used to save his life because he was taken to a hospital that legally had the right to refuse him treatment.

African-American folk medicine therefore took roots not only as an offshoot of African cultural heritage, but also as a necessity when African Americans could not gain access to the traditional health care delivery system. Furthermore, some African Americans turned to African-American folk medicine because they either could not afford the cost of medical assistance or were tired of the insensitive treatment by caregivers in the health care delivery system (Bullough & Bullough, 1982). Today African Americans have access to the health care delivery system through legal channels. Some African Americans still refuse to use the system, however, citing reasons such as past experiences, the escalating cost of health care, and the sometimes insensitive treatment on the part of non-Black caregivers in regard to the physiological and psychosocial differences evidenced among African Americans.

Some African Americans have a strong religious orientation, and most African Americans belong to the Protestant faith. Although folk medicine and folk practices are widely documented in the literature as being common practices for the treatment of illnesses among African Americans, the most common and frequently cited method of treating illness remains prayer (Spector, 1979). According to Snow (1977), many of her informants found it impossible to separate religious beliefs from medical ones.

Implications for nursing care

Cultural health practices are often considered efficacious, neutral, or dysfunctional (Pillsbury, 1982). Practices that are considered efficacious are recognized by Western medicine as beneficial to health regardless of whether they are different from scientific practice. Practices that are regarded as beneficial by the nurse should be actively encouraged. The nurse should keep in mind that a treatment plan that is congruent with the client's own beliefs has a better chance of being successful. For example, some African Americans believe that certain herbs and spices are essential in the treatment of certain disequilibriums in the body. In this case an herbal decoction could be used in place of water and might be just as beneficial for the treatment of specific conditions such as dehydration. Neutral practices (such as putting a knife under the bed to cut pain) are considered to be of no significance one way or the other to the health of an individual. However, psychological benefits may have a profound effect on the perception of pain. Dysfunctional health practices are viewed as harmful from a health point of view. For example, it is considered a dysfunctional health practice in Western medicine to use sugar and over-refined flour excessively. Dysfunctional health practices found among some African Americans include such practices as using boiled goat's milk and cabbage juice for stomach infection.

Because some African Americans tend to equate good health with luck or success, an illness may be viewed as undesirable and equated with bad luck, poverty, domestic turmoil, or even unemployment. As indicated previously, illnesses may be classified as natural or unnatural. Natural illnesses occur because a person is affected by natural forces without adequate protection. The nurse may be able to help the client more readily understand how these natural illnesses, such as colds and flu, can be avoided. Unnatural illnesses, which are believed to be the direct result of evil influences, are much more difficult for the nurse to combat. If the nurse has a client who believes that unnatural illness has resulted from witchcraft or voodoo or is a punishment from God, it may be very difficult to convince the client that a treatment can be implemented that will minimize or eliminate the problem. For example, a client may view breast cancer as a punishment from God. In this instance the client should be encouraged to seek medical treatment because unnecessary delay can have serious consequences. Although the nurse may not subscribe to cultural healing beliefs, it is essential that the nurse recognize their existence and their importance for some African-American clients. It is also important for the nurse to remember that effective nursing care cannot be implemented until the nurse acknowledges certain cultural health beliefs that have an effect on the client's behavior and recovery.

Among some African Americans it is believed that the maintenance of health is strongly associated with the ability to read the signs of nature. Subsumed in this belief is the idea that natural phenomena such as the phases of the moon, the seasons of the year, and the planetary positions all either singly or in combination affect the human body and human physiological functioning. Some African Americans believe that the best days to wean babies, for example, or to have dental or surgical procedures done, can be found in the *Old Farmer's Almanac* (Snow, 1974). To the nurse such beliefs may seem peculiar; however, the nurse must acknowledge the existence of such beliefs before culturally appropriate nursing care can be given. The nurse must also recognize that, although some of these beliefs may be helpful, others may be neutral, and still others may be extremely dangerous for the client. The nurse must be able to sort beliefs into these three categories and be able to assist the client in recognizing beliefs that may be dangerous.

Some African Americans believe that cultural healing remedies help a person psychologically in dealing with discomfort. However, when these things fail, they believe a physician should be consulted. These same African Americans may also believe that the nurse should recognize these cultural beliefs and use remedies based on these beliefs that prove to be helpful to the client (Bloch, 1976a). When an African-American client does arrive for professional health care, the nurse might assume that the client has tried all the cultural healing remedies known. While doing the initial assessment, the nurse needs to find out what the client has been using at home to minimize illness symptoms. This initial assessment will assist the nurse in determining whether these home remedies will interact or interfere with ortho-dox medical approaches. If the client has been using harmless home remedies, such remedies may con-tinue to be used in the client's treatment. Other harmless remedies might be added to the client care plan at the client's suggestion (Bloch, 1976a).

Religion for some African Americans has func-tioned primarily as an escape mechanism from the harsh realities of life. The African-American church functions to promote self-esteem among its mem-bership. The African-American church also acts as a curator for maintaining the culture of many African Americans. Therefore the nurse cannot overlook the importance of the African-American minister and the African-American church in the recovery of the client. If there is no African-American minister within the hospital facility, the nurse should contact the client's own minister. It is essential for the nurse to remember that the African-American minister can essentially bridge the gap between the African-American client and other health care workers be-cause the African-American minister understands the rituals, folk ways, and difference in the mores of African Americans (Smith, 1976).

BIOLOGICAL VARIATIONS

Until recently, the education of health care practitio-ners was based on the biopsychosocial characteris-tics of the dominant White culture. The lack of an in-depth understanding of biological and cultural differences resulted in less than optimum health care for persons who were not members of the dominant culture. When providing care to African-American clients, the nurse must realize that racial differ-ences involve more than skin color and hair texture. African-American people have distinctive genotypes and phenotypes that characterize them as a racial

group and as different from other racial groups. Moreover, the nurse must understand that African Americans also have ethnic and cultural differences that distinguish them from other ethnic and cultural groups.

Birth weight

Data from previous epidemiological reports con-sistently reveal that there is a difference in the mean birth weight of approximately 200 g between African-American infants and White infants, with White infants weighing more. These differences persist even when socioeconomic status, maternal age, parity, and smoking are controlled for (Hulsey, Levokoff, & Alexander, 1991). Davis, Cutter, Golden-berg, et al. (1993) used ultrasound examinations to compare biparietal diameter (BPD), head circumfer-ence (HC), abdominal circumference (AC), and fe-mur length in 5405 African-American and White fe-tuses. They found no significant difference in the BPD, HC, and AC; however, the femur length in African-American fetuses was significantly longer. The birth weights of the infants were also compared, and these data again revealed differences in birth weight between African-American and White infants (3331 versus 3135, $p < 0.001$), with White infants be-ing heavier.

It is clear that prematurity, which is defined as a birth weight under 2500 g, is twice as common for African Americans as it is for Whites (Morton, 1977), and it has been suggested that the definition for prematurity be lowered from 2500 to 2200 g for African Americans (Morton, 1977). The gestational period for African Americans tends to be 9 days shorter than that for Whites, and a slowing down of gestational growth occurs in African-American infants after 35 weeks. Before 35 weeks of gesta-tion, African-American infants are usually larger than White infants (Giger, Davidhizar, & Wieczorek, 1993; Pratt, Janus, & Sayal, 1977). The reasons for these differences in birth weights remain vague.

Growth and development

African-American children tend to mature faster than White children. Today African-American chil-dren are more mature at birth in both the musculoskeletal and the neurological systems (Falkner & Tanner, 1978). Neurologically, African-American children tend to be more advanced until about 2 or 3 years of age, and in the musculoskeletal system they tend to be more advanced until puberty (Roche, Roberts, & Hamell, 1978). The differences in skeletal maturity are attributed to genetic and environmental factors.

Body size, height, weight, bone length, and body structure of African Americans and Whites have been extensively studied in the United States. Studies done by Abraham, Clifford, and Najjar (1976) revealed that the average height and weight of African-American and White men 18 to 74 years of age are approximately the same; White men tend to be 0.5 cm taller than African-American men. The average height for African-American and White women is the same; however, African-American women are consistently heavier than White women at every age, and between 35 and 64 years of age they are typically an average of 20 pounds heavier than their White counterparts.

Body proportion

The body proportions of African Americans differ from those of Whites, Orientals, and Native Americans. There are definitive differences in bone length that are obvious on study. African Americans have shorter trunks than Whites and tend to have longer legs than Whites, Orientals, and Native Americans. African-American men tend to have wider shoulders and narrower hips than Orientals, who tend to have narrow shoulders and wide hips. The long bones of African Americans are significantly longer and narrower than those of Whites (Farrally & Moore, 1976). The bones of African Americans are also denser. African-American men have the densest bones, followed by African-American women, White men, and finally, White women, who have the least bone density of the two races. The greater bone density explains why osteoporosis is rare in African Americans and why White women have a greater incidence of osteoporosis. Bone curvature also varies among the different races. The femurs of African Americans are quite straight, compared with those of Native Americans, whose femurs are anteriorly

convex, and those of Whites, who have intermediate curvature. This characteristic appears to be genetically determined, but weight also seems to be a factor because obese African Americans and Whites tend to demonstrate more curvature than other individuals do (Gilbert, 1977).

Body fat

The amount and distribution of body fat is another area where there are pronounced differences by virtue of race and ethnic group. The racial differences are mostly related to socioeconomic status. Persons from the lower socioeconomic class tend to have more body fat than those from the middle class, and persons from the middle class tend to have more body fat than those from the upper class. There is some evidence indicating that fat distribution may vary according to race. African-American people tend to have smaller skin-fold thickness in their arms than Whites have, but the distribution of fat on the trunk is similar for both Whites and African Americans (Bagan, Robson, & Soderstrom, 1971). Whites have a larger chest volume than African Americans; hence they have greater vital capacity and forced expiratory volume (Oscherwitz, 1972). African Americans, on the other hand, have a larger chest volume than Native Americans and Orientals and thus greater vital capacity and forced expiratory volume than members of these racial groups (Oscherwitz, 1972).

Skin color

Skin color, or pigmentation, is the most distinguishing physical difference among the various races and is determined by melanin. All people have some melanin, but some racial groups have more melanin than others. The greater the amount of melanin an individual has, the darker the skin pigmentation will be. The skin color of persons who are classified as African Americans ranges from "white" to very dark brown or perhaps even black. Melanin provides protection from the effects of the sun; thus African Americans and other dark-skinned individuals have a lower incidence of skin cancer. African Americans do get sunburned but not so easily as Whites do (Overfield, 1995).

The skin coloring should be uniform, but areas that are not exposed to the sun may be lighter, such as the buttocks, abdomen, and thorax. The exceptions to this rule for African-American people are the skin folds in the groin, the genitalia, and the nipples, which tend to be darker than the rest of the body. (An old wives' tale suggests that to determine the true color of a newborn infant, one should look at the ears, which tend to be darker at birth than the rest of the body.) Except for the areas just mentioned, hypopigmentation and hyperpigmentation (unless it is a birthmark) are abnormal (Bloch, 1983). Pigmentation of the lips, nail beds, palmar surfaces, creases of the hands, and plantar surfaces and creases of the feet may vary, just as skin coloring does. The range of coloring for the lips of African Americans may vary from pink to plum. The palmar and plantar surfaces may range from light pink to dark pink to a brown, and the creases may range from dark pink to dark brown, depending on the amount of pigmentation (Bloch, 1976b). The gums may have areas of hyperpigmentation, and the sclerae may have scattered areas of brown pigmentation that appear to be freckles.

Mongolian spots are a common variance found in African-American infants. They are migratory leftovers of melanocytes that have lingered in the lumbosacral region at a greater than normal depth, which accounts for their dark blue-green appearance. Mongolian spots occur in 90% of African Americans, 80% of Orientals and Native Americans, and only 9% of Whites (Jacob & Walton, 1976). Normally found on the buttocks, thighs, ankles, and arms, mongolian spots usually disappear in the first year of life and should not be mistaken for a bruise.

Birthmarks appear to be most common in African-American individuals, occurring in 20% of African Americans, compared with 2% to 3% of Whites, Mexicans, and Native Americans. These pigmented marks appear as sharply demarcated macules that vary from light tan to dark brown, depending on the skin color. They may be present anywhere on the body (Overfield, 1995).

Black skin is also more susceptible to an overgrowth of connective tissue in response to injury, or keloid formation. Keloids are raised areas of scar tissue that can result from minor injuries such as skin tears or punctures, from more major injuries such as burn injuries or traumatic lacerations, or from surgical incisions (Rook, 1970).

Normal, healthy skin should be warm, dry, and elastic. There should be a red glow present in Black skin. Color changes associated with abnormal conditions are rashes, which may be difficult or impossible to detect in the individual who is darkly pigmented. Darkly pigmented lips and nail beds with melanin deposits make nursing assessment even more difficult. When possible, the nurse should become familiar with the client's normal coloring to establish a baseline value. The skin assessment should be done in a well-lighted room. Sunlight is the best lighting; if artificial lighting is used, it should be nonglaring (Bloch & Hunter, 1981). When assessing the darkly pigmented individual for specific color changes such as pallor, jaundice, or cyanosis, the nurse should inspect the conjunctivae and oral membranes of the buccal mucosa. Jaundice also appears as a yellowish discoloration of the sclerae if they are not pigmented. The mucous membranes of the buccal mucosa and the palmar and plantar surfaces may also be inspected for yellow discoloration.

The nurse may also rely on palpations and the client's history to detect the presence of bruises in the darkly pigmented client. The nurse should use the dorsal surface of the hand to assess for areas of increased warmth and tenderness. Questioning should include a history of recent trauma. The petechiae cannot be readily visualized on the dark-skinned individual. The nurse should inspect the sclerae for dark blue spots. The client history should include questioning about symptoms of conditions in which petechiae would be present. Palpation and the client history may also be used to detect the presence of a macular rash on the client who is dark skinned (Bloch, 1983).

Enzymatic variations

Biochemical variations and their effects on health vary according to race. As with other racial variations, biochemical variations are attributed to genetic factors and environmental influences. Lactose intolerance is a well-known condition that is correlated with race: 90% of African Blacks and 75% of African Americans are affected with lactose intolerance (Giger, Davidhizar, & Cherry, 1991; McCrackin, 1971). Individuals with lactose intolerance lack the enzyme to convert lactose to glucose and galactose, and as a result, gastrointestinal symptoms of bloating, cramping, and diarrhea occur. The condition is genetically transmitted, though the specific gene has not been identified (Johnson, Cole, & Abner, 1981). There appear to be two periods in life during which symptoms occur: infancy shortly after weaning and the teen years or early twenties. The condition is diagnosed on the basis of signs or symptoms that occur after the ingestion of milk or other products containing lactose. Treatment is by having the individual avoid these products, with appropriate substitution of other products. In addition, there are products available on the market that can be taken to assist in the alleviation of symptoms associated with this condition. Some people report a degree of success with such products, whereas other people report little benefit from their use. The nursing implications for nurses caring for African-American clients include (1) knowledge of the condition and its prevalence among African Americans and (2) education of clients with the condition to avoid products containing lactose. The education of these clients should include encouraging them to read labels and make appropriate food substitutions (Bloch, 1974).

Susceptibility to disease

Cardiovascular disease Cardiovascular disease remains the leading cause of morbidity and mortality in the United States for all demographic groups. Cardiovascular disease includes coronary heart disease, congenital heart disease, rheumatic fever, valvular heart disease, dysrhythmias, and cerebrovascular disease. The major causes of death attributable to cardiovascular disease are myocardial infarction, which is number one, and cerebrovascular accident, which is third (National Center for Health Statistics, 1998). The incidence of hypertension among African Americans was discussed in Chapter 7. However, hypertension is an extremely important consideration for the African American (development of coronary heart disease). Coronary heart disease was once perceived as a disease that most commonly afflicted men. This perception was probably because the condition strikes men more often in the middle years of life. This perception had been reinforced by the Framingham study, which was initiated in 1948. In this classic study, the data indicated that, on the average, women develop the symptoms of heart disease a decade later than men. Work relative to this study continues, and the data may indicate that the incidence of the disease continues to be disproportionately higher among men than in women. Woods (1998) reported that 6% of women in the United States have had a coronary event by 60 years of age compared to 20% of men of the same age. After 60 years of age both men and women have a 25% risk of death from coronary heart disease.

According to Lerner and Kannel (1985), the incidence of coronary heart disease is three times higher in men than in women between 45 and 54 years of age. After 65 years of age this gap narrows, and by 75 years of age, the incidence of the disease is essentially equal for both sexes. A major flaw in earlier studies of cardiovascular disease is that the majority of subjects were White males, and therefore data relevant for this specific population may not be an accurate reflection of the pathological processes of coronary heart disease in women and individuals from different racial groups.

For more than a decade research findings have consistently revealed that the mortality for coronary heart disease in African-American males and females is higher than that of White males and females. Liao and Cooper (1995) noted that for the first time since the category of coronary heart disease had been recorded in vital statistics, the age-adjusted mortality for myocardial infarction in Black males exceeded that of Whites. Further findings from this study indicate that in 1980 the mortality for White males was 11% higher than that for Black males (218.0 versus 196.0, per 100). In 1989 this contrast was reversed, with the mortality for Black males higher (144.5 per 100,000 compared to 139.7) than that for White males. For Black females the mortality was consistently higher than that for White females throughout the 10-year period, with the absolute gap steadily increasing from +18.7 in

1980 to + 21.9 in 1991. More recent data support the fact that more African-Americans males and females are dying from coronary heart disease than their White counterparts are. Data from the 1997 Heart and Stroke Statistics Update indicated that the age-adjusted death rate from myocardial infarction was highest for African-American males and females (267.9 and 190.3 per 100,000) compared to that for white males and females (165.3 and 99.2 per 100,000). According to Woods (1998), African-American women tend to develop coronary heart disease much earlier than White women do. In addition, the death rate for African-American women under 55 years of age is twice that of White women. Finally, until 75 years of age the mortality from coronary heart disease is higher in African-American women compared to women of other racial backgrounds (Woods, 1998).

Major risk factors associated with the development of coronary heart disease include smoking, hypertension, and elevated serum cholesterol. Other risk factors that have been attributed to coronary heart disease are diabetes, obesity and heredity (MMWR, 1998). Smoking is prevalent among women, with the highest prevalence of smoking found among Native-American women. In stark contrast, the prevalence of hypertension is highest among African-American women at all age groups. Approximately 35% of African-American women between 25 and 44 years of age have been classified as hypertensive (Stokes, Kannel, Wolf, et al., 1986).

Hypertension is a major risk factor for cardiovascular disease (Wieck, 1997). According to results of NHANES III Examination Survey, 1988-1991, the age-adjusted prevalence of hypertension in African Americans was 32.4%, almost 40% higher than that of non-Hispanic Whites and Hispanics. For African-American women the incidence of hypertension increases significantly with age, diabetes, and obesity (Wieck, 1997). Of the four leading causes of death in African Americans, hypertension can be associated with at least three of the four disease states. For example, coronary heart disease is the leading cause of death among African Americans, cerebrovascular accidents are listed as third, and diabetes is listed as the fourth leading cause of death. Coronary heart dis-

ease and cerebrovascular accidents can occur or are exacerbated as a result of hypertension. Individuals with diabetes have a higher risk of coronary heart disease and hypertension, and both conditions are exacerbated by diabetes.

A serum cholesterol level greater than 240 mg/dL is generally associated with the increased risk of mortality and morbidity from coronary heart disease (Kannel, 1983). Low-level, high-density lipoprotein is an excellent indicator for predicting morbidity caused by coronary heart disease (National Center for Health Statistics, 1991). The data available are suggestive that the prevalence of serum cholesterol levels is high in African-American women (25%), and that for all women, regardless of race or ethnicity, serum cholesterol levels rise steadily with age (National Center for Health Statistics, 1990).

Throughout the years, data available have reinforced the ideology that there are notable differences between Whites and African Americans for the prevalence of many cardiovascular conditions such as hypertension, renal failure, and stroke (American Heart Association, 1991). Recently, however, significant differences have been noted in the incidences of sudden cardiac arrest found among African Americans. Data from this study indicate that not only are African Americans more likely to experience sudden cardiac arrest, but they are also more likely to succumb to the arrest. In fact, among African Americans in all age groups, both men and women have higher rates of cardiac arrests than their White counterparts have. The survival rate for African Americans, compared with Whites, was remarkably different (0.8% versus 2.6%). Three plausible explanations have been offered for differences between the rates and lethality of sudden cardiac arrest for African Americans and their White counterparts, as follows: (1) inexperience and lack of familiarity with basic CPR techniques of the persons at the site; (2) response time of the emergency ambulance to the site, particularly in "African-American neighborhoods"; and (3) response time of the hospital emergency team to the African-American client in full cardiac arrest (Becker, Han, Meyer, et al., 1993). Because the findings from this study indicate that the incidence of cardiac arrest is significantly higher among African Americans in every age group, early intervention and prevention techniques to reduce the chronicity of coronary heart disease appears to be a plausible mechanism to prevent cardiac arrest among this population.

AIDS (HIV) risk In 1995 Approximately 90% of adults and adolescents with AIDS were male. Currently, men who have sex with men still represent the largest group of individuals with HIV/AIDS in the United States (Ward & Duchin, 1998). However, since the first reported case in 1981, HIV/AIDS has become a major cause of morbidity and mortality among African Americans. Ward and Duchin (1998) report that for the first time the number of African Americans with the diagnosis of AIDS was approximately equal to the number of reported cases in whites. Since 1995, HIV infection has become the leading cause of death in persons ages 24 to 44 years of age (Muma & Borucki, 1994). A disproportionate number of individuals with AIDS in this age range are African American. Ward and Duchin (1998) report that the death rate from AIDS was about 129% greater for African-American males (178.0 per 100,000) than that for White males (138.0 per 100,000). African-American females fare even worse (53 per 100,000), with a death rate of 8833 times greater than that for White females (6 per 100,000) (Ward & Duchin, 1998). Statistical data from the Centers for Disease Control and Prevention, in Atlanta, supports the fact that a greater percentage of African Americans are infected with HIV and are dying from AIDS compared to individuals of other races. According to demographic data from the CDC

AIDS hotline a total number of 612,078 persons have died from AIDS (Table 8-1).

A study reported in *Scope* (1989), a quarterly publication of the Institute of Black Chemical Abuse, verified other research findings that high-risk behaviors tend to cluster together and that behavioral factors, rather than biological variables, account for the racial differences in HIV infection rates.

Moore, Stanton, Gopalan, and Chaisson (1994), researchers at Johns Hopkins University, School of Medicine, conducted a study on HIV-positive individuals to determine if there were notable differences in the administration of antiretroviral drugs among Black and White clients. Findings from this study are suggestive that Black HIV-positive individuals are less likely than their White counterparts to be given antiretroviral drugs, including medication to prevent *Pneumocystis carinii* pneumonia (PCP). Of the number of Blacks surveyed, only 58% of those medically eligible received drug therapy, compared with 82% of their White counterparts. Researchers found no significant differences in receipt of drug therapy with respect to such moderating variables as age, gender, mode of HIV transmission, type of insurance, income, education, or place of residence.

Guidelines published by the U.S. Public Health Service (PHS) suggest that to effectively treat HIV-infected persons antiretroviral therapy should begin when the client's CD4 cell count falls to 500 cells per cubic millimeter or less. The PHS guidelines also suggest that prophylactic treatment for PCP should begin when the CD4 count reaches 200 cells per cubic millimeter or less. Because CD4 cells are integral

---

Table 8-1 Demographic data from the Centers for Disease Control AIDS hotline: mortalities from June 1981 through June 1997.

	Male	**Female**	**Pediatric**
NON-HISPANIC WHITE	256,353	21,319	1400
NON-HISPANIC BLACK	160,984	51,411	4586
HISPANIC	88,756	18,663	1873
ASIAN–PACIFIC ISLANDER	3850	449	41
NATIVE AMERICAN	1390	261	26
UNKNOWN ORIGIN	601	10	16

From the Centers for Disease Control and Prevention, Atlanta, Georgia.

to the body's immune defense, reduction in CD4 cells is generally associated with a weakening in the immune system. This reduction, particularly among HIV-positive individuals, generally signals an onset of disease symptoms, including PCP (Moore et al., 1994). Moore et al. (1994) also noted that among those clients with a CD4 cell count of 500 or less, only 48% of Blacks, compared to 68% of Whites, received antiretroviral therapy. Despite the PHS guidelines for administration of prophylactic therapy to all clients with a CD4 cell count of 200 or less, researchers found an even greater disparity between Blacks and their White counterparts with Blacks invariably receiving little intervention when CD4 cell counts dropped to 200 or less.

Psychological characteristics

Some studies depict the pattern of interaction in the African-American family as being pathological and unstable. Findings from one study indicate that if there is stability in the African-American family it is attributable to the presence of a controlling, domineering mother. The pathological family interaction that occurs in some African-American families is said to affect the male son so profoundly that in later life he is unable to adjust to the role of husband and father. Consequently, in unstable African-American families the African-American male is unable to form mature, lasting relationships with others (Culture of Poverty Revisited, n.d.). In studies done on African-American male alcoholics, these individuals were found to have the lowest scores on tests of personality integration, with a more passive and compliant coping style than any other ethnic group of male alcoholics (Carroll, Klein, & Santo, 1978). It is believed that this passive and compliant coping style was rooted in the slavery era. During slavery, African-American mothers were forced to teach their male children to be passive if they were to survive the authority of the slave master because to be "uppity" meant possible physical punishment or even death. Today it would seem essential that the African-American male display the same survival skills because the authority figure still remains (police, educators, employers, and so forth).

In a study done on African-American boys from father-absent homes, it was found that dependency and a passive coping style were evident among these boys (Barclay & Cusumano, 1967). Other studies suggest that boys from father-absent homes tend to be more dependent on their peer groups, display fewer aggressive behaviors, have lower self-esteem, and are more likely to display overt masculine behavior. In some studies looking at psychological issues of father-absent homes, social class appeared to be an intervening variable. A more deleterious effect on sex-role orientation was found in boys who lived in father-absent homes before 5 years of age (Covell & Turnbull, 1982). Because there is a probability of an African-American male being reared in a female-headed household, it has become necessary for African-American mothers to encourage masculine traits in their sons. In an earlier study it was found that mothers who encouraged masculine traits in their sons had more of an effect in father-absent homes than in father-present homes (Biller, 1969).

Some social scientists and health care providers contend that African Americans are at risk for the development of mental health problems. Corrective steps have been taken to alleviate the development of mental health problems; however, the mental health system continues to struggle to meet the emotional needs of African Americans (Snowden, 1982; Snowden & Todman, 1982). Bullough and Bullough (1982) reported that admission rates to mental health hospitals are higher and the hospital stay is longer for African-Americans than for any other ethnic group in the United States. However, it was found that when socioeconomic status was carefully controlled, psychosis rates among Whites and African Americans appeared similar.

Chemical abuse Alcoholism is one of the major health problems in the African-American community, contributing to reduced longevity. There are high incidences of acute and chronic alcohol-related diseases among African Americans, such as alcoholic fatty liver; hepatitis; cirrhosis of the liver; heart disease; cancer of the mouth, larynx, tongue, esophagus, and lung; and unintentional injuries and homicide (Ronan, 1987).

Harper and Dawkins (1976) reported that, of 16,000 articles on alcohol abuse published from 1944 to 1974, only 77 included references to African

Americans and only 11 were specifically about African Americans. King (1982) reported that most studies between 1977 and 1980 dealt only with patterns of alcohol use. Only one study (Stalls, 1978) explored racial differences in patterns of alcohol metabolism. Stalls (1978) found an increasing incidence of alcohol abuse among African-American youth and women, with serious implications for fetal alcohol syndrome. Drinking appeared to peak between 16 and 23 years of age, and, among women, drinking was highest for divorced women younger than 45 years of age. Brisbane (1987) noted that women who drank were typically younger than 45 years of age, were employed, and considered themselves middle class. Williams (1986) noted a contradiction in the high incidence of alcohol-related diseases and drinking patterns reported in African Americans: when age and socioeconomic levels were controlled, African Americans actually abstained more, drank less frequently, and consumed less alcohol than their White counterparts. African-American women were the exception, with 11% of African-American women drinking heavily, compared with 4% of White women.

Several causes of alcohol abuse and misuse in African Americans have been identified in the literature. A primary factor is economics. Many African-American men drink as a result of unemployment, which leads to depression and frustration because of the inability to meet financial commitments. Williams (1986) concluded that unemployment is correlated with a high risk for alcohol problems among African Americans. Availability is also a factor (Parker & Harman, 1978). Brown and Tooley (1989) have reported that in Los Angeles there are approximately three liquor stores per city block. African-American peer pressure is also reported as a contributing factor; peers expect heavy drinking, and brand names and quantity are often status identifiers. Finally, heavy alcohol use may be related to a desire to escape unpleasant feelings. Sterne and Pittman (1972) have also pointed out themes that seem to be present in African-American alcohol use. They linked being paid on the weekend to Saturday relaxation and thus drinking. A second theme is the prevalence of taverns in the African-American community that serve as social centers. Finally, alcohol appears to be used as an escape from personal problems.

African Americans are less likely to seek treatment for problem drinking than any other ethnic group in the United States (Lawson & Lawson, 1989). Research indicates that several areas must be addressed to increase the likelihood of successful treatment outcomes. The first step is to get the African-American alcoholic into a treatment program. Programs that are located within the community and are accessible to public transportation are more likely to be used, except by the upwardly mobile African-American person, who is more likely to seek private services outside the community. The African-American church can and in some instances does serve a dual role in this first step because it can provide a facility and at the same time act as a referral source. Most African-American churches are centrally located within the African-American community, and even as members relocate, they tend to maintain their roots in the African-American church. Also, prayer has been associated with the treatment modality and overall success rate for the recovering alcoholic. The church continues to be the mainstay of the African-American family, and rather than seeking outside help for alcoholism, the family often attempts to resolve problems by going to the minister. Some African Americans have reported that they stopped drinking before seeking professional help because of their spirituality, which assisted with the transition (Brisbane, 1987; Hudson, 1986; Knox, 1986; Westermeyer, 1984).

When treating the recovering alcoholic, the nurse must remember that the family can often provide assistance in the form of shelter, food, money, or clothing. The extended family may also take on counseling roles that close relatives find too painful (Brisbane & Womble, 1986). The nurse must also have an awareness of the socioeconomic context and its effect on intrapsychic processes. The elimination of stereotypical bias by both the nurse and the client and the inclusion of social values and traditions are necessary to maximize intervention, give culturally appropriate nursing care, and affect recovery rates (Institute of Black Chemical Abuse, 1988).

Posttraumatic stress disorder Many studies have been conducted that indicate that minority Vietnam veterans have experienced a greater degree of mal-adjustment after the Vietnam War than their White counterparts (Allen, 1986; Laufer, Gallops, & Frey-Wouters, 1984). Some of these studies have given a variety of reasons for this maladjustment, including the fact that minorities felt more conflict about participating in the war because they had less to gain than persons in the dominant culture. Another reason postulated by the researchers was that minorities were more likely to be identified with the enemy, who were also different in skin color from White Americans. Perhaps the most significant reason for posttraumatic stress disorder (PTSD) among minority Vietnam veterans was that the status of minorities declined in the United States during the turbulence of the 1960s at the same time that African Americans were fighting for the United States in Vietnam (Allen, 1986; Laufer, Gallops, & Frey-Wouters, 1981).

In a more recent study, Penk, Robinowitz, Black, et al. (1989) also found that, among Vietnam combat veterans, African Americans appeared to be more maladjusted than their White counterparts. One conclusion of this study is that ethnicity emerges as a significant parameter in studies of PTSD, but the exact contributions of ethnicity have not been explained fully by current findings on the subject. Many researchers have postulated that significant increases in PTSD in African-American Vietnam veterans may be attributable in part to the fact that during the Vietnam War years (1964 to 1975) African Americans suffered the major loss of a leader (through the assassination of Martin Luther King, Jr., in 1968) and experienced the racial conflicts evidenced by rioting in Washington, D.C., Watts (in Los Angeles), and other cities throughout the country (Karnow, 1983).

Other psychological characteristics The psychiatric literature on psychological characteristics of African Americans and treatment of African Americans by mental health professionals is controversial. The psychiatric literature has reported increased psychopathological disorders among African Americans (Pasamanick, 1964). Anatomical, neurological, and endocrinological differences have been cited as signs of African-American inferiority (Thomas & Sillen, 1972; Tobias, 1970). Research has been done on African Americans that would not have been considered for other ethnic groups. For example, in the Tuskegee project, African-American men with syphilis were intentionally denied treatment without being informed of their disease (Cave, 1975; Jones, 1982). Research on IQs has been used to support statements of genetic inferiority and justify social policies such as selective immigration laws and school segregation (Hirsch, 1981). Such psychological research has added to racial stereotyping and bias among some mental health professionals.

According to Meyers and Weissman (1980-1981), some differences in phobias have been found between African Americans and Whites. Robins, Helzer, Croughan, and Ratcliff (1981) noted that the lifetime prevalence of acrophobia was significantly higher for African Americans than for Whites. Vernon and Roberts (1982) found that African Americans, compared with Whites, had a significantly lower lifetime rate of both major and minor depression but had a rate of bipolar depression that was twice that of Whites. A possible explanation for the discrepancy in findings is the lack of national data on racial differences in diagnostic analogs. It is now widely accepted that on the Minnesota Multiphasic Personality Inventory (MMPI) African Americans tend to score higher on the paranoia and schizophrenia scales than Whites because the instrument was not standardized on an African-American population (Bell & Mehta, 1981; Gynther, 1981; Jones, Gray, & Parson, 1981). When standardized diagnostic systems are used today, African Americans do not differ from Whites in the prevalence of most psychiatric disorders. Robins, Helzer, Croughan, and Ratcliff (1981) and Meyers and Weissman (1980-1981) have reported finding no significant race differences for schizophrenia or affective disorders (Adebimpe, 1981; Lawson & Lawson, 1989; Mukherjee, Shukla, & Woodle, 1983; Spurlock, 1985).

Snow (1978) found that a belief in witchcraft was shared by a third of the African-American clients who were treated at a southern psychiatric center. African Americans who believe they have a folk illness may use the services of a root worker, reader, spiritualist, or voodoo priest. It is important for the nurse to know that the client may have used the services of a folk practitioner before or with scientific mental health therapy. Wintrob (1973) has promoted the idea that individuals who believe in folk remedies such as root work or obeah (Black ritual) may regard scientific treatment only as palliative because curing the total condition requires neutralization by a specially skilled folk healer. Wintrob (1973), Kreisman (1975), Weclew (1975), and Sandoval (1977) have suggested that mental health professionals should attempt to complement use of scientific medicine with folk practices for clients who believe mental disorders are attributed to folk causes.

Implications for nursing care

The best reason for including the concept of biological variations in nursing practice is that knowledge of scientific facts aids the nurse in giving culturally appropriate care. It is also essential for the nurse who cares for people from other cultures to know certain biological concepts not only to give culturally appropriate nursing care, but also to give nonharmful nursing care.

Important biological variations that the nurse should be aware of are related to body size, birth weight, and body proportion. It is important for the nurse who works with African-American children to remember that at birth African-American children tend to weigh less and be shorter than their White counterparts and that these variations may be attributable in part to socioeconomic status. Therefore the nurse, whether in a hospital or in a clinic setting, must carefully evaluate growth status in terms of height and weight for African-American children. Some nurses believe that, because growth charts are White normed, data gleaned from these charts lack implications in regard to African-American children. It is important for the nurse to recognize that even for African-American children serious growth deviation can have implications for intervention for nutritional deficiencies. These variations between African-American and White children may continue as the child grows. For example, African-American preschoolers are neurologically more advanced than their White counterparts. In addition, African-American children tend to have less subcutaneous fat than White children but are taller and heavier by 2 years of age (Owen & Lubin, 1973). The fact that African-American pre-

schoolers are taller and heavier may indicate a need for appropriate client teaching about nutritional needs of the growing child.

Because the average weight for an African-American woman is consistently higher than that for her White counterpart at every age, the nurse must teach African-American clients the value of serving nutritiously sound meals. In addition, the nurse must emphasize the importance of exercise, not only to maintain ideal weight, but also for cardiovascular purposes.

It is essential that the nurse develop a sensitivity for and familiarity with physical features that are common to African Americans as well as with African-American–related illnesses and diseases. If the nurse is unable to develop a familiarity with physical features common to African Americans and with African-American illnesses or diseases, the nurse cannot possibly hope to recognize or diagnose conditions that may cause disequilibrium in the body. In addition, the nurse must be prepared to deal promptly, efficiently, and appropriately with clinical variables that are common to all African-American clients and yet have significant variability in some African-American clients, such as hypertension or sickle cell anemia. There is no clear correlation between hypertension and obesity in African Americans, as there is with other ethnic groups such as Whites. On the other hand, there appears to be a direct correlation between the amount of skin pigmentation and the frequency of hypertension. Therefore, because it has been suggested that there is a direct relationship between skin pigmentation and hypertension, the nurse should emphasize the need for the African-American client to undergo hypertension screening (Boyle, 1970).

Because G-6-PD deficiency is a hematological problem that is present in 35% of African Americans, it is essential that the nurse stress the importance of the fluorescent spot test as a screening tool in diagnosing this deficiency. The nurse can serve as a client advocate and insist or mandate that this test be a routine part of laboratory testing for all African-American clients. Also, precautions should be taken to eliminate the transfusion of G-6-PD–deficient blood, particularly in transfusions for infants (Beutler, 1972). In addition, the nurse should exercise precaution when planning diets for African-American clients, particularly African-American infants, because they may be lactose intolerant. In these cases the nurse should plan diets that allow substituting more compatible products with the same nutritional value for milk and milk products (Bloch, 1981).

SUMMARY

It is important for the nurse to remember that if help is requested in regard to an African-American client it generally will come from within the family system and that it is important to include the family system when planning and implementing nursing care. Failure to do so may result in failed interventions. The nurse who is attempting to help the client problem-solve also needs to remember that problem solving tends to be action oriented; the African-American client may become impatient if it appears that nothing is actually happening to alleviate the present problem (Bloch, 1983).

In caring for the African-American client, the nurse must recognize and acknowledge the client's racial, cultural, and ethnic background because it is in these areas that the client's experiences occur. Not only is it important for the nurse to consider necessary adjustments in client care when the client is from a different racial origin, but it is also important that the racial origin of the nurse be considered. In a classic and innovative study by Remington and DaCosta (1989), the effects of ethnocultural differences between supervisor and caregiver are dramatically illustrated. The nurse who denies or does not believe race is a factor denies a significant part of the client's being.

Case Study

Mr. Willie Lee, a 51-year-old male, resides with his wife and 5 children in a small city in South Carolina. Early this morning Mr. Lee came to the emergency room with his wife complaining of indigestion and was not being able to get his breath. Mr. Lee told the nurse that for the past 2 or 3 months he has times when he couldn't "catch his breath." He also stated that he has had experienced what he believed to be indigestion for a couple months and that he had been using baking soda for relief. Mrs. Lee told the nurse that her husband has "high blood" and has not been taking his Cardizem for about 3 months.

Physical assessment yields the following vital signs: BP, 204/110; pulse, 100; respirations, 36; oxygen saturation, 86%; temperature, 97.1°. On auscultation of lungs, expiratory wheezes audible throughout and fine bibasilar crackles. Skin cool and diaphoretic. Oral mucosa pink. nailbeds pale, capillary refill >3 seconds.

Mr. Lee is diagnosed with congestive heart failure. He is given 40 mg of furosemide IV and placed on 40% oxygen per mask. A chest radiograph, electrocardiogram, and chemistry profile are ordered. Within an hour Mr. Lee's symptoms improve, and he is admitted to a medical unit for diagnostic values and further treatment.

Results of laboratory tests and diagnostic results are as follows:

Potassium   3.8
Creatinine   2.0
Glucose   140
Sodium   137
BUN   30

Chest radiograph: interstitial pulmonary edema, cardiac enlargement
Electrocardiogram: normal sinus rhythm with left ventricular hypertrophy

Mr. Lee was discharged 5 days later with prescription for Vasotec and Dyazide. He was also given instructions to limit sodium intake to 2 g/day.

CARE PLAN

 Nursing Diagnosis   Fluid-volume excess related to sodium and water retention, decreased glomerular filtration

Client Outcomes	*Nursing Interventions*
1. Client's vital signs, breath sounds, intake and output, weight, and laboratory values are consistent with normovolemia.	1. Administer supplemental oxygen as ordered.
	2. Assess respiratory rate, pattern, and breath sounds q4h and prn.
	3. Balance activity with periods of rest.
	4. Monitor intake and output every shift.
	5. Monitor weight daily.
	6. Assess client and family knowledge of signs and symptoms of fluid retention.
	7. Teach patient and family importance of reporting signs and symptoms of fluid-volume excess.
	8. Teach client and family the symptoms that require immediate medical attention.

 Nursing Diagnosis   Altered health maintenance related to lack of knowledge of pathological condition, complications, and management of hypertension

Client Outcomes	*Nursing Interventions*
1. Client and family will verbalize understanding of pathological condition, complications, and importance of lifelong management of hypertension	1. Discuss the complications of uncontrolled hypertension.
	2. Elicit client and family input in achieving compliance with lifelong therapy.
	3. Explain pathology of hypertension.
	4. Explain to client that there is no cure for hypertension.
	5. Stress the importance of lifelong therapy for hypertension.
	6. Explain the actions and indications of antihypertensive medication (Vasotec).
	7. Explain the actions and indications of diuretic (Dyazide).

 Nursing Diagnosis   Altered sexuality related to effects of antihypertensive medication

Client Outcomes	*Nursing Interventions*
1. Client will verbalize understanding that impotence is a side effect of antihypertensive medications and the importance of notifying physician of symptoms rather than stopping medication.	1. Provide client with privacy and opportunity to discuss problems related to sexuality.
	2. Explore client's concerns related to sexual function.
	3. Discuss actions, indications, and potential side effects of antihypertensive medications with client.
	4. Stress the importance of notifying the physician of side effects rather than stopping the medication abruptly.

 Nursing Diagnosis   Anxiety related to complexity of therapeutic regimen, life-style changes, lack of control of condition, and potential complications of hypertension

Client Outcomes	*Nursing Interventions*
1. Client will experience physiological and emotional comfort and a sense of well-being	1. Explore client's perception of hypertension related to life-style changes.

2. Ask client and family to discuss how hypertension has affected their life-style.
3. Assess stressors in client's life and effective coping mechanisms.
4. Assess family resources and support systems.
5. Involve client and family in goals to reduce anxiety and to develop effective coping methods.

 Nursing Diagnosis   Knowledge deficit related to pathophysiological state and therapeutic regimen for hypertension

Client Outcomes

Client will be able to define hypertension; state the complications of hypertension; explain the actions, indications, and side effects of medications and the necessity for lifelong compliance with therapy.

Nursing Interventions

1. Assess client's knowledge of hypertension.
2. Assess client's knowledge of hypertensive therapy.
3. Provide oral and written instructions related to hypertension including therapeutic management.
4. Discuss the possibility of rebound hypertension if medication is abruptly discontinued
5. Discuss the complications of uncontrolled hypertension.
6. Elicit client and family input in measures to achieve compliance with lifelong therapy.

STUDY QUESTIONS

1. Discuss the cause of the symptoms of dyspnea and chest discomfort in patients with congestive heart failure.
2. Explain how uncontrolled hypertension can precipitate congestive heart failure.
3. List the complications of uncontrolled hypertension.
4. Explain why it is important for the nurse to get a detailed health history from Mr. Lee.
5. Identify measures for the nurse to use to help Mr. Lee to discuss problems related to noncompliance with medications.
6. List several strategies that may help health care providers communicate better with African Americans.
7. Describe ways in which health care providers may show sensitivity and acceptance of African-American folk health care practices.
8. Compare and contrast the social organization of African Americans, especially in the South, from the 1940s to the present.
9. List several practices from ancient African ancestry that are a part of modern nursing philosophy.
10. Describe the importance of folk medicine practices and folk healers to African Americans in the rural setting.

References

Abraham, S.J., Clifford, L., & Najjar, M.F. (1976, Nov.). Height and weight of adults 18-74 years of age in the United States. *Advance Data, 3,* 1-18.

Adebimpe, V. (1981). Overview: White norms and psychiatric diagnosis of Black patients. *American Journal of Psychiatry, 138,* 279-285.

Albertson, C. (1982). *A night in the life of Bessie Smith.* New York: Steine & Day.

Allen, I.M. (1986). Post-traumatic stress disorder among Black Vietnam veterans. *Hospital and Community Psychiatry, 37,* 55-61.

American Heart Association (1991). Cardiovascular disease and stroke in African-Americans and other racial minorities in the United States: a statement for health professionals. *Circulation, 83,* 1462-1480.

Anderson, S.V., & Bauwens, E.E. (1981). *Chronic health problems: concepts and application.* St. Louis: Mosby.

Angelou, M. (1989). Maya Angelou (personal interview and portrait). In Lanker, B. (Ed.), *I dream a world: portraits of Black women who changed America.* New York: Stewart, Tabori, & Chang.

Bagan, M., Robson, J., & Soderstrom, R. (1971). Ethnic differences in skin fold thickness. *American Journal of Clinical Nutrition, 24,* 864-868.

Barclay, A., & Cusumano, D.R. (1967). Father absence, cross sex identity, and field-dependent behavior of male adolescents. *Child Development, 38,* 343-350.

Becker, L., Han, B., Meyer, P., et al. & CPR Chicago Project (1993). Racial difference in the incidence of cardiac arrest and subsequent survival. *New England Journal of Medicine, 329*(9), 600-607.

Bell, C., & Mehta, H. (1981). The misdiagnosis of Black patients with manic depressive illness: second in a series. *Journal of the National Medical Association, 73,* 101-107.

Beutler, E.H. (1972). Glucose-6-phosphate dehydrogenase deficiency. In Williams, W.J. (Ed.), *Hematology* (pp. 291-308). New York: McGraw-Hill.

Biller, H.B. (1969). Father absence, maternal encouragement, and sex role development in kindergarten boys. *Child Development, 40,* 539-546.

Bloch, B. (1974, May 3-4). A look at nursing intervention and Black patient care. In Bloch, B. (Coordinator), *Care of the Black patient on the job: an on the job look at health care needs of the Black patient.* Conference presented by Continuing Education in Nursing, University of California, San Francisco, School of Nursing.

Bloch, B. (1976a). *Health care from a minority viewpoint.* Unpublished study, University of California, San Francisco, School of Nursing.

Bloch, B. (1976b). Nursing intervention in Black patient care. In Luckraft, D. (Ed.), *Black awareness: implications for Black patient care* (pp. 27-35). New York: American Journal of Nursing Company.

Bloch, B. (1981). Black Americans and cross-cultural counseling experiences. In Marsella, A.J., & Pedersen, P.B. (Eds.), *Cross cultural counseling and psychotherapy.* New York: Pergamon Press.

Bloch, B. (1983). Bloch's assessment guide for ethnic/cultural variations. In Orque, M.S., Bloch, B., & Monrroy, L.S.A. (Eds.), *Ethnic nursing care: a multicultural approach* (pp. 49-75). St. Louis: Mosby.

Bloch, B., & Hunter, M. (1981). Teaching physiological assessment of Black persons. *Nurse Educator, 6,* 24-27.

Boyle, E., Jr. (1970). Biological pattern in hypertension by race, sex, body weight, and skin color. *Journal of the American Medical Association, 213,* 1637-1643.

Brisbane, F.L. (1987). Divided feeling of Black alcoholic daughters. *Alcohol Health and Research World, 12,* 48-50.

Brisbane, F.L., & Womble, M. (1986). Afterthoughts and recommendations. *Alcoholism Treatment Quarterly, 2* (3-4), 249-270.

Broderick, J., Brott, T., Kothari, R., et al. (1998). *The Greater Cincinnati/Northern Kentucky Stroke Study.* Cincinnati, Ohio: University of Cincinnati Medical Center.

Brown, F., & Tooley, J. (1989). Alcoholism in the Black community. In Lawson, G., & Lawson, A. (Eds.), *Alcohol and substance abuse in special populations.* Rockville, Md.: Aspen.

Bullough, V.L., & Bullough, B. (1982). *Health care for the other Americans.* East Norwalk, Conn.: Appleton-Century-Crofts.

Carroll, J.F., Klein, M.I., & Santo, Y. (1978). Comparison of the similarities and differences in the self-concepts of male alcoholics and addicts. *Journal of Consulting Clinical Psychology, 46,* 575-576.

Cave, V. (1975). Proper uses and abuses of the health care delivery system for minorities with special reference to the Tuskegee syphilis study. *Journal of the National Medical Association, 67,* 82-84.

Centers For Disease Control AIDS Hotline (1997). *National Center for Health Statistics Monthly Vital Statistics Report (1996), 45*(3), 10 (DHHS Publication No. PHS 3, 10). Hyattsville, Md.: Public Health Services.

Centers for Disease Control and Prevention (1988). Mortality patterns: United States, 1988. *Morbidity Mortality Weekly Report 1991, 40,* 493-502.

Covell, K., & Turnbull, W. (1982). The long-term effects of father absence in childhood on male university students' sex-role identity and personal adjustment. *Journal of Genetic Psychology, 141,* 271-276.

Culture of poverty revisited (no date). New York: Mental Health Committee Against Racism.

Davis, R.O., Cutter, G.R., Goldenberg, R.L., et al. (1993). Fetal biparietal diameter, head circumference, abdominal circumference and femur length: a comparison by race and sex. *Journal of Reproductive Medicine, 38,* 201-206.

Dillard, J.L. (1972). *Black English: its history and usage in the United States.* New York: Random House.

Falkner, F., & Tanner, J. (1978). *Human growth I: principles and prenatal growth.* New York: Plenum Press.

Farrally, M., & Moore, W. (1976). Anatomical differences in the femur and tibia between Negroids and Caucasians. *American Journal of Physiology and Anthropology, 43*(1), 63-69.

Giger, J., Davidhizar, R., & Cherry, B. (1991, April-May). Biological variations in the Black patient. *Imprint, 38*(2), 95, 97-98.

Giger, J., Davidhizar, R., & Wieczorek, S. (1993). Culture and ethnicity. In Bobak, I., & Jensen, M. (Eds.), *Maternity and gynecologic care* (ed. 5) (pp. 42-67). St. Louis: Mosby.

Gilbert, B.M. (1977). Anterior femoral curvature: its probable basis and utility as a criterion for racial assessment. *American Journal of Physical Anthropology, 45*(3), 601-604.

Gutman, H. (1976). *The Black family in slavery and freedom: 1750-1925.* New York: Vintage Books/Division of Random House.

Gynther, M. (1981). Is the MMPI an appropriate assessment device for Blacks? *Journal of Black Psychology, 7,* 67-75.

Hall, E.T. (1966). *The hidden dimension.* New York: Doubleday.

Hall, E.T. (1976). *Beyond culture.* New York: Anchor Books.

Harper, F., & Dawkins, M. (1976). Alcohol and Blacks: survey of periodical literature. *British Journal of Addiction, 71,* 327-334.

Henderson, G., & Primeaux, M. (1981). *Transcultural health care.* Reading, Mass.: Addison-Wesley.

Hirsch, J. (1981). To "unfrock the charlatans." *Sage Race Relations Abstracts, 6,* 1-65.

Hudson, H.L. (1986). How and why Alcoholics Anonymous works for Blacks. *Alcoholism Treatment Quarterly, 2*(314), 11-29.

Hulsey, T.C., Levkoff, A.H., & Alexander, G.R. (1991). Birth weight of infants of Black and White mothers without pregnancy complications. *American Journal of Obstetrics and Gynecology, 164,* 1299-1302.

Hymes, D. (Ed.) (1970). *Pidginization and creolization of languages.* London: Cambridge University Press.

Institute of Black Chemical Abuse (1988). *Annual report.* Minneapolis: the institute.

Institute of Black Chemical Abuse (1989, spring). *Scope.* Minneapolis: the institute.

Jackson, J., Neighbors, H., & Gurin, G. (1986). Findings from a national survey on Black mental health: implications for practice and training. In National Institute of Mental Health: *Mental health research and practice in minority communities.* Rockville, Md.: U.S. Department of Health and Human Services.

Jacob, A.H., & Walton, R.G. (1976). Incidence of birthmarks in the neonate. *Pediatrics, 58,* 218-222.

Jacques, G. (1976). Cultural health traditions: a Black perspective. In Branch, M.F., & Paxton, P.P. (Eds.), *Providing safe nursing care for ethnic people of color.* East Norwalk, Conn.: Appleton-Century-Crofts.

Johnson, R., Cole, R., & Abner F. (1981). Genetic interpretation of social/ethnic differences i. lactose absorption and tolerance. *Human Biology, 53*(1), 1-3.

Jones, B., Gray, B., & Parson, E. (1981). Manic-depressive illness among poor urban Blacks. *American Journal of the National Medical Association, 72,* 141-145.

Jones, L. (1966). *Home: social essays* (pp. 105-115). New York: Morrow.

Jones, L. (1982). *Bad blood: the Tuskegee syphilis experiment.* New York: Free Press.

Jordan, W.C. (1975). Voodoo medicine. In Williams, R.A. (Ed.), *Textbook of Black-related diseases* (pp. 115-138). New York: McGraw-Hill.

Jordan, W.C. (1979). The roots and practice of voodoo medicine in America. *Urban Health 8,* 38-48.

Kamin, L.J. (1974). *The science and politics of IQ.* Hillsdale, N.J.: Lawrence Erlbaum.

Kannel, W.B. (1983). High density lipoproteins: epidemiologic profile and risks of coronary artery disease. *American Journal of Cardiology, 52,* 9B-12B.

Kannel, W.B. (1985). Lipids diabetes and coronary heart disease: insights from the Framingham study. *American Heart Journal, 110,* 1100-1107.

Karnow, S. (1983). *Vietnam: a history.* New York: Viking Press.

King, L.M. (1982). *Alcoholism—studies regarding Black Americans: 1979-1980.* Alcohol and Health Monograph 4: Special Population Issues, 385-407.

Kluckhohn, C. (1976). The gifts of tongues. In Samovar, L.A., & Porter, R.E. (Eds.), *Intercultural communication: a reader.* Belmont, Calif.: Wadsworth.

Knox, D.H. (1986). Spirituality: a tool in the assessment and treatment of Black alcoholics and their families. *Alcoholism Treatment Quarterly, 2*(3-4), 313-343.

Kreisman, J. (1975). The curandero's apprentice: a therapeutic integration of folk and medical healing. *American Journal of Psychiatry, 132,* 81.

Laufer, R.S., Gallops, M.S., & Frey-Wouters, E. (1984). War stress and trauma: the Vietnam veteran experience. *Journal of Health and Social Behavior, 25,* 65-85.

Laufer, R.S., Yager, T., Frey-Wouters, E., et al. (1981). *Legacies of Vietnam.* Washington, D.C.: U.S. Government Printing Office.

Lawson, G., & Lawson, A. (1989). *Alcoholism and substance abuse in special populations.* Rockville, Md.: Aspen.

Leininger, M. (1978). *Transcultural nursing.* New York: John Wiley & Sons.

Lerner, D.J., & Kannel, W.B. (1985). Patterns of coronary heart disease morbidity and mortality in the sexes: a 26-year follow-up of the Framingham population. *American Heart Journal, 111,* 383-390.

Liao, Y., Cooper, R., (1995). Continued adverse trends in coronary heart disease mortality among Blacks, 1980-1991, *Public Health Reports, 110,* 572-578.

LoBiondo-Wood, G., Zimmerman, L.M., & Gatson-Johansson, F.J. (1989, April 2). *Pain descriptors selected by different ethnic groups.* Paper presented at the 13th Annual Midwest Nursing Research Society Conference, Cincinnati, Ohio.

Mbiti, J. (1970). *African religions and philosophies.* New York: Anchor Books.

McCrackin, R. (1971). Lactose deficiency: an example of dietary evaluation. *Current Anthropology, 12*(4-5), 479-517.

McKenzie, J., & Chrisman, N. (1977). Healing herbs, gods, and magic. *Nursing Outlook, 25*(5), 325-327.

Meyers, J., & Weissman, M. (1980-1981). *The prevalence of psychiatric disorders (DSM-III in the community: 1980-1981).* Unpublished manuscript.

Mitchel, F. (1978). *Voodoo medicine: Sea Islands herbal remedies.* Berkeley, Calif.: Reed, Cannon, & Johnson.

Moore, R., Stanton, D., Gopalan, R., & Chaisson, R. (1994). Racial differences in the use of drug therapy for HIV disease in the urban community. *New England Journal of Medicine, 330*(11), 763-768.

Morbidity and Mortality Weekly Report (1997). *47,* 20-28.

Morbidity and Mortality Weekly Report (1998). *47,* 22-27.

Morbidity and Mortality Weekly Report (1998). *47,* 91-93.

Morton, N.E. (1977). Genetic aspects of prematurity. In Reed, D.M., & Stanley, F.J. (Eds.), *Epidemiology of prematurity.* Baltimore: Urban & Schwarzenberg.

Mukherjee, S., Shukla, S., & Woodle, J. (1983). Misdiagnosis of schizophrenia in bipolar patients: a multiethnic comparison. *American Journal of Psychiatry, 140,* 1571-1574.

Muma, R., & Borucki, M. (1994). Epidemiology. In Muma, R., Lyons, B., Borucki, M., & Pollard, R. (Eds.), *HIV manual for health care professionals.* East Norwalk, Conn.: Appleton & Lange.

Murray, R.B, & Huelskoetter, M.W. (1991). *Psychiatric/mental health nursing.* East Norwalk, Conn.: Appleton & Lange.

National Center for Health Statistics (1985, Sept.). *Monthly Vital Statistics, 34* (suppl. 2), 1-24.

National Center for Health Statistics (1990). *Health, United States, 1989* (DHHS Publication No. PHS 6, 93-1232). Hyattsville, Md.: Public Health Services.

National Center for Health Statistics (1991). *Health, United States, 1990* (DHHS Publication No. PHS 6, 93-1232). Hyattsville, Md.: Public Health Services.

National Center for Health Statistics, Healthy People 2000 Review (1993). *Health, United States, 1992* (DHHS Publication No. PHS 93-1232). Hyattsville, Md.: Public Health Services.

National Center for Health Statistics (1998). *Health, United States, 1998,* Socioeconomic status and Health Chartbook (DHHS Publication No. PHS 6, 98-1232). Hyattsville, Md.: Public Health Services.

Oscherwitz, M. (1972). Differences in pulmonary function in various racial groups. *American Journal of Epidemiology, 96*(5), 319-327.

Overfield, R.T. (1995). *Biologic variations in health and illness: race, age and sex differences* (ed. 2). Reading, Mass.: Addison-Wesley.

Owen, G.M., & Lubin, A. (1973). Anthropometric differences between Black and White preschool children. *American Journal of Diseases in Children, 126,* 168.

Parker, D., & Harman, M. (1978). The distribution of consumption model of prevention of alcoholic problems: a critical assessment. *Journal of the Study of Alcohol, 39,* 377-399.

Pasamanick, B. (1964). Myths regarding prevalence of mental disease in the Negro. *Journal of the National Medical Association, 58,* 6-17.

Penk, W.E, Robinowitz, R., Black, J., et al. (1989). Ethnicity: post-traumatic stress disorder (PTSD) differences among black, white, and Hispanic veterans who differ in degrees of exposure to combat in Vietnam. *Journal of Clinical Psychology, 45*(5), 729-735.

Pillsbury, B. (1982). Doing the month: confinement and convalescence of Chinese women after childbirth. In Kay, M. (Ed.), *Anthropology of human birth.* Philadelphia: F.A. Davis.

Ploski, H., & Williams, J. (1989). *The Negro almanac: a reference work on the African-American* (ed. 5). Detroit: Gale Research.

Poussaint, A., & Atkinson, C. (1970). Black youth and motivation. *Black Scholar, 1,* 43-51.

Pratt, M.W., Janus, Z.L., & Sayal, N.C. (1977). National variations in prematurity (1973 and 1974). In Reed, D.M., & Stanley, F.J. (Eds.), *The epidemiology of prematurity* (pp. 53-74). Baltimore: Urban & Schwarzenberg.

Preliminary first-ever and total incidence rates of stroke among blacks. *Stroke, 29,* 415-421.

Remington, G., & DaCosta, G. (1989). Ethnocultural factors in resident supervision: black and white supervisors. *American Journal of Psychotherapy, 43*(3), 343-355.

Robins, L.N, Helzer, J.E, Croughan, J., & Ratcliff, K.S. (1981). National Institutes of Mental Health Diagnostic Interview Schedule: its history, characteristics, and validity. *Archives of General Psychiatry, 38,* 381-389.

Roche, A.F., Roberts, J., & Hamell, P.V. (1978). Skeletal maturity of youths 12-17 years of age: racial, geographic and socioeconomic disproportions. *National Health, 11*(167), 1-98.

Ronan, L. (1987). Alcohol-related health risks among Black Americans. *Alcohol Health and Research World, 12,* 36-39.

Rook, A. (1970). *Racial and other genetic factors in dermatology.* Philadelphia: F.A. Davis.

Sandoval, M. (1977). Santería: Afro-Cuban concepts of disease and its treatment in Miami. *Journal of Operational Psychiatry, 8*(52), 48-53.

Scope; refer to Institute of Black Chemical Abuse (1989).

Scott, N., Kelsey, S., Detre, L., et al. and the NHLBI PTCA Registry Investigators (1994). Percutaneous transluminal coronary angioplasty in African-American patients (The National Heart Lung and Blood Institute 1985-1986 Percutaneous Transluminal Coronary Angioplasty Registry). *American Journal of Cardiology, 73,* 1141-1146.

Smith, J.A. (1976). The role of the Black clergy as allied health care professionals in working with Black patients. In Luckraft, D. (Ed.), *Black awareness: implications for Black care* (pp. 12-15). New York: The American Journal of Nursing Company.

Snow, L.E. (1974). Folk medical beliefs and their implications for care of patients: a review based on studies among Black Americans. *Annuals of Internal Medicine, 81,* 82-96.

Snow, L.E. (1977). Popular medicine in a Black neighborhood. In Spicer, E.H. (Ed.), *Ethnic medicine in the Southwest.* Tucson: University of Arizona Press.

Snow, L.E. (1978). Sorcerers, saints, and charlatans: Black folk healers in urban America. *Culture, Medicine, and Psychiatry, 2,* 69.

Snow, L.E. (1983). Traditional health beliefs and practice among lower class Black Americans. *Western Journal of Medicine, 139*(6), 820-828.

Snowden, L. (1982). *Reaching the underserved: mental health needs of neglected populations.* Newbury Park, Calif.: Sage Publications.

Snowden, L., & Todman, P.A. (1982). The psychological assessment of Blacks: new and needed developments. In Johns, E.E., & Korchin, S.J. (Eds.), *Minority mental health* (pp. 193-226). New York: Praeger.

Spector, R.E. (1979). *Cultural diversity in health and illness.* East Norwalk, Conn.: Appleton-Century-Crofts.

Spurlock, J. (1985). Psychiatric states. In Williams, R.A. (Ed.), *Textbook of Black-related diseases.* New York: McGraw-Hill.

Stalls, F.A. (1978). Racial differences in alcohol metabolism. *Alcohol Clinical and Experimental Research, 2*(1), 10.

Stanhope, M., & Lancaster, J. (1988). *Community health nursing.* St. Louis: Mosby.

Staples, R. (1976). *Introduction to Black sociology.* New York: McGraw-Hill.

Sterne, M., & Pittman, D.J. (1972). *Drinking practices in the ghetto.* St. Louis: Washington University Social Science Institute.

Stokes, J., III, Kannel, W.B., Wolf, P.A., et al. (1987). The relative importance of selected risk factors for various manifestations of cardiovascular disease among men and women from 35 to 64 years old: 30 years of follow-up in the Framingham study. *Circulation, 75*(6 pt. 2), V65-73.

Stokes, L.G. (1977). Delivering health services in a Black community. In Reinhardt, A.M., & Quinn, M.B. (Eds.), *Current practice in family-centered community nursing* (pp. 51-65). St. Louis: Mosby.

Sue, D. (1981). *Counseling the culturally different: theory and practice.* New York: John Wiley & Sons.

Thomas, A., & Sillen, S. (1972). *Racism and psychiatry.* New York: Brunner/Mazel.

Tobias, P. (1970). Brain-size, grey matter, and race: fact or fiction. *American Journal of Physical Anthropology, 32,* 3-26.

Turner, L. (1948, April). Problems confronting the investigation of Gullah. *American Dialect Society Publications, 9,* 78-84.

Trotter, D. (1996). Nursing role in management of hypertension. In Lewis, S., Collier, I., & Heitkemper, M. (Eds.), *Medical surgical nursing assessment and management of clinical problems* (ed. 4) (867-870). St. Louis: Mosby.

U.S. Department of Commerce, Bureau of the Census (1982). *Current population reports, divisions and states: 1980* (1980 Census of Population, Doc. No. P.C. 80-51-1. Superintendent of Documents). Washington, D.C.: Government Printing Office.

U.S. Department of Commerce, Bureau of the Census. (1992). *The Black population in the United States, March 1991* (Publication No. P20-464). Washington, D.C.: Government Printing Office.

U.S. Department of Commerce, Bureau of the Census (1993a, June 12). News Release, Washington, D.C.: Commerce News.

U.S. Department of Commerce, Bureau of the Census (1993b). *We the American Blacks.* Washington, D.C.: Racial Statistical Branch: Bureau of the Census.

Vernon, S., & Roberts, R. (1982). *Use of the SADS-RDC in a triethnic community survey.* Springfield, Mass.: Merriam-Webster.

Ward J., & Duchin, J. (1998). US epidemiology of HIV and AIDS. In Volberding, P.A, & Jacobson, M.A. (Eds.), *AIDS clinical review* (10-32). New York: Marcel Dekker Publications.

Weclew, R. (1975). The nature, prevalence, and level of awareness of *curanderismo* and some of its implications for community health. *Community Mental Health Journal, 11,* 145.

Westermeyer, J. (1984). The role of ethnicity in substance abuse. In Stimmel, B. (Ed.), *Cultural and sociological aspects of alcoholism and substance abuse* (pp. 9-18). New York: Haworth Press.

White, E.H. (1977). Giving health care to minority patients. *Nursing Clinics in North America, 12,* 27-40.

Wieck, K.L., (1997). Hypertension in an inner city minority. *Journal of Cardiovascular Nursing, 11,* 41-49.

Williams, M. (1986). Alcohol and ethnic minorities: Native Americans—an update. *Alcohol Health and Research Works, 11*(2), 5-6.

Wintrob, R. (1973). The influences of others: witchcraft and rootwork as explanations of behavior disturbances. *Journal of Nervous and Mental Disorders, 156,* 318.

Wolfram, W.A., & Clark, H. (Eds.) (1971). *Black-White speech relationships.* Washington, D.C.: Center for Applied Linguistics.

Woods, S. (1998). Can aspirin prevent coronary heart disease in women? *Women's Health in Primary Care, 1,* 210-214.

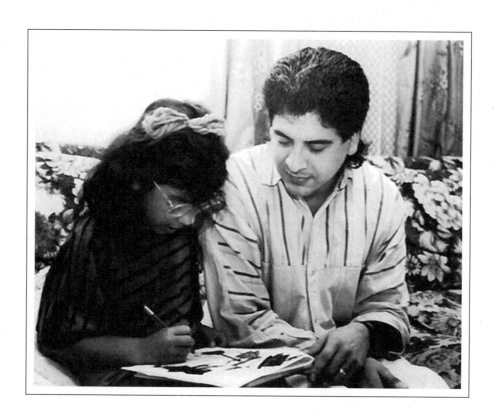

Joan Kuipers

CHAPTER 9 Mexican Americans

BEHAVIORAL OBJECTIVES

After reading this chapter, the nurse will be able to:

1. Discuss the influence of Spanish-language usage by Mexican Americans in adapting to the mainstream United States culture.
2. Explain the distance and intimacy behaviors of Mexican Americans.
3. Describe the organization of the Mexican-American family unit.
4. Explain the Mexican-American orientation to time.
5. Identify Mexican-American beliefs regarding the ability to control the environment.
6. Describe how the "hot-cold" beliefs of Mexican Americans influence their health and illness beliefs.
7. Explain the health care beliefs, diseases, and practices within the *curanderismo* folklore system.
8. Identify the biological variations of Mexican Americans.
9. Identify implications or precautions for providing effective nursing care to Mexican Americans.

OVERVIEW OF MEXICO

Mexico, or what is officially referred to as the United Mexican States *(Estados Unidos Mexicanos)*, is a country in the southern part of North America. Mexico consists of 31 states and a federal district. The boundaries of Mexico extend southward from the United States to Guatemala and Belize in Central America. The western coast of Mexico borders on the Pacific Ocean, which includes the Gulf of California and the Gulf of Tehuantepec. The eastern coast of Mexico fronts on the Caribbean Sea and the Gulf of Mexico, which includes the Bay of Campeche. Mexico, which includes several outlying islands, has a total area of 761,604 square miles and is the third largest Latin-American nation after Brazil and Argentina. Mexico is about a fifth the size of the United States.

Most Mexicans are *mestizos,* that is, of mixed Spanish and Indian descent. They trace their native heritage back to Indian groups that built great civilizations in Mexico long before the Spanish explorers arrived in the 1500s (Falicov, 1982). When the Spaniards came to Mexico in 1519, they found Indians who were skilled in writing, mathematics, astronomy, painting, sculpture, and architecture. Indian pottery, metalwork, and textiles were very highly developed for the time period. Spain's discovery and eventual conquest of Mexico marked the start of the destruction of many elements of long-standing civilization (Villarruel & Leininger, 1995). Missionaries were sent to convert the Indians to Christianity. Many of the riches of the land were carried back to Spain. Many of the native beliefs about medicinal plants were incorporated into the Spanish medicinal system. The use of the native herbal remedies by the Spaniards may be one explanation for the contemporary cultural commitment of this type of health treatment (Villarruel & Leininger, 1995).

In 1997, the population of Mexico was estimated to be 97,563,374 (Information Please Almanac, 1998). During 1983 and 1984, Mexico suffered its worst financial crisis in 50 years, leading to critically high unemployment and an inability to pay its foreign debt. The collapse of oil prices in 1986 cut into Mexico's export earnings and worsened the situation. Political and governmental conflict since that time has resulted in an unstable situation that has contributed to many Mexicans seeking economic gain in the United States. In February 1995, agreement was reached with the United States to prevent the collapse of Mexico's private banks. However, strict provisions gave the United States virtual veto power over key elements in Mexico's economic policy. As a consequence of the terms for receiving international support, the Mexican economy suffered a severe recession in 1995 and the peso fell drastically.

In 1997 it was estimated Mexico had a population of 97,563,374 with an average annual rate of natural increase of 2.12%. The birth rate of Mexico is estimated to be 25.8 births per 1000 persons, whereas the infant mortality is estimated to be 23.9 per 1000 persons (Information Please Almanac, 1998). For every child between 1 and 4 years of age who dies in the United States, approximately 23 die in Mexico (U.S. Department of Commerce, Bureau of the Census, 1993b). One of the leading causes of death among children is malnutrition. Approximately 50% to 75% of the Mexican population suffer from malnutrition. Although the problem of malnutrition in Mexico is believed to be primarily economic, it may also have an educational component. The life expectancy at birth has increased from 35 to 62 years of age over the last 4 decades. The gross domestic product (1995 estimate) is $721.4 billion with a $7700 per capita income (Information Please Almanac, 1998).

MEXICAN AMERICANS

The southwest region of the United States was settled by Spaniards in 1598 in what is today New

Mexico. Later, citizens of the United States began settling in what was then Mexican territory. Mexicans helped establish many southwestern cities and taught the settlers skills in mining, farming, and ranching. After the Mexican-American War (1846-1848) in the Treaty of Guadalupe Hidalgo (1848) the United States assumed what is today Arizona, California, Texas, New Mexico, Utah, parts of Colorado, Nevada, and Wyoming. A treaty provided those of Mexican descent land and cultural rights. Unfortunately these rights were never honored, and Mexican Americans living in these areas tended to become an economically segregated working-class group (Moore & Pachon, 1985).

Over the years numerous socioeconomic and political conditions in Mexico and the United States have contributed to the movement of Mexicans to the United States including the Mexican Revolution of 1910, the demand for cheap agricultural and industrial labor in the United States, and, most recently, the North American Free Trade Agreement (Villarruel & Leininger, 1995; Althaus, 1997). Because of the geographical closeness of Mexico and the United States and the permeability of the border, some Mexicans move back and forth between Mexico and the United States legally and some illegally. This movement allows them to remain in contact with their families and native customs while at the same time seeking economic opportunities in the United States. Mexican Americans who have immigrated have tended to move into the southwestern section of the United States, where the majority reside in Texas and California. Most Mexican Americans have rural agricultural backgrounds (U.S. Department of Commerce, Bureau of the Census, 1993b). However, it is difficult to generalize about geographical location and the occupational background of people in this ethnic group. The diversity in Mexican Americans ranges from rural villagers in New Mexico and Colorado (Saunders, 1954; Weaver 1970), to agricultural laborers in Texas (Rubel, 1966), to low-income residents in Arizona, to urban low-class individuals in California (Clark, 1970). Just as the people are diverse, so too are the many studies that represent different populations of Mexicans and offer differing definitions of Mexican

Americans. Therefore any discussion of Mexican Americans is further complicated by the problem of precisely defining this population.

The proximity of Mexico to the United States has resulted in a noteworthy amount of drug trafficking. The practice of smoking *Cannabis* leaves came to the United States with Mexican immigrants who came North during the 1920s (Musto, 1991). Today, much of the cocaine that reaches the United States from Colombia comes by way of Mexico (Booth, 1996). Along with the drugs has come an increase in violence for border cities. Law-enforcement officials say the violence is a direct result of Mexico's drug organizations though others say that drug problems in the United States are not simply from Mexico (Lee, 1997). However, the increase in violence in border cities and cities on the West coast is in contrast to the general decrease in crime rates across the United States (LaFranchi, 1997). This is also creating problems for the judicial system by packing jail cells and for the inner city health care provision because the health care system is not prepared for the influx of health and socially related problems (Lynn, 1997; Nugent, Linares, Brykczynski, Crawford, Fuller, & Riggs, 1988).

Use of the health care system in America has been problematic for many Mexican Americans (Hahn, 1995). Ross (1995) noted that job-based insurance is possessed by 63% of Whites in the United States, 57% of Asians, 46% of Blacks, but only 37% of Hispanics. Explanations for lack of insurance is partly related to communication difficulties and lack of understanding that insurance is needed. Lack of health insurance is also related to culture because most Hispanics who have immigrated recently do not understand the competitive health care market and that they need insurance, and many still place their trust in traditional herbal remedies (Ross, 1995; Villarruel & Leininger, 1995). Additionally complicating the use of the health care system is that many Mexican Americans lack work skills, have low-paying jobs, and live in crowded substandard city housing, which has limited access to quality health care facilities (García, 1988; Ross, 1995).

Immigration of Mexicans to the United States has created difficulties in some schools in the western United States. Some schools have not adapted to handle the influx of Mexican Americans and the special needs of teaching children who do not have English-speaking skills (Serrano, 1997). In California funds are not provided for educating children who are illegal aliens.

According to the U.S. Department of Commerce, Bureau of the Census (1993b), the Mexican-American population nearly doubled in size between 1970 and 1980. The Mexican-American population continues to grow. Between 1980 and 1990, the number of Mexican Americans residing in the United States doubled again in size. Today there are 13,495,938 Mexican Americans residing in the United States composing 5.4% of the general population (U.S. Department of Commerce, Bureau of the Census, 1993a). Mexican Americans, or Chicanos, are also the largest Hispanic group residing in the United States, representing 61% of the 22.3 million Hispanic people (U.S. Department of Commerce, Bureau of the Census, 1993b). Cubans (5%), Puerto Ricans (13%), Central and South Americans (12%), and other Hispanics make up the other 39% (U.S. Department of Commerce, Bureau of the Census, 1993a). It is projected that by the year 2000 there were be over 31 million Hispanics in the United States and will outnumber all other minority groups in the United States (Caudle, 1993; Ross, 1995). Although 9.0% of the United States population were Hispanic American in 1990, it is projected that by the year 2021 the Hispanic-American population will triple (U.S. Department of Commerce, Bureau of the Census, 1992). Contributing to the population growth is the youthfulness and high fertility among Hispanics (de León Siantz, 1994). In 1998, the number of Mexican Americans residing in the United States numbered 18,039,000 (U.S. Department of Commerce, Bureau of the Census, 1998). If the current population estimates hold constant by the year 2010, Hispanics will outnumber African Americans (41,139,000 to 40,109,000 (U.S. Department of Commerce, Bureau of the Census, 1998).

"Cultural uniqueness" is not academic nomenclature for Mexican Americans. The phrase is used to describe physical, emotional, and behavioral distinctions unique to many Mexican Americans (Chávez,

1986). Unlike European immigrants who often hasten to absorb the culture found in the United States, many Mexican Americans have not. Even today, Mexican Americans try to retain a cultural identity within the dominant population (Chávez, 1986). In *Megatrends*, John Naisbitt (1982) states that "none of the new groups individually can begin to match the numbers and the potential influence of Spanish-speaking Americans." Concepts such as *machismo* (manliness), *confianza* (confidence), *respeto* (respect), *vergüenza* (shame), and *orgullo* (pride) predominate in the culture, and traditional gender and family roles continue to be part of the heritage that separates Mexican Americans from other cultural groups. Unfortunately and perhaps because of the desire to retain cultural identity, many Mexican Americans have experienced discrimination in education, jobs, and housing. Skin color, language differences, and Spanish surnames have all contributed to discrimination. For some Mexican Americans, feelings of isolation, persecution, and discrimination have resulted in acute paranoid reactions and post-traumatic stress disorder (PTSD) (Cervantes, Snyder, & Padilla, 1989; Murphy, Giger, & Davidhizar, 1994; Rivera, 1978).

Although some Mexican Americans are well educated (Favazza, 1983), according to Bonilla (1973), the educational achievement of most Mexican Americans is extremely low. For example, in the early 1970s the average Mexican-American child completed only a seventh-grade education; only 27% of Mexican Americans completed high school; and only 2.5% of Mexican-American men and 1% of Mexican-American women graduated from college (Statistical Abstracts, 1988). In 1986 Mexican Americans who had less than 5 years of schooling encompassed a total population of 15.5%: in the 25- to 34-year-old age group, approximately 6% had less than 5 years of schooling; in the 35- to 44-year-old age group, 10.2% had less than 5 years of schooling; in the 45- to 64-year-old age group, 17.5% had less than 5 years of schooling; and in the 65-year-old or older age group, 33.1% had less than 5 years of schooling. In contrast, in 1986 Mexican Americans who had completed 4 years of high school or higher education encompassed a total population of 37.6%:

in the 25- to 34-year-old age group, 54.7% had completed high school or more; in the 35- to 44-year-old age group, 47% had completed high school or more; in the 45- to 64-year-old age group, 33.5% had completed high school or more; and in the 65-year-old or older age group, approximately 9.8% had completed high school or more (Statistical Abstracts, 1988). Gradually, Mexican Americans have learned the English language, and as they have begun to speak English more fluently, the level of education has increased. In 1990, 44% of Mexican Americans had completed high school, and 6.2% had obtained a college degree (U.S. Department of Commerce, Bureau of the Census, 1993b). Consequently, problems of some Mexican Americans are dissipating as they become more active in seeking solutions to poor housing, jobs, and discrimination.

A major issue for some Mexican Americans is lack of citizenship, which is a barrier to gaining education, skills, stable jobs, decent living conditions, and government benefits. Mexican Americans who are illegal aliens frequently experience tension regarding discovery and deportation back to Mexico. Preoccupation with possible discovery and deportation for illegal aliens serves to further augment the symptoms of PTSD (Cervantes, Snyder, & Padilla, 1989). The plight of the illegal alien has been expanded since enactment of the Immigration and Reform and Control Act of 1986 (Gelfand & Bialik-Gilad, 1989). In an attempt to control illegal immigration into the United States, employers are now required to verify citizenship status within 24 hours after hiring an employee. Sanctions are being placed against employers who fail to meet this requirement or who hire illegal aliens knowingly. Noncitizens who apply for public assistance funds must verify that they are not undocumented aliens. It is now very difficult for these people to obtain health care except from church-related agencies. Because of diagnostic-related group requirements, hospitals are not so willing to treat uninsured, indigent people. Also, undocumented aliens do not qualify for Medicare or Medicaid funds. There are some states (such as California) where health care is not provided for undocumented aliens. Nonetheless, it is feared that, as this group ages without adequate health care, chronic and costly medical conditions will develop. Because of employer sanctions, aliens are forced into low-paying jobs, which limit even more their ability to support the costs of their own health care needs or those of their aged relatives (West & Moore, 1989). Many employers have been accused of knowingly hiring illegal workers because they are willing to work for less compensation (Taylor & Smith, 1997). However, although immigration officers may sweep through a plant, picking up illegal aliens and deporting them, many are soon back. Meanwhile the cost to the United States taxpayer for this process and the economic hardship on both the illegal aliens and the employers leave this an unsolved international problem (Taylor & Smith, 1997).

In 1990, 73.0% of Mexican-American families were married couple families, 8.8% were single male householder families, and 21.0% were female-headed households. Of the total number of Hispanic males in the work force, 28.1% held jobs as operators, fabricators, and laborers; 19.7% held jobs in precision, production, craft, and repair; 16.1% held jobs in services; 16.7% held jobs in technical, sales, and administrative support; 12.0% held jobs in managerial and professional specialties; and 7.4% held jobs in farming, forestry, and fishing (U.S. Department of Commerce, Bureau of the Census, 1993b). Despite the shift from jobs related to agriculture for the general population of Hispanics residing in the United States, in 1990 the median family income for Hispanics was only $25,064, compared with $35,225 for the general population (U.S. Department of Commerce, Bureau of the Census, 1993b). Although Mexican Americans have not been broken out of the labor statistics thus far reported by the Census Bureau, they have fared better than some Hispanics regarding median family income (that is, Puerto Ricans, $21,941; Dominicans, $19,726). In fact, for all Mexican-American families, the median income is $24,119. However, Mexican-American female householders have not fared so well, with a median income of $12,714 (U.S. Department of Commerce, Bureau of the Census, 1993b).

In stark contrast to the data presented by the Census Bureau, in a presentation for the National Conference on Migrant and Seasonal Farmworkers (May 11, 1993) and other data that describe the migrant population as a variety of ethnic and racial backgrounds, including Hispanic/Latino, Black/African American, Jamaican, Haitian, Hmong, and Anglo among others (National Commission to Prevent Infant Mortality, 1993), Kissam reported that, except for southern Florida, 80% to 90% of all the migrant and seasonal labor force were foreign born and almost all were of Mexican origin (Mines, Gabbard, & Samardick, 1992). Kissam reported the following developments in the migrant Mexican labor force: (1) diffusion into other geographical areas of the United States, (2) greater ethnic and linguistic diversity than earlier workers, (3) increasing numbers of unaccompanied males supporting families who remain at home, (4) changing characteristics of reunited families settling in the United States after the father had migrated for 5 to 10 years (Children of these families transfer to U.S. schools after years of school in Mexico, rather than having K-12 schooling in the United States. These families experience a high level of stress in assimilating as a united family and as immigrants.), (5) increasing numbers of very young and very old migrant workers, and (6) growing numbers of female-headed households. The changing demographics of Mexican migrant farmworkers present many challenges to U.S. agencies in adequately meeting their needs. Although the majority of migrant and seasonal farmworkers are U.S. citizens or legal residents of the United States, most experience prejudice and hostility in the communities in which they live and work (National Center for Farmworker Health, 1995). Most migrant farmworkers earn an annual income below the poverty level and half earn wages below $7500 per year (National Center for Farmworker Health, 1995). Most migrant farmworkers have a Third World health status despite living in one of the richest nations on earth (Anderson & Murphy, 1996).

COMMUNICATION

Spanish, the primary language for many Mexican Americans, is the third most commonly used language in the world and one of the six languages used by the United Nations (Monrroy, 1983).

Dialect

The Spanish language is spoken in many dialects; Mexican Americans who have an Indian heritage may speak one of more than 50 Spanish dialects. Fortunately, however, most of the words spoken have the same meaning (Monrroy, 1983). Differences in dialect may be found in certain communities. Dialects may also be identified by their proximity to the Mexican border.

Touch

Adult Mexican Americans can be characterized as tactile in their relationships. Although female Mexican Americans may initiate more tactile behavior in communicating, there is a contradiction where modesty is concerned. There is a strong social value that women do not expose their bodies to men or even other women. During a pelvic examination a female Mexican-American client may express "feeling hot" because of the embarrassment from the examination (Brownlee, 1978). Some Mexican Americans will even avoid touching their own genitalia (Clark, 1970). Although religious beliefs may explain lack of birth control, extreme discomfort with certain areas of the body may also explain why some Mexican-American women avoid the use of a diaphragm. Men also have strong feelings about modesty and may feel threatened if expected to have a complete physical examination (Murillo, 1978). This modesty may explain the reluctance of some Mexican-American men to use condoms (Monrroy, 1983).

Context

When being interviewed, Mexican Americans may engage in "small talk" before approaching the business of the interview. It is important for the nurse to remember that small talk will often facilitate accomplishing nursing objectives for the interview and is therefore not a "waste of time."

Murillo (1978) has noted that in communicating with others, Mexican Americans use diplomacy and tactfulness. There is also pride in verbal expression, which is likely to be elaborate and indirect. Direct confrontation and arguments are considered rude and disrespectful. Self-disclosure is reserved for those whom the individual knows well. The Mexican American may appear agreeable on the surface regarding an issue because of the value of courtesy. However, later the nurse may be surprised and disappointed because agreements are not being carried out. Kidding is seen as rude, deprecating, and offensive and is likely to generate a negative response (Monrroy, 1983). In communicating, Mexican Americans use all the physiological senses such as smelling, tasting, touching, feeling, and hearing. Intensified use of the senses in communication has been related to the Mexican American's love of sounds, bright colors, action, and even spicy food (Murillo, 1978).

Kinesics

Eye behavior is important to Mexican Americans, especially when children are involved. *Mal ojo* ('evil eye') is a folk illness described as a condition that affects infants and children (Dorsey & Jackson, 1976) and occurs because an individual who is believed to possess a special power voluntarily or involuntarily injures a child by looking at and admiring but not touching the child (Foster, 1978). With this condition the child cries, develops a fever, vomits, and loses its appetite. This disorder may be prevented by touching or patting a child when admiring the child. The spell is broken when the individual who has given the "evil eye" touches the child. Therefore the nurse should touch the child when giving care because in the minds of Mexican Americans this action can both prevent and treat the illness.

English as a second language

Most Mexican Americans can also speak some English. However, the inability to speak English fluently has led to a high failure rate for school-aged Mexican Americans. Lack of language fluency has also limited the ability to improve job status and in turn the quality of life. Laosa (1975) reported that the longer Mexican immigrants stay in the United States, the less likely they are to retain the mother language, which probably is most directly attributable to the fact that English is the language used in schools and at work. Increasing attention is being given to the need for bilingual education for Mexican-American students, and as a result, more

Mexican Americans are becoming bilingual. However, a reverse problem is sometimes encountered where young Mexican children learn English as their primary language and then are not able to communicate with older relatives who speak only Spanish (Gonzales, 1997).

Communication by Mexican Americans is also complicated because many Mexican Americans learn a language that blends English and Spanish. Mexican-American adults use this blended form of language more often than children do. Consequently, a nurse who may know both English and Spanish may still have difficulty understanding this blended language.

Some Mexican Americans still use English selectively. In an extensive study on language loyalty among various ethnic groups residing in the United States, it was found that Spanish remains the most persistent of all foreign languages. Thus, because of its persistent use, Spanish seemingly has the greatest prospects of survival (Fishman, 1967). Although other ethnic groups have become disillusioned with the use of their mother tongue, Mexican Americans have been more likely to retain their mother language in succeeding generations in the United States. Even today, some fluency in Spanish characterizes most Mexican Americans at all income levels. Another reason for the persistence of Spanish among Mexican Americans is that in the United States the mass media for information and entertainment is permeated with Spanish. Today Spanish accounts for approximately 66% of the total foreign-language broadcasting in the United States. The demand for more Spanish-language media has led to the development of two national Spanish-language television networks. During the 1980s, 200 U.S. radio stations broadcasted in Spanish. There has been a dramatic increase in Spanish-language newspapers, magazines, and journals (Galván, 1993). This is significant for the provision of improved health care for these people.

It is not uncommon for people who speak different languages to use each language in different contexts or for different purposes. Perhaps the most frequent situation is that of Mexican Americans who use English in their work and Spanish at home or with their friends (Marcos, 1988). There are several rather isolated villages in northern New Mexico where the only English spoken is for official occasions such as conferring with a government agency. Because of the remoteness of these communities, these Mexican Americans may retain Spanish as their principal language.

Implications for nursing care

Because some Mexican Americans rely on Spanish to communicate with other people, it is very frightening for them to participate in the American health care system, and it is frustrating for the nurses giving them care. Hahn (1995) noted that some White Americans are ethnocentric and although they work with Mexican Americans they may think that it is unimportant to learn the language. On the other hand, some health care professionals realize that clients may feel more comfortable receiving care from someone with a similar ethnic background and are working to recruit Mexican-American students (Ludwig-Beymer, Blankemeier, Casas-Byots, & Suarez-Balcazar, 1996). Another way to assist in the comfort level of clients is to encourage students preparing to serve the Mexican population to study Spanish because clients could be encouraged to communicate in the language most comfortable to them. This is particularly true in areas of the country like southern California, where the Mexican population is growing (Gonzales, 1997). When professional staff cannot speak Spanish and professional translators or a bilingual family is not available, Hahn (1995) also noted that it may be necessary to have the housekeeping staff translate, a less-than-ideal situation.

It is important for the nurse to remember that language is a cultural factor that influences health care practices. The nurse who works with bilingual Mexican Americans must remember that often under stress these persons may revert to their first language, Spanish. The nurse should avoid scolding the client who communicates in Spanish. Rather, the nurse should emphasize that the nurse can be more helpful if the client communicates in the language that both the nurse and the client understand. When this is impossible because of high levels of stress on the part of the client, the nurse should find a translator. Family members may provide invaluable assistance both in reducing stress and in translating the client's needs. Using family members could also promote the building of trust in the nurse to facilitate compliance on the part of the client.

Understanding the profound effect of bilingualism on the client also requires appreciation of the dimension of language independence—the capacity to acquire, maintain, and use two separate language codes, each with its own lexical, syntactic, phonetic, semantic, and ideational components. Many Mexican Americans who are proficient in both Spanish and English operate parallel language codes, each with its own associations between message words and events in their ideational system (Marcos & Alpert, 1976). A good example of language compartmentalization can be found in the saying of Emperor Charles V: "To God I speak in Spanish, to women in Italian, to men in French, and to my horse in German" (Oxford Dictionary of Quotations, 1980). In certain situations a client may speak to his or her family in Spanish, to the nurse in English, and, when extremely stressed, to both family and nurse in a combination of both English and Spanish. This tendency for bilingualism can become extremely alarming for the client as well as for health care providers. For the nurse caring for a Mexican-American surgical client, Burden (1986) provided a useful Spanish translation guide to assist in implementing individualized care. In addition, Murphy, Giger, and Davidhizar (1994) have suggested strategies for teaching non–English speaking clients through the use of culturally relevant client education material. The nurse may also find the Short Acculturation Scale for Hispanics (SAS) useful in providing information on the client's level of acculturation in order to provide culturally competent care (Marín, Sabogal, Marín, et al., 1987).

It is also important for the nurse to keep in mind that Mexican Americans tend to describe emotional problems by using dramatic body language. In addition, research has shown that when Mexican Americans are interviewed in English, or across their language barrier, they are usually judged by experienced clinicians as showing a more severe degree of symptoms than when they are interviewed in their mother tongue (Favazza, 1983; Marcos, Alpert, Urcuyo, & Kesselman, 1973).

The nurse must guard against the use of idioms and abstractions when dealing with clients who do not completely understand the language. The nurse should also avoid responding to the client in a joking manner. For example, a nursing assistant working with a Mexican client who needed a bath jokingly used the phrase "dirty Mexican." The client reported this to the nursing supervisor, stating that this was a racial comment and therefore fell under the state statutes against client abuse. The nursing assistant countered that the phrase was used in a nonharmful manner to cajole the client into taking a bath because he was dirty. When working with a Mexican-American client who lacks understanding of the language, statements using slang or colloquialisms should be avoided because they may be interpreted literally.

One of the most important roles of the nurse in caring for the Mexican-American client is that of teacher. Teaching should begin with an assessment of the client's ability to communicate and understand, which will guide the nurse in deciding which other family members should be included in the teaching process. The home situation must be carefully evaluated to adapt care to the reality of the living situation. Instruction should include all aspects of the client's condition and treatment and should be communicated in simple, concrete terms with ample opportunity to raise questions and validate understanding. There should be continuous evaluation of learning by questioning and return demonstrations, and problem solving should be encouraged. Throughout this process the nurse must continue to build a trusting relationship with the client so that follow-up care will be maintained, helping to ensure that the client will seek medical care before future situations get out of control.

SPACE

Kluckhohn (1976) categorized people and the modalities of relationships as individualistic, collateral, or lineal. Some Mexican Americans are categorized as both collateral and lineal, implying that there may be a patron-peon system, such as a boss-worker relationship, or a family-versus-individual relationship.

Mexican Americans value physical presence, including that of family members. It is important for Mexican Americans to see relatives face to face, embrace, touch, and just be with each other (Keefe, 1984). Mexican Americans as a group demonstrate a great need for group togetherness. Ford and Graves (1977) found that when Mexican-American second-graders related to others, there was closer interpersonal distance and more touching among girls. Touching was of longer duration when spatial distances were closer. Boys tended to be less tactile when relating to others. It is believed that this pattern of socialization begins with the parent-child relationship and continues into adulthood. During the early years the parents are permissive, warm, and caring with all their children. However, in later years, the girls remain much closer to home and are protected and guarded in their contacts. In contrast, the boys are allowed to be with other boys in informal social groups where they develop their *machismo* (Murillo, 1978).

Implications for nursing care

Despite the fact that Mexican Americans like consistent, close relationships and physical touching, female nurses should always assist a male physician in examining a female client and guard against exposing body parts other than those that are the focus of the examination (Murillo-Rohde, 1977). Male clients may refuse to allow a complete examination because of their modesty.

The nurse who plans care delivery for Mexican-American clients must keep in mind that Mexican Americans may resist care provided by those perceived as being different or from a different ethnic background (Monroy, 1983). Some Mexican Americans may also have cultural biases that prohibit care being administered by persons of the opposite sex. For example, a male student nurse was assigned to a Mexican-American client in labor. This assignment precipitated problems because the client, husband, and family were all very uncomfortable because "only her husband should see her like that." It was necessary to change the assignment in order to provide care.

SOCIAL ORGANIZATION

The foundation of the Mexican community is the nuclear family (parents and children). It is generally believed that Mexican Americans are familistic. For some Mexican Americans familism has been perceived as curtailing mobility by sustaining emotional attachment to people, places, and things. In the Mexican-American culture, familism has been identified as the prime cause not only of low mobility, but also of resistance to changes of all kinds. For Mexican Americans, familism, along with the specially assigned male role, is a source of collective pride. Nevertheless, Mexican Americans are believed to be deterred from collective and individual progress because of familism.

For Mexican Americans extended family relationships have special significance, and the family is perhaps the most significant social organization (Murillo, 1978). The major dominating theme of the traditional Mexican-American family is the need for collective achievement of the family as a group. Thus the need for family collectivity and other family needs supersede the needs of individual members. Also, any dishonor or shame that may occur for an individual member is considered a reflection on the entire family. The Mexican-American family takes pride in family endeavors and generally does not seek help from outsiders to solve problems or meet needs. Mexican-American families place a great deal of value on having many relatives live nearby. The local extended family is tightly integrated, has frequent face-to-face encounters, and provides one another with mutual aid (Keefe, 1984). Lantican and Corona (1989) have reported that Mexican Americans have a mean network size of 5.78, which may include in-laws, grandparents, and a substantial number of other relatives. Some 69% of the Mexican Americans studied reported that most of their support was provided by immediate family members. One interesting aspect of this study revealed that for the Mexican-American primigravidas studied, pregnancy was most likely to be discussed with the husband first. There are frequent expressions of affection, trust, and respect among kin. Members of extended families are concerned about how their behaviors and actions will affect (either positively or negatively) their families. The Mexican-American client who is hospitalized often desires the presence of the family. Family members come to the hospital willingly and expect to be part of the decision-making process.

Villarruel and Denyes (1997) reported that the importance and obligation of Mexican Americans in meeting the needs of others indicates that there may be a higher priority placed on promoting and supporting the development of abilities to care for others than on abilities to care for self. Two other patterns, the "accepted obligation to perform roles within the family" and the "willingness to bear the burden so as not to cause pain for others" further indicate that caring for others is both expected and rewarded (Villarruel & Denyes, 1997; Villarruel, 1995). Tran and Dhooper (1996) noted that when Mexicans, Puerto Ricans, and Cubans elders were compared the level of education and sex was significant in identified patterns of social service needs. Cubans generally reported a lower rate of needs than the other two groups. Ethnic differences were more likely to appear among less educated respondents. Embry and Russell (1996) also studied elderly Mexicans. They noted a culturally prescribed definition of old and the use and sometimes over-reliance on the family as the support system. Sahud (1989) supported the pattern of Mexican elderly for reliance on support. However, Sahud noted that in the United States Mexican-American elderly tend to expect psychological support whereas in Mexico the expectation of support is all encompassing.

Most Mexican Americans have nuclear families that live separately, though some extended family or other relatives often live in the same household (Miller, 1986). According to Chávez (1986), new immigrants (especially those who are undocumented) tend to live in a multiple-family arrangement, which offers the advantages of social and economic support. As the length of residency increases and the family becomes more financially independent, the nuclear family tends to find a singular arrangement for its household.

There is a high incidence of teenage pregnancy found among Mexican Americans. Fitzpatrick et al.

(1990) found that, among United States teenage girls, Mexican Americans have the highest teenage pregnancy rate. In 1989, the birth rate for Mexican-American women 15 to 19 years of age was 94.5 per 1000 population, compared with 85.8 per 1000 for African-American women, and 66.0 per 1000 for White women (National Center for Health Statistics, Healthy People 2000 Review, 1993).

Within the family the father has the dominant role, assuming responsibility for being head of the house and the decision maker (Monrroy, 1983). For the male family member, there is a strong sense of *machismo* that is incompatible with the loss of self-esteem or authority. The mother of the family has a primary role of keeping the family cohesive. Although the mother may influence family decisions, she does not have a dominant role in the family. Increasing numbers of Mexican-American women are finding work outside the home. Women who live in a rural setting often help with the family farming activities. Divorce is uncommon, but stable out-of-wedlock relationships are common in the lower socioeconomic levels. Meleis, Douglas, Eribes, et al. (1996) reported that when a group of employed, low-income Mexican women who worked in urban hospitals were studied, role overload and stress was experienced. There appeared to be difficulty reconciling the traditional cultural expectations of a woman's role in the changing society, which added the role of working outside the home.

The entire family may contribute to the financial welfare of the family. Parental control in Mexican-American families is strong. Older children contribute by caring for younger family members or animals or by helping with the production of food or other family enterprises. Children in migrant families often earn money by working along with other family members. The elderly are respected and live with married children if they are not self-sufficient. The elderly also pass down cultural and folk medicine beliefs.

Váldez (1980) found that Mexican-American families of a lower socioeconomic class tended to show more ethnic identification than those of a higher socioeconomic class. This phenomenon served to provide support for Mexican Americans of lower socioeconomic classes and a more positive adaptation to the mainstream United States culture.

An important institution in the Mexican heritage is the Catholic practice of *compadrazgo,* or coparenthood (godparenthood), which was introduced to Mexico by the Spaniards. Godparents accept coresponsibilities for a child along with the parents. This kinship begins with the baptism of the child and continues throughout the child's life; it is used for religious purposes and becomes an important resource for coping with the stresses of life (Kemper, 1982). Frequently, a godparent is chosen from a higher socioeconomic level, which enables the child to have social resources that are more extensive than what the family could provide.

Another important tradition for many Mexican-American families is the way in which holidays are celebrated with Mexican traditions. Others continue to celebrate Mexican holidays. During the celebration of the Mexican Christmas, called *Las Posadas,* the children are fond of breaking a *piñata,* a papier-mâché container filled with candy and gifts. Other important holidays are Cinco de Mayo (May 5) and Guadalupe Day (December 12), which is Mexico's most important religious holiday. Affluent Mexican Americans often spend significant amounts of money on special food and drink, decorations, and fireworks for a holiday festival. Holidays provide an opportunity for Mexican Americans to share with others.

Death beliefs and practices

Many Mexican Americans believe that whatever the cause of death it is the will of God. For example, Kalish and Reynolds (1981) found that 72% of Mexican Americans believed that accidental death was attributable to divine will as compared with 56% of Anglo-Americans. Kalish and Reynolds (1981) also found that 27% of Mexican Americans thought of their own death daily compared to 13% of Anglo-Americans. Whereas none of the Anglo-Americans believed that individuals should be allowed to die when they feel unproductive or unhappy, 3% of Mexican Americans reported they believed this should be allowed. Seventy-six percent of the Mexican Americans in this study reported that they are likely to touch the body of a deceased family member compared to 51% of Anglo-Americans. Additionally 59% reported they would likely kiss the body of the deceased compared to 33% of Anglo-Americans. In addition, 59% of Mexican Ameraicans believe that a person should visit the grave of his or her spouse at least six times during the first year compared to 35% of Anglo-Americans.

Implications for nursing care

Of primary importance for the nurse caring for Mexican-American clients is the concept that family values and roles are paramount to the client's treatment and recovery. The nurse should remember that the male head of the family should be consulted in health care decision making for other family members. It is also important that the nurse include the entire family, both immediate and extended members, in the assessment, planning, and implementation of nursing care if treatment is to be effective (Hough, 1985). Rather than viewing a large family who wishes to be with the client as an annoyance and frustration to staff, the nurse should discuss with the family how visits can be planned so that care can still be delivered and the client can obtain needed rest.

Murillo-Rohde (1977) has suggested that nurses use the family to help with the client's care. She says the family could feed, bathe, or walk the client, thus decreasing the anxiety and guilt of the family and of the client. In addition, the nurse could be relieved of some of the work load. Allowing the family to participate in the client's care builds trust and respect and encourages compliance and support for discharge planning and teaching. However, the nurse should be aware that in one study by researchers at the University of California, only two thirds (65%) of the Mexican Americans in the study believed that the patient should be told if there was a diagnosis of metastatic cancer. The other respondents believed that the giving of information and the decision-making responsibility and information should rest with the family (Ethics; 1995). Thus, Mexican clients and families may not agree on who has the right to have medical information.

When the nurse is experiencing difficulty in getting a client to follow a particular medical regimen, the nurse may suggest that the client solicit the opinions of other family members regarding proposed actions. Suggesting family consultation will demonstrate that the nurse understands the importance of the family in regard to health matters. Nurses can encourage Mexican-American clients to use health-promoting behaviors with the rationale that the family cares about their health and will support them in meeting their goals (Kerr & Ritchey, 1990). Furthermore, the nurse's actions should help to build a relationship of trust between the nurse and the client. Burk, Wieser, and Keegan (1995) note that to facilitate provision of culturally sensitive care to Mexican Americans at a birthing center on the Mexican border, prospective CNMs (certified nurse-midwifes) are evaluated for their understanding of and desire to work with this particular population. New staff are required to read culture-specific information and are encouraged to attend Spanish classes to develop a familiarity with the language. Knowledge of the client's culture has been found to be a positive dimension in the client-provider process and important in providing culturally appropriate care.

When caring for a younger client, the nurse may encounter the *compadrazgo*, or godparent, who provides important support to the child and family. The godparent may want to assume some of the care of the client because of a sense of divine responsibility for the child's welfare. Allowing this assistance can reduce fear and anxiety and enhance adjustment to the health care facility.

TIME

Mexican Americans are usually characterized as having a present orientation of time and being unable or reluctant to incorporate the future into their plans. An example of this orientation is that some Mexican Americans may spend several years' savings on an important religious festival. Also, the Mexican custom of the siesta in some ways represents the belief that rest (or the present) has a priority over continued work that could produce monies to safeguard the future. Individuals with this present orientation of time may appear to lack practical concern about the future or the need for deferring gratification to a future time. Many investiga-

tors believe that this orientation restrains Mexican Americans from upward social mobility. In addition, some regard the present orientation of time as a barrier to assimilation and integration into the mainstream of American culture.

Khoury and Thurmond (1978) found few differences in the time perceptions of Mexican-American and White American college students, despite the fact that the Mexican-American students in the study were still maintaining cultural ties with the Mexican-American culture. However, these findings cannot be generalized to Mexican Americans who are more immersed in their culture and less educated.

Implications for nursing care

It is important for the nurse to remember that personal ethnocentric attitudes toward time may negatively affect the planning of care for clients with a different time orientation. Because Mexican Americans have been characterized as being present-time oriented, they may not share the nurse's attitude concerning matters related to time, particularly if the nurse is from a future-oriented cultural group. A Mexican-American client may be late for an appointment not because of reluctance or lack of respect but because the client may be more concerned with a current activity than with the activity of planning ahead to be on time. This concept, known as "elasticity," implies that future-oriented activities can be recovered but present-oriented activities cannot.

Because Mexican Americans are likely to be present-time oriented, the nurse may experience difficulties in planning and implementing health care measures such as long-term planning. In addition, the nurse may experience difficulties in explaining why and when medications should be taken. When working with a client who has a condition such as hypertension, it is important for the nurse to emphasize the effects of this condition as well as short-term problems that can occur if the medication is not taken on time. Emphasis on short-term problems is more likely to be beneficial because it is more likely to get results.

Because Mexican Americans are present-time oriented, their perceptions and understanding of acute and chronic illness may be affected. Mexican Americans may first seek out the most accessible and affordable care, which may be folk healing with a folk practitioner.

ENVIRONMENTAL CONTROL
Locus of control

Mexican Americans are more likely to believe in an external locus-of-control than persons in the dominant culture are. This belief that the outcome of circumstances is controlled by external forces is conveyed socially. Some Mexican Americans perceive life as being under the constant influence of the divine will. There is also a fatalistic belief that one is at the mercy of the environment and has little control over what happens. Associated with this view is the belief that personal efforts are unlikely to influence the outcome of a situation; thus, some Mexican Americans do not believe that they are personally responsible for present or future successes or failures. This belief may precipitate feelings of hopelessness regarding future and positive change. The effect of this fatalistic belief was noted in a study by Sennott-Miller (1994) of Hispanic women who had difficulty maintaining cancer-prevention activities.

Effect on personal control Data from transcultural studies have found that people with a belief in external control can be expected to have more distress as an outcome of this view (Hough, 1985). On the other hand, Mirowsky and Ross (1984) noted that distress was not observed in the Mexican culture as an outcome of a belief in an external locus of control. They also suggested that although distress can result from strong family ties it is offset by the family's strong support and responsibility to the individual. A consequence of strong family ties is that the individual may have a greater feeling of personal control, which in turn deters anxiety. When Mexican Americans experience pain, they value stoicism and self-control. Calvillo and Flaskerud (1991) suggest that crying and moaning in these clients may serve the purpose of relieving pain rather than communicating that the pain is intolerable and intervention is desired.

Duffy, Rossow, and Hernandez (1996) reported that when the Health-Promoting Lifestyle Profile (HPLP) was administered Mexican women had the highest total scores of all minority groups but lower scores than all predominantly White groups. HPLP self-actualization and interpersonal support were the highest subscale scores. Although Mexican-American women in this study tended to practice more health-promoting life-style behaviors when compared to other minority groups, it was also noted that a high number of the women worked in professional health care–related fields. However, their scores were lower than those reported for predominantly White groups, an indication that Mexican-American women may lag substantially behind their White counterparts in the practice of "heart-healthy" life-styles, even when the influence of socioeconomic status was removed. The exercise subscale was the lowest score for all groups, including minorities. Age, education, self-efficacy, health locus of control (internal and powerful others), and current health status made statistically significant contributions to the HPLP subscale scores. The finding that Mexican-American women who experienced declining health had a low practice of regular exercise supports Duffy's (1993) and Weitzel and Waller's (1990) findings that reported that health status is directly related to engaging in exercise, an area that is under personal control. Kuster and Fong (1993) also found that age, education, income, length of residence in the United States, and perceived health status correlated significantly and positively with the Spanish HPLP total and subscale scores, with age most highly correlated with the total score. Additionally the Mexican-American sample reported a less-frequent practice of health responsibility, nutrition, and stress-management behaviors, which when viewed together may cause a serious predisposition to conditions found to be more prevalent in Mexican-American women such as obesity, non–insulin dependent diabetes and hypertension and other cardiovascular problems (Hazuda, Haffner, Stern, & Eifler, 1983; Stern, Rosenthal, Haffner, et al., 1984). Interestingly, the Mexican-American women have relatively high scores on self-actualization and interpersonal support scores, and as respondents got older, they reported engaging in a greater number of health-promoting, self-actualizing, health-responsible, stress-management, and nutritional behaviors. These findings have significant implications for health professionals in terms of education related to health-promotion activities for Mexican Americans.

Health care beliefs

The cultural belief in external locus of control influences the manner in which some Mexican Americans view health. Some Mexican Americans believe that health may be the result of good luck or a reward from God for good behavior. For some Mexican Americans health represents a state of equilibrium in the universe wherein the forces of "hot," "cold," "wet," and "dry" must be balanced. This concept is believed to have originated with the early Hippocratic theory of health and the four humors. According to the Hippocratic theory, the body humors—blood, phlegm, black bile, and yellow bile—vary in both temperature and moisture (Harwood, 1971). Persons who subscribe to this theory believe that health exists only when these four humors are in balance. Thus health can be maintained by diet and other practices that keep the four humors in balance. Illness, on the other hand, is believed to be misfortune or bad luck, a punishment from God for evil thoughts or actions, or a result of the imbalance of hot and cold or wet and dry. Cox (1986) found that a large number of elderly Hispanics attributed their health problems to old age and therefore did not seek any type of intervention.

Theory of hot and cold and perception of illness

One category of disease is hot and cold imbalance, in which illness is believed to be caused by prolonged exposure to hot or cold. To cure the illness, the opposite quality of the causative agent is applied to assimilate the hot or cold. Included in this category are illnesses that, rather than being caused by temperature itself, are associated with hot or cold aspects of substances found in medicines, elements, air, food, and bodily organs (Richardson, 1982). Treatment is focused on such things as suggestions, practical advice, prayers, or indigenous herbs, with the goal of reestablishing balance (Ruiz, 1985).

Headaches may have a causative agent that is believed to have a hot or cold quality. If the causative agent for a headache is believed to have a hot qual-ity, cold herbs may be placed on the temples to absorb the heat; if the causative agent is believed to have a cold quality, hot herbs are applied (Ingham, 1970). As another example of hot and cold imbalance, a person who has eaten unripened fruit may complain that "the cold of the fruit has gotten me in the stomach" (Currier, 1966).

Other illnesses such as paralysis, rheumatism, and earaches are believed to be caused when cold *aires* enter the body. These illnesses are disabling and painful (Currier, 1966). People are believed to be more susceptible to cold *aires* when going from a warm place to a cold place, or when they have just eaten because eating is believed to cause a warm state. When people with these illnesses have a high fever, a hot poultice is administered to the legs to draw the fever out of the head to the cool legs. The origin of these cold *aires* is believed to be in dark places such as river bottoms, ant hills, and caves, particularly those dark places "where the devil lives." The cure for *los aires* is for the individual to be cleansed with hot herbs and eggs and then covered with cigarette smoke (Ingham, 1970). Cleansing may also be done with black and red clay whistle dolls and combined with an offering of hot black chicken, unsalted *mole*, tamales, alcohol, and cigarettes that is made to an ant hole. These practices are also described as witchcraft.

Although cold is believed to harm the body from without, excesses of heat developed from within the body itself and extending outward are believed to be related to such diseases as cancer, rheumatism, tuberculosis, and paralysis (Wilson & Kneisl, 1992) (Box 9-1). The focus of heat in the body is the stomach, whereas the head, arms, and legs are believed to be cool. Hot illnesses such as skin ailments and fever may be visible to the outside world. Many of the disorders caused by hot and cold imbalances are digestive in nature, which is related to the fact that an imbalance of hot and cold foods is believed to be damaging and is suggestive that to ensure good health both hot and cold foods must be taken into the body (Currier, 1966). The quality of the food eaten determines whether diarrhea is a hot or cold condition. If the stool is green or yellow, the diarrhea is hot and the remedy is cold tea, whereas if

---

Box 9-1

HOT-COLD CONDITIONS AND THEIR CORRESPONDING TREATMENT

HOT CONDITIONS
Fever
Infections
Diarrhea
Kidney problems
Rashes
Skin ailments
Sore throat
Liver problems
Ulcers
Constipation
HOT FOODS
Chocolate
Cheese
Temperate-zone fruits
Eggs
Peas
Onions
Aromatic beverages
Hard liquor
Oils
Meats such as beef, waterfowl, mutton
Goat's milk
Cereal grains
Chili peppers
HOT MEDICINES AND HERBS
Penicillin
Tobacco
Ginger root
Garlic
Cinnamon
Anise
Vitamins
Iron preparations
Cod-liver oil
Castor oil
Aspirin

COLD CONDITIONS
Cancer
Pneumonia
Malaria
Joint pain
Menstrual period
Teething
Earache
Rheumatism
Tuberculosis
Colds
Headache
Paralysis
Stomach cramps
COLD FOODS
Fresh vegetables
Tropical fruits
Dairy products
Meats such as goat, fish, chicken
Honey
Cod
Raisins
Bottled milk
Barley water
COLD MEDICINES AND HERBS
Orange flower water
Linden
Sage
Milk of magnesia
Bicarbonate of soda

Adapted from Wilson, H., & Kneisl, C. (1992). *Psychiatric nursing.* Reading, Mass.: Addison-Wesley.

the stool is white, the diarrhea is cold and the remedy is hot tea.

Hot and cold are also associated with other aspects of life. Symbolically, cold is related to things that menace the individual, whereas hot is related to warmth and reassurance. In addition to air, water is seen as a source for cold. If an individual has participated in an activity that is considered hot, this person will not go near water because of its association with death (at death, blood is believed to be turned into water). The effort to balance hot and cold forces in the Mexican-American belief system reflects the relationship between the individual and the environment. It is a symbolic attempt to attain a social order that is equitable (Ingham, 1970).

Theory of hot and cold and effects on growth and development Hot and cold have symbolic significance for the nature and process of reproduction. During pregnancy a woman may be advised not to eat hot foods. On the other hand, during menstruation or after childbirth a woman might be told to avoid cold foods or taking a bath. Infertility is associated with a "cold" womb, lack of intimacy, and rejection. A pregnant woman is believed to have an especially warm body, and to dissipate the warmth, she should bathe often and take short walks (Currier, 1966). The idea that warmth relates to intimacy follows in the relationship of mother and child. If a mother rejects her child, she is subject to an emotionally based disease called *bilis,* which can cause the infant to have chronic headaches and permanent injury. This belief indicates that the child may display chronic malnutrition, which Currier (1966) relates to a lack of affection and support. Nursing of the child is also related to hot and cold characteristics. A diminished milk flow is believed to result from coldness, whereas warmth is believed to increase the flow. An excess of warmth causes the child to become ill because the milk curdles and becomes indigestible.

During the first year of life, a child is kept physically close to the mother either by being wrapped in her shawl or by sleeping in a bed next to her. When the child is weaned and starts walking, the mother deprives the child of this physical contact; and when the child experiences the cold floors and lack of physical attachment, he or she may experience rage and depression. This condition is related to a lack of support and physical warmth (Currier, 1966).

Folk medicine

The belief that health is a matter of chance and controlled by forces in nature is the basis of folk medicine. Folk medicine as practiced by Mexican Americans combines elements of the European Roman Catholic view and of the original Indians of Mexico. These beliefs have led to unique ways of accounting for physical and mental illnesses, their consequences, and unique methods of dealing with illnesses. This belief and practice system regarding health care is indigenous to the Mexican-American community and is known as *curanderismo* (Rivera & Wanderer, 1986). Within this folk medicine system, the *curandero* is the folk healer. The *curandero* views illness from a religious and social context, rather than the medical-scientific perspective of the dominant Western society (Applewhite, 1995).

The concept of balance dominates much of the Mexican-American world view regarding the cause and treatment of illness. Good health infers that one is in proper balance with God, family, fellow human beings, and church (Weclew, 1975). Illness is often believed to be a result of an imbalance in the social or spiritual aspects of life.

Types of folk practitioners Operating within the *curanderismo* folklore system of beliefs and practices are several levels of healers. The first healer sought out is a member of the family; if the case is or becomes more complicated, healers within the community are sought out. Several levels of folk healers are described here, beginning with the lowest level, the family healer.

Family folk healer. The first person to be consulted at the time of illness is a key family member who is respected for her knowledge of folk medicine. This individual may be a wife, mother, grandmother, or other revered elderly relative. The healing practices are passed down in the family from mother to daughter. If the client does not improve, an intermediary person usually directs the client to the *curandero.*

Yerbero. The *yerbero* (or *herbero*) is a folk healer who specializes in using herbs and spices for preventive and curative purposes. This person grows and distributes herbs and spices and explains how to use them effectively (Richardson, 1982).

Curandero and curandera. The more serious physical and mental or emotional illnesses are brought to the *curandero* (folk healer). If the practitioner is a woman, she is referred to as a *curandera.* The *curandero* perceives life as being under the consistent influence of the divine will. People are believed to be born as sinners, with death being the result of their sins. The central focus of these healers' treatment is relieving clients of their sins. Suffering is seen as a component of illness, and death is seen as failure to be cured of sin (Ruiz, 1985). The *curandero* believes that water, food, and air are important to the maintenance of health. Imbalance of these elements, imbalance between God and man, and imbalance between hot and cold are believed to contribute to illness.

Weclew (1975) and Ness and Wintrob (1981) have reported that *curanderos* see clients with a wide range of both physical and psychological symptoms, such as gastrointestinal distress, back pain, headache, fever, depression, anxiety, irritability, fatigue, hostility, shame, guilt, sexual problems, alcoholism, and the common folk diseases. The diagnosis is made after a thorough assessment of all aspects of the client's life, including the family and even the supernatural. The treatment is provided in a room in the *curandero*'s home that is decorated with much religious paraphernalia. Treatments used include massage, diet, rest, suggestions, practical advice, indigenous herbs, prayers, magic, and supernatural rituals. Although *curanderos* generally use white magic, there are times when they may resort to black magic because the cure is difficult.

The *curandero*, who is believed to have the "God-given" gift of healing and is a full-time specialist, is often consulted before medical contact is made or may be consulted concomitantly with a medical contact. The effectiveness of *curanderos* seems to be in their ability to use their personality and healing regalia to encourage hope and trust on the part of the client. The beliefs and practices of this healer are supported by the family and the community, which tends to strengthen the client's sense of control over the situation. *Curanderos* are often preferred over the medical community because they are personal, are less dehumanizing, know the family, and are an integral part of the Mexican-American community. *Curanderos* in most cases have power over witches because they are believed to heal through the power of God.

Brujos and brujas (witches). The level of healers called "witches" may not be sought out until other forms of healing have been tried. The practitioners of witchcraft utilize several kinds of magic. Black magic is practiced by both male witches *(brujos)* and female witches *(brujas),* and red magic and green

magic are believed to empower a witch to solve love problems by assuming an animal form. As mentioned previously, white magic is practiced by a *curandero,* is considered good magic, and is used in folk healing (Wanderer & Rivera, 1986).

A motive for witchcraft may be hatred, jealousy, or envy. To cure, witches may use food or drink, imitative magic (such as dolls), evil air, or animal metamorphosis to bewitch (Wanderer & Rivera, 1986). There are many superstitions adhered to in this healing mode; for example, keeping black animals protects against witchcraft.

Health and folk beliefs specific to children In addition to the childhood illnesses believed to be caused by *aires,* several other folk-defined childhood illnesses are well known in the literature on *curanderismo* (Rivera & Wanderer, 1986).

Caída de la mollera. Caída de la mollera refers to a fallen fontanel in infants caused by a fall, by bouncing the child roughly, or by removal of the nipple from the baby's mouth with too much force. This condition is viewed as an imbalance between the fontanel and the palate that blocks the passage of foods and liquids. Associated with *caída de la mollera* are the symptoms of inability to suck or grasp the nipple, vomiting, diarrhea, fever, restlessness, and crying spells.

Before seeking out a physician, mothers often seek out older women in the community who seem to know how to treat this problem. The following remedies have been noted by Ruiz (1985): pressing against the palate from inside the mouth, praying, applying eggs to the head and then pulling hairs, and holding the child with the head down. Reinert (1986) has noted that this condition is usually caused by severe dehydration and correct medical treatment with intravenous fluids is essential.

Mal ojo (evil eye). As mentioned earlier, *mal ojo* occurs when an individual who is believed to possess a special power admires or covets the child of another and looks at but does not touch the child. *Mal ojo* at times is associated with witchcraft and black magic. This condition is characterized by headaches, high fever, crying, diarrhea, restlessness, irritability, loss of weight and sleep, and sunken eyes (Rivera & Wanderer, 1986; Ruiz, 1985). The cure for the problem is to mix a hen's egg with water and place this under the head of the child's bed, which supposedly drives the bad influence out of the child's body. Another remedy is to have the person believed to be the source of the "evil eye" touch the afflicted individual. It is believed that the child will deteriorate, with severe coughing and vomiting, and possibly die if not treated. Families are known not to bring children with this problem to physicians because they fear the physician will misdiagnose the child and the child's condition will worsen.

Folk-related diseases of both children and adults

Susto (magical fright). Susto is caused by a frightening experience or event and leads to the temporary loss of one's spirit from the body. This condition may even affect an unborn child if the mother is frightened. *Susto* is associated with childhood epilepsy, is seen more often in females, and if left untreated is believed to develop into tuberculosis or can even be fatal. Symptoms of *susto* include crying, insomnia, anorexia, restlessness, nightmares, stomachache, diarrhea, high fever, and being afraid of just about anything.

Susto is treated by getting the client on the floor, outstretching the hands, and then having a healer sweep the client with indigenous herbs while praying. This treatment attempts to get the individual's spirit back into the body (Rivera & Wanderer, 1986; Ruiz, 1985).

Empacho. Patients suffering from *empacho* ('obstacle') are believed to have a chunk of food that they are unable to pass, causing a lot of abdominal pain. They are taken to an older woman who possesses the knowledge to treat this problem. To diagnose the illness, the client is held face down by the skin of the back. During this procedure, if a crack is heard, the diagnosis is *empacho,* and the following treatment is instituted: body massages around the back and waist are given to restore the body's balance of hot and cold, which in turn, allows the food chunk to pass through the intestine (Ruiz, 1985).

Religious views Roman Catholicism is the predominant religion practiced by Mexican Americans. Common religious practices are baptism, confirmation, communion, weddings, and funerals. During times of crisis, Mexican Americans may rely on the priest and family for prayers. When a family member is ill, rituals that are practiced include making promises, lighting candles, visiting shrines, and offering prayers (Logan & Semmes, 1986). Death and grief are considered "God's will" and are usually accompanied by saying the rosary. Grief behaviors tend to be demonstrative (Lawson, 1990). The religious views are heavily influenced by the folk beliefs.

Roman Catholic Mexican Americans may have beliefs that are influenced by ancient Indian practices of witchcraft and voodoo. As a result, some Mexican Americans may believe in demons. Incorporated in this system is a belief in witchcraft practices to manipulate evil forces (Wanderer & Rivera, 1986). Wanderer and Rivera (1986) have noted that in the Mexican American community witchcraft is called *brujería* and is seen as a magical or supernatural illness and occasionally as an emotional illness. *Brujería* has no scientific basis and is believed to be precipitated by opponents using the evil forces of hexes and spells. Symptoms of *brujería* include paranoia, delusions, hallucinations, feelings of being controlled by another person, mania, perverted and fitful behavior, depression, suspicion, and anxiety. Motives for witchcraft include envy, vengeance, hatred, and jealousy (Kiev, 1968; Madsen & Madsen, 1969).

Implications for nursing care

It is important for the nurse to be aware that use of alternative therapies from Mexico is very prevalent among Mexican Americans. Keegan (1996) reported that 44% of Mexican Americans in a study in the Texas Rio Grande Valley reported using alternative practitioners one or more times during the previous year. The most commonly sought therapies were herbal medicine, spiritual healing and prayer, massage, relaxation techniques, chiropractic, and visits to a Mexican folk healer, or *curandero.* The majority (66%) indicated that they never reported visits to alternative practitioners to their established primary health provider.

The belief held by many Mexican Americans that the outcome of circumstances is controlled by external forces can influence compliance with traditional health care recommendations. The belief that they do not have control over their lives can influence Mexican Americans to be less compliant regarding traditional health care recommendations. This perspective may negatively affect the acceptance of wellness programs in the United States health care system such as smoking cessation, addiction programs, prenatal care, health-promotion activities, and chronic disease treatment. Because the Mexican-American healing system of *curanderismo* incorporates religious beliefs, some Mexican Americans may also believe that they are more in touch with the divine will and therefore the origin and healing of illness, when they enter the health care system. The nurse should understand that Mexican Americans will have more respect for the caregiver who accepts the spiritual and folk basis of their health beliefs.

The healers in the folk medicine system are people with whom the Mexican Americans have established relationships and with whom they can easily communicate. These healers know and can treat the folk illnesses that the uninitiated health care worker may not recognize. It is helpful for the nurse to understand the respect this culture has for the *curandero,* who is often consulted simultaneously with the physician or nurse. The long-term goal of a nurse working in a Mexican-American community should be to understand the folk medicine beliefs and to try to establish a relationship with the *curandero* in the hope of influencing acceptance and understanding of the rationale for modern health care practices and thereby gaining the community's confidence.

The nurse should recognize that the *curandero* is involved in relieving people of their sins so that they can experience healing and that a spiritual perspective is usually an integral part of the U.S. health care system. One might compare the healer's influence in this ethnic group to that of the clergy in the dominant U.S. society, wherein mutual cooperation is focused on meeting clients' spiritual and physical needs. Mexican-American clients also need to be encouraged to practice their religious beliefs and to receive supportive visits from the clergy. Acknowledging the client's reliance on the folk health care system as well as on his or her religious beliefs and medical assistance will promote a more holistic focus for nursing care.

It is important to recognize the strong influence of hot and cold imbalance in folk beliefs. Some of these healing beliefs and practices are practical such as massage, prayer, listening, or the application of cold for a fever. However, some practices can lead to missed clues for serious conditions that do not respond to these remedies such as prolonged diarrhea, vomiting, dehydration, parasites, or malnutrition in children. For example, the nurse should suspect that malnutrition in a 1-year-old child may be caused by the practice of separating the child from the mother at the time of weaning. Teaching the mother about the child's physical and emotional needs may improve the malnutrition. When dealing with children, Leininger (1978) warns the nurse to touch the children so that if the parents fear the "evil eye," the cultural remedy of touch will cure the condition.

Beliefs regarding hot and cold characteristics will affect on how the client accepts some of the treatment plan. The nurse should notice how the client is accepting treatment, and if there is noncompliance, the nurse should talk with the client and family to determine if the basis for noncompliance is folk beliefs. For example, the nurse might inquire if the condition is considered a hot or cold disease. The client may have some definite beliefs about this and about whether the medical treatment can restore the hot-cold balance within the body. If the treatment is in contradiction to folk beliefs, the nurse should use solid scientific evidence to support the importance of the treatment. One can expect the older client or first-generation immigrant to be more attached to these beliefs; therefore, focusing health teaching on younger family members may be more useful in establishing compliance.

In dealing with folk-related diseases, the nurse needs to understand perceived causes for these conditions, for example, environmental influences, such as *caída de la mollera* or *empacho,* or evil influences, such as *mal ojo* or *susto.* Because these diseases are considered indigenous to the culture, they are usually seen and treated first by the *curandero.* Patients coming to the nurse's attention with these conditions probably have had these symptoms for a while and have already been treated unsuccessfully by the *curandero.* The nurse's physical assessment needs to be thorough. Cultural variables should be included in the assessment. In managing pain, Calvillo and Flaskerud (1991) believe that the important variables to assess are cultural, psychological, and social factors that affect attitudes and responses to pain and how pain is reported. Rather than showing disrespect for the folk healer, the nurse should develop the relationship with the client in such a way as to maintain the support of the folk healer. Respect should also be shown for amulets that the client might wear to protect against the evil eye or evil spirits. For example, the *mano milagroso* ('miraculous hand') is worn by many people of Mexican origin for luck and the prevention of evil. The *mano milagroso* is worn by some people of Mexican background to ward off evil. Amulets worn by persons from Mexico may have red yarn attached (Spector, 1996a). The nurse should allow the client to continue to wear the amulet rather than attempting to take it away. The nurse should appreciate that eating eggs and bread, drinking tea, and sleeping are methods that some persons from Mexico believe are effective to maintain health, and these beliefs should be respected (Spector, 1996b).

BIOLOGICAL VARIATIONS
Skin color

The skin color of Mexican Americans can vary from a natural tan to dark brown. Persons with lighter color have more Spanish ancestry, whereas darker-skinned persons have more Indian ancestry. It is more difficult to recognize vasodilatation or vasoconstriction in the darker-skinned client in whom vasoconstriction and anemia are manifested as an ashen color rather than a bluish coloration. The mongolian spots (areas of darker skin found on the sacral area) found on infants usually disappear by 4 years of age. The hair of Mexican Americans is usually dark and may be curly and woolly, straight, or wavy (Monrroy, 1983).

Susceptibility to disease

Several categories of diseases occur with high incidence in Mexican Americans. Reinert (1986) cited a report from the Texas Special Committee on Diabetes Service, which states that in Mexican Americans not only is the incidence of diabetes five times the national average, but complications are also more frequent. Hispanic Americans suffer primarily from adult-onset diabetes with diabetes ranking as the third leading cause of death for Hispanic women between 45 and 74 years of age (Vásquez, 1997). In a study using census figures from 1969 to 1971 and 1979 to 1981, Stern, Bradshaw, Eifler, et al. (1987) reported less decline in the death rates of Mexican-American men from total ischemic heart disease and myocardial infarction than in the death rates of other men. Hypertension is also found with increased prevalence among Mexican Americans (National Center for Health Statistics, Healthy People 2000 Review, 1993). Pernicious anemia, most often seen in the elderly, has been shown to occur in those of Latin America origin at a younger age than in White patients (Carmel, Johnson, & Weiner, 1987). There is evidence that a low socioeconomic status has a strong effect on hemoglobin and hematocrit levels than the middle and upper class classes have. There is also some evidence that given similar socioeconomic conditions, Mexican Americans tend to have higher hematocrit levels than their White counterparts have (Overfield, 1995). Hispanics in the Southwest were found to have a poorer prognosis with melanoma because such melanoma arose from the palms, sublingual regions, mucous membranes, and soles; were more advanced in stage; occurred in older people; and metastasized (Black, Goldhahn, & Wiggins, 1987).

Hispanic Americans in the San Antonio Heart Study were found to be less knowledgeable about preventing heart attacks and not engaging in risk-reducing behaviors as often as non-Hispanic Whites (Hazuda, Stern, Gaskill, et al., 1983). Derenowski (1990) noted that cardiovascular risk reduction and changes in lifestyle are necessary components of education for some Mexican Americans. In providing this education, however, the nurse must remember to address cultural differences such as health values, ethnic care practices, family life patterns, and dietary practices. The whole family should be committed to developing and sustaining the life-style changes if they are to be successful.

It is essential for the nurse working with Mexican Americans to realize that approximately 85% of the health problems common to Mexican Americans involve communicable diseases (Anthony-Tkach, 1981; National Center for Health Statistics, Healthy People 2000 Review, 1993), including respiratory tract infections, diarrhea, skin disorders, nutritional problems (particularly during the first year of life), macroscopic parasitosis, and amebiasis. One of the most severe medical problems facing nations throughout the world is tuberculosis, which is believed to occur in areas where there are crowded living conditions, low income, substandard housing, and inadequate health care such as that which existed for many in Mexico. In the United States the population that is most at risk for the incidence and transmittal of tuberculosis includes newly arrived immigrants, including Mexicans (Hood & Jackson, 1989; Phipps, 1993). Because there is a high prevalence of tuberculosis in Mexico, it is believed that Mexican Americans may have a predisposition to a higher prevalence of tuberculosis than other Americans have (Phipps, 1993). Findings from a study of 845 African-American, Mexican-American, and White adolescents in San Diego indicate that, among the subjects surveyed, Mexican American adolescents had a higher rate of positive tuberculin tests, necessitating treatment (Fitzpatrick, Fujii, Shragg, et al., 1990). In a similar study, 310 Florida migrant workers were surveyed for prevalence of communicable disease. Of the number of subjects surveyed, 53% were Hispanic. Data from this study indicated that there was a high prevalence of syphilis, HIV-1 infections, and tuberculosis found among the subjects (Centers for Disease Control and Prevention, 1992a). In another study by the CDC, 44% of farmworkers screened had positive TB skin-test results (National Center for Farmworker Health, 1996). Barriers to health access among migrant communities where workers are stationary parallel those found among migrants who relocate. In both cases cultural differences have been found to prevent these individuals from accessing health care (Bechtel, Shepherd, & Rogers, 1995; Morrison, Rienzo, & Frazee, 1995; Eshleman & Davidhizar, 1997).

Hepatitis C has also been found to occur at a higher rate among Mexican Americans. Although the rate among Whites in the United States is 1.5% among Mexican Americans it is 2.1% (Cronin, 1997). Although an estimated 3.9 million persons in the United States have hepatitis C, this blood-borne virus, which can kill, was not identified until 1989. Since blood banks began screening for hepatitis C in 1990, the rate of new infections have declined. Although half the number of persons who obtained the disease before 1990 are believed to have received it from blood, the other half likely did so by sharing needles or straws to inject drugs (Cronin, 1997). It is estimated that more people could die from the complications of hepatitis C than from AIDS (Cronin, 1997). Some 70% of the cases result in liver damage that leads to death. Once the disorder is diagnosed, life-style changes such as avoiding alcohol can prolong length and quality of life for persons with hepatitis C.

There is a growing incidence of childhood obesity noted among Mexican Americans. Alexander and Blank (1988) suggest that the increasing incidence of obesity in Mexican-American children may be a result of mothers believing that a fat baby is a healthy baby. The mothers in this study had a greater body mass index than mothers in a control group did. These subjects also had "pushier" feeding practices with their children. To prevent the complications of adult obesity stemming from childhood obesity, nurses should identify mothers and their children who are at risk for obesity and encourage a weight-reduction program. The nurse should make an assessment of the potential need for nutritional education among Mexican-American clients. Hispanic women may have cultural dietary variations prenatally. For example, antepartal cravings including that for clay are not denied. In the postpartum period warm tea, broth, and corn gruel are acceptable foods, whereas citrus fruits, port (a wine), and tomatoes are avoided. It is believed harmful to eat and breastfeed simultaneously. The mother may believe stress and anger makes bad milk and makes a breastfeeding infant ill. Some Hispanics neutralize the bowel when weaning from breast to bottle by feeding only anise tea for 24 hours (White, Linhart, & Medley, 1996).

The two leading causes of death in Mexico are pneumonia and gastrointestinal diseases that are related to bacteria and parasites. Accidents and violence are believed to be the third leading cause of death among Mexicans, and cardiovascular disease is believed to be the fourth leading cause of death

(Anthony-Tkach, 1981). Up to 78% of all farmworkers suffer from parasitic infection compared to 2% to 3% of the general population (National Center for Farmworker Health, 1996).

In a recent study of 19 low-income, Mexican-American women diagnosed as having non–insulin dependent diabetes mellitus (NIDDM), Luyas (1989) found that the clients or their informants explained diabetes onset in terms of economic and family problems, whereas health providers explained diabetes onset mainly in biological terms. This study illustrates the importance of knowing the client's perspective on a medical diagnosis to provide culturally appropriate and sensitive nursing care. Urban, elderly Mexican Americans are at risk for many age-related chronic health conditions associated with migrant status, decreased levels of education and of nutrition, and poverty. Because of the stressful urban environment, they need assistance with alleviation of stress and language barriers, transportation, eligibility requirements, and positive self-perceptions (McKenna, 1989).

Nationwide, AIDS cases among Hispanics are occurring at triple the rate of non-Hispanics (Caudle, 1993). Mexican Americans are not listed separately. Because of the unsanitary working and housing conditions of migrant farmworkers and limited opportunity to protect themselves, the opportunity for higher risk for HIV infection exists (Aplemis, 1996). A study of farmworkers in Florida found the rate of HIV infection to be 5%, 10 times higher than that of the general population (HIV infection, 1992). Rates of infection found in other studies among farmworkers working in the eastern migrant stream have ranged from a low of 2.5% in North Carolina to 13% in rural South Carolina (HIV seroprevalence, 1987; Jones, Rion, Hollis, et al., 1991; Lyons, 1992). In a study of 587 subjects interviewed in Harris County, Texas, community health centers, only 58% of Hispanics indicated that they understood that the use of condoms during sexual intercourse decreased the risk of contracting AIDS (Aruffo, Coverdale, & Vallbona, 1991).

Psychological characteristics

According to Reinert (1986), Mexican Americans often encounter serious health problems resulting from the stress of coping with poverty. These problems include being overweight and an increased risk for suicide. Because of their belief that alcohol consumption is a way of celebrating life, alcohol is consumed in all aspects of life and contributes to the increased incidence of accidents and violence. Arrendondo, Weddige, Justice, and Fitz (1987), in reviewing the literature, found that, for Mexican Americans, alcoholism is possibly the most crucial health problem. Research on substance abuse among Hispanics indicates that alcohol is the most frequently abused intoxicant. Edmondson (1975) has suggested that Mexican-American adult men have an alcoholism rate that is significantly higher than the national norm for other American men. Other researchers have also reported high levels of alcoholism within the American Hispanic community (García, 1976; Ruiz, Vásquez, & Vásquez, 1973.) Men are most often affected because the male role may be correlated with being able to ingest large amounts of alcohol. The family pride protects this behavior as long as the man provides for the family. Some research has been reported that indicates that children who have alcoholic parents or grandparents are at higher risk for alcoholism because of their physiological relationship (Lawson, Ellis, & Rivers, 1984). Arrendondo, Weddige, Justice, and Fitz (1987) noted that Mexican Americans have a higher death rate from illnesses related to chronic alcohol consumption, such as cirrhosis of the liver.

In a study on the prevalence of psychiatric disorders, Karno, Hough, Burnam, et al. (1987) reported that Mexican Americans had fewer drug-abuse problems than non-Hispanics had. Other research has found, however, that when rates of substance abuse are considered among Mexican Americans marijuana is the second most abused drug, with heroin and cocaine being the third most abused drugs (Eden & Aguilar, 1989). Inhalants are also frequently abused among young Hispanics (Eden & Aguilar, 1989).

Some studies have indicated that there is less incidence of mental illness among Spanish-speaking people. This is believed to be because there are fewer role conflicts in Mexican American families because the rules of behavior of the culture are clearly defined (Murillo, 1978). In Mexican-American families, the family may also serve as a buffering mechanism that encourages individual members to share, thereby reducing anxiety and stressful situations. The Mexican American's view of the world also enables some Mexican Americans to blame external forces for failures, thereby reducing guilt. Mexican Americans are also unlikely to seek treatment in hospitals and other clinical facilities for mental illnesses. Mexican American women have been found to have slightly more dysthymic disorders, panic disorders, and phobias than other women (Murillo, 1978). Social and cultural differences between the Mexican American and the dominant American society appear to be a recurring theme among Mexican-American clients with symptoms of psychological disorders. Feelings of social isolation may serve to increase personal feelings of isolation. It is important for the nurse to be aware of self-image problems that are socially created and those that are personal. Knowledge of these factors will assist the nurse in making the diagnosis and planning nursing care that will help lower the client's psychological risk.

Implications for nursing care

Nurses must be aware that cultural differences are important to client care and therefore must be considered when providing care. A health intervention that opposes a particular cultural practice may not be successful even if it is considered a good health measure. For nursing care to be effective, the nursing and health measures implemented must be considered culturally relevant. This same awareness must be developed by the nurse regarding biological variations. A nurse who lacks understanding of biological variations may actually contribute to the promotion of ill health.

It is important for the nurse to recognize that the informal health care system in Mexico is generally composed of several elements, one of which is self-medication. In the early 1980s in Mexico, just as in the United States, prescriptions were required for all medications such as antibiotics and steroids. However, during this time the sale of drugs in Mexico was uncontrolled, except for narcotics, barbiturates, and other addictive drugs. The pharmacist was, in effect, the chief physician's surrogate, and many Mexican-American immigrants have been accustomed to receiving medication from a pharmacist without a prescription. In addition, some Mexican Americans consider medication to be always necessary and may not believe their illness is being treated unless a particular medication is ordered.

The massive scale to which self-medication is practiced in Mexico is potentially dangerous (Anthony-Tkach, 1981). To illustrate this point, in 1974 an outbreak of typhoid fever that was considered to cause the worst incidence in the century occurred in and around Mexico City. The causative agent was identified as chloramphenicol-resistant *Salmonella typhi*. Health officials in Mexico City believed that the indiscriminate use of antibiotics may have caused the organism to become resistant to the effects of chloramphenicol. It is important for the nurse to assess whether a Mexican-American client with a communicable disease is practicing self-medication for treatment. The assessment of the potential for self-medication as well as close follow-up study may be beneficial in reducing the drug-resistant causative organisms that can ensue from self-medication. The nurse who works with Mexican-American clients with communicable diseases needs to emphasize that communicable diseases are preventable and that prompt care is essential to reducing exposure to as well as morbidity and mortality from communicable diseases.

When working with the Mexican-American client, the nurse should be knowledgeable about the effects of the bacillus Calmette-Guérin (BCG) as opposed to the purified protein derivative (PPD) skin test for tuberculosis. BCG is a strain of *Mycobacterium bovis* that is widely used in countries with a high incidence of tuberculosis, such as Mexico. When an individual is inoculated with BCG and then later given a PPD skin test, there generally is an intense reaction to the combination of the BCG and the PPD, resulting in possible skin necrosis and subsequent scarring of the infected area (Anthony-Tkach, 1981). Therefore the nurse who works with Mexican-American clients must ascertain whether the client has had a tuberculosis skin test and, if so, whether the test was the BCG. If in doubt about which type of skin test was given, the nurse should recommend that the client have a chest radiograph instead of a skin test. Because of the rise in tuberculosis, syphilis, and AIDS in Hispanic migrant workers, nurses should assess for these diseases and urge appropriate follow-up care. Nurses should be reminded that the initial use of folk remedies can allow these diseases to spread and cause the delay of medical treatment.

Treatment of chemical dependency among Mexican Americans is a major challenge because of three central factors that inhibit treatment: integration of alcohol consumption within the Hispanic culture, the psychology of the Hispanic culture, and the family dynamics of the traditional Hispanic. Drinking behavior is so ingrained in the Mexican culture that social functions ranging from baptisms to funerals generally include the serving of alcoholic beverages (Arrendondo, Weddige, Justice, & Fitz, 1987). Drinking occurs among Mexican Americans when the individual is coping with negative feelings as well as when the individual is experiencing positive feelings. The nurse must remember that the fatalistic element of Hispanic psychology helps to incorporate and at the same time augment drinking problems among Mexican Americans. When a drinking problem is described by a Mexican American in an intake interview, it may be followed by the client saying, "That's life" or "This is our cross to bear." For the most part, this external locus of control serves to block the identified alcoholic, and the family as well, from assuming a more active role in the recovery process.

Rather than seeking outside professional help for the treatment of alcohol abuse, Mexican Americans may collaborate with the *curandero* in treating the alcoholism or may try self-medication. The nurse must assess whether the client who is a substance abuser is using a *curandero* or is self-medicating with other drugs because these factors may further intensify the problem. The nurse must also assess carefully whether a client with a drug-abuse problem would be best suited for individual, group, or family therapy. This determination can only be made after a thorough intake interview. Because the Mexican-American family is built on a system of family orientation, it is believed that perhaps the best mode of treatment for Mexican Americans is family therapy. The initial purpose of family therapy for Mexican-American substance abusers should be to evaluate the family's influence on the client's chemical-dependency problems. The nurse should

incorporate both the nuclear and the extended family in the evaluation.

To plan safe, effective, individualized nursing care for members of the Mexican-American community that is appropriate and congruent with their lifestyles and cultural beliefs, nurses must know and understand the cultural patterns and belief systems of this ethnic group (Murillo-Rohde, 1977). Conway and Carmona (1990) caution nurses that Mexican-American beliefs in traditional health and home remedies are often perceived by Mexican Americans as a wealth of options that decreases their need for using the modern health care system.

Mexican-American farm workers face many health problems because of their alienation, poverty, and ongoing seasonal mobility. O'Brien (1983) relates that if they have worked as migrants since childhood they frequently experience debilitating back pain and arthritis. In addition to other chronic health problems, short-term illnesses present problems (such as hemorrhaging after childbirth or abortion, dental problems), and nutritional illnesses occur because of inadequate food supplies. Nurses should be aware of local migrant programs that can assist in meeting their various health needs.

Kerr and Ritchey (1990) suggest that Mexican-American migrant farm workers have the following potential needs for improved health: improved access to health resources, improved knowledge of health-promoting behaviors, and fewer language barriers. Taking portable equipment (such as cholesterol screening equipment) to the migrant camps would improve accessibility. Health-promoting behaviors could be improved by assessment of the migrants for their current knowledge and healthful practices. Language barriers could be decreased if English classes were taught and if nutritional labeling in Spanish were instituted.

It is important for the nurse to remember that Mexican Americans differ from other cultural groups in their expression of symptoms and in how the ill person is perceived and treated by others. For example, in the Mexican American culture, epilepsy carries a far lesser social stigma than in other ethnic and cultural groups. Mexican Americans incorporate Hippocratic explanations when describing this particular disease and believe it is caused by a physical imbalance; thus treatment is reported to be medicinal and herbal (Kiev, 1972).

SUMMARY

To provide appropriate health care for the Mexican-American population, it is crucial for nurses to be aware of the stereotypes that commonly are held in viewing minority groups. This is especially true for Mexican Americans who are often stereotyped as "Hispanic" despite the fact that there are many Hispanic subgroups with their own demographic characteristics and beliefs (Hahn, 1995). It is critical for the culturally sensitive nurse to evaluate each client as a unique individual despite cultural group. Bond and Jones (1997) and Davidhizar (1997) note that one way to develop cultural sensitivity in nursing students is through cross-cultural experiences. By intense short-term immersion experiences in Mexico nursing students not only develop skill in the language but have the opportunity to reflect on personal cultural values and to develop sensitivity in providing culturally appropriate care.

Mexican-American immigrants present many special needs and potential problems in adjustment. There are many males who have left their families in Mexico and face the difficulty of separation. Some families are reunited after separation but experience difficulty in readjusting as a family and in negotiating the U.S. educational system, health care system, and other aspects of the new American culture. Because some Mexican American are migrants, it is also important to be aware that the composition of the migrant farm workers is also diverse and subject to stereotyping by health care professionals (Kissam, 1993). Nurses must understand that ethnic and language diversity presents new challenges.

The Mexican-American community in the United States is rich in cultural beliefs and values. This group has adhered to traditional beliefs and values more than other minority groups have. Because this group is growing rapidly in size and now is gradually moving to areas of the country other than the Southwest, more nurses will be coming into contact with Mexican Americans through community and health care systems and need to respond to the challenges this presents. Rooda (1993), Bonaparte (1979), and Joseph (1997) all reported that when the nurse does not understand the culture of the Hispanic client personal attitude toward the client is likely to be negative and consequently less effective. By understanding the cultural diversity unique to Mexican Americans and accepting their beliefs, especially those relating to health care, the nurse can plan effective, culturally appropriate care.

Case Study*

George García, a 23-year-old migrant farm worker, and his wife, Anita, age 20, bring their 4-month-old daughter to the emergency room of a small community hospital. They speak only broken English. They have another small child with them as well as two older women. They are very worried about the infant, who they say has been unable to retain feedings of diluted cow's milk. Now, because of poor sucking and increased sleeping, the infant has not had anything by mouth for the past 24 hours. When asked, the parents indicate that the infant has had only three wet diapers since yesterday. The nurse notices that the infant's eyes are sunken, she is listless, and her fontanels are depressed. When asked, the parents say the infant has been sick for 3 or 4 days. One of the older women makes a pushing-up motion with her hand as she points to the infant's mouth. Further assessment reveals a rectal temperature of 103° F. The family has not taken the temperature at all in the past 3 to 4 days. Skin turgor is good; mucous membranes are tacky. There has been no diarrhea. The infant's heart rate is 120 and regular, but thready. Respirations are 12 per minute at rest. The infant does not cry during rectal temperature taking or when touched with a cold stethoscope.

*I wish to acknowledge Stacie Hitt, R.N., M.S.N., for assistance in developing the case study and care plan.

CARE PLAN

 Nursing Diagnosis   Fluid-volume deficit related to diarrhea

Client Outcome

1. Infant will exhibit signs of adequate hydration.

Nursing Interventions

1. Offer appropriate fluids as tolerated.
2. Maintain accurate record of intake.
3. Weigh daily.
4. Assess all parameters (such as vital signs, skin character).
5. Apply urine collection device if indicated.
6. Measure urine volume and specific gravity.

 Nursing Diagnosis   Nutrition, altered, less than body requirements

Client Outcome

1. Infant will consume and retain appropriate number of calories per weight per day.

Nursing Interventions

1. Gradually reintroduce foods as indicated.
2. Observe infant's response to feedings.
3. Describe feeding behavior.

 Nursing Diagnosis   Diarrhea resulting in alteration in bowel elimination as evidenced by hypoactive bowel sounds

Client Outcome

1. Infant will resume normal peristaltic and elimination patterns.

Nursing Interventions

1. Record fecal output: number, volume, characteristics.
2. Observe and record presence of associated signs: tenesmus, cramping, vomiting.

Nursing Diagnosis   Body temperature, altered

Client Outcome	*Nursing Interventions*

Client Outcome

1. Infant will regain and maintain a body temperature within normal limits.

Nursing Interventions

1. Reduce environmental temperature.
2. Place infant in lightweight clothing and bed linen.
3. Encourage cool liquids.
4. Take rectal temperature every 4 hours.

 Nursing Diagnosis   Sensory alteration as evidenced by listlessness

Client Outcome

1. Infant will respond to a full range of stimuli.

Nursing Interventions

1. Record intervals of sleep and wakefulness; observe infant's level of activity when awake.
2. Assess ease of arousal.
3. Encourage family to participate in holding, caring, and talking with client.

 Nursing Diagnosis   Communication, impaired verbally, related to foreign-language barriers

Client Outcome

1. Family will be able to communicate basic needs and understanding of infant's condition and care

Nursing Interventions

1. Assess language spoken best by family.
2. Assess family's ability to comprehend English.
3. Talk slower than normal to family.
4. Use gestures or drawings for clarity.
5. Be careful to touch children after looking directly at them.
6. Make a conscious effort to address father when explaining care.
7. Show respect to older women.
8. Obtain a fluent, consistent translator.

 Nursing Diagnosis   Health maintenance, altered, related to lack of health information

Client Outcome

1. Family will demonstrate understanding and ability to perform skills necessary for care of infant at home.

Nursing Interventions

1. Determine information family needs.
2. Determine folklore beliefs related to health care.
3. Initiate the teaching.
4. Determine influence older women have on family's health care beliefs.
5. Determine equipment needed for home care.
6. Seek social service referral.
7. Seek assistance from agencies.

STUDY QUESTIONS

1. Which family member is likely to make the decision about whether to allow the infant to be hospitalized?
2. What might the nurse do to encourage the best communication with this family?
3. What kinds of data should be obtained in the history?
4. What folk disease does the family likely believe the infant has?
5. How should the nurse explain to the family why the infant needs to be hospitalized?
6. Why would it be advantageous for the nurse to touch both the infant and the other child while relating to them?
7. How could the nurse show acceptance of the folk remedies that may have already been tried with the infant?
8. The infant is admitted to the hospital. What could be expected in terms of family visitation?
9. What teaching goals should the nurse have for this family?

References

Alexander, M., & Blank, J. (1988). Factors related to obesity in Mexican American preschool children. *Image: Journal of Nursing Scholarship, 20*(2), 79-82.

Althaus, D. (1997, May 25). Maquiladoras hold out thin hope for better life. *Houston Chronicle,* 1.

Anderson, C., & Murphy, A. (1996). Will elderly seasonal nomads need health service? *Public Health Reports, 111*(1), 55-56.

Anthony-Tkach, C. (1981). Care of the Mexican American patient. *Nursing and Health Care, 2,* 424-427.

Aplemis, L. (1996, Fall). Migrant health care: creativity in primary care. *Advanced Practice Nursing Quarterly,* 45-49.

Applewhite, S. (1995). *Curanderismo:* demystifying the health beliefs and practices of elderly Mexican Americans. *National Association of Social Workers, 20,* 247-253.

Arrendondo, R., Weddige, R., Justice, C., & Fitz, J. (1987). Alcoholism in Mexican Americans: intervention and treatment. *Hospital and Community Psychiatry, 38*(2), 180-183.

Aruffo, J., Coverdale, J., & Vallbona, C. (1991). AIDS knowledge in low-income and minority populations. *Public Health Report, 106*(2), 115-119.

Bechtel, G., Shepherd, M., & Rogers, P. (1995). Family, culture, and health practices among migrant farmworkers. *Journal of Community Health Nursing, 12,* 15-22.

Black, W., Goldhahn, R., & Wiggins, C. (1987). Melanoma within a southwestern Hispanic population. *Archives of Internal Medicine, 123*(10), 1331-1334.

Booth, C. (1996, Feb. 26). Caribbean blizzard. *Time,* 46-48.

Bonaparte, B. (1979). Ego defensiveness, open-closed mindedness, and nurses' attitude toward culturally different patients. *Nursing Research, 28*(3), 166-170.

Bond, M., & Jones, M. (1997). Creating culturally competent professionals. *Reflections, 23*(2), 18-19.

Bonilla, E.S. (1973). Ethnic and bilingual education for cultural pluralism. In Stent, M.D., Hazard, W.R., & Rivlin, H.H. (Eds.), *Cultural pluralism in education: a mandate for change* (pp. 115-122). East Norwalk, Conn.: Appleton-Century-Crofts.

Brownlee, A.T. (1978). *Community, culture, and care.* St. Louis: Mosby.

Burk, M.E., Wieser, P.C., & Keegan, L. (1995). Cultural beliefs and health behaviors of pregnant Mexican-American women: implications for primary care. *Advances in Nursing Science, 17*(4), 37-52.

Burden, N. (1986). A translation guide for postanesthesia nurses. *Journal of Post Anesthesia for Nurses, 1*(2), 112-116.

Calvillo, E., & Flaskerud, J. (1991). Review of literature on culture and pain of adults with focus on Mexican-Americans. *Journal of Transcultural Nursing, 2*(2), 16-23.

Carmel, R., Johnson, C., & Weiner, J. (1987). Pernicious anemia in Latin Americans is not a disease of the elderly. *Ethnology, 147*(11), 1995-1996.

Caudle, P. (1993). Providing culturally sensitive health care to Hispanic patients. *Nurse Practitioner, 18*(12), 40-51,

Centers for Disease Control and Prevention, U.S. Department of Health and Human Services. (1992a). HIV infection, syphilis, and tuberculosis screening among migrant farm workers—Florida. *Morbidity and Mortality Weekly Report, 41*(39), 723-725.

Cervantes, R., Snyder, S., & Padilla, A. (1989). Posttraumatic stress in immigrants from Central America and Mexico. *Hospital and Community Psychiatry, 40*(6), 615-619.

Chávez, N. (1986). Mental health services delivery to minority populations: Hispanics—a perspective. In Miranda, M., & Kitano, H. (Eds.), *Mental health research and practice in minority communities.* Rockville, Md.: National Institute of Mental Health.

Clark, M. (1970). *Health in the Mexican American culture.* Berkeley: University of California Press.

Conway, F., & Carmona, P. (1990). Cultural complexity: the hidden stressors. *Journal of Advanced Medical-Surgical Nursing, 1*(4), 65-72.

Cox, C. (1986). Physican utilization by three groups of ethnic elderly. *Medical Care, 24*(8), 667-676.

Cronin, M. (1997, July 30). Billboard campaign spotlights growing hepatitis C epidemic. *The Seattle Times,* A1.

Currier, R. (1966). The hot-cold syndrome and symbolic medicine. *Ethnology, 5*(3), 251-263.

Davidhizar, R. (1997, Nov. 7). Personal conversation. R. Davidhizar is Dean of Nursing at Bethel College School of Nursing, Mishawaka, Indiana

de León Siantz, M. (1994, March). The Mexican-American migrant farmworker family: mental health issues. *Nursing Clinics of North America, 29*(1), 65-72.

Derenowski, J. (1990). Coronary artery disease in Hispanics. *Cardiovascular Nursing, 4*(4), 13-21.

Dorsey, P., & Jackson, H. (1976). Cultural health traditions: the Latino-Chicano perspective. In Branch, M.F., & Paxton, P.P. (Eds.), *Providing safe nursing care for ethnic people of color* (pp. 41-80). Norwalk, Conn.: Appleton-Century-Crofts.

Duffy, M. (1993). Determinants of health-promoting lifestyles in older persons. *Image: The Journal of Nursing Scholarship, 25,* 23-28.

Duffy, M., Rossow, R., & Hernandez, M. (1996). Correlates of health-promotion activities in employed Mexican American women. *Nursing Research, 45*(1), 18-24.

Eden, S., & Aguilar, R. (1989). The Hispanic chemically dependent client: considerations for diagnosis and treatment. In Lawson, G., & Lawson, A. (Eds.), *Alcoholism and substance abuse in special populations.* Rockville, Md.: Aspen.

Edmondson, H.A. (1975, Feb. 7). Mexican American alcoholism and deaths at L.A.C. and U.S. Medical Center. Testimony before the Subcommittee on Alcoholism to the California State Health and Welfare Committee, Los Angeles, California.

Embry, D., & Russell, N. (1996, Winter). Silver strands of Mexico: support systems for the elderly. *Journal of Multicultural Nursing and Health, 2*(2), 343-348.

Eshleman, J., & Davidhizar, R. (1997). Life in migrant camps for children—a hazard to health. *Journal of Cultural Diversity, 4*(1), 13-16.

Ethics (1995, Nov.). Cultures diverge on patient autonomy. *American Journal of Nursing, 95,* 10.

Falicov, C. (1996). Mexican families. In McGoldrick, M., & Pearce, J.K., & Giordano, J. (Eds.), *Ethnicity and family therapy.* New York: Guilford Press.

Favazza, A. (1983). Cultural factors in diagnosis and treatment. In *ACP psychiatric update.* New York: Medical Information Systems.

Fishman, J. (1967, April). Bilingualism with and without diglossia: diglossia with and without bilingualism. *Journal of Social Issues, 23,* 29-38.

Fitzpatrick, S.B., Fujii, C., Shragg, G.P., et al., (1990). Do health care needs of indigent Mexican American, black, and white adolescents differ? *Journal of Adolescent Health Care, 11*(3), 128-132.

Ford, J., & Graves, J. (1977). Differences between Mexican American and White children in interpersonal distance and social touching. *Perceptual and Motor Skills, 45*(3), 779-785.

Foster, G. (1978). Relationship between Spanish and Spanish American folk medicine. In Martínez, R.A. (Ed.), *Hispanic culture and health care: fact, fiction, folklore* (pp. 183-202). St. Louis: Mosby.

Galván, M. (1993). Hispanic Americans. In *World Book Encyclopedia* (pp. 244-259). Chicago: World Book.

García, D. (1988). Mexican Americans. In Nault, W. (Ed.), *World Book Encyclopedia* (pp. 446-449). Chicago: World Book.

García, L. (1976, February 4). Spanish speaking alcoholism problems and needs. Testimony before the Subcommittee on Alcoholism and Narcotics to the U.S. Senate, Washington, D.C.

Gelfand, D., & Bialik-Gilad, R. (1989). Immigration reform and social work. *Social Work, 34*(1), 23-27.

Gonzales, J. (1997, May 26). Relearning a lost language. *Los Angeles Times,* A-1.

Hahn, M. (1995, Nov.). Providing health care in a culturally complex world. *Advance for Nurse Practitioners, 3,* 43-45.

Harwood, A. (1971). The hot-cold theory of disease. *Journal of the American Medical Association, 216*(7), 1153-1158.

Hazuda, H.P., Stern, M.P., Gaskill, S., et al. (1983). Ethnic differences in health knowledge and behaviors related to the prevention and treatment of coronary heart disease. *American Journal of Epidemiology, 117,* 717-728.

HIV infection, syphilis, and tuberculosis screening among migrant farm workers—Florida (1992). *Morbidity and Mortality Weekly Report, 41,* 39.

HIV seroprevalence in migrant and seasonal farmworkers—North Carolina, 1987 (1988). *Morbidity and Mortality Weekly Report, 41,* 34.

Hood, L., & Jackson, N. (1989). Caring for the patient with TB. *Advancing Clinical Care, 4*(4), 14-18.

Hough, R. (1985). Life events and stress in Mexican-American culture. In *Stress and Hispanic mental health: relating research to service delivery* (pp. 110-146). Rockville, Md.: U.S. Government Printing Office.

Information please almanac (1997). Boston: Houghton Mifflin Co.

Information please almanac (1998). Boston: Houghton Mifflin Co.

Ingham, J. (1970). On Mexican folk medicine. *American Anthropologist, 72*(1), 76-87.

Jones, J.L., Rion, P., Hollis, S., et al. (1991, Sept.). HIV-related characteristics of migrant workers in rural South Carolina. *Southern Medical Journal 84,* 1088-1090.

Joseph, H. (1997). Attitudes of army nurses toward African American and Hispanic patients. *Military Medicine, 162*(2), 96.

Kalish, R., & Reynolds, D. (1981). *Death and ethnicity: a psychocultural study.* Farmingdale, N.Y.: Baywood Publishing Co.

Karno, M., Hough, R., Burnam, M., et al. (1987). Psychiatric disorders among Mexican Americans and non-Hispanic Whites in Los Angeles. *Archives of General Psychiatry, 44*(8), 695-700.

Keefe, S. (1984). Real and ideal extended familism among Mexican Americans and Anglo Americans: on the meaning of "close" family ties. *Human Organization, 43*(1), 65-70.

Keegan, L. (1996, Dec.). Use of alternative therapies among Mexican Americans in the Texas Rio Grande Valley. *Journal of Holistic Nursing, 14*(4), 277-294.

Kemper, R. (1982). The *compadrazgo* in urban Mexico. *Anthropological Quarterly, 55*(1), 17-30.

Kerr, M., & Ritchey, D. (1990). Health-promoting lifestyles of English-speaking and Spanish-speaking Mexican-American migrant farm workers. *Public Health Nursing, 7*(2), 80-87.

Khoury, R., & Thurmond, G. (1978). Ethnic differences in time perception: a comparison of Anglo and Mexican Americans. *Perceptual and Motor Skills, 47*(3), 1183-1188.

Kiev, A. (1968). *Curanderismo: Mexican American folk psychiatry.* New York: Free Press.

Kiev, A. (1972). *Transcultural psychiatry.* New York: Free Press.

Kissam, R. (1993, May 11). *Everyday realities and effective public policy: the case of migrant and seasonal farmworkers.* Paper presented at the meeting of the National Conference on Migrant and Seasonal Farmworkers, Denver, Colorado.

Kluckhohn, F. (1976). Dominant and variant value orientations. In Brink, P.J. (Ed.), *Transcultural nursing: a book of readings* (pp. 63-81). Englewood Cliffs, N.J.: Prentice Hall.

Kuster, A.E., & Fong, C.M. (1993). Further psychometric evaluation of the Spanish language health-promoting lifestyle profile. *Nursing Research, 42*(5), 266-269.

LaFranchi, H. (1997, June 17). US awakes to drug violence spilling north from Mexico. *Christian Science Monitor,* 1.

Lantican, L., & Corona, D. (1989, November 14). A comparison of the social support networks of Filipino and Mexican American primigravidas. Paper presented at the Sigma Theta Tau International Conference, Indianapolis, Indiana.

Laosa, L.M. (1975). Bilingualism in three United States Hispanic groups: contextual use of language by children and adults and their families. *Journal of Educational Psychology, 67*(5), 617-627.

Lawson, G., Ellis, D.C., & Rivers, P.C. (1984). *Essentials of chemical dependency counseling.* Rockville, Md.: Aspen.

Lawson, L. (1990). Culturally sensitive support for grieving parents. *Journal of Maternal Child Nursing, 15*(2), 76-79.

Lee, L. (1997, June 2). Reyes holds the line. *El Paso (Texas) Herald-Post,* 1.

Leininger, M. (1978). *Transcultural nursing: concept, theory, and practice.* New York: John Wiley & Sons.

Logan, B., & Semmes, C. (1986). Culture and ethnicity. In Logan, B., & Dawkins, C. (Eds.), *Family centered nursing in the community* (pp. 112-113). Reading, Mass.: Addison-Wesley.

Ludwig-Beymer, P., Blankemeier, J.R., Casas-Byots, C., & Suarez-Balcazar, Y. (1996, July-Dec.). Community assessment in a suburban Hispanic community: a description of method. *Journal of Transcultural Nursing 8*(1), 19-27.

Luyas, G. (1989, Nov. 14). An explanatory model of diabetes by Mexican American woman. Paper presented at the Sigma Theta Tau International Conference, Indianapolis, Indiana.

Lynn, A. (1997, May 27). Packing them in at the jail. *The Spokesman-Review,* 1. Spokane, Washington.

Lyons, M. (1992, March-April). Study yields HIB prevalence for New Jersey farmworkers. *Migrant Health Clinical Supplement.*

Madsen, W., & Madsen, C. (1969). *A guide to Mexican witchcraft.* Mexico: D.F. Minutiae.

Marcos, L.R. (1988). Understanding ethnicity in psychotherapy with Hispanic patients. *American Journal of Psychoanalysis,* 48(1), 35-42.

Marcos, L.R., & Alpert, M. (1976). Strategies and risks in psychotherapy with bilingual patients: the phenomenon of language independence. *American Journal of Psychiatry,* 133, 1275-1278.

Marcos, L.R., Alpert, M., Urcuyo, L., & Kesselman, M. (1973). The effect of interview language on the evaluation of psychopathology in Spanish-American schizophrenic patients. *American Journal of Psychiatry,* 130, 549-553.

Marín, G., Sabogal, F., Marín, B.V., et al. (1987). Development of a short acculturation scale for Hispanics. *Hispanic Journal of Behavioral Sciences, 9,* 183-205.

McKenna, M. (1989). Twice in need of care: a transcultural nursing analysis of elderly Mexican Americans. *Journal of Transcultural Nursing,* 1(1), 46-52.

Meleis, A., Douglas, M., Eribes, C., et al. (1996). Employed Mexican women as mothers and partners: valued, empowered, and overloaded. *Journal of Advanced Nursing,* 23(1), 82-90.

Miller, F. (1986). The people. In Cayne, B., & Holland, B. (Eds.), *Encyclopedia Americana* (pp. 819-830). Danbury, Conn.: Grolier.

Mines, R., Gabbard, S., & Samardick, R. (1992, Sept.). *Harvest worker analysis.* Commission on Agricultural Workers.

Mirowsky, J., & Ross, C. (1984). Mexican culture and its emotional contradictions. *Journal of Health and Social Behavior,* 25(1), 2-13.

Monrroy, L.S.A. (1983). Nursing care of Raza/Latina patients. In Orque, M.S., Bloch, B., & Monrroy, L.S.A. (Eds.), *Ethnic nursing care: a multicultural approach* (pp. 115-148). St. Louis: Mosby.

Moore, J., & Pachon, H. (1985). *Hispanics in the United States.* Englewood Cliffs, N.J.: Prentice Hall.

Morrison, S., Rienzo, B., & Frazee, C. (1995). Developing health education for Hispanic migrant preschool youth. *Journal of Health Education, 26,* 207-210.

Murillo, N. (1978). The Mexican American family. In Hernández, C.A., Haug, M.J., & Wagner, N.N. (Eds.), *Chicanos: social and psychological perspectives* (pp. 15-25). St. Louis: Mosby.

Murillo-Rohde, I. (1977). Care for all colors. *Imprint,* 24(4), 29-32, 50.

Murphy, J., Giger, J.N., & Davidhizar, R. (1994). Strategies for designing culturally relevant client education materials. *American Society for Healthcare Education and Training of the American Hospital Association,* 8(3), 8-12.

Musto, D. (1991, July). Opium, cocaine and marijuana in American history. *Scientific American,* 40-47.

Naisbitt, J. (1982). *Megatrends.* New York: Warner Books.

National Center for Farmworker Health, Inc. (1995). *Facts about America's migrant farmworkers.* Austin, Texas: National Center for Farmworker Health, Inc.

National Center for Farmworker Health, Inc. (1996). *Fact sheet: basic health.* Austin, Texas: National Center for Farmworker Health, Inc.

National Center for Health Statistics, Healthy People 2000 Review (1993). *Health United States, 1992.* Hyattsville, Md.: Public Health Service.

National Commission to Prevent Infant Mortality (1993). *HIV/AIDS: a growing crisis among migrant and seasonal farmworker families.* Washington, D.C.: National Commission to Prevent Infant Mortality.

Ness, R., & Wintrob, R. (1981). Folk healing: a description and synthesis. *American Journal of Psychiatry,* 138(11), 1477-1481.

Nugent, K., Linares, A., Brykczynski, K., et al. (1988, July-Aug.). A model for providing health maintenance and promotion to children from low-income ethnically diverse backgrounds. *Journal of Pediatric Health Care,* 2(4), 175-180.

O'Brien, E. (1983). Reaching the migrant worker. *American Journal of Nursing,* 83a(6), 895-897.

Overfield, T. (1995). *Biologic variations in health and illness: race, age, and sex differences* (ed. 2). New York: CRC Press.

Oxford dictionary of quotations (1980). New York: Oxford University Press.

Phipps, W. (1993). The patient with pulmonary problems. In Long, B.C., Phipps, W.J., & Cassmeyer, V. (Eds.), *Medical surgical nursing: concepts and clinical practice.* St. Louis: Mosby.

Reinert, B. (1986). The healthcare beliefs and values of Mexican Americans. *Home Healthcare Nurse, 4*(5), 23-27, 29-31.

Richardson, L. (1982). Caring through understanding: part 2. Folk medicine in the Hispanic population. *Imprint, 29*(2), 21, 72-77.

Rivera, G.K., & Wanderer, J. (1986). Curanderismo and childhood illnesses. *The Social Science Journal, 23*(3), 361-372.

Rivera, J. (1978). *The new faces of racism: the Chicano case.* Report to the Association for Humanist Sociology, New York, N.Y.

Rooda, L. (1993, May). Knowledge and attitudes of nurses toward culturally different patients: implications for nursing education. *Journal of Nursing Education, 32*(5), 209-213.

Ross, J. (1995, Oct. 5). Who are they, where are they and how do we talk to them? Hispanic Americans. *Hospitals and Health Networks, 69*(19), 65.

Rubel, A. (1966). *Across the tracks: Mexican Americans in a Texas city.* Austin, Texas: University of Texas Press.

Ruiz, P. (1985). Cultural barriers to effective medical care among Hispanic-American patients. *Annual Review of Medicine, 36,* 63-71.

Ruiz, P., Vásquez, W., & Vásquez, K. (1973). The mobile unit: a new approach in mental health. *Community Mental Health Journal, 9,* 18-24.

Sahud, A. (1989). *Attitudes about aging and the aged in Mexico and the United States.* Doctoral dissertation University of California, Berkley.

Saunders, L. (1954). *Cultural difference and medical care.* New York: Russell Sage Foundation.

Sennott-Miller, L. (1994, Nov.). Using theory to plan appropriate interventions: cancer prevention for older Hispanic and non-Hispanic White women. *Journal of Advanced Nursing, 20*(5), 809-814.

Serrano, B. (1997, June 1). A lesson in inequality: districts in wealthy areas, where school levies are common, often have better schools. *The Seattle Times,* A1.

Spector, R. (1996a). *Cultural diversity in health and illness.* Stamford, Conn.: Appleton & Lange.

Spector, R. (1996b). *Guide to heritage assessment and health traditions.* Stamford, Conn.: Appleton & Lange.

Statistical abstracts of the United States (1988). Washington, D.C.: U.S. Department of Commerce, Bureau of the Census.

Stern, M.P., Bradshaw, B., Eifler, C.W., et al. (1987). Secular decline in death rates due to ischemic heart disease in Mexican Americans and non-Hispanic Whites in Texas, 1970-1980. *Circulation, 76*(6), 1245-1250.

Stern, M., Rosenthal, M., Haffner, S., et al. (1984). Sex differences in the effects of sociocultural status on diabetes and cardiovascular risk factors in Mexican Americans. *American Journal of Epidemiology, 120,* 831-851.

Taylor, M., & Smith, D. (1997, July 19). INS sweeps round up 211 Tarrant workers. *Fort Worth Star-Telegram,* 1.

Tran, T., & Dhooper, S. (1996). Ethnic and gender differences in perceived needs for social services among three elderly Hispanic groups. *Journal of Gerontological Social Work, 25*(3/4), 121-147.

U.S. Department of Commerce, Bureau of the Census (1992). *Population projections of the United States by age, sex, race, and Hispanic origins: 1990 to 2050,* Washington, D.C.: U.S. Government Printing Office, 25-1095.

U.S. Department of Commerce, Bureau of the Census (1993a, June 12). *News Release,* Commerce News.

U.S. Department of Commerce, Bureau of the Census (1993b, Nov.). *We the Americans . . . Hispanic people.* Washington, D.C.: U.S. Government Printing Office.

U.S. Department of Commerce, Bureau of the Census (1998). *March 1996 CPS: Age by race—ethnicity, both sexes.* Internet release, Feb. 3, 1998.

Váldez, A. (1980). *Ethnic maintenance among Mexicans and Puerto Ricans.* Report to Southwestern Sociological Association, Waco, Texas.

Vásquez, S. (1997, May 20). Diabetes alert: high-fat, genetics make Hispanics prone to the disease. *Rocky Mountain News,* 3d.

Villarruel, A., & Denyes, M. (1997). Testing Orem's theory with Mexican American's. *Image: Journal of Nursing Scholarship, 29*(3), 283-288.

Villarruel, A., & Leininger, M. (1995). Culture care of Mexican Americans. In Leininger, M. (Ed.), *Transcultural nursing.* New York: McGraw-Hill.

Wanderer, J., & Rivera, G. (1986). Black magic beliefs and white magic practice: the common structures of intimacy, tradition and power. *The Social Science Journal, 23*(4), 419-430.

Weaver, T. (1970). Use of hypothetical situations in a study of Spanish-American illness referral systems. *Human Organisms, 29,* 140.

Weclew, R. (1975). The nature, prevalence, and level of awareness of "curanderismo" and some of its implications for community mental health. *Community Mental Health Journal 11*(2), 145-154.

Weitzel, M., & Waller, P. (1990). Predictive factors for health-promotive behaviors in white, Hispanic and black blue-collar workers. *Family and Community Health, 13*(1), 23-33.

West, M., & Moore, E. (1989). Undocumented workers in the United States and South Africa: a comparative study of changing control. *Human Organization, 48*(1), 1-9.

White, J., Linhart, J., & Medley, L. (1996, Sept.). Culture, diet and the maternity. *Advance for Nurse Practitioners, 4,* 26-28.

Wilson, H., & Kneisl, C. (1992). *Psychiatric nursing.* Reading, Mass.: Addison-Wesley.

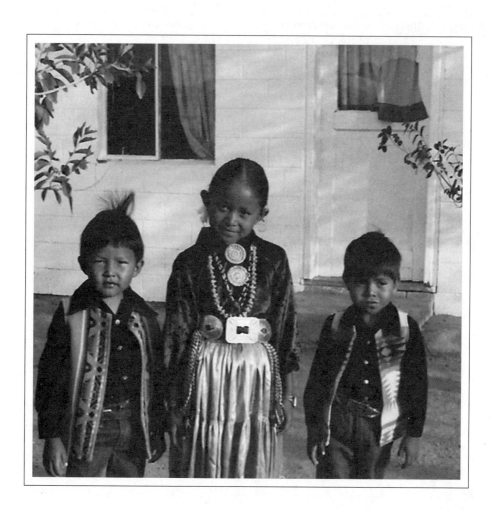

CHAPTER 10 Navajos

Catherine E. Hanley

BEHAVIORAL OBJECTIVES

After reading this chapter, the nurse will be able to:

1. Identify ways in which the Navajo culture influences Navajo individuals and health-seeking behaviors.
2. Recognize physical and biological variances that exist in and across Navajo groups to provide culturally appropriate care.
3. Develop a sensitivity and understanding for communication differences as evidenced within and across Navajo groups to avoid stereotyping and to provide culturally appropriate nursing care.
4. Develop a sensitivity and understanding for psychological phenomena that influence the functioning of a Navajo when nursing care is being provided.
5. Describe the influence of traditional Navajo folk medicine and the relationship to health-seeking behaviors.

OVERVIEW OF THE NAVAJOS

Archeological evidence places Navajos in the Gobernador Canyon area of northwestern New Mexico by the late 1400s or early 1500s. By the early 1600s some Navajos had migrated as far as the Black Mesa country of northern Arizona (Iverson, 1990). The first written historical observations of the Navajos (Navahos) have been attributed to Arate Salmerón (1626) and Father Benavides (1630).

According to Iverson (1990), the various Pueblo peoples exerted a tremendous influence on the evolution of the Navajo culture in the new region. There is historical evidence indicating that the Navajos and Pueblos were at times foes. However, Brugge (1968) suggested a number of instances when Navajo and Pueblo villages allied themselves against the Spanish and other outside groups. Young (1961) concluded that the Navajos and the Pueblos existed together in a more peaceful rather than hostile relationship. Re-

gardless of whether the Pueblos and the Navajos lived peacefully, the Pueblos probably did influence change in the Navajo life-style in some critical ways. For example, the Navajos have a matrilineal clan system that still exists today and dictates that a Navajo inherits the clan and thus the lineage from the mother (Iverson, 1990). The implication is that people from the same clan are considered relatives with varying responsibilities to one another.

For the western Pueblos the clan traditions were strong, and it is probable that they influenced the Navajos in the direction of clan formation (Iverson, 1990). In addition, the Pueblo people were very sedentary and had agricultural ways that undoubtedly also had some effect on the Navajos. As a consequence of these influences, the Navajos gradually adopted a way of life that was significantly less nomadic, with less emphasis on hunting than that of other Apachean groups. Seemingly, the Navajos learned trades such as weaving, pottery making, silversmithing, and agriculture from the Pueblo people en route to the Southwest. According to Iverson (1990), the Navajos credit "Spiderwoman" with their instruction in weaving. Differences existed in that Pueblo men traditionally were weavers, whereas Navajo men very rarely became weavers.

During the sixteenth, seventeenth, and eighteenth centuries, the Navajo people underwent tremendous expansion, cultural acquisition, and social change. According to Young (1961), the Navajos have always had a great capacity to absorb and elaborate on cultural traits adopted from other people. For example, the Pueblo weaving tradition is responsible for producing the Navajo blanket, which is unmistakably the product of the *Diné* (the Navajo word for 'people'). The language, though distinctively Navajo (from the entirely different Athapaskan family of languages), was learned by other Indians; however, few Navajos attempted to master a foreign tongue (Young, 1961). The Navajo people lived freely on the land of their forefathers, located between the four sacred mountains: Mount Blanca (Colorado) to the east, Mount Taylor (New Mexico) to the south, San Francisco Peak (Arizona) to the west, and Mount Hesperus (Colorado) to the north. Four directional colors were associated with the four sacred mountains: white with Mount Blanca, blue with Mount Taylor, yellow with San Francisco Peak, and black with Mount Hesperus. To understand the history of the Navajo people, it is important to understand the significance of the four sacred mountains, which historically were considered the cardinal boundary peaks surrounding the Navajo country. Even today, Navajo people believe that the four sacred mountains were gifts from the "Holy People" *(diyín dine'é, or haashch'ééh dine'é);* therefore, traditions, prayers, songs, and sacred trust are embodied in these mountains (Navajo Health Systems Agency, 1985).

Perhaps one of the most significant periods of Navajo history occurred during 1864, when over 9000 Navajo people were captured in what is now Arizona and were forced to journey to Fort Sumner on the Bosque Redondo Reservation in what is now New Mexico. During this long journey (known in Navajo history as the "long walk") and internment at Fort Sumner, over 2000 Navajo men, women, and children died of respiratory tract diseases, gastrointestinal disorders, and exhaustion.

During May 1868, the fourth year of their forced internment, the Navajos' elected leader, Chief Barboncito, said to a Washington delegation appointed by President Andrew Johnson, "I hope to God you will not ask me to go to any other country except my own." In speaking these words, Chief Barboncito expressed the feelings, beliefs, traditions, and desires of the Navajo people. On May 28, 1868, the United States of America and the Navajo tribe entered into a treaty that was ratified on August 12, 1868, by President Andrew Johnson (Treaty, 1973).

After the signing of the 1868 treaty, the Navajos moved progressively in the direction of the Four Sacred Mountains. Gradual as it might have seemed, the call from the Four Sacred Mountains for the return to Navajo ways reflected the futuristic response of self-determination, self-governance, and self-actualization (Hanley, 1987). Although the treaty signed at Fort Sumner was not the first treaty but the eighth treaty made between the Navajo people and the United States in 22 years, it was historically significant because it led to their release from Fort Sumner and to the establishment of their first reservation at Fort Defiance, Arizona. (At that time Arizona was a separate territory; it became the forty-eighth state in 1912.) After the Navajo people were released from their internment at Fort Sumner, they began to develop a diversified economy. For the Navajo, raising livestock was an important element of the economy but not the only element. From early and later historical accounts, it appears that the Navajos have always been perceived as great farmers. A reemerging question about the Navajo people concerns why they traditionally needed such a diverse economy; another reemerging question concerns why livestock took on a more essential role within the Navajo economy. The answers to these questions seemingly overlap and are mutually reinforcing: for the Navajo people, a diversified economy made more thorough and efficient use of the different opportunities provided by various soils, altitudes, and vegetations.

Three different climatic zones exist in the area in which the Navajo people live. The humid, or mountain, zones account for roughly 8% of the total Navajo area, the mesas and high plains, with their intermediate steppe climate, account for roughly 37% of the Navajo area, and the comparatively warm desert regions account for roughly 55% of the Navajo area. Winter temperatures in these regions range from an average minimum of 4° to 15° F in the humid zone, to 10° to 25° F in the steppe zone, to 11° to 30° F in the desert zone. Summer temperatures in these regions range from an average maximum of 70° to 80° F in the humid zone, to 80° to 88° F in the steppe zone, to 100° F or higher in the desert. The average rainfall in all three areas is concentrated in the late summer period, which extends from July to September, with great variation in amount within each zone. The desert and humid zones each receive an additional 41% of precipitation in the form of winter snow.

The soils in the Navajo region may be classified as excellent, good, or fair in terms of runoff, grass-producing ability, and erosion. Only about a third of the area is considered excellent or good in terms of soil productivity, and about 15% of the soil is unproductive, with little vegetation cover. The vegetation includes grassland, meadows, sagebrush, browse (shrub), and woodland (which is inaccessible and barren in some places). More Navajo land is covered with coniferous timber than with sagebrush (Young, 1961).

It was believed that the conflicts between the Navajos and their neighbors were contributing factors to their economic diversification. For example, historical accounts suggest that as raiding by and against the Navajo people grew in intensity, it consequently complicated agricultural pursuits and led to an increased need for mobility. In addition, the steady growth of the Navajo population figured greatly in the economic diversification: as the Navajo tribe grew in number, so did the quantity of livestock. Two principal periods of growth occurred in the Navajo tribe. The first period came in the last years of the eighteenth century and in the early years of the nineteenth century before the White American campaign against the Navajos. The second principal period of growth followed the Navajo return from Bosque Redondo. It was during the first period

of expansion that livestock was established as an economically important commodity (Brugge, 1964).

The spectacular growth of the Navajo population began during the post–Fort Sumner era. In 1870 the Navajo population numbered 15,000 (Boyce, 1942). By 1900 the Navajo population had grown to 21,000, and by 1935 the population had grown to 35,500. The population has grown steadily ever since. In 1981 there were approximately 151,000 Navajo Indians, who resided primarily in rural areas on or near the 27,000-square-mile reservation that is located in Arizona, New Mexico, Colorado, and Utah (U.S. Department of Commerce, Bureau of the Census, 1992). By 1986 the Navajo population had grown to 171,097, making the Navajo tribe the largest Indian tribe in the continental United States. Today, however, the Navajo are the second largest tribe in the United States with a population of 225,298 (U.S. Department of Commerce, Bureau of the Census, 1995), with the first being Cherokees at about 310,000.

Today there are approximately 500 Indian tribes (2,337,391 people) residing in 26 states, with most Native Americans residing in the western part of the United States as a consequence of the forced western migration of the tribes. It should be noted that there is a clear distinction between American Indian (AI) and the Alaska Natives (AN). The term "Native American" is intended to imply tribes residing in the continental United States (in contrast to "Native Canadians"). Today, although many Native Americans remain on reservations and in rural areas, an equal number also reside in cities, especially in Oklahoma, California, New Mexico, and Alaska (Henderson & Primeaux, 1981; U.S. Department of Commerce, Bureau of the Census, 1995).

In 1990, the median family income for the Navajo was $13,940 as compared to $21,519 for the general American Indian population and $35,225 for the general U.S. population (U.S. Department of Commerce, Bureau of the Census, 1995). Similarly, the per capita income for the Navajo was $4,788 as compared with $8,284 for the general American Indian population and $14,420 for the general U.S. population (U.S. Department of Commerce, Bureau of the Census, 1995). In 1990, 21,204 (47.3%) Navajo families live at or below the poverty level as compared to 19,100 of Cherokee (19.4%) ; 8,939 of Sioux (39.4%); and 7,814 of Chippewa (31.2%) (U.S. Department of Commerce, Bureau of the Census, 1995).

The Navajo tribe derives revenue from oil, coal, uranium, and federal grants and contracts. Nevertheless, high unemployment rates continue to be a major problem among the Navajos (Heraldson, 1988).

COMMUNICATION
Dialect and style

The Navajo language is classified as Athapaskan because historically it has been shown to be derived from the languages used by the people of Lake Athabasca in northwestern Canada. The Navajo language is also similar to the languages spoken by some peoples living in Alaska, some on the northern coast of the Pacific Ocean, and some in northern California (such as the Hupas). In addition, Navajo and the 12 groups of Apache dialects form a dialect continuum of one single language. These separate groups speaking a language similar to the Navajo language are referred to as "Athapaskans."

The language of the Navajo people involves a tonal speech in which pitch is of great importance. Every vowel and consonant is fully sounded regardless of how many times they are doubled or tripled in the same word. Vowels are often interchanged, creating several variations and meanings of the same word.

The Navajo language is believed to reflect a concept of the universe that is constantly in motion. In the Navajo language, position is defined as a withdrawal from motion. For example, a person speaking English says "on," whereas a Navajo person says something directly opposite in meaning for the word "on": the Navajo speaker says, "at rest." Whereas an English speaker says, "I dressed" or "One dresses," the Navajo speaker says, "I moved into my clothes" or "One moves into clothes." The language directly parallels mythological thought in that not only is the language in motion, but so too are cultural and spiritual heroes (Sobralske, 1985).

When Navajo people speak, most of the sentences contain the concept "good." For some Navajo people the concept "good" may be defined as a favorable or desirable quality that promotes prosperity and happiness. Therefore the word "good" is synonymous

with other words such as "agreeable, attractive, or beautiful" (*nizhóni*). The concept of goodness is directly related to the ideology of health and is even found in the Blessingway healing ceremony. This ceremony is viewed by the Navajos as a "good" event because it promotes everlasting harmony or perfection.

Even today the majority of Navajo people still speak the native language. Although many Navajo Indians are fluent in both the Navajo language and the English language, there are also many who do not speak English and therefore require the assistance of a Navajo interpreter when seeking or receiving health care. The Navajo language does not always have an equivalent single word for an English word; instead, the language uses a description of all occurrences affecting what is being said.

Until recently the Navajo language was unwritten. In World War II a special branch of the U.S. Marine Corps was developed for Navajos who served as Navajo code talkers. It has been estimated that this highly esteemed group saved millions of lives because the enemy was unable to understand the Navajo language or infiltrate its code.

Touch

Instead of shaking hands on meeting another person, as it is practiced in the dominant United States culture, Navajos extend their hand and lightly touch the hand of the person they are greeting. Other examples of the use of touch in the Navajo culture include the tradition of massaging a newborn baby as a bonding experience between mother and baby and the tradition of giving a small gift and preparing a small feast for the family when the baby laughs for the first time because this token of esteem touches the heart of all the people around the baby. Another example is the taboo against touching a dead person or an animal killed by lightning, which is extended to touching articles associated with the deceased individual or animal. This taboo is not extended to animals whose death resulted from the other natural causes.

Use of silence and the importance of names

On initially meeting strangers, Navajo people may appear silent and reserved. Once the Navajo individual becomes familiar with the other person, warm behavior is usually demonstrated. In addition, when introducing themselves by name, Navajos give honor to ancestors by stating the clan and the location of the home.

Kinesics

Kinesics practiced within the Navajo culture includes the avoidance of eye contact. In dominant cultures in the United States, eye contact is considered important and if not present may cause suspicion. However, the opposite is true in the Navajo culture, where eye contact is considered a sign of disrespect.

In earlier days Navajo people frowned on pointing anything at another person because pointing was considered insulting. Some Navajos believed that an object being passed to another person should be held upright so that an end would not point at the other person.

Language lateralization

In a study of language lateralization in Navajo reservation children, one group of Navajo children was tested by a researcher who spoke only Navajo (McKeever, Hunt, Wells, & Yazzie, 1989). Another group of Navajo and White children was tested by a researcher who spoke only English. Findings from the study indicate that there appeared to be a strong right-ear advantage for the White children tested by the English-speaking researcher. A similar right-ear advantage was found in the Navajo children when they were tested by the Navajo-speaking researcher, whereas the Navajo children tested by the English-speaking researcher revealed minimal, nonsignificant right-ear advantage. Most of the previous research has suggested that Navajos and other Native Americans have an absence of right-ear advantage. The results of this study were found to be inconsistent with the view that Navajos and other Native Americans are right-brain-hemisphere dominant and thus have a left-ear advantage as a function of the appositional mode of language and thought (McKeever, Hunt, Wells, & Yazzie, 1989).

Implications for nursing care

Because the Navajo language does not always have one single word that is similar to one English word in meaning, to do a nursing assessment and develop a nursing diagnosis, goals, and interventions, the nurse must remember that what is being said must be interpreted by approximation. Because some Navajo people do not speak English, it may be necessary to provide a person who is fluent in the Navajo language. When a Navajo interpreter is utilized, this person must be knowledgeable about medical terminology as well as the cultural aspects of the Navajo lifestyle.

It is also important to remember that the first encounter is not always made to deal with official matters. It is meant to provide an opportunity for the nurse to become acquainted with the family and vice versa. Future rapport with the family is based on this consideration.

Navajo individuals who enter the profession of nursing may experience a cultural shock when care must be provided for a dying patient because of the taboo against touching a dead or dying person and items associated with death. Because of the taboos associated with death, some Navajo nurses may have a healing ceremony performed after contact with a dead person.

SPACE

Time and space are bound to each other; therefore, it must be remembered that the elimination of time alters spatial concepts (Hall, 1966). For some Navajo people there is no such thing as imaginary space. Space is so real a concept that it may not be located in any dimension other than real space. For example, space may not be located in the realm of thought; there is no abstract space. For the Navajo Indian a space such as that found in a room or a house is the same as a small universe (Hall, 1966).

For the Navajo people, personal living space, or that of the traditional Navajo dwelling (hooghan, 'hogan'), is surrounded with many traditions and superstitions or taboos. The hogan is a round open room with distinct functional areas. Many Navajo people believe that shared space provides a spiritual security and a sense of trust. Sheepskins, with the head facing the fire, are used for sleeping. A wood-burning stove, situated center front with the vent pipe extending through the ceiling, provides a means of cooking food. Taboos associated with death in a hogan include the need to seal the entry, warning other Navajos to stay away, and frequently the need to abandon or burn the hogan when a death has occurred. Another event that renders a hogan unusable is lightning striking in proximity; even wood from such a hogan is never used for any purpose by a Navajo, except for a Navajo medicine man in relation to ceremonies. Before a new hogan is occupied, it is usually blessed by a hired Navajo medicine man, who either strews pollen along the cardinal points or performs a formal ceremony. The hogan is so important to the Navajo culture that all Navajo ceremonies are performed in it. Although the hogan is often crowded with members of both nuclear and extended families, the Navajo need for extension of space is demonstrated by the fact that miles often separate one hogan from another or one camp from another.

Implications for nursing care

Because personal space is so important and has no imaginary boundaries, it is important for the nurse to remember that some Navajo clients may have difficulty adapting to situations that place them in spaces that are not familiar. It is important for the nurse to familiarize the client with the space provided during hospitalization and when personal space is limited during health care administration. The nurse should be sensitive to the fact that a hospital might be unfamiliar to some Navajo people, with new things and experiences such as different types of food, different buildings and equipment, different varieties of uniforms, different types of health professionals and support staff, and different types of communication. This situation is particularly true when Navajo clients are hospitalized off the reservation where Navajo interpreters are unavailable or when great distances from their home prevent visitation from their extended family.

The nurse may encounter other health concerns and problems related to life in the cramped environment of a hogan, such as infectious diseases from the lack of indoor plumbing and water supply and burns related to the indoor stoves. Lack of food and food storage may contribute to nutritional deficiencies. In addition, the distance between hogans has a public health implication because isolation from the mainstream creates barriers in the delivery of

health care. One main barrier is the lack of public transportation. Non–Navajo speaking public health nurses cope with this barrier with the assistance of Navajo interpreters traveling as a team in a four-wheel-drive vehicle over treacherous terrain and unpaved roads.

SOCIAL ORGANIZATION
Family

The Navajo culture is extremely family oriented, but the term "family" has a much broader meaning than just referring to the nuclear family of father, mother, and children. The biological family is the center of social organization and includes all members of the extended family. The Navajo people are traditionally a matriarchal society, which means that when a couple marry, the husband makes his home with his wife's relatives, and his family becomes one of several units that live in a group of adjacent hogans or other-type dwellings.

There is no set number or type of relatives limiting the extended family, and their focus is to help one another grow, to collaborate on resources that will provide an adequate livelihood, and to participate in daily life occurrences. Assistance with ceremonies, particularly those associated with birth, death, marriage, or sickness, is shared and has great importance. Usually a male family member looked on as having the greatest amount of prestige will rise as leader for the extended family and provide necessary direction. However, in settling issues, all sides are listened to and the entire group determines the outcome.

The family is considered so important in the Navajo culture that to be without relatives is to be really poor; children learn from infancy that the family and the tribe are of paramount importance. In the Navajo culture, being available for a family member is extremely important, and it is common practice for many members of the extended family to come to the hospital and stay with the client or in proximity to the client until discharge. This situation is particularly true of mothers who have a child in the pediatric unit. All efforts should be made to provide overnight accommodations for the mother in the same room with the child if this is not medically contraindicated.

Family roles and structure

In the traditional nuclear family, the mother is responsible for the domestic duties associated with the home. The father, on the other hand, is responsible for any outside work necessary to maintain the family and the home. Children are responsible for assisting both parents (Roessel, 1981). Within Navajo families children are viewed as assets, not liabilities. Navajo Indian children are rarely told they cannot do something but instead are frequently told of the consequences of doing a particular thing (Primeaux, 1977). Children are encouraged by their parents and members of the extended family to live and learn by their decisions. Because the Navajo traditions are passed down by the elderly, Navajo children are taught to respect tradition and to honor wisdom (Primeaux, 1977).

Marriage

Even today, some Navajo marriages are still arranged. In any case, marriage and the family are considered the foundation of Navajo life. In Navajo society, women are expected not to excel or achieve more success than their husbands (Roessel, 1981). This is even the case among some Navajo nurses who may be cautious about excelling in the profession at the risk of their marriage. In earlier times divorce among traditional Navajos occurred when the wife placed her husband's belongings outside the hogan (Roessel, 1981).

Traditional Navajo dress

The dress of traditional Navajo women has been adapted from the dress of the Spaniards encountered during the internment of the Navajo people at Fort Sumner. The dress usually consists of long, gathered calico skirts and brightly colored velveteen blouses. Because of the harsh terrain and large amount of walking done by Navajo women to get from one place to the other, sneakers and socks are the primary type of footwear.

Traditional Navajo men have adapted the western type of garb, which includes jeans, cotton western shirts, boots, and wide-brimmed hats. Both men and women commonly carry woolen blankets and wear large amounts of turquoise, coral, and silver jewelry as well as ornate buttons and belts. Also, both men and women traditionally wear their long hair tied in a knot behind their head; the knot is covered with rows of white woolen yarn.

Religion

Historically the Navajo people have been guided by sacred myths and legends that describe the tribe's evolution from inception to the present. Supernatural beings portrayed in these stories symbolize the Navajo culture, in which religion and healing practices are blended with each other. Values and beliefs intrinsic to their culture and religion form the Navajo day-to-day living experiences.

Implications for nursing care

It is important for the nurse to remember that both the nuclear and the extended family are of paramount importance to the Navajo client. Because Navajo people believe that family members are responsible for each other, it is not uncommon for many relatives to come to the hospital to care for the Navajo client. Restrictive hospital rules that allow only two visitors at a time or only immediate relatives have no meaning for some Navajo people. The nurse and other members of the health care team should be sensitive to the reality that hogans and camps are at times located a great distance from one another and that visiting a sick relative in the hospital may necessitate travel for many miles, with other family sacrifices needed to obtain funding for this journey. Referral to appropriate available resources will have a positive influence on family-centered care. The presence of family members also provides an ideal opportunity for their inclusion in discharge-planning sessions. Flexibility in scheduling follow-up clinic appointments should also be considered.

Because the Indian kinship or clan system is unfamiliar to most nurses in the United States, it is important for the nurse to develop a sensitivity to and an understanding of the significance of Indian clanships. For example, not only does one inherit lineage from one's mother, but also it is not uncommon for a Navajo child to have several sets of grandparents, uncles, cousins, brothers, and sisters. Among the Navajo people first cousins may be treated as brothers and sisters, and great aunts and uncles as grandparents. The whole system of clanship may prove to be thoroughly confusing to the nurse because several sets of grandparents, brothers, sisters, uncles, and aunts may show up at the hospital, all claiming close relationship to the client.

TIME

The cultural interpretation of time has a temporal focus that views human life as existing in a three-point range that includes past, present, and future (Kluckhohn & Strodtbeck, 1961). Navajo Indians are viewed as being primarily present-time oriented. However, it should be noted that some Navajo Indians are perceived as being both past- and present-time oriented. The common orientation regarding the man-nature theme is a mixed perception that espouses that man is subjugated to nature and at the same time is suggestive that man should learn to live in harmony with nature. In a classic study by Kluckhohn and Strodtbeck (1961), it was noted that the present-time orientation was the preferred mode of time orientation for the population of Rimrock Navajos sampled. The findings of the study also suggested that past-time orientation was somewhat more preferable than future-time orientation but that the difference in preference was not statistically significant. In the study it was also noted that although some of the respondents preferred to be perceived as being subjugated to nature the one significant preference was a perception of being in harmony with nature.

Implications for nursing care

Most people in the dominant culture in the United States are regulated by clocks and are therefore very time conscious. Future-oriented individuals may have a great deal of difficulty with some Navajo people because of their present-time orientation. It is important for the nurse to remember that because Navajo Indians are perceived as being present-time oriented, time is viewed as being on a continuum with no beginning and no end (Primeaux, 1977). In some Navajo homes there are no clocks because Navajo time is casual, present oriented, and relative

to present needs that must be accomplished in a present-time frame. Because certain tasks are associated with present needs, it may be difficult for the nurse to counsel and advise a Navajo client about crucial future events such as taking medications. The present-time orientation of a Navajo client may cause this person to eat two meals today, four meals tomorrow, no meals the next day, and three meals the day after. This becomes an important nursing implication if a client is told to take the medicine with meals, particularly if the medication is to be taken three times a day. Another indication of the Navajo present-time orientation is related to the failure to keep clinical appointments.

ENVIRONMENTAL CONTROL

Some Navajo Indians are perceived as having an external locus of control; although they believe that man is not subjugated to the effects of nature, they also believe that it is essential for man to live in harmony with nature and its elements. As mentioned earlier, Kluckhohn and Strodtbeck (1961) noted that the Rimrock Navajos sampled preferred the orientation theme of "man in harmony with nature." One conclusion from the study was that some Navajo Indians had a mixed locus of control that was suggestive of both a "being"-oriented and a "doing"-oriented culture.

In the past, self-esteem and a health-oriented locus of control have been postulated as predictors of attitudes and behaviors directly related to children's health. Lamarine (1987) conducted a study to measure the relationship between self-esteem, a health-oriented locus-of-control, and health attitudes of Navajo children in the fourth to sixth grades. The analysis of the data indicates that there is a statistically significant relationship between self-esteem and positive attitudes toward health. In addition, the study found that self-esteem was a modest predictor of health attitudes and health behavior intentions among Navajo and Pueblo children.

A craniofacial team at the University of New Mexico Medical Center at Albuquerque has been successful in the treatment of a large population of Navajos because of team awareness of the Navajo concept of health (Smoot, Kucan, Cope, & Asse, 1988). This understanding of the Navajo concept of health in which man is viewed as being in balance with the environment (and therefore an understanding of the Navajo concerns with ghosts, "skinwalkers," and rules for orderly living) allowed team members to integrate the family, as well as the Navajo medicine man, into the care and treatment of children with craniofacial diseases. In addition, to provide culturally appropriate care, the craniofacial team had to develop an understanding of traditional Navajo healing ceremonies and the need for special handling of disposed body parts during surgery.

Illness and wellness behaviors

Traditional Navajo concepts espouse the need for the Navajo people to be in harmony with the surrounding environment and with the family. Some Navajo Indians have a perception of health that is not limited to the physical body but encompasses congruency with the family, environment, livestock, supernatural forces, and community. To maintain spiritual health, some Navajo people believe that it is essential to be in harmony with supernatural forces. Iverson (1990) concluded that health and religion cannot be separated in the Navajo world; rather, the link between traditional religion and healing ceremonies found among Navajo Indians is obvious.

Traditional Navajo concepts of health and disease have a fundamental place in the Navajo concept of man and his place in the universe. Native healing ceremonies encompass traditional Navajo medicine and general native healing practices and form the foundation of Navajo culture. These ceremonies are central to the attitudes, beliefs, values, and perceptions of the Navajo people.

Blessingway is the main philosophy from which over 35 major and minor ceremonial variations are derived. This Navajo practice attempts to remove ill health by means of stories, songs, rituals, prayers, symbols, and sand paintings (Sobralske, 1985). In the Blessingway ceremony the importance of family and clan members is emphasized in the healing process. The mother is considered particularly important because she can relate prenatal incidents of ill nature that affect health.

Native healers

Navajo medicine men and medicine women spend many years learning their skills and serving as apprentices. There are several types of medicine men and women:

1. Diagnosticians, or those who diagnose illness or the cause of disharmony. Their title may be "crystal gazer" or "hand trembler," depending on the method used in diagnosing the patient.
2. Singers (*hataałii,* an undifferentiated singular-plural noun), or those who perform and direct the elaborate and complex healing ceremonies.
3. Herbalists, or those specialized practitioners who use herbs to treat patients and who may also diagnose illness and causes of ailments.

Medicine men and medicine women have *jish,* or medicine bundles, containing symbolic and sacred items, including corn pollen, feathers, stones, arrowheads, and other instruments used for healing and blessing. Many of these sacred objects and plants are found on the sacred mountains that border the Navajo reservation and are gathered by medicine people only (Navajo Health Systems Agency, 1985).

There is great effort on the part of the Indian Health Service and the traditional Navajo healers to work together in a collaborative and cooperative way. It is not uncommon to observe a medicine man or medicine woman in the hospital speaking with a physician regarding the care of a client. When medically indicated, clients may also receive passes to participate in a healing ceremony held outside the hospital. There has been a continued and sustained mutual respect on the part of these two groups for the expertise of the other (Navajo Health Systems Agency, 1985).

In 1984 the Navajo Health Systems Agency conducted a research study to investigate the types of traditional healing services being provided and the types of cultural orientation to traditional healing practices being provided for newly hired Indian Health Service care providers. The conclusions of the survey reiterated the need for continued and improved collaboration and cooperation between traditional medicine people and Western physicians. For example, serious cases of injury and illness are often referred to the hospital by medicine people, and physicians have sent clients to medicine people when deemed appropriate, particularly in cases of psychological or behavioral disorders (Navajo Health Systems Agency, 1985).

Implications for nursing care

To a Navajo Indian the concept of being is a fundamental concept; as mentioned earlier, Navajos are considered more "being" oriented than achievement oriented. Individuals are perceived as being more important than possessions, wealth, or other material things. If something is perceived as good, it is only as good as its value to other people. It is important, therefore, for the nurse to remember that some Navajo Indians believe that goodness is found only when one is in complete harmony with the surrounding environment. The nurse should also keep in mind that if a Navajo is to have the perception of being in harmony with the environment the environment must be structured in such a way that harmony is promoted. If a nurse were to deny or not allow the client the opportunity to achieve harmony with other people, animals, plants, nature, weather, and supernatural forces, the client would not be able to obtain a sense of assuredness in relation to physical, social, psychological, and spiritual health.

It is important for the nurse to determine which cultural health practices are beneficial, neutral, or harmful to the client to provide culturally appropriate care. If a cultural practice is considered either beneficial or neutral, the practice should be incorporated into the plan of care. However, if a cultural practice is considered harmful, the nurse should devise a teaching strategy that will assist the client in developing an understanding of the implications of the practice on continued health maintenance. For example, after delivery the umbilical cord is taken from the newborn, dried, and buried near an object or place that symbolizes what the parents want for the child's future. Burial close to the home of the infant signifies the continued tie or relationship with

the child's home and Mother Earth. Because this neutral practice does not negatively affect health care, it should be acknowledged, accepted, and incorporated into the plan of care. Also, to provide culturally appropriate nursing care, it is essential that the nurse respect the need for Navajo people to maintain traditional rituals even when hospitalized. For example, it would not be uncommon for a Navajo individual to sprinkle certain foods such as corn and cornmeal around the bedside during a curative ritualistic ceremony. The nurse who comes in the room and finds cornmeal around the bedside may initially be disturbed and insist that it be removed. However, the nurse should keep in mind that this cornmeal (as well as other rituals) is extremely important in the ritual and that, because it does not have any negative health-related implications, it should be left at the bedside until the client and the family desire its removal (Primeaux, 1977).

The United States government has passed numerous acts and implemented numerous programs specifically to address health-related issues among the Navajo people and their involvement in the determination of their health care. The 1975 Indian Self-Determination Act provides that any federal program serving the health needs of Navajo people may be either self-determined or contracted for by the Navajo tribe or its designee. Services contracted for must be comparable to or exceed existing services under the direction of federally operated programs such as the Indian Health Service. Through collaborative efforts the commitment to improve the health status of the Navajo population and to increase tribal involvement in health care management has been enhanced, reconfirmed, and extended to other components of health care (Hanley, 1987).

The basic authority for health care for American Indians and Alaskans is provided by the Snyder Act of 1921. The Bureau of Indian Affairs assumed responsibility as a federal branch for providing health care services for the Navajo people until 1954. At that time, the responsibility was transferred to the Indian Health Service as a result of the U.S. Transfer Act of 1954. In 1967 the Navajo area of the Indian Health Service was established to address the health care needs of Navajos. Today, the Navajo area is one of 12 areas within the Indian Health Service and has its administrative location in Window Rock, Arizona.

BIOLOGICAL VARIATIONS

Many Native Americans are faced with a number of health-related problems. Some of the contributing factors include the fact that many of the old ways of diagnosing and treating illness have not outlasted the migration and changing ways of most Native Americans. It has been estimated that at least one third of all Native Americans live in a state of absolute poverty. As a direct result of this poverty, the compounded problems of lost skills and economic endeavors, and the increased complexity of disease entities, many Native Americans are in a health-related crisis. In addition, as a result of poverty, many illnesses and diseases are related to such factors as poor living conditions and malnutrition. Native Americans are believed to be at risk for tuberculosis, maternal and infant deaths, diabetes, and malnutrition.

In the past, Native Americans continuously had the highest infant mortality in the United States; however, infant mortality for Native Americans from 1983 to 1991 (5.9 deaths per 1000 live births) was below the national level of 10.4 deaths per 1000 live births for all persons in the United States in 1985 (U.S. Department of Health and Human Services, Indian Health Service, 1998). (The birth rate for Native Americans is almost double that of the general U.S. population.) Although the neonatal death rate for Native Americans has been reduced, the postneonatal death rate is 2.3 times that for infants from the general U.S. population, including all other ethnic groups (U.S. Department of Health and Human Services, Indian Health Service, 1992). The high postneonatal death rate is believed to be attributable to the pronounced incidence of diarrhea among young babies and to the harsh environment.

In 1996 the ratio of the age-adjusted death rates for all causes of deaths for the Native-American population to that of the general U.S. population was 491.6 per 100,000 population. This figure includes all races and may indicate that American Indians are no longer dying at a faster rate than the U.S. population in general. American Indians still have higher death rates from specific causes; for example, death rates from accidents and diabetes are more than twice those of the general U.S. population and death rates from tuberculosis and liver diseases are more than three times those of the general U.S. population (U.S. Department of Health and Human Services, Indian Health Service, 1992: National Center for Health Statistics, 1998). The life expectancy at birth for most Native Americans is 71.1 years, which is an increase of at least 6 years from the expectancy figure for 1969 to 1971. However, although Native Americans have had an increase in life expectancy, their life expectancy still lags behind that for all other races in the United States (National Indian Health Board, 1984; U.S. Department of Health and Human Services, Indian Health Service, 1992).

From 1984 to 1992, the leading causes of death in the Native-American population included (1) heart disease, (2) accidents, (3) malignant neoplasms, (4) cerebrovascular disease, (5) chronic liver disease, (6) diabetes, (7) pneumonia and influenza, (8) homicide, (9) suicide, and (10) chronic obstructive pulmonary disease (U.S. Department of Health and Human Services, Indian Health Service, 1992). In 1988 the leading causes of death among the Navajo population included (1) heart disease, (2) all accidents, including motor vehicle accidents, (3) malignant neoplasms, (4) pneumonia and influenza, (5) homicide, (6) chronic liver disease, including cirrhosis, and cerebrovascular disease, (7) suicide, congenital anomalies, and diabetes, (8) chronic obstructive pulmonary disease, (9) nephritis, and (10) septicemia (U.S. Department of Health and Human Services, Indian Health Service, 1988). The leading causes of hospitalization for Navajo clients during 1988 included (1) obstetrical deliveries, (2) all accidents, including motor vehicle accidents, (3) upper respiratory tract infections, (4) diseases of the genitourinary system, (5) ill-defined conditions, (6) mental disorders, (7) supplementary conditions, (8) diseases of the circulatory system, (9) skin diseases, and (10) diseases of the endocrine system

(U.S. Department of Health and Human Services, Indian Health Service, 1992).

Body size and structure

Navajo children tend to have low length-for-age and high weight-for-length measures. These reference indicators are suggestive that there is a suboptimal nutritional status among Navajo Indians. Navajo children with birth weights of less than 2500 g tend to be shorter, lighter, and thinner than children with birth weights of over 2500 g. In a study by Peck, Marks, Kibley, et al. (1988), the analysis of the data indicates that much of the nutritional risk, as indicated by growth abnormality among Navajo infants, is most directly attributable to the persistent effects of intrauterine growth retardation and low birth weights.

Skin color

Skin color is perhaps the most recognizable way in which people are categorized. Although other surface characteristics subtly add to this categorization, skin color is perhaps one of the most obvious ways in which people vary across ethnic and cultural barriers. Skin-color variability is caused by a pigment that is produced by the melanocytes located in the epidermal layer of the skin. According to Wasserman (1974), the melanocytes originate in the neural crest, which is near the embryonic central nervous system and seemingly migrate into the fetal epidermis. This origin explains the significance of pigmentation. Mongolian spots are therefore leftovers that somehow linger in the lumbosacral region at a somewhat greater than ordinary depth and causes the bluish effect seen on the skin surface. Mongolian spots are obvious in 90% of Blacks, 80% of Orientals and Native Americans, and 9% of Whites (Jacobs & Walton, 1976). Mongolian spots are commonly found on the buttocks and back and occasionally on the abdomen, thighs, and arms. Mongolian spots appear so ominous on inspection that a nurse who is unfamiliar with this type of discoloration may easily mistake them for child abuse. The neural origin of melanocytes explains the shape. Mongolian spots resemble neurons with dendritic appendages that insert themselves well up into the epidermal cells. These append-

ages inject melanosome granules containing melanin pigments into the epidermal cells (Szabó, 1975).

Dark-skinned individuals are seemingly protected from the effects of sunlight to a greater degree than light-skinned individuals are. One reason for this may be the dispersal of the melanosomes from the basal cells directly to the stratum granulosum. Therefore, when inspecting the skin of Whites, Orientals, and Native Americans, the nurse will find that melanosomes are incorporated singly (Szabó, Gerald, Pathak, & Fitzpatrick, 1969).

Other visible physical characteristics

One visible physical difference that appears to be a startling finding for the nurse is the cleft uvula, wherein the uvula may be separated at the tip, thereby giving it a fishtail appearance. Although this is the most common variation, the separation can also occur as a complete separation into two uvulas (Meskin, Gorlin, & Isaacson, 1964). Although this condition is rare in Blacks and Whites, it occurs in about 10% of Orientals and as high as 18% of Native Americans (Schaumann, Peagler, & Gorlin, 1970).

Another visible physical difference is related to age-related increases in earlobe creasing. A recent study of Eskimos, Navajos, and Whites by Overfield and Call (1983) found no differences among the groups in the frequency of age-related earlobe creasing. However, findings from the study did indicate a difference in relation to age and onset of earlobe creasing across ethnic and cultural barriers. Whites were found to have earlobe creases at least a decade earlier than Navajos were.

Enzymatic variations

Lactose intolerance occurs among the majority of the populations of the world. In fact, it affects 94% of Orientals, 90% of African Blacks, 79% of Native Americans, 75% of American Blacks, 50% of Mexican Americans, and 17% of White Americans (Bose & Welsh, 1973; Leichter & Lee, 1971; McCracken, 1971; Sowers & Winterfeldt, 1975).

Susceptibility to disease

Tuberculosis The role of socioeconomic factors in the incidence of tuberculosis, which includes conditions such as overcrowding and poor nutrition, cannot be disregarded. However, ethnicity also appears to be an important factor in the incidence of tuberculosis. Numerous studies suggest a high incidence of tuberculosis among Native Americans (Delien, 1951; Heath, 1980). The incidence of tuberculosis varies among tribes from a low of 2% for Apaches to 4.6% for Navajos (Reifel, 1949). In the 1980s the previously high incidence of tuberculosis among Native Americans was greatly decreased, but the incidence is still considered high compared with the general population.

Diabetes Non–insulin dependent diabetes (NIDDM), or type II diabetes mellitus, is a major health problem for Native Americans, occurring as early as the teens or early twenties. The earlier onset has led to an earlier onset of complications as well as excessive mortality in the early and midadult years. Age-specific death rates for diabetes appear to be 2.6 times higher for Native Americans between 25 and 54 years of age, compared with the rest of the general U.S. population (U.S. Department of Commerce, Bureau of the Census, 1995). The age-adjusted death rate for diabetes as the single underlying cause among American Indians was 34.8 as compared to 19.5 for White Americans; 26.9 for Hispanics; and 13.1 for Asian Americans (Diabetes surveillance report, 1997). In addition, the complications from diabetes among Native Americans are appearing with distressing frequency. The National Diabetes Advisory Board noted in May 1982 that complications such as amputations have a rate of occurrence 2 to 3 times that of the general U.S. population and a renal failure rate 20 times that of the general U.S. population. In a recent study of the Ute Indians, the prevalence of diabetes among this tribe was noted to be 4 times the statewide rate and that the rate of diabetic neuropathy is at least 43 times that of the diabetic population in the general Utah population.

According to the U.S. Department of Health and Human Services (1982), 33% of outpatient visits in some facilities for Indian health services are for diabetes-related problems. In addition, in some Indian tribes the rate of newly diagnosed diabetes is as high as 25%. (It is interesting to note, however, that

before the 1940s the incidence of diabetes among Indians was rare [Tom-Orme, 1984]). The highest prevalence rates of diabetes among Native Americans are found among the Pimas of Arizona, the Senecas of Oklahoma, and the Cherokees of North Carolina; the lowest rates are found in the Navajos, Hopis, and Apaches (Tom-Orme, 1984).

It is uncertain as to why diabetes mellitus is so prevalent among Native Americans. One hypothesis suggests that some Native Americans have a genetic predisposition for diabetes that is seemingly triggered by changes in dietary practices and increasing obesity (Neel, 1962). Another hypothesis, called the "thrifty-gene" hypothesis, suggests that during the centuries when Native Americans lived a migratory life, which was characterized by periods of feast and famine, a "thrifty gene" developed as a result of natural selection. It has been proposed that this gene might have possibly affected carbohydrate metabolism and storage so that, during times when food was readily available, carbohydrates could be more readily stored in the body to be used during periods of scarcity. This theory proposes that, even today, some Native Americans continue to store carbohydrates in excess, but because periods of food scarcities or famine no longer occur in the propensity that they once did, Native Americans tend to become obese, which ultimately leads to the development of diabetes (Andrews & Boyle, 1998).

Numerous studies support the idea that Native Americans have a predisposition for diabetes mellitus. In a study by Sugarman (1989), 177 cases of gestational diabetes and 13 cases of preexisting diabetes were identified in a retrospective analysis of 4094 deliveries among Navajo women. The findings of the study therefore suggest a prevalence of 4.6% for gestational diabetes. The study also noted that, when women with preexisting diabetes or who had documented gestational diabetes were excluded, the prevalence of gestational diabetes was 3.4%. Although each data source independently failed to identify 20% to 40% of diabetic pregnancies, more than 97% of cases were identified when the data sources were used collectively (Sugarman, 1989).

In a similar study, 181 pregnant Navajo women were screened for gestational diabetes (Massion,

O'Connor, Gorab, et al., 1987). The findings of this study indicated that the 50 g oral glucose screening test was greater than 7.2 mmol/L or 130 mg/dL in 44 of the subjects, or approximately 24.3% of the subjects. In addition, the test was greater than 8.3 mmol/L or 150 mg/dL in 23 of the subjects, or approximately 12.7%. Using standard oral glucose tolerance testing, the incidence of gestational diabetes in the study population was 6.1%. Therefore the study concluded that universal screening of gestational diabetes is recommended among Navajo women because they are perceived as a high-risk population (Massion, O'Connor, Gorab, et al., 1987).

Sugarman and Percy (1989) noted an age- and sex-adjusted prevalence of NIDDM of 10.2% among approximately 76% of Navajo adults living on reservations. This figure was approximately 60% greater than the estimated prevalence of 6.4% for the general U.S. population. In addition, findings from the study suggest that Navajo people are overweight, compared with the general U.S. population (Sugarman & Percy, 1989).

O'Connor, Fragneto, Coulehan, and Crabtree (1987) conducted a cross-sectional study to assess the association of various demographics and medical care variables with metabolic outcomes in Navajos with NIDDM. In the study, the dependent variable was identified as metabolic control and was measured as the mean of all random plasma glucose values obtained at scheduled clinic visits for diabetes over a 2-year period. Using multivariant analysis, the researchers noted that better metabolic control was most strongly associated with compliance with appointments. In addition, the study noted an association between the mode of treatment and metabolic control.

Hypertension Hypertension is rapidly becoming an increasingly important health problem among American Indians and in particular the Navajos. Percy, Freedman, Gilbert, et al. (1997) conducted a community-based study in 1991 and 1992 that included three standardized measurements of blood pressure on the Navajo reservation. Findings from this study indicated that the overall age-standardized prevalence of hypertension among the 780 adults

examined (systolic >140 mm Hg; diastolic >90 mm Hg) was 19%, with a 24% prevalence noted among men and a 15% prevalence noted among women. Further findings from this study are suggestive that among the subjects surveyed the prevalence of hypertension increased with age and relative weight, was more prevalent among men, and was associated with diabetes mellitus (Percy, Freedman, Gilbert, et al., 1997).

Shigella The resistance to trimethoprim-sulfamethoxazole (TMP-SMX) emerged among *Shigella* isolates from the Navajo reservation in the southwestern United States in 1985 and consequently was of paramount importance to health care workers (Griffin, Tauxe, Redd, et al., 1989). In 1983 TMP-SMX resistance was noted at a rate of 3%; however, by 1985 this rate had increased significantly to 21%. The findings of the study indicated that all the respondents who were studied and examined were resistant to ampicillin and streptomycin and had minimal inhibitory concentrations resistant to sulfamethoxazole. The findings also indicated that polyclonal, highly TMP-SMX–resistant *Shigella* emerged through transfer of trimethoprim-resistant genes from aerobic bowel flora to endemic *Shigella* strains. Therefore the findings indicated that the use of antimicrobials can lead to symptomatic shigellosis.

Myocardial infarction Klain, Coulehan, Arena, and Janett (1988) noted that the myocardial infarction attack rate for Navajo men had more than doubled in comparison with an earlier study by the researchers. In addition, they noted that there was a gradual increase in myocardial infarctions among Navajo women. The study concluded that the majority of the Navajos who sustained acute myocardial infarctions were hypertensive (51%), diabetic (50%), or both (31%). However, it was noted that very few of the respondents in the study admitted that they smoked cigarettes.

Arthritis There appears to be a high prevalence of arthritis, including rheumatoid arthritis, among selected American Indian tribes as compared with non-Indian populations (Hill & Robinson, 1969; Rosenberg, Petty, Oen, et al., 1982). Rheumatoid arthritis was found at a rate of 6.8% in Chippewa Indians, and Willkens, Hansen, Malmgren, et al. (1982) noted in a study on Yakima Indians in Washington State that Chippewa women had an arthritis incidence of 3.4%. Although it has been suggested that Navajo Indians have a unique form of arthritis, the findings of one study suggest that Navajos have the same type of arthritis as that of the rest of the U.S. population (Rate et al., 1980). Nurses should also be aware that there have been notable findings of arthritis in the presence of negative blood studies in the Navajo population. Although it has been suggested that geographical location is one major contributing factor to the problem of arthritis, tribes that reside in one location and then move to another do not exhibit any changes in prevalence rates (Overfield, 1995).

HIV and AIDS Native Americans and Alaska Natives, in a 13-state area, had twice the reported gonorrhea and syphilis morbidity, compared with the rest of the general population. In addition, in some states, they also had the highest incidence of hepatitis B. Among these populations, there was also an increase in epidemic intravenous methamphetamine use in one rural American Indian–Alaska Native community. The number of persons who are HIV seropositive is reported to be low in these groups. However, it is believed that this low number is somewhat distorted because of the racial misclassification of these individuals (U.S. Department of Health and Human Services, Indian Health Service, 1992). From 1982 to 1991, the total number of American Indians and Alaska Natives reported with AIDS was 322. Of this number, 278 were male and 48 were female. This number accounts for 16 cases of AIDS per 100,000 American Indians and Alaska Natives, compared with 206,070 cases or 84 per 100,000 for the general U.S. population. It is important to remember, however, that although there has been a relatively lower number of cumulative AIDS cases among American Indians and Alaska Natives the incidence of AIDS is steadily increasing among this population (U.S. Department of Health and Human Services, Indian Health Service, 1992). In 1996, there were 97 total AIDS deaths across all age groups among American Indian and Alaska Natives, bringing the cumulative death total for AIDS to 942 (HIV surveillance report, 1997).

Nutritional preferences

Because there are more than 500 different American Indian tribes, American Indian dietary practices vary widely. However, it should be noted that contemporary American Indian diets combine foods indigenous to the areas with modern processed foods. Food practices are also influenced by tribal beliefs and practices, geographical area, and local availability of selected foods. In certain tribal areas where game and fish are plentiful, these foods are important food sources in the diet. Although fruits, berries, roots, and wild greens are perceived to have important nutritional value, they are scarce in many federally defined Indian geographical regions. They are also scarce in urban centers such as large cities except when found in season in supermarkets (Andrews & Boyle, 1998; U.S. Department of Agriculture, Food, and Nutrition Service, 1984).

Foods preferred by many Navajos include meat and blue cornmeal. Milk, on the other hand, is usually not listed by Navajo people as a preferred food, and this lack of preference for milk has contributed to protein malnutrition among Navajos. One study reporting protein malnutrition among elderly Navajo clients indicates that protein malnutrition is present and is more common in males, hospitalized clients, and the elderly (Williams & Boyce, 1989). The importance of cultural dietary preferences among Navajos in relation to client teaching has been identified by Koehler, Harris, and Davis (1989). According to these researchers, dietitians and nutritionists should be aware of the rich ethnic diversity that exists among Native Americans and use this knowledge accordingly in nutritional counseling.

After 6 months of ethnographic research, Wolfe and Sanjur (1988) conducted a study on 107 Navajo women who for the most part were in the food assistance program. With its primary purpose being to describe and evaluate the contemporary Navajo diet, the study was done on the basis of a 1-day dietary recall. Using data from this 1-day dietary recall, mean nutrient intakes were found to be below the recommended daily allowances for calcium, phosphorus, iron, and vitamin A. Analysis of the data also suggested that 63% of the women in the sample were overweight or obese. Although overall percentages of energy from fat, carbohydrates, and protein were closer to those recommended in the dietary allowances than the percentages found in the general U.S. population were, the fat intake appeared to be primarily saturated, and fiber intake was lower than the average for the rest of the general U.S. population. In addition, among the Navajo women sampled in the study, traditional foods were infrequently consumed. Another significant finding indicated that women with higher incomes tended to have better diets. The study also noted that commodity foods supplied by the U.S. Department of Agriculture's food distribution program provided approximately 43% of caloric intake and 37% to 57% of the intake of all nutrients exception for fat and vitamin C for 72% of the population sampled. Thus a significant finding of the study was the important contribution that the food distribution program makes to the contemporary Navajo diet.

Alcohol metabolism

For many years behavioral scientists have been searching for the biological reason why certain racial or ethnic groups such as Orientals and Native Americans react to alcohol differently than the way other racial or ethnic groups do, and they have noted that alcohol metabolism varies as a result of ethnic heritage. For example, some Orientals and Native Americans have reported physical symptoms such as profound facial flushing and other vasomotor symptoms after drinking alcohol. Wolff (1973) noted that most Whites do not experience similar symptoms. It has also been suggested that a high incidence of alcoholism is found in some ethnic groups such as Native Americans, Blacks, and Whites (Klatsky, Friedman, Siegelaub, et al., 1977).

As indicated in Chapter 7, there are two different enzymes involved in alcohol metabolism, both of which are variations of alcohol dehydrogenase (ADH): a high-activity type of ADH, which converts alcohol to acetaldehyde rapidly, and a low-activity

variant, which converts it slowly (Kalow, 1982, 1986, 1989; Stamatoyannopoulos, Chen, & Fukui, 1975). The enzyme involved in metabolism of acetaldehyde to acetic acid also has several varieties, including acetaldehyde dehydrogenase 1 through 4. Acetaldehyde dehydrogenase 1 (ALDH-1) is considered "normal"; other types are considered "deficient" in their ability to metabolize acetaldehyde (Goedde, 1983, 1986; Keltner, 1994).

In Whites, alcohol is metabolized "fairly efficiently" by the liver enzyme alcohol dehydrogenase, whereas in Native Americans and Asians it is metabolized by acetaldehyde dehydrogenase, which works faster, often causing circulatory and unpleasant effects such as facial flushing and palpitations (Kudzma, 1992). Studies have indicated that American Indians and Orientals experience noticeable facial flushing and other vasomotor symptoms after ingesting alcohol as compared with their White and African-American counterparts, who experience less severe reactions.

Although attempts have been made to explain biological variations of metabolic absorption of alcohol in different racial or ethnic groups, it is not meant in this context to explain the causes of alcoholism. Alcoholism exists among Native Americans in very high percentages.

Psychological characteristics

There appears to be one interesting racial difference in brain development in regard to cerebral speech-lateralization differences noted among Orientals, Native Americans, and other races. It has been suggested that Hopi, Navajo, and Japanese individuals either process linguistic information in both hemispheres or have right-hemisphere dominance (Overfield, 1995; Scott, 1979). Among Navajos this finding is very demonstrable, particularly when one is given a dichotic listening task. Navajos appear to have a left-ear advantage, which is suggestive of right cerebral hemisphere dominance, as opposed to their White counterparts, who have the usual right-ear advantage suggestive of left cerebral hemisphere dominance. For the nurse who is working with an aphasic client, possible racial differences in cerebral dominance cannot be overlooked (Overfield, 1995).

Implications for nursing care

It is important for the nurse to remember that although many researchers have implicated socioeconomic factors as a causative agent in tuberculosis other researchers have related ethnicity to the high incidence of tuberculosis. Regardless of the causation, nurses need to assist Navajo people in learning about the significance of tuberculosis. Teaching should be clear and should attempt to clarify any misunderstandings about tuberculosis. The nurse should use straightforward and easy-to-understand language. For example, the nurse might teach the client and the family how tuberculosis is spread and demonstrate how the organism can actually be seen through a microscope. The nurse should also make every effort to explain the symptoms of tuberculosis in simple terms so that the client and the family develop an understanding of the condition. For example, the nurse might begin by telling the client and the family that the symptoms begin with the client beginning to lose weight, then developing a cough, and then starting to spit up blood. In addition, the nurse might lessen the anxiety created by the need for radiographs by saying that the taking of radiographs is just like the taking of photographs (Wauneka, 1962).

Harris, Davis, Ford, and Tso (1988) designed and tested a cardiovascular health education curriculum using 215 fifth-grade students from rural New Mexico, including Navajo, Pueblo, and Hispanic children. The teaching effort of the program was augmented by materials, examples, and exercises relevant to these particular cultures. The findings of the study suggested a significant increase in knowledge among these students about the cardiovascular system; obesity; tobacco use; and the need for exercise, nutrition, and habit change. The study concluded that a culturally oriented program can be valuable in promoting a healthful life-style in minority children.

SUMMARY

Today, the Navajo nation is a culture in transition. As changes occur in educational levels, employment, and environment, the Navajo people find themselves assimilating more with the dominant culture of the United States. The need to be able to blend their traditional culture with the dominant culture of the United States is creating conflict for some Navajo people. When providing health care to Navajo clients, nurses are being challenged to seek ways to bridge the gap between traditional cultural practices and Western medical practices to provide culturally appropriate nursing care.

Case Study

Mary Littlejohn, a 20-year-old Navajo Indian, is admitted to the hospital for a high-risk pregnancy related to gestational diabetes. This is Mrs. Littlejohn's second pregnancy. She is married and has a 2-year-old daughter at home. She lives in a hogan with her daughter, husband, mother, father, and two aunts. There is no running water, electricity, or plumbing in the home. When Mrs. Littlejohn arrives at the hospital for admission, 12 of her family members are with her. Once she has been admitted to her room and is in bed, her grandmother sprinkles cornmeal around her bed. When the nurse takes the client's history, Mrs. Littlejohn relates that she had the same problem the last time she was pregnant. Mrs. Littlejohn also relates to the nurse that she has felt tired and very weak, has had some spots before her eyes, and has had headaches. In addition, she has had to urinate very frequently at night and does not appear to be able to get enough water or food. The nurse notes on examination that the client's blood pressure is 140/88, her temperature is 99.8° F, her pulse is 102, and her tongue appears coated. The laboratory test done at Mrs. Littlejohn's last clinic visit 1 week ago revealed that her serum glucose level was 160 mg/dL.

CARE PLAN

 Nursing Diagnosis   Health maintenance, altered, related to high-risk pregnancy

| *Client Outcomes* | *Nursing Interventions* |

Client Outcomes

1. Client and family will verbalize a desire to learn more about high-risk pregnancies, diabetes, gestational diabetes, and appropriate techniques to reduce symptoms.
2. Client and family will verbalize a willingness to comply with a medical therapeutic regimen to control gestational diabetes.
3. Client and family will verbalize an understanding of the need to comply with routine, scheduled follow-up care to prevent an at-risk delivery.

Nursing Interventions

1. Identify with client and family sociocultural factors that influence health-seeking behaviors.
2. Determine client's and family's knowledge level about diabetes, gestational diabetes, and implications for high-risk pregnancies.

 Nursing Diagnosis   Communication, impaired, related to sociocultural variables

Client Outcomes

1. Family will be able to communicate personal and family-related needs to health care personnel.
2. Family will be able to communicate feelings about diabetes, gestational diabetes, and treatment regimen.
3. Each family member will be able to send precise, understandable messages to one another through appropriate verbal and nonverbal communication.

Nursing Interventions

1. Assist family in developing adequate communication techniques to communicate feelings and anxieties to one another and to health care personnel.
2. Assist family in developing the ability to determine discrepancies in communicated verbal and nonverbal behavior.
3. Assist family in developing appropriate language skills and nonverbal perception to decrease the possibility of faulty perception.

 Nursing Diagnosis   Family processes, altered, related to gestational diabetes and high-risk pregnancy

Client Outcomes

1. Family will participate in care and maintenance of client.
2. Family will assist nurse in helping client return to a high level of wellness.
3. Family will verbalize difficulties encountered in seeking appropriate external resources.

Nursing Interventions

1. Determine family's understanding of client's condition.
2. Determine support systems available to family from external resources.
3. Determine with family supportive networks of friends and extended family members.
4. Involve family in care and management of client.
5. Encourage family to verbalize fears and anxieties.

STUDY QUESTIONS

1. List several factors that may contribute to diabetes among Navajos.
2. Identify at least one reason why Mrs. Littlejohn's grandmother sprinkled cornmeal around client's bed.
3. Describe at least two communication barriers encountered by nurses in the dominant society when providing care to Navajo clients.
4. Describe at least one health practice that Mrs. Littlejohn may adhere to that may be perceived as negative.
5. Describe the structure of the traditional Navajo family and the relationship to health-seeking behaviors.
6. Identify the possible negative effects of the environment and spatial relationships in a hogan on health and health-seeking behaviors.

References

Andrews, M.M., & Boyle, J.S. (1998). *Transcultural concepts in nursing care* (ed. 3). Philadelphia: Lippincott-Raven Publishers.

Bose, D.P., & Welsh, J.D. (1973). Lactose malabsorption in Oklahoma Indians. *American Journal of Clinical Nutrition, 26,* 1320-1322.

Boyce, G. (1942). *A primer of Navajo economic problems.* Mimeographed material. Window Rock, Ariz.: Navajo Service, Bureau of Indian Affairs.

Brugge, D. (1964). Navajo land usage: a study in progressive diversification. In Knowlton, C.S. (Ed.), *Indian and Spanish adjustments to arid and semiarid environments.* Lubbock, Texas: Texas Technological College Committee on Desert and Arid Zone Research, Contribution No. 7.

Brugge, D. (1968, Spring). Pueblo factionalism and external relations. *Ethnohistory,* pp. 191-200.

Delien, H. (1951). Continuity of program—a necessity of tuberculosis control among American Indians. *Lancet, 71*(4), 136-137.

Diabetes surveillance report (1997). Atlanta, Ga.: Centers for Disease Control and Prevention, U.S. Department of Health and Human Services.

Goedde, H. (1983). Population genetic studies on aldehyde dehydrogenase isozyme deficiency and alcohol sensitivity. *American Journal of Human Genetics, 35,* 769-772.

Goedde, H. (1986). Ethnic differences in reactions to drugs and other xenobiotics: outlook of a geneticist. In Kalow, W., Goedde, H.W., & Agarwal, D.P. (Eds.), *Ethnic differences in reactions to drug and xenobiotics* (pp. 9-20). New York: Alan R. Liss.

Griffin, P.M., Tauxe, R.V., Redd, S.C., et al. (1989). Emergence of highly trimethoprim-sulfamethoxazole–resistant *Shigella* in a Native American population: an epidemiologic study. *American Journal of Epidemiology, 129*(5), 1042-1051.

Hall, E. (1966). *The hidden dimension.* New York: Doubleday.

Hanley, C.E. (1987, April). Changing patterns of health care on the Western Navajo reservation. Unpublished thesis, Chicago, Ill.: American College of Healthcare.

Harris, M.B., Davis, S.M., Ford, V.L., & Tso, H. (1988). The checkerboard cardiovascular curriculum: a culturally oriented program. *Journal of School Health, 58*(3), 104-107.

Heath, C. (1980). *A descriptive and evaluative study of the tuberculosis occurring in American Indians residing in Shannon and Washabaugh Counties, South Dakota, 1970 through 1978.* Master's thesis, Houston, Texas: University of Texas, Houston.

Henderson, G., & Primeaux, M. (1981). *Transcultural health care.* Reading, Mass.: Addison-Wesley.

Heraldson, S.S. (1988). Health and health services among the Navajo Indians. *Journal of Community Health, 13*(3), 129-142.

Hill, R.H., & Robinson, H.S. (1969). Rheumatoid arthritis and ankylosing spondylitis in British Columbia Indians. *Canadian Medical Association Journal, 100,* 509-511.

HIV surveillance report (1997). *Estimated incidence of AIDS and deaths of persons with AIDS, adjusted for delays in reporting, by quarter-year of diagnosis/death, United States, January 1985 through June 1997.* Atlanta, Ga.: Centers for Disease Control and Prevention.

Iverson, P. (1990). *The Navajos.* New York: Chelsea House Publishers.

Jacobs, A.H., & Walton, R.G. (1976). Incidence of birthmarks in the neonate. *Pediatrics, 58,* 218-222.

Kalow, W. (1982). The metabolism of xenobiotics in different populations. *Canadian Journal of Physiological Pharmacology, 60,* 1-19.

Kalow, W. (1986). Outlook of a pharmacologist. In Kalow, W., Goedde, H.W., & Agarwal, D.P. (Eds.), *Ethnic differences in reactions to drugs and xenobiotics.* New York: Liss.

Kalow, W. (1989, March). Race and therapeutic drug response. *New England Journal of Medicine, 320*(9), 588-589.

Keltner, N. (1994, Nov.). Personal communication with J. Giger.

Klain, M., Coulehan, J.L., Arena, V.C., & Janett, R. (1988). More frequent diagnosis of acute myocardial infarction among Navajo Indians. *American Journal of Public Health, 78*(10), 1351-1352.

Klatsky, A.L., Friedman, G.D., Siegelaub, A.B., & Gérard, M.J. (1977). Alcohol consumption among white, black, or oriental men and women: Kaiser-Permanente multiphasic health examination data. *American Journal of Epidemiology, 105*(4), 311-323.

Kluckhohn, F., & Strodtbeck, F. (1961). *Variations in value orientations.* Elmsford, N.Y.: Row, Peterson.

Koehler, K.M., Harris, M.B., & Davis, S.M. (1989). Core, secondary, and peripheral foods in the diets of Hispanic, Navajo, and Jemez Indian children. *Journal of American Dietary Association, 89*(4), 638-640.

Kudzma, E. (1992, Dec.). Drug responses: all bodies are not created equal. *American Journal of Nursing, 92,* 48-50.

Lamarine, R.J. (1987). Self-esteem, health locus of control, and health attitudes among Native American children. *Journal of School Nursing, 57*(9), 371-374.

Leichter, J., & Lee, M. (1971). Lactose intolerance in Canadian West Coast Indians. *Journal of Digestive Diseases, 16*(9), 809-813.

Massion, C., O'Connor, P., Gorab, R., et al. (1987). Screening for gestational diabetes in a high-risk population. *Journal of Family Practice, 25*(6), 569-575.

McCracken, R. (1971). Lactase deficiency: an example of dietary evolution. *Curriculum Anthropology, 12*(4-5), 479-517.

McKeever, W.F., Hunt, L.J., Wells, S., & Yazzie, C. (1989). Language laterality in Navajo reservation children: dichotic test results depend on the language context of the testing. *Brain Language, 36*(1), 148-158.

Meskin, L.H., Gorlin, R.J., & Isaacson, R.J. (1964). Abnormal morphology of the soft palate: the prevalence of cleft uvula. *Cleft Palate Journal, 1,* 342-346.

National Center for Health Statistics (1998). *Health United States, 1998 with socioeconomic status and health chartbook.* Hyattsville, Md.: the center.

National Indian Health Board. (1984). A research agenda for Indian health. *NIHB Reporter, 3*(12), 4.

Navajo Health Systems Agency (1985). *Report on traditional medicine survey.* Window Rock, Ariz.: Navajo Health Systems Agency.

Neel, J.V. (1962). Diabetes mellitus: a "thrifty" genotype rendered detrimental by progress. *American Journal of Human Genetics, 14,* 353-362.

O'Connor, P.J., Fragneto, R., Coulehan, J., & Crabtree, B.F. (1987). Metabolic control in non–insulin-dependent diabetes mellitus: factors associated with patient outcomes. *Diabetes Care, 10*(6), 697-701.

Overfield, T. (1995). Biologic variation in health and illness (ed. 2). Reading, Mass.: Addison-Wesley.

Overfield, T., & Call, E.B. (1983). Earlobe type, race, and age: effects on earlobe creasing. *Journal of American Geriatric Society, 31*(8), 479-481.

Peck, R., Marks, J., Kibley, M., et al. (1988). Birth weight and subsequent growth among Navajo children. *Public Health Reports, 33,* 88.

Percy, C., Freedman, D.S., Gilbert, T.J., et al. (1997). Prevalence of hypertension among Navajo Indians. *Journal of Nutrition, 127*(10 suppl.), 2114S-2119S.

Primeaux, M. (1977). Caring for the American Indian patient. *American Journal of Nursing, 77*(1), 91-94.

Rate, R.G., Morse, H.G., Bonnell, M.D., & Kuberski, T.T. (1980). Navajo arthritis reconsidered: relationship to HLA-B27. *Arthritis Rheumatism, 23*(11), 1299-1302.

Reifel, A. (1949). Tuberculosis among Indians of the United States. *Diseases of the Chest, 16,* 234-249.

Roessel, R. (1981). *Women in Navajo society.* Rough Rock, Navajo Nation, Ariz.: Navajo Resources Center.

Rosenberg, A.M., Petty, R.E., Oen, K.G., & Schroeder, M.L. (1982). Rheumatic diseases in western Canadian Indian children. *Journal of Rheumatology, 9*(4), 589-592.

Schaumann, B.F., Peagler, F.D., & Gorlin, R.J. (1970). Minor orofacial anomalies among a Negro population. *Oral Surgery, 29*(4), 566-575.

Scott, S. (1979). Cerebral speech lateralization in the Native American Navajo. *Neuropsychologia, 17*(1), 89-92.

Smoot, E.C., Kucan, J.O., Cope, J.S., & Asse, J.M. (1988). The craniofacial team and the Navajo patient. *Cleft Palate Journal, 25*(4), 395-402.

Sobralske, M. (1985). Perceptions of health: Navajo Indians. *Topics in Clinical Nursing, 7*(3), 32-39.

Sowers, M., & Winterfeldt, E. (1975). Lactose intolerance among Mexican Americans. *American Journal of Clinical Nutrition, 28,* 704-705.

Spector, R. (1985). Cultural diversity in health and illness. East Norwalk, Conn.: Appleton-Century-Crofts.

Stamatoyannopoulos, G., Chen., S., & Fukui, M. (1975). Liver alcohol dehydrogenase in Japanese: high population frequency of atypical form and its possible role in alcohol sensitivity. *American Journal of Human Genetics, 27,* 789-796.

Sugarman, J.R. (1989). Incidence of gestational diabetes in a Navajo Indian community. *Western Journal of Medicine, 150*(5), 648-651.

Sugarman, J.R., & Percy, C. (1989). Prevalence of diabetes in a Navajo Indian community. *American Jounal of Public Health, 79*(4), 511-513.

Szabó, G. (1975). The human skin as an adaptive organ. In Damon, A. (Ed.), *Physiological anthropology.* New York: Oxford University Press.

Szabó, G., Gerald, A.B., Pathak, M.A., & Fitzpatrick, T.B. (1969). Racial differences in the fate of melanosomes in human epidermis. *Nature, 222,* 1081-1082.

Tom-Orme, L. (1984). Diabetes intervention on the Uintah-Ouray reservation. In Carter, M. (Ed.), *Proceedings of the Ninth Annual Transcultural Nursing Conference.* Salt Lake City, Utah: Transcultural Nursing Society.

Treaty between the United States of America and the Navaho tribe of Indians (1973). Las Vegas: KC Publications.

U.S. Department of Agriculture, Food, and Nutrition Service (1984). *Native Americans: a guide for nutrition educators.* Washington, D.C.: U.S. Government Printing Office.

U.S. Department of Commerce, Bureau of the Census (1992). *American Indian population by tribes in the United States: 1990* (Publication No. 1990 CPH-L-99). Washington, D.C.: U.S. Government Printing Office.

U.S. Department of Commerce, Bureau of the Census (1995, Aug.). *Top 25 American Indian tribes for the United States: 1990 and 1980.* Internet release.

U.S. Department of Health and Human Services, Indian Health Service (1988). Indian Health Service chart book series. Washington, D.C.: U.S. Government Printing Office.

U.S. Department of Health and Human Services, Indian Health Service (1992). Prevalence of HIV and AIDS in American Indians and Alaska Natives. *The IHS Primary Care Provider, 17*(5), 66-69.

U.S. Department of Health and Human Services, Public Health Service, National Institutes of Health (1982). *Diabetes in the 80's. Report of the National Diabetes Advisory Board.* Washington, D.C.: U.S. Government Printing Office.

Wasserman, H.P. (1974). *Ethnic pigmentation: historical, physiological and chemical aspects.* New York: Elsevier.

Wauneka, A. (1962). Helping a people to understand. *American Journal of Nursing, 62*(2), 88-96.

Willkens, R.F., Hansen, J.A., Malmgren, J.A., et al. (1982). HLA antigens in Yakima Indians with rheumatoid arthritis. *Arthritis and Rheumatism, 25*(12), 1435-1439.

Williams, R., & Boyce, W.T. (1989). Protein malnutrition in elderly Navajo patients. *Journal of American Geriatrics and Sociology, 37*(5), 397-406.

Wolfe, W.S., & Sanjur, D. (1988). Contemporary diet and body weight of Navajo women receiving food assistance: an ethnographic and nutritional investigation. *Journal of American Dietary Association, 88*(7), 822-827.

Wolff, P. (1973). Dietary habits and cancer epidemiology. *Cancer, 43,* 1955-1961.

Young, R. (1961). The origin and development of Navajo tribal government. In Young, R.W. (Ed.), *The Navajo yearbook* (vol. 8, pp. 371-411). Window Rock, Ariz.: Bureau of Indian Affairs.

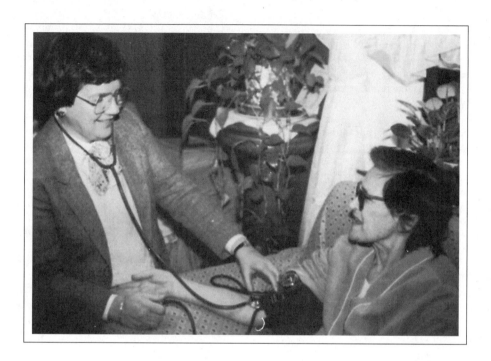

CHAPTER 11 Appalachians

Cynthia C. Small

BEHAVIORAL OBJECTIVES

After reading this chapter, the nurse will be able to:

1. Describe the communication style used by Appalachians.
2. Explain the Appalachian orientation to both time and space.
3. Explain the health care benefits, values, behaviors, and medical and folk practices of persons from the Appalachian culture.
4. Describe how the attitude of Appalachians affects the use of conventional medical health care services.
5. Identify how beliefs of persons from Appalachia affect feelings of environmental control.
6. Develop a culturally sensitive care plan for persons from Appalachia or with an Appalachian background.

OVERVIEW OF APPALACHIA

According to the United States Department of Commerce, Bureau of the Census (1998), approximately 23.7 million people live in the federally defined Appalachian regions spanning 1000 miles across 400 counties in 13 states, including all of West Virginia and selected counties in Alabama, Georgia, Kentucky, Maryland, Mississippi, New York, North Carolina, Ohio, Pennsylvania, South Carolina, Tennessee, and Virginia. These 13 states were set forth in a bill that was enacted by the U.S. Congress in 1965, titled the Appalachian Regional Act. Today, data collected on the Appalachian region is done with federal authority by the Appalachian Regional Commission (U.S. Department of Commerce, Bureau of the Census, 1993).

In the past, it has been difficult to make numerical statements about Appalachia because most statistical facts were tabulated on a statewide rather than a regional basis. However, it was possible to make some generalizations about the Appalachian region based on pooled data. For example, the population within

the federally defined region has always been largely White, primarily of Scottish-Irish or British descent, and predominantly fundamentalist Protestant. For the most part, the Appalachian region is classified as a rural, nonfarming area. In Appalachian areas such as West Virginia, less than 10% of the population is in settlements of more than 2500 persons (Durrance & Shamblin, 1976; Lewis, Messner, & McDowell, 1985; Tripp-Reimer & Friedl, 1977).

Today, however, the scope of the Appalachian Regional Commission has been expanded. As a result, in the 1990 Census, efforts were made to more precisely identify this population. In 1990, the per capita income of persons described as Appalachian was $15,800, compared with $14,143 for the rest of the general population. Although the per capita income is slightly higher than the national average, the poverty rate is significantly higher at 15.3% for Appalachians, compared with 13.1% for the rest of the general U.S. population. In concert with the poverty rate is the infant mortality, which is 9.3% (U.S. Department of Commerce, Bureau of the Census, Statistical Abstract, 1997).

In 1990, of the number of Appalachians in federally defined Appalachian regions, 14.4% of persons 25 years of age or older had less than an eighth-grade education; 31.6% had some high school education but no diploma; 68.4% held a high school diploma or GED; and 14.3% held a 4-year college degree or higher (U.S. Department of Commerce, Bureau of the Census, 1993). Although many Appalachians tend to value education, there have been some problems noted on formal IQ tests among Appalachian children. In a study cited by Borman and Stegelin, findings suggested that among Tennessee mountain children, the greatest improvement in overall IQ test performance occurred in children 6 to 15 years of age particularly those students who had access to larger schools. Further findings from this study indicate that, when formal education was stopped, children who had an average IQ of 94.7 by 6 years of age had experienced a dramatic drop to 73.5 by 16 years of age. It was postulated that this drop may be attributable to decreased educational stimuli particularly in a rural environment. It has been suggested that the IQ test scores of children in Appalachia has increased by at least 10 points (Purnell & Counts, 1998). Although fewer children in Appalachia drop out of school than those in the past, the high school drop-out rate is 17%, which is significantly higher than the drop-out rate for children of other racial and ethnic groups (Penn, Borman, & Hoeweler, 1994; Obermiller & Maloney, 1990). There has been very little change in the graduation rates from 4-year colleges, which remain at 36% as compared to 45% for their non-Appalachian counterparts (Penn, Borman, & Hoeweler, 1994).

In 1991, the unemployment figure for persons identified as Appalachian was 7.5% (U.S. Department of Commerce, Bureau of Labor, 1991). Predominant industries in many of the Appalachian regions include mining, timber, and textiles. Steinman (1970) noted that the Appalachian population, rather than being characterized by a single condition, is noteworthy for geographical and sociocultural isolation. Although persons who are considered Appalachian generally reside in the Appalachian

region, some have migrated to various parts of the United States. On the other hand, some mainstream Americans have also migrated to the Appalachian regions to work primarily in service-oriented professions; however, migration to the region does not in itself result in classification as an Appalachian.

Because of the isolation, lack of definitive physical characteristics, and low visibility of the people, the Appalachian subculture has been relatively overlooked as an American ethnic minority. This is in contrast to most minority groups, which have received a great deal of attention and tend to be outwardly distinguishable from the mainstream or majority of Americans. Although Appalachians have been referred to as "mountaineers" or "hillbillies," they infrequently identify themselves by such classifications and have not tended to identify themselves as belonging to an ethnic or minority group. The largest operating unit of social organization among Appalachians tends to be the family; therefore, the people tend to maintain a family group identity and loyalty as opposed to an Appalachian group identity.

The forefathers of many Appalachian people came from countries such as England, Wales, Scotland, Germany, and France to seek religious freedom (Tripp-Reimer, 1982). Traditionally, the population was overwhelmingly White with only 3.2% of the population being African-American (Obermiller & Maloney, 1990). Over the last 30 years, the number of ethnically and culturally diverse persons moving to the federally defined Appalachian areas has proliferated (Purnell & Counts, 1998). Historically the quest for freedom from oppression was made evident by the particular pattern in which the Appalachian people settled and by their use of space to distance themselves from outsiders. Although many of these individuals, who later would be called "Appalachians," were literate when they arrived in the United States, formal education was stopped when the isolation from the mainstream of society began (Jones, 1983). It appeared that these Europeans who fled to the United States in search of religious freedom and solitude chose to reject the accouterments of civilization. Today, life in the wilderness and the continuing isolation of Appalachians, particularly southern mountaineers, has distinguished Appalachians from the mainstream of American society. For many Appalachians, continued isolation has led to a disparity not only in formal education, but also in health status.

Because of their continued isolation, Appalachians have continued to be the brunt of discriminatory jokes, cartoon strips, and television programming depicting them as shiftless, lazy, irresponsible, toothless, and preoccupied with making "moonshine" and fighting to protect their families from intruders. As with much labeling of minority groups, this stereotyping has emphasized negative behaviors and perpetuates the continued isolation. However, the nurse must keep in mind that identification of Appalachians as a subcultural group, without the negative stereotyping, is essential because a large majority of Appalachians do share similar values, beliefs, behaviors, and health care needs. It is also essential to identify Appalachians as a subcultural group because of the approximately 3.5 million Appalachian people who have migrated to major urban areas of the north central United States since 1950. People who have migrated from the Appalachian regions for the most part have remained at the poverty level and often tend to congregate with other persons from Appalachia, thus further perpetuating the Appalachian subculture in many areas (Tripp-Reimer, 1982).

Many Appalachian persons live in and around the rocky, mountainous terrain, and the roads to their homes are long, rough, steep, narrow, and often impossible to navigate. In addition, many of the homes are small and overcrowded, with inadequate plumbing and sewage systems, which promotes the spread of disease (Schwartz, 1973). Other contributing factors that augment poor health status among Appalachians include low-paying jobs, lack of employment, low educational attainment levels, and increased poverty levels. It is believed that the employment of Appalachians in coal mines and textile factories further increases the risk of respiratory disorders and other medical problems among these people.

COMMUNICATION

Appalachians are English-speaking people; however, the meaning of words used by Appalachians may differ from their meaning when used by individuals in the mainstream of American society. Also, in various Appalachian regions people use different dialects, some of which are quite dissimilar to Standard English, both in vocabulary and pronunciation. A distinguishing feature of these various dialects is that they contain numerous items of Scottish or Elizabethan English heritage. Some of these distinctions are only minor variations in pronunciation and are rapidly learned, such as *deef* for *deaf, welks* for *welts, whar* for *where, hit* for *it, your'n* for *your,* and *heerd* for *heard.*

In some Appalachian regions different dialects used by the people are similar to those of the cultural heritage. Other distinctions involve phrases that convey meanings different from the same phrases as they are used in Standard English (Dial, 1974). Thus phrases used by some Appalachians may be interpreted entirely differently by non-Appalachians. For example, an Appalachian person may say "running off," which may be interpreted by a non-Appalachian as 'leaving home', 'going on tour', or 'running away', but for an Appalachian person this term implies 'diarrhea'. Although these examples of basic difficulties in communicating with Appalachian people are not indicative of a health threat, it is important for the nurse to remember that among Appalachians some folk beliefs are expressed in distinct idioms, which therefore have highly significant clinical application.

Snow (1976) concluded that one of the major concerns of southern folk medicine is the state of the blood. The characteristics or ranges of the blood for some Appalachians include thick to thin, good or bad, and high or low. Among Appalachians the characteristic of high or low is a measure of blood volume, and it is believed that the variations of high or low blood can be regulated through diet. If symptoms of high blood occur, such as headaches, vision problems, palpitations, and dizziness, certain foods and drinks are omitted and others are consumed. Significant clinical problems might arise if an Appalachian were told that there was a problem with "high blood pressure." The patient more than likely would interpret high blood pressure as 'high blood', which would be harmful because the Appalachian folk remedy for "high blood" is drinking brine from pickles or olives. The assumption behind this remedy is that the excess blood volume will be drawn from the cells.

Appalachians are people oriented and are very accepting of other Appalachian persons who have health-related problems. This people-oriented value can be seen in the way in which individuals from Appalachia communicate regarding health problems. For example, it is unacceptable among Appalachians to use the term "crazy" in reference to an individual with a mental health deviation. However, it is acceptable to say that such an individual has "bad nerves" or is "quite turned." It is important for the nurse to be aware of differing language meanings when interacting with Appalachian people to communicate effectively.

Some Appalachians rely on nonverbal communication techniques such as avoiding eye contact with the nurse or any other outside person to communicate needs (Finney, 1969). Although avoidance of eye contact in other regions of the United States may be regarded as shyness, depression, or untruthfulness, to the Appalachian person, maintaining eye contact (or "staring") is viewed as being impolite or lacking good manners (Mullen & Phillips, 1998; Hicks, 1969). In addition, direct eye contact is viewed by some Appalachians as aggressive or hostile behavior (Murray & Huelskoetter, 1987). It is only when an Appalachian person becomes angry or upset that direct eye contact is observed in a relationship. Appalachians are also considered to be a context culture group (Helton, 1995).

Many Appalachian people tend to use a verbal pattern that is much more concrete than the patterns displayed by middle-class Americans, who tend to be more abstract. In other words, Appalachians tend to use fewer adverbs and adjectives and less precise descriptions of emotions or discrete body sensations. For example, it would be quite difficult for the nurse to elicit from an Appalachian client specific information on the type of pain experienced, that is, dull or sharp. Appalachians are a private people who do not generally interfere in other people's business because they do not want to offend anyone. Also, some Appalachians may tell others

what they want to hear rather than what they should hear. Their intent is not to distort the truth but to avoid hurting another person's feelings.

Implications for nursing care

As the textile, mining, and lumber industries began to grow in the Appalachian regions, many Appalachian persons were stripped of their land and other natural resources. Therefore it became difficult for them to trust outsiders. Before positive interactions can occur between an Appalachian person and an outsider, it is essential that a trusting relationship be established. One of the best ways to gain the confidence of an Appalachian person is to use tact and to take the time to listen and talk about matters that relate to the individual and the family. It is also important that the nurse use the approach of dropping hints as opposed to giving orders. Another useful technique is to solicit the opinion and advice of the Appalachian person before taking any action. This technique is useful because it may increase the self-worth and self-esteem of the Appalachian person and because it promotes the feeling that the nurse considers the individual and his or her beliefs important.

Hicks (1969) reported that Appalachians demonstrate what is termed an "ethic of neutrality," which is evidenced in four behavioral imperatives: (1) avoiding aggression or assertiveness, (2) not interfering in another person's business unless requested to do so, (3) avoiding domination over other people, and (4) avoiding arguments and seeking agreement.

Again, the nurse should be aware that some Appalachians may tell nurses what they want to hear rather than what they need to hear, thus augmenting the difficulties encountered when the nurse attempts to develop a culturally appropriate nursing care plan. Perhaps one reason for this is that most health care professionals in the Appalachian regions are more than likely to be cultural outsiders and may be viewed as being unfamiliar with the needs of Appalachian people. Foreign-born nurses and physicians have an even greater difficulty establishing rapport with Appalachians because of language, skin color, and cultural differences. Regardless of the cultural heritage that a nurse may bring to the health care arena, it is essential that the nurse allow ample opportunity for establishing rapport and developing a working relationship with the client. The nurse can establish this relationship by taking time to listen and to converse with the client and the family, using language that is understandable to them and soliciting, when possible, their advice (Lewis, Messner, & McDowell, 1985).

SPACE

Personal space is a very important concept to Appalachian individuals. For the most part, Appalachians have preferred to live apart from the rest of society in social and physical isolation. Although this separation originally developed out of a desire to escape religious persecution, the desire for isolation persisted after migration to the United States, with Appalachian families living on small farms or homes some distance from their neighbors or "up the holler." Thus family relationships are often the only social contact.

Implications for nursing care

In contrast to the typical behavioral characteristic of Appalachians, which is to be family oriented and concerned with the well-being of others, when an Appalachian is ill, personal space collapses inwardly (Simpkins, 1979), meaning that the Appalachian person expects to be waited on and cared for by others. Thus the focus of both the individual and the members of the family is on the ill person. In a hospital setting this may create obstacles to planning and executing nursing care because it is not unusual for a large number of family members to arrive with the client and to expect to maintain proximity with the client throughout the duration of the hospitalization. This desire for proximity is also evidenced when a client is scheduled for a clinic appointment, even if the condition is perceived by the health care professionals as minor.

SOCIAL ORGANIZATION
Family

Appalachians are extremely family-oriented people (Jones, 1983). The nuclear and extended family are both very important to the Appalachian persons.

Relatives may even help an individual determine which job to take and which church to attend. Some Appalachians are so intensely loyal that they feel a personal responsibility for in-laws, nieces, and nephews, as well as other distant family members. Appalachians tend to place a greater importance on the extended family than most middle-class Americans do; the extended family is considered important regardless of the economic level of the individual. Thus relatives are sought for advice, validation, and support on all matters, particularly those pertaining to health and illness (Culture of Poverty Revisited, 1977; LaFargue, 1980). For the Appalachian person, the consideration of the extended family is important because kinship groups are the major social-organizing force in the region. Therefore it is difficult to organize an entire community because some Appalachians do not consider the community a working level of social organization. Rather, these people perceive the most inclusive working level of social organization to be the extended family (Tripp-Reimer & Friedl, 1977). The concept of family is of such paramount importance to most Appalachians that Purnell and Counts (1998) noted that most Appalachians rarely move no more than 30 miles from their families.

The extensive ties to the nuclear and extended family are evident when a family member or relative becomes ill or dies, in that members of the entire family may be absent from their jobs to be with the ill or dying relative during the duration of the crisis. This tendency to miss work because a family member is ill has a negative effect for some Appalachians at the work place. If a family member is chronically ill or if many members are ill, continued employment may be sacrificed for the "good" of the family (Jones, 1983). This intense loyalty for family members remains long after an Appalachian person has migrated from the region, and many supervisors in northern industries become frustrated with Appalachian employees when they are absent from their jobs because of the funeral of a cousin or other distant relative or because the employee needed to "take his wife to the doctor." This loyalty is also carried over into housing in northern areas; a landlord may find a property deserted with all personal belongings intact because the tenant had an urgent need to return to the Appalachian region to be with a sick relative.

Appalachian families are closely knit. It is not unusual for the family to take in relatives for long periods of time, thus creating or increasing the problem of overcrowding. This tendency to take in family members for an extended period of time is seen even in Northern areas. In fact, one of the foremost problems found among Appalachians in northern cities is overcrowding because the Appalachian migrants take in relatives until they get a job or a place of their own. Appalachians are so fiercely loyal to their family that although members of the immediate family may not approve of taking in additional relatives it is difficult for them to ask the relative to leave. James Stills (1978) gives an excellent example of this type of familism in *River of Earth*:

A father may bring in a relative regardless of whether or not there is food, and the mother may become so disgusted that she burns down the house and moves the family into a tiny smoke house in order to get rid of the relatives whom her husband could not ask to leave.

According to Stills, among Appalachians blood is very thick. The Appalachian family is basically patriarchal (Murdock, 1971; Tripp-Reimer, 1982). The father is generally responsible for determining whether a family member should see a doctor. However, "grandmas" have a lot of clout in health care matters, especially if there is a concern about which home remedy is best to use for a particular illness. In the case of pregnancy, the family tends to become more cohesive and provide love and security to the expectant mother. Children are very important to the Appalachian family, and a great deal of importance is placed on having children. Having children implies that a man is "really a man" and that a woman is "fulfilled." Appalachians begin having children at an earlier age and tend to have very large families. Children are often cared for by the grandparents, particularly if both parents work. The children appear to have a sense of who they are and a greater sense of belonging. Appalachian children are accepted regardless of what they do. For the most part, Appalachians do not wish to have their lives or

the lives of their children influenced by mainstream America (Murray & Huelskoetter, 1991).

Elderly family members are respected and either live with their children or at a nearby location. The attitude among Appalachians toward the elderly is one of honor because the culture is transmitted through teachings passed down through the generations. Rowles (1983) found that spatial separation of the elderly from children when the children relocated generated critical dilemmas for the current generation of elderly Appalachians who have difficulty reconciling fear of leaving the familiar environment (with its physical, social, and emotional support) with their desire to be close to the family. The study was based on a 4-year observation of elderly persons in a rural northern Appalachian community and was done primarily to explore the tensions between factors that reinforced inertia and factors that encouraged relocating to the homes of children residing outside the Appalachian region.

The Appalachian family prefers to be independent. At a time when most people hire others to fix their cars or build their homes, Appalachians take pride in doing things for themselves. This may explain the difficulty encountered by many Appalachian persons when it is necessary to ask for financial help or welfare. However, there are conflicting opinions on this issue. Although some Appalachian professionals report that Appalachians would rather work than accept welfare, some non-Appalachian professionals contend that Appalachian people do not like to work, are benefit oriented, and are basically unmotivated (Tripp-Reimer, 1982).

Religion

Appalachians tend to be very religious, not in the sense that they go to church regularly, but in the sense of value. Initially on arrival in the United States, many Appalachian persons were Presbyterians, Episcopalians, or belonged to some other formally organized denomination. However, these churches required educated clergy and a centralized organization, both of which proved to be impractical in the wilderness. As a result, locally autonomous sects sprang up and began to grow in the Appalachian regions. For the most part, these individualistic churches stressed the fundamentals of the faith and depended largely on local resources and leadership. Many social reformers have viewed the local sect churches found in the Appalachian regions as a hindrance to social progress. However, it has been said by some Appalachians that what these social reformers have failed to see is that the church has helped the Appalachian people and made life worth living in grim situations (Jones, 1983).

For the most part, religion has shaped the lives of the Appalachian people; at the same time, however, the Appalachian people have shaped their religion. Culture and religion are intertwined among Appalachians. Religion has become fatalistic for these people and for the most part stresses rewards in another life. There are few Appalachian atheists because the harshness of the terrain seems to demand a spiritual belief in a life in the hereafter. The findings of a study on the effects of religious variables (Schiller & Levin, 1988) indicate that, although it is difficult to isolate any consistent trends in regard to religious variables, low-ordered analysis would tend to indicate that because of their religious values, Jews are higher utilizers of health care than non-Jews. On the other hand, the findings of the study in regard to religion and health care utilization among Appalachians were inconclusive.

Implications for nursing care

It is important for the nurse to remember that because Appalachians tend to be family oriented it is essential to solicit family opinions and attitudes in regard to health care. If the family's ideas and opinions are not incorporated into the plan of care, it is likely that the client may not accept or value the health care services provided. The nurse must also keep in mind that regardless of the acuity level of the client it is possible that the entire family may congregate at one time to be with the client to lend support. Rather than becoming frustrated by this situation, the nurse should use family members to improve client-teaching techniques. For example, if an Appalachian is admitted to the hospital for diabetes, not only should the client be given instructions on diabetic care, but the family members should also be given the same level of instruction because they can shape or alter the client's perception of illness and Western medical treatment.

The nurse must also remember that because religion and culture are intertwined in most cases, it is important that an assessment of the client's religious beliefs be done on admission to the health care system. Because some Appalachians tend to be very fundamental and fatalistic in their religious beliefs, it is essential that the nurse consider that this belief is an influencing variable that may determine whether a client will elect to seek conventional medical advice.

TIME

Appalachians are considered present oriented. They believe that because tomorrow is not promised, they must live for today. Their life-style is laid back and unhurried, which is reflected in the inability of some Appalachians to adhere to a set schedule or time. For example, it is not uncommon for a client to arrive 2 days early or 2 days late for a health clinic appointment. However, if the client cannot be seen that day, he or she may never return.

In a comparison of time perceptions of Appalachians and non-Appalachian health care professions, Tripp-Reimer (1982) found a strong difference in interpretations of time perceptions. The analysis of the data indicates that non-Appalachian professionals view present-time orientation as a negative value. These professionals concluded that Appalachians have no concept of time and that they lack the concepts and skills needed for both long-term and short-term planning and frequently do not keep appointments. According to these professionals, present-time orientation is so interwoven with the day-to-day routine of Appalachians that it is a wonder these people are able to get through a day. On the other hand, the Appalachian professionals concluded that Appalachians tend to live for today because they cannot be sure of what tomorrow will bring.

Another finding of the study was that Appalachians often miss appointments during the day because they are afraid of being fired if they take off from work. Although these findings may not be representative of all people with present-time orientation, they do illustrate the need for the nurse to be culturally sensitive when working with clients with present-time orientation (Tripp-Reimer, 1982).

Implications for nursing care

Because some Appalachians have a present time–oriented outlook, they tend to live at a more easygoing pace that facilitates an awareness of body rhythms as opposed to time schedules and clocks. Because some Appalachians are present time oriented, it is best and often necessary for the nurse to spend a few minutes visiting "a spell" with the client before an examination or treatment is to be done. Although the nurse may be concerned about the time constraints and may not wish to engage in a time-consuming activity such as small talk, it is best to remember that present-oriented people, such as Appalachians, value such activities. Another consideration for the nurse is that it is quite common for some Appalachian clients to arrive for an appointment when they feel ready as opposed to when the appointment is scheduled. If a doctor or nurse refuses to see a client because he or she is late, the client and the client's family may not utilize the services again. One way to facilitate the client arriving at an appointment on time is to make the necessary transportation arrangements.

ENVIRONMENTAL CONTROL
Locus of control

Appalachians tend to have an external locus of control. The dominant value orientation of Appalachians is a deviation from those value orientations held by middle-class Americans, who have been classified as "doing," or achievement, oriented. Appalachians, on the other hand, tend to be "being" oriented, which means that they tend to be oriented toward spontaneous activity and have a more relaxed pace of life. Simpkins (1979) concluded that the "being" orientation held by some Appalachians forms a "toot" work pattern; that is, they may work for a time and then engage in other activities to reestablish equilibrium. This "being" orientation, when coupled with the present-time orientation, tends to block a preventive orientation toward health care while promoting and enhancing a crisis orientation. Therefore it is very likely that the nurse's initial encounter with an Appalachian

client may be an emergency situation, such as a birth.

The external locus of control demonstrated by some Appalachians is viewed as one of fatalism and is believed to have a strong link to religion. Appalachians believe that God has control over their lives and that however things turn out, it is the "Lord's will." In addition, they tend to see their rewards in the life to come. This orientation as developed by Kluckhohn and Strodtbeck (1961) is termed "man to nature." Some middle-class Americans believe that man has control over nature, whereas some Appalachians do not believe that they have control over their future. It is this fatalistic belief that results in the failure of some Appalachians to seek preventive medical advice. However, not all Appalachians respond to their fatalism in this manner. In a classic study by Ford (1967), the data indicate that although 70% of the Appalachians surveyed believed that the time of death is predetermined more than 80% would seek medical care in the case of a dire illness.

The lineal-collateral relational orientation for some Appalachians possibly serves as the basis for some of the most dramatic deterrents to the use of health care services (see Chapter 6). The lineal-collateral orientation indicates that an individual's most significant relationships are with family-related groups, kinship groups, or close neighbors. Many middle-class Americans tend to seek self-actualization through their jobs and other personal involvements, whereas Appalachians tend to seek fulfillment through kinship and neighborhood interactions. Fatalism or fatalistic attitudes may cause individuals to become complacent with their condition or health problem and not attempt to improve their life or seek health care. On the other hand, fatalistic attitudes may help the Appalachian person handle disappointments in life. Associated with this outlook of fatalism is the belief that an individual lives under certain rules and regulations in life; therefore, the total belief system could be classified as fundamental and fatalistic.

Illness and wellness behaviors

The way in which an Appalachian person views health is influenced by beliefs in an external locus of control. The belief that life is controlled by nature is a major factor in the practice of folk medicine for some Appalachians and has led to some unusual ways of coping with illness. The Appalachian folk medicine system has folk healers commonly referred to as "granny women" or "herb doctors." These folk healers are used because they are familiar with the culture, because they are mountain people themselves, because they have a similar religious background, and because they are trusted. They use herbs such as ginseng, foxglove, and yellow root, all of which have been shown to have some medicinal value. However, the strength of the drugs that are used in home remedies may be considerably weaker than the drugs used in pharmaceutical preparations (Lewis, Messner, & McDowell, 1985). Nevertheless, there is a tendency on the part of some Appalachians to utilize folk practitioners rather than physicians. In such cases an individual may actually stop taking medication prescribed by a physician and begin taking herbal medication.

The Appalachian view of illness differs from the traditional mainstream American view of illness. According to the Appalachian view, sickness is the will of God. Also, in the Appalachian view there is a very clear distinction between the role of the well (that is, as a self-sufficient mountaineer) and the role of the ill. The nurse should remember that during illness personal space for some Appalachians has a tendency to collapse inwardly, resulting in a reversal of the role that is typically considered normal for the Appalachian people (Simpkins, 1979).

The Appalachian region has a deficiency in health care resources and practitioners. However, even if resources were available, it is unlikely that some Appalachians would use them because some Appalachians maintain a general distrust of health care organizations and professionals. Numerous other reasons for lack of use of available services have been cited, including a general dislike of impersonal, formal relationships and a fear of being "cut on" or "going under the knife." Thus some Appalachians tend to seek conventional medical health care only when extreme situations arise.

Some Appalachians, like some other individuals in the mainstream of American society, will try home remedies when they first become ill. However, for some Appalachians this first stage of illness be-havior is likely to last longer and consist of a wider range of therapeutic treatments such as herbal decoctions, poultices, and tonics. This situation can have serious adverse effects because some Appalachian clients will wait a long time before seeking even a lay practitioner such as a "granny woman" or an "herb doctor" (Lewis, Messner, & McDowell, 1985; Messner, Lewis, & Webb, 1984). The lay practitioner will be consulted during the second stage of illness, and it is this delay in seeking conventional Western medical treatment that augments even the most minor physical ailments.

Horton (1984) found that the incidence of headaches in Appalachian women and backaches in Appalachian men are not within the normal patterns of medical statistics. The findings of Horton's study further indicate that the Appalachian perception of disability may be in considerable contrast with that of the predominant society. It is a common belief among some Appalachians that disability is inevitable and accompanies age. Some Appalachians view all incapacity as disabling but believe that to be a "deserving" disabled person one must be moral and physically active. The study also found that it is a common belief among Appalachians that good Christian members of the community are called as servants to minister to the disabled and their families. Therefore medical rehabilitation is not viewed as a feasible option.

Nations, Camino, and Walker (1985) conducted a study to determine if ethnomedical beliefs and practices play an important role in primary care. In their study, 33 of 73 clients from a rural Appalachian area who presented themselves at a university primary care internal medicine program had 54 ethnomedical complaints. Of the ethnomedical complaints presented, 24.1% were of high blood pressure, 22.2% were of feeling weak and dizzy, 16.7% were of "nerves," 5.6% were of "sugar," and 3.7% were of "falling out." These 33 clients also had biomedical complaints, and the remaining 40 clients had biomedical complaints without evidence of ethnomedical complaints. No clients presented ethnomedical complaints alone. In the study, approximately two thirds of the clients consulted nonmedical personnel, including family members and friends, for their complaints, and at least 70% engaged in self-treatment before any clinical consultation. Those clients who presented ethnomedical complaints along with biomedical complaints sought advice from nonphysicians significantly more often than those clients who presented biomedical complaints only (with an alpha set of 0.02). However, no statistical differences were found in the self-treatment practices among the groups. Approximately 130 biomedical complaints were presented and recorded by the client's physicians; however, none of the 54 ethnomedical complaints was formally recorded. The high incidence of ethnomedical complaints among Appalachians and the failure of physicians to recognize these complaints mandate that health care providers be taught improved history-taking skills and the essentials of ethnomedical illnesses if culturally sensitive client care is to be provided.

Health care beliefs, diseases, and practices within the folklore system

Appalachians depend greatly on other family members to the point where it is difficult to consider hospitalization. Furthermore, Appalachians generally dislike hospitals because many believe that one enters a hospital to die.

Findings from one study are suggestive that Appalachian women with respect to how experience and spirituality are described in general tended to have a strong belief in a God or a Supreme Being (Burkhardt, 1993). Further findings from this study suggested that these individuals also had a sense of connectedness with self, nature, and others. In this regard, the subjects studied also appear to have a sense of self-reliance and inner strength (Burkhardt, 1993). Elnicki, Douglas, Morris, and Shockcor (1995) studied Appalachians to examine perceptions of any of these individuals regarding barriers to access of preventive measures. Findings from this study are suggestive that 85% of the participants were lacking in at least one preventive measure and thus identified lack of knowledge and costs as primary reason for omitting the measures. Further findings from this study are also suggestive that 72% of those persons who indicated that they lacked at least one preventive measure indicated that if the barriers were removed they would obtain the measure (Elnicki, Douglas, Morris, and Shockcor, 1995).

Similarly, Reed, Wineman, and Bechtel (1995) surveyed Appalachians utilizing a health risk–appraisal tool to diagnose perceived community health needs. Findings from this study are suggestive that, although these participants generally perceived their health as good, overall their health practices were poor. These researchers concluded that the health risk–appraisal tool was perhaps not culturally sensitive to specific health and social needs of this at-risk population. Rosswurm, Dent, Armstrong-Persily, et al. (1996) found that among Appalachians, although culture, age, gender, and rural residence affected responses to illness and recovery, traditional values and roles persisted.

Mullen and Phillips (1998) utilized Giger and Davidhizar's Transcultural Assessment Model as the overarching theoretical framework to explore the cultural beliefs of Southeast Ohio Appalachians. The primary purpose of this qualitative ethnographic study was to identify cultural beliefs of Southeast Appalachians as a means of providing culturally competent nursing care. Giger and Davidhizar's Transcultural Assessment Model was used to identify cultural beliefs from six phenomena of interest, which include (1) communication, (2) space, (3) social organization, (4) space, (5) time, (6) environmental control, and (7) biological variations. Subjects were 14 adults who were native to southeastern Ohio who had resided in the area their entire life. Giger and Davidhizar's Transcultural Assessment Model, which also included interview questions and observational guidelines, was used for structured interviews. Findings from this study are suggestive that these individuals were more socially inclined, communicate more openly, have more of an internal locus of control, have fewer personal space needs, are more future oriented, use no significant home remedies, are more conscientious about getting to appointments on time, and are more likely to follow medical protocols than Appalachians in general. However, findings also are suggestive that these individuals still resembled the mainstream Appalachian population in that they tended to have a strong character, tended to be stoic and nonassertive, and also tended to have a strong belief in a Supreme Being. Figure 11-1 illustrates some of these findings.

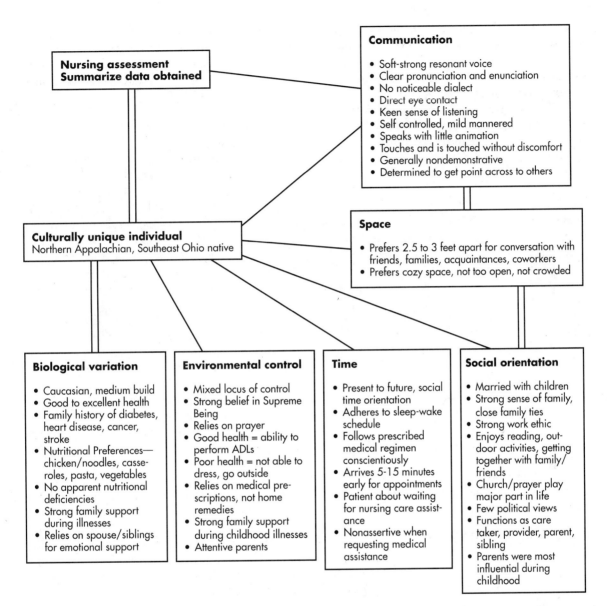

Nursing assessment
Summarize data obtained

Communication

- Soft-strong resonant voice
- Clear pronunciation and enunciation
- No noticeable dialect
- Direct eye contact
- Keen sense of listening
- Self controlled, mild mannered
- Speaks with little animation
- Touches and is touched without discomfort
- Generally nondemonstrative
- Determined to get point across to others

Culturally unique individual
Northern Appalachian, Southeast Ohio native

Space

- Prefers 2.5 to 3 feet apart for conversation with friends, families, acquaintances, coworkers
- Prefers cozy space, not too open, not crowded

Biological variation

- Caucasian, medium build
- Good to excellent health
- Family history of diabetes, heart disease, cancer, stroke
- Nutritional Preferences—chicken/noodles, casseroles, pasta, vegetables
- No apparent nutritional deficiencies
- Strong family support during illnesses
- Relies on spouse/siblings for emotional support

Environmental control

- Mixed locus of control
- Strong belief in Supreme Being
- Relies on prayer
- Good health = ability to perform ADLs
- Poor health = not able to dress, go outside
- Relies on medical prescriptions, not home remedies
- Strong family support during childhood illnesses
- Attentive parents

Time

- Present to future, social time orientation
- Adheres to sleep-wake schedule
- Follows prescribed medical regimen conscientiously
- Arrives 5-15 minutes early for appointments
- Patient about waiting for nursing care assistance
- Nonassertive when requesting medical assistance

Social orientation

- Married with children
- Strong sense of family, close family ties
- Strong work ethic
- Enjoys reading, outdoor activities, getting together with family/friends
- Church/prayer play major part in life
- Few political views
- Functions as care taker, provider, parent, sibling
- Parents were most influential during childhood

Figure 11-1 Giger and Davidhizar's Transcultural Assessment Model applied to Southeast Ohio Appalachians.
(From Mullen, S. & Phillips, C. [1998]. *Cultural beliefs of South Eastern Ohio Appalachians,* Proceedings of the Fourth Interdisciplinary Health Research Symposium, 1998, Health Care and Culture, April 29-30, Morgantown, West Virginia.)

Appalachians have a tendency to be noncompliant in following medical regimens and treatment but expect to be helped directly when seeking episodic treatment in the medical system because of illness. For example, if the physician applies some ointment to a sore, the client will generally be confident that help has been given. However, if the physician gives the ointment to the client with instructions for use, this may be viewed by the client as a refusal to provide care.

Implications for nursing care

Because some Appalachians tend to have an external locus of control, which may foster a fatalistic attitude, the nurse must be willing to recognize that some less-than-conventional medical treatment can have beneficial effects. Those folk beliefs and practices that have neutral or beneficial effects should be incorporated into the plan of care. In the case where folk medicine beliefs and practices are not only inconsistent but may also prove to be harmful, it is essential that the nurse provide health information that is congruent with the client's frame of reference. The relevance of providing health information to Appalachians is evidenced in the findings of a study by Chovan and Chovan (1985) to determine the ways in which men and women cope with stressful situations. They found that when coping responses were characterized in four modes—intrapsychic, inaction, direct action, and information seeking—Appalachian individuals used the information-seeking mode.

BIOLOGICAL VARIATIONS

Unsanitary conditions that were prevalent in the 1970s continue today in many Appalachian regions. Schwartz reported in 1973 that 60% of the houses in Appalachia had inadequate plumbing, only one out of four communities had a water system, and only one out of eight communities had a sewage system. In 1985 Lewis, Messner, and McDowell (1985) reported living conditions for some elderly Appalachians that remained below standard by middle-class values, lacking running water, electricity, and indoor plumbing. Many Appalachians suffer from parasitic diseases that are more than likely related to the unsanitary conditions.

These conditions augment the water and air pollution that is further enhanced by the mining and textile industries. In addition, the crowding of large families and the intense poverty serve to augment the prevalence of disease.

Susceptibility to disease

Respiratory tract diseases Mortality from tuberculosis is 50% higher than the national average among Appalachians (National Center for Health Statistics, Healthy People 2000 Review, 1993). In addition, the incidence of other respiratory tract diseases such as pneumonia, influenza, and black lung disease is far greater than the national average. High-risk occupations, as in the mining, timber, and textile industries, increase the number of respiratory and other disabling physical health problems. Steinman (1970) reported an increased prevalence of early childhood diseases in a screening program in a rural area of Kentucky. For example, 30% of the children surveyed had upper respiratory tract diseases, 24% had hypochromic anemia, and 34% had ear ailments such as otitis media.

Coronary artery and coronary heart disease The incidence of coronary artery and coronary heart disease among Appalachians has also been reported to exceed the national average. Leaverton, Feinleib, and Thom (1984) noted that among White men and women the recent decline in mortality from coronary disease has not been uniform by state; rather, some clustering regarding coronary disease has emerged. When the data regarding certain Appalachian states were reviewed, similarities that tended to indicate a slower decline and thus a worsening of mortality from coronary heart disease appeared.

Diabetes Leichter, Hernandez, Fisher, et al. (1982) studied the social and economic effect of diabetes mellitus and its complications in Kentucky and found that diabetes is a more serious public health problem than previously believed. According to the study, diabetes afflicts 4.4% of the population in Kentucky; borderline forms of diabetes affect an additional 2.4% of the population in Kentucky and appear to be especially prevalent in the Appalachian regions and in rural western Kentucky. In general, an average of 5.23% of all hospitalizations in Kentucky occur because the client has diabetes.

Infant mortality

Spurlock, Moser, and Flynn (1989) conducted a study to analyze differences in postnatal mortalities between the southeastern Appalachian region of Kentucky and the remainder of the state. The primary purpose of the study was to identify factors related to increased infant mortality in the Appalachian region. The findings of the study are suggestive that the relative risk of postnatal death in the Appalachian region compared with the remainder of Kentucky was 1.38 (95% confidence = 1.15 to 1.65). Even when adjustments for birth weight, maternal age, and marital status of the parents were made, no appreciable effects on the risk ratio were evidenced. It was interesting to note, however, that adjustments for maternal education negated the increased risk of postnatal deaths among births in the Appalachian region. When causes of postnatal deaths were examined, three specific disease groupings were found that were disproportionately represented among infants in the Appalachian region: sudden infant death syndrome, congenital malformations, and infections.

Nutritional deficiencies

Ezell, Skinner, and Penfield (1985) studied the snacking patterns of adolescents selected from four metropolitan and three rural schools in eastern Tennessee. According to the study, 89% of the respondents ate at least one snack on the day of the survey, and boys and girls were similar in their snacking habits and patterns. Morning snacks, which more than likely were purchased from the school store or the school vending machine, including items such as candy and salty foods; afternoon and evening snacks included items such as bread and cereals; and carbonated beverages and desserts were popular during all periods. The nutrients that were present in the lowest amounts in these snacks included iron, calcium, and vitamin A.

Skinner, Salvetti, Ezell, et al. (1985) also studied the snacking patterns of male and female adolescents in a southern Appalachian state. They noted that breakfast was skipped by 34% of the respondents and that 27% either skipped lunch or ate a snack lunch. The evening meal was eaten by 94% of the boys and 89% of the girls, and snacks accounted for about one third of the daily caloric intake. The mean intake of nutrients for girls indicated a deficiency in vitamin A, calcium, and iron at all the meals throughout the day. The mean intake of nutrients, particularly iron, for boys was low at breakfast and lunch and in snacks.

Blondell (1988) studied urban rural factors associated with cancer mortality in Kentucky to develop a hypothesis on cancer prevention. The data from Blondell's study are suggestive that subsistence farming, where most of the farm produce is kept for home use rather than marketed, was the single best indicator of low overall cancer rates for males and females in rural and Appalachian Kentucky. The study also noted that the subsistence farming diet was based largely on milk and whole grains, which are reported to be rich in anticarcinogens, including selenium, magnesium, calcium, protease inhibitors, fiber, phenols, and allelopaths.

Psychological characteristics

It is important for the nurse to be aware that people in Appalachia tend to define illness as a state requiring the presence of subjective symptoms. What is defined by others as mental illness may be referred to as a "case of nerves" (Tripp-Reimer & Friedl, 1977) or a person "getting old" or being "odd-turned" (Lewis, Messner, & McDowell, 1985). In other words, an elderly Appalachian seen as functioning quite normally in the hills by neighbors may be diagnosed as severely depressed if taken to a psychiatric clinic outside Appalachia. Behaviors often associated with mental illness may be referred to by the Appalachian as laziness, immorality, or being "psychic" or criminal. Rather than psychiatric treatment or in fact any sort of medical treatment, Appalachians view the appropriate response for these problems as either toleration by the family or punishment by the legal system (Flaskerud, 1980).

Banziger and Foos (1983) conducted a study to determine the association between income factors, such as welfare and unemployment, and utilization of community mental health centers in rural Appalachia. A multiple-regression analysis indicated that compared with other independent variables such as life satisfaction, demographics, and other personal and social factors, users of mental health care services were more likely to be recipients of food stamps. This relationship was noted to be considerably stronger when the more rural areas were separated out for analysis. Some relationship between employment and the need to use mental health services was also found. In a similar study done by Banziger, Smith, and Foos (1982), the relative predictive strengths of selected economic factors such as welfare, banking activity, and unemployment were reviewed for utilization of mental health services. A regression analysis indicated that economic factors accounted for considerable variations in mental health factors. The findings also indicate that welfare may be a primary factor and an excellent predictor of utilization of mental health services.

Critchley and Cantor (1984) studied the authenticity of Charcot's original description of hysteria, which has been questioned in the popular media. The findings of this study indicate that it is possible to encounter florid forms of hysteria in culturally deprived communities such as those in Appalachian regions.

Implications for nursing care

Most of the health problems found in Appalachian regions are partially the result of factors found in the environment, including occupational hazards specific to the region. Because of the remoteness of some of the areas, lack of available health care services, and poor sanitary conditions, some health problems that have been alleviated in the more progressive parts of the United States, such as tuberculosis, remain prevalent among the population in the Appalachian regions. Another factor that contributes to health-related problems in the Appalachian regions is that there are 34% fewer physicians and 20% fewer dentists practicing in these areas than in other parts of the United States (Tripp-Reimer & Friedl, 1977). The limited number of licensed physicians and dentists has resulted in a major portion of primary health care being delivered by nurses. Nurses in Appalachian regions provide comprehensive family-oriented care, whether as nurse-midwives, school or community health nurse practitioners, or staff nurses in outreach clinics.

A recurrent theme among Appalachians is the lack of available health information and the desire for more health information on the part of the people. It is essential that the nurse devise health teaching plans and strategies for implementation that will reach across the Appalachian regions regardless of remoteness.

SUMMARY

The Appalachian people have a rich heritage that can offer the nurse and other health care providers insight into the cultural beliefs. For generations these cultural beliefs and values have been passed down and have persevered. In recent years, some Appalachians have moved to urban areas, and nurses and health care providers are now more likely to come into contact with Appalachian people through the conventional medical system. When working with persons from the Appalachian region, the nurse can use some of the positive aspects inherent to the people, such as strength, independence, sensitivity, and faith, all of which will facilitate a therapeutic nurse-client relationship. In addition, knowledge of the culture and acceptance of health care beliefs can serve to assist the nurse in giving culturally sensitive, individualized nursing care.

Case Study

Sarah James, an 89-year-old widow who lives alone next door to one of her sons in Sweetwater, Tennessee, is seen at the clinic by the family clinical nurse specialist because she "feels bad." She arrives at the clinic with her three sons and their families, who are concerned because Sarah has been "running off" several times a day and will not eat. The clinical nurse specialist visits "for a spell" and then begins to take a health history. When the clinical nurse specialist asks what has brought Mrs. James to the clinic, the eldest son reveals that Sarah has "run off" six or seven times since yesterday and cannot drink her tea. Also, according to the eldest son, Mrs. James has not recently traveled out of Sweetwater, does not have proper refrigeration, and has recently eaten some "tater" salad that had set out all day in the hot weather. It is determined that the diarrhea is watery, brown, and nonodorous. Mrs. James has also had dry heaves but has not vomited and does not verbalize symptoms of pain.

Further assessment by the clinical nurse specialist reveals that Mrs. James has generalized weakness, poor skin turgor, dark circles around the eyes, sticky mucous membranes, pale skin, rectal temperature of 101° F, generalized abdominal tenderness, hyperactive bowel sounds, thready but regular heart rate of 100, blood pressure of 110/60, respirations of 24, and weight of 110 pounds.

After a complete physical examination, the clinical nurse specialist orders a stool culture, electrolytes, and a complete blood cell count. After collaboration with the clinic physician the eldest son approves Mrs. James's admission to the hospital with her entire family in attendance. Mrs. James is crying as she enters the hospital. A diagnosis of dehydration and *Salmonella* poisoning is made. Arrangements are made for follow-up examination after discharge from the hospital.

CARE PLAN

 Nursing Diagnosis   Diarrhea related to inadequate refrigeration of food, resulting in six to seven watery brown stools per day

Client Outcomes

1. Client will resume normal elimination and peristaltic action within the next 24 to 48 hours.

Nursing Interventions

1. Measure daily weight.
2. Record amount, character, and volume of stools.
3. Obtain stool culture.
4. Assess pain status.
5. Explain specific reason for problem (that is, lack of refrigeration of potato salad and other foods that need refrigeration).
6. Note results of CBC and electrolytes.

Nursing Diagnosis   Communication, impaired verbal, related to cultural differences, resulting in possible misinterpretation on the part of the nurse and other health care providers

Client Outcomes

1. Communication will be established between client, nurse, and family to understand health condition and needs.

Nursing Interventions

1. Determine meaning of verbal and nonverbal cues.
2. Establish rapport with client and family.
3. Be aware of cultural factors such as avoiding eye contact.
4. Communicate with client in an unhurried manner.
5. Communicate in specific terms.
6. Learn the form of language used by Appalachians.
7. Ask client and family for their advice.
8. Avoid criticism and spend extra time with client.
9. Communicate on a first-name basis.

 Nursing Diagnosis   Home maintenance management, impaired, related to lack of refrigeration, resulting in inadequate food storage

Client Outcomes

1. Family will obtain proper refrigeration for client before hospital discharge.

Nursing Interventions

1. Determine beliefs related to assistance from government agencies.
2. Determine specific information family should learn and know.
3. Understand role reversal that occurs during illness.
4. Use Appalachians from client's community.
5. Include family in decision making.

 Nursing Diagnosis   Anxiety related to cultural belief that people go to the hospital to die, resulting in episodes of crying

Client Outcomes

1. Client will show signs of decreased anxiety.

Nursing Interventions

1. Utilize the clergy.
2. Exhibit a calm and unhurried manner.
3. Reassure client.
4. Be flexible in visiting regulations.
5. Be accepting of client's cultural differences.
6. Explain procedures to client in specific terms.
7. Involve family in nursing care.
8. Provide arrangement for one family member to stay during the night.

Nursing Diagnosis   Fluid volume deficit related to six to seven watery stools per day, resulting in poor skin turgor, dark circles around the eyes, sticky mucous membranes, rapid thready pulse, and weakness

Client Outcomes	*Nursing Interventions*
1. Client will exhibit signs of adequate hydration within 24 hours.	1. Offer fluids such as tea from home when tolerated.
	2. Maintain balanced intake and output.
	3. Measure daily weight.
	4. Specifically explain reason for and effect of IV therapy and medications.
	5. Increase fluids as indicated.
	6. Monitor vital signs.
	7. Keep items in reach to prevent accidents.

 Nursing Diagnosis   Nutrition, altered: less than body requirements, related to frequent loose stools, resulting in absence of food intake for the past 48 hours and possible weight loss

Client Outcomes	*Nursing Interventions*
1. Client will consume a balanced diet for body size and maintain present weight before discharge.	1. Monitor weight.
	2. Provide nutritionally balanced diet at times client feels like eating.
	3. Document food intake.
	4. Explain necessity for proper diet in specific terms.
	5. Determine what foods Appalachians like to eat.
	6. Encourage rest.

STUDY QUESTIONS

1. List some strategies that may help the nurse communicate with an Appalachian family.
2. Describe the prevailing attitude of Appalachians toward hospitals and hospitalization.
3. Compare and contrast the differences in illness behaviors between middle-class Americans and Appalachians.
4. Describe the orientation and significance of the extended family and the relative role within the Appalachian family structure.
5. Describe the possible importance of folk medicine practices and folk healers to persons from Appalachian regions.
6. Describe ways in which the nurse and other health care professionals may develop sensitivity toward and acceptance of Appalachian folk medicine practices.
7. Indicate resources that health care providers can use to facilitate wellness.
8. List at least three major health problems that place many Appalachians at risk.

References

Banziger, G., & Foos, D. (1983). The relationship of personal financial status to the utilization of community mental health centers in rural Appalachia. *American Journal of Community Psychology, 11*(5), 543-552.

Banziger, G., Smith, R.K., & Foos, D.T. (1982). Economic indicators of mental health service utilization in rural Appalachia. *American Journal of Community Psychology, 10*(6), 669-686.

Blondell, J.M. (1988). Urban-rural factors affecting cancer mortality in Kentucky. *Cancer Detection Preview, 11*(3-6), 209-223.

Borman, K., & Stegelin, D. (1994). Youth at risk. In Borman, K., & Obermiller, P. (Eds.), From mountain to metropolis: Appalachian migrants in American cities.

Burkhardt, M. (1993). Characteristics of spirtuality in the lives of women in a rural Appalachian community. *Journal of Transcultural Nursing, 4*(2), 12-18.

Chovan, M.J., & Chovan, W. (1985). Stressful events and coping responses among older adults in two sociocultural groups. *Journal of Psychology, 119*(3), 253-260.

Critchley, E.M., & Cantor, H.E. (1984). Charcot's hysteria renaissant. *British Medical Journal, 289*(6460), 1785-1788.

Culture of poverty revisited (1977). A critique by the Mental Health Committee Against Racism. New York: Mental Health Committee Against Racism.

Dial, W. (1974). The dialect of the Appalachian people. In Maurer, B. (Ed.), *Mountain heritage*. Morgantown, W.Va.: Morgantown Printing & Binding.

Durrance, J., & Shamblin, W. (1976). *Appalachian ways.* Washington, D.C.: The Appalachian Regional Commission.

Elnicki, D., Douglas, K., Morris, M., & Shockcor, W. (1995). Patient-perceived barriers to preventive health care among indigent, rural Appalachian patients. *Archives of Internal Medicine, 155*(4), 421-424.

Ezell, J.M., Skinner, J.D., & Penfield, M.P. (1985). Appalachian adolescents' snack patterns: Morning, afternoon, and evening snacks. *Journal of American Dietetics Association, 85*(11), 1450-1454.

Finney, J. (1969). *Culture, change, mental health and poverty.* New York: Simon & Schuster.

Flaskerud, J. (1980). Perceptions of problematic behaviors by Appalachians, mental health professionals and lay non-Appalachians. *Nursing Research, 29*(3), 140-149.

Ford, T. (1967). The passing of provincialism. In Ford, T. (Ed.), *The southern Appalachian region.* Lexington: University of Kentucky Press.

Hicks, G. (1969). *Appalachian valley.* New York: Holt, Rinehart, & Winston.

Horton, C.F. (1984). Women have headaches, men have backaches: patterns of illness in an Appalachian community. *Social Science Medicine, 19*(6), 647-654.

Jones, L. (1983). Appalachian values. In Whisnant, D. (Ed.), *All that is native and fine: the politics of culture in an American region.* Chapel Hill, N.C.: University of North Carolina Press.

Kluckhohn, F.R., & Strodtbeck, F.L. (1961). *Variations in value orientations.* Evanston, Ill.: Row, Peterson.

LaFargue, J.P. (1980). A survival strategy: kinship networks. *American Journal of Nursing, 80*(9), 1636-1640.

Leaverton, P.E., Feinleib, M., & Thom, T. (1984). Coronary heart disease mortality rates in United States blacks. 1968-1978: interstate variation. *American Heart Journal, 108*(3), 732-737.

Leichter, S.B., Hernandez, C., Fisher, A., et al. (1982). Diabetes in Kentucky. *Diabetes Care, 5*(2), 126-134.

Lewis, S., Messner, R., & McDowell, W. (1985). An unchanging culture. *Journal of Gerontological Nursing, 11*(8), 20-26.

Messner, R., Lewis, S., & Webb., D.D. (1984). Unique problems and approaches in Appalachian patients with Crohn's disease. *The Society of Gastrointestinal Assistants Journal, 7,* 38-46.

Mullen, S., & Phillips, C. (1998). Cultural beliefs of southeastern Ohio Appalachians. *Proceedings of the Fourth Interdisciplinary Health Research Symposium, 1998 Health Care and Culture,* April 29-30, Morgantown, West Virginia.

Murdock, G. (1971). *Outline of cultural materials.* New Haven, Conn.: Human Relations Area Files.

Murray, R.B., & Huelskoetter, M.W. (1991). *Psychiatric/mental health nursing.* East Norwalk, Conn.: Appleton & Lange.

National Center for Health Statistics, Healthy People 2000 Review (1993). *Health, United States, 1992.* Hyattsville, Md.: Public Health Service.

Nations, M.K., Camino, L.A., & Walker, F.B. (1985). "Hidden" popular illnesses in primary care: resident's recognition and clinical implications." *Culture, Medicine, and Psychiatry, 9*(3), 223-240.

Obermiller, P.J., & Maloney, M. (1990, Dec.). The current status and future prospects of urban Appalachians. *Urban Advocate* (n2), 7.

Penn, E.M, Borman, K.M., & Hoeweler, F. (1994). Echoes from the hill: urban Appalachian youths and educational reform. In Borman, K.M., & Obermiller, P.J. (Eds.), *From mountain to metropolis: Appalachian migrants in American cities* (pp. 83-92). Westport, Conn.: Bergin & Garvey.

Purnell, L., & Counts, M. (1998). Appalachians. In Purnell, L., & Paulanka, B. (Eds.), *Transcultural health care: a culturally competent approach.* Philadelphia: F.A. Davis.

Reed, B., Wineman, J., & Bechtel, G. (1995). Using a health risk appraisal to determine an Appalachian community's health care needs. *Journal of Cultural Diversity, 2*(4), 131-135.

Rosswurm, M., Dent, D., Armstrong-Persily, C., et al. (1996). Illness experience and health recovery behaviors of patients in Southern Appalachia. *Western Journal of Nursing Research, 18*(4), 441-459.

Rowles, G.D. (1983). Between worlds: a relocation dilemma for the Appalachian elderly. *International Journal of Aging Human Development, 17*(4), 301-314.

Schiller, P.L., & Levin, J.S. (1988). Is there a religious factor in health care utilization? A review. *Social Science and Medicine, 27*(12), 1369-1379.

Schwartz, J. (1973). Rural health problems of isolated Appalachian counties. In Nolan, R., & Schwartz, J. (Eds.), *Rural and Appalachian health.* Springfield, Ill.: Charles C. Thomas, Publisher.

Simpkins, O. (1979). Appalachian culture. In Mauerer, B. (Ed.), *Mountain heritage.* Morgantown, W.Va.: Morgantown Printing & Binding.

Skinner, J.D., Salvetti, N.N., Ezell, J.M., et al. (1985). Appalachian adolescents' eating patterns and nutrient intakes. *Journal of American Dietetics Association, 85*(9), 1093-1099.

Snow, L. (1976). High blood is not high blood pressure. *Urban Health, 5,* 4-55.

Spurlock, C.W., Moser, M., & Flynn, L.J. (1989). Regional differences in death rates among postneonatal infants in Kentucky, 1982-1985. *Journal of the Kentucky Medical Association, 87*(3), 119.

Steinman, D. (1970). Health and rural poverty. *American Journal of Public Health, 60,* 1813-1823.

Stills, J. (1978). *River of earth.* Lexington, Ky.: University of Kentucky Press.

Tripp-Reimer, T. (1982). Barriers to health care: variations in interpretation of Appalachian client behavior by Appalachian and non-Appalachian health professionals. *Western Journal of Nursing Research, 4*(2), 179-191.

Tripp-Reimer, T., & Friedl, M.C. (1977). Appalachians: a neglected minority. *Nursing Clinics of North America, 12*(1), 41-54.

U.S. Department of Commerce, Bureau of the Census (1993). *Population profiles of the United States: 1993* (Economics and Statistics Administration. Publication No. P23-185). Washington, D.C.: U.S. Government Printing Office.

U.S. Bureau of the Census, *Statistical Abstract of the United States: 1997* (ed. 117). Washington, D.C.: U.S. Government Printing Office.

U.S. Department of Commerce, Bureau of the Census (1998). *Population profiles of the United States: 1998, June.* Internet update.

U.S. Department of Commerce, Bureau of Labor. (1991). *Labor profiles of the United States: 1991.* Washington, D.C.: Government Printing Office.

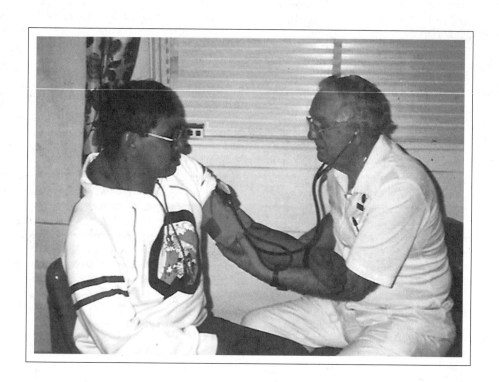

CHAPTER 12 American Eskimos

Dolly Lefever and Ruth Elaine Davidhizar

BEHAVIORAL OBJECTIVES

After reading this chapter, the nurse will be able to:

1. Describe the stressful effect of acculturation of the Eskimo people into Western society, whether in Alaska or in the mainland United States.
2. Understand verbal and nonverbal communication barriers that may affect health care for Eskimo people.
3. Describe attitudes and beliefs of Eskimos that relate to health and illness.
4. Identify the shift in health and illness patterns as Eskimo people have adopted the Western diet and life-style.
5. Describe the problems related to providing health care to Eskimos residing in widely scattered and isolated villages in Alaska.

Settlements of Eskimos are found in diverse locations, including the northern territories of Canada, Alaska, Russia, and Greenland. Although Eskimos may be found throughout the world, this chapter focuses on Alaskan Eskimos who have remained in their native land and those who have migrated to the mainland United States. However, comments are also made about Canadian Eskimos, whose health needs are very similar. To provide culturally appropriate nursing care, it is necessary for the nurse to understand the culture and heritage of the Eskimo people.

OVERVIEW OF ALASKA
The land

Alaska is often described in superlatives. One fifth the size of the continental United States, Alaska has more coastline than the other 49 states combined and is by far the largest state in the continental United States; it is more than double the size of Texas, which by any standards is considered a large state. Alaska is larger than all but 16 of the nations in the world. Everything in Alaska appears to be on a grand scale. It is the home of the largest mountain in North America, Mount Denali (Mount McKinley), which rises to a height of 20,320 feet and is joined by six other peaks that are over 14,500 feet high. Furthermore Alaska also is the home of Malaspina, a great glacier that is larger than Rhode Island. There are more than 100,000 glaciers in Alaska, and these generally cover more than 28,000 square feet each, providing Alaska with 125 times more glacier area than the rest of the United States combined (Kimble & Good, 1955). Alaska is a land where airplanes track icebergs the size of Cleveland and great brown bears, polar bears, and other wild animals roam relatively undisturbed.

The chief influences on the climate in Alaska are its northern latitude, its large land mass, and its coastal waters. Winters are long and bitterly cold, except for the region along the southeast coast. Summers throughout the state are short and cool. The temperature varies by virtue of the season and geographical region; for example, the average temperature at Juneau, in the south of Alaska, is about 25° F in January and 55° F in July, whereas in Nome, in the north of Alaska, the average temperature is only about 4° F in January and 49° F in July. Because of its northern latitude, an unusual feature of Alaska's terrain is permafrost, or permanently frozen ground. In the Arctic region continuous permafrost underlies surface dirt in depths of about 2000 feet. Some buildings and highways have been erected on permafrost. This has created some problems because, as the permafrost thaws, the structures may sink. In addition, in regions where there is permafrost, aboveground cemeteries are commonplace.

Parts of Alaska beyond the Brooks range fall beyond the treeline. Thus in the far north only willows grow, and only in parts of the valleys protected from the wind. Lack of light, warmth, and water; the permafrost; and chilling winds cause the tundra in the far north to be covered with only a flat matting of short, ancient willows and birches (López, 1986). Annual snowfall over most of the subarctic is light, often no more than 4 to 6 inches, and actual snowstorms are rare. Ground blizzards frequently occur in coastal areas, however, where most settlements are located. High winds and a furious swirling of dry snow already on the ground often persist for days and are commonly referred to as a "blizzard." The windchill factor, (−1° F for every 1 mph in winter, causes rapid skin freezing (Morris, 1985). When caught in a blizzard, an Eskimo can cut out a circle in the icy crust of snow covering the ground, dig a hole in the snow, crawl in, replace the icy lid, and remain there until the storm has passed (Holderman, 1993). Because of the freezing temperatures, wind, and blizzards, which are experienced in some areas throughout the winter, both natives and nonnatives still may wear native garb, including parkas and footgear (mukluks) made of animal skins (López, 1986). However, today, mukluks are rarely seen except for traditional dancing and most Eskimo people wear Western clothes, such as Down's Synthetics. Formerly, Eskimos near the windy sea coast areas

preferred sealskin because it has no pores and is warmer (Holderman, 1993). Cost influences what is worn today even more than warmth.

In 1969, the largest auction in the history of mankind was held in Anchorage, Alaska. Some of the world's largest oil companies and consortiums gathered for the sale or lease of some 450,000 acres of the North Slope oil fields. Today one of the most amazing construction projects in American history, the Trans-Alaska Pipeline System spans the entire length of the 49th state from north to south. The pipeline is so revered in the northern state that some Alaskans even refer to it as America's "Great Wall of China" (Brown, 1997). Since its origin, some 70,000 workers have spent at least some time on the job. The many jobs and large percentage of the state budget from the oil has directly benefited the quality of life of the Eskimos. The largest refinery is found just 15 miles outside of Fairbanks, in the small town of North Pole. The Tulsa-based company now operates the majority of convenience and service stores in Alaska (Brown, 1997). Just at the time when the large oil fields were believed to be tapped out, a stunning array of North Slope finds indicated that there may yet be 5.5 billion barrels of oil buried beneath the permafrost. New technology and expedited studies ordered by the Alaskan governor launched exploratory drilling in 1997 on the first 4.6 million acres in an Arctic National Wildlife Refuge (Murphy, 1997). In the sale of just 3253 acres of land in 1997 from the Refuge the Kenai Natives Association Inc. received $4.4 million from the Exxon Valdez Oil Council (Loshbaugh, 1997)

The people

Alaska is a land with many diverse populations. The native population is divided culturally into three groups: Indians, Aleuts, and Eskimos. For centuries the native people of Alaska lived in isolated regions and were undisturbed by outside cultures. In 1741, the Aleuts were brutally exploited by Russians after the fur trade. Alaska was purchased from Russia in 1867 and was governed as a federal district without representation until 1912. Congress was reluctant to spend taxpayer's money on an unknown and seemingly worthless territory a world away from Washington. Beginning in 1883 missionaries began to convert the Native population and introduced limited health services (Nord, 1995). In the early 1900s when outsiders discovered the wealth of Alaska's natural resources, the long-undisturbed culture at last came face to face with elements of the Western culture brought by Alaska's new occupants, the "outsiders." The gold rushes in the early 1900s brought miners and their families. In the 1940s and 1950s military personnel came to Alaska because of its strategic geographical location. Between 1941 and 1945 over 1 billion dollars was pumped into Alaska by the federal government to develop transportation systems: the railroad, highways, airfields, docks, and breakwaters. The most recent onset of Westerners arrived after 1969, with the sale of land to oil companies. In 1970 the population of Alaska was 302,173, which represented approximately a 33.6% increase in the population since the 1960s and made Alaska one of the largest growth areas in the United States. However, during the 1970s only 22% of the population was non-White.

Most of the non-Whites in Alaska in the 1970s were aborigines, including Indians, Aleuts, and Eskimos. In the 1970s almost 50% of the population and most of the aborigines lived in rural and isolated communities. Even natives in the rural areas, however, were not immune to the onslaught of Westerners and the concomitant cultural shock that continues today (López, 1986).

In 1995, there were 603,617 people residing in Alaska (World Almanac, 1997; Information Please Almanac, 1998). Of this number, 75.5% were White; 4.1% were Black, 15.6% were American Indian, Eskimo, or Aleut; 3.6% were Asian or Pacific Islander; and 3.2% were Hispanic (World Almanac, 1997; Information Please Almanac, 1998). Of the number of Asian, Pacific Islander, American Indian, Aleut, or Eskimo residing in Alaska, 21,869 are American Indian, 10,052 are Aleut, 44,401 are Eskimo, 1595 are Japanese, 522 are Chinese, 3092 are Filipino, 1536 are Korean, 241 are Asian Indian, 383 are Vietnamese, 402 are Hawaiian, 149 are Guamanian, 134 are Samoan, and 6323 are of other nationalities (U.S. Department of Commerce, Bureau of the Census, 1993b; Statistical Reports, 1991). Eskimos constitute 77.7% of the

total *native* population in Alaska, and other Alaskan Natives, including Aleuts and American Indians, constitute about 43.9% (U.S. Department of Commerce, Bureau of the Census, 1993b). From 1980 to 1991 the American Indian, Eskimo, and Aleut population increased 3.6% per year. The rapid growth of this population was a result of natural increase, though there was an apparent increase in the reporting of this racial category between the two censuses (Hollmann, 1993). The mean age for this group in the same 10-year period increased from 27.3 to 28.5, with the median age increasing from 23.2 to 26.0. The number of American Indians and Alaska Natives reached 1,161,625 in the 1990 census with the largest population age group from 5 to 9 years of age with 132,017 (U.S. Department of Health and Human Services, Indian Health Services, 1992a).

OVERVIEW OF THE ABORIGINES

The Athapaskan people who reside in Alaska and Canada comprise several different tribes, including the Tsimshian, the Haida, the Tlingit, and seven small tribes belonging to the Athapaskan language family. The ancestors of the Tsimshians, the Haidas, and the Tlingits migrated to Alaska from Canada in the eighteenth and nineteenth centuries (Galens, Sheets, & Young, 1995). Many of the Tsimshians live along the Nass and Skeena rivers. The Haidas are located on the Prince of Wales Islands, and the Tlingits originally settled along the coastal region, which extended from Ketchikan to Katalla. The Haidas and the Tlingits are distantly related. Both tribes, but particularly the Haida, are noted for their totem pole carving. Today, many of the southeastern Indians of that area are fisherman or work in fish canneries. For the most part these people have abandoned their former tribal customs. The Athapaskan Indians live along the wide, flat river valleys west and east of Fairbanks from the Yukon River to the Alaskan highway. The mainstay of these tribes is hunting and trapping. Many Indians lived on the caribou herds and followed them as they roamed the northland.

The Aleuts inhabit the Aleutian Islands and the Alaskan peninsula. The Aleuts are closely related to the Eskimos because both groups are descendants from Asian migrants who came to what is now known as Alaska about 10,000 to 15,000 years ago. The Aleuts have their own unique customs, traditions, and language. For survival the Aleuts engage in sealing, with fishing as the main industry (Lefever, 1993). Because the land is permafrost, there is no opportunity to grow food and farm.

The Eskimo people are found along the Bering Sea and the Arctic Ocean coasts, as well as along the lower Yukon and Kuskokwim River regions. Archaeologists believe that the ancestors of the Eskimos came across the Bering Strait from Asia about 10,000 to 15,000 years ago (Dunbar, 1968). Archaeologists have estimated that during the period from 1750 to 1800, 48,000 Eskimos lived along the Arctic region of North America. Nearly one half (26,000) lived in the area now known as Alaska. Approximately two fifths of these early Alaskans spoke Yupik. These Eskimos lived in southwestern Alaska, with the Yukon River as the natural dividing line between this group and the more northern coastal Inupiak (Milan, 1980).

Although customs, traditions, and some heritage are shared among the aborigines, these groups have traditionally been enemies. Disputes over territorial rights to land or game resulted in the development of an animosity that has been carried on through the generations. For example, it has been reported that some Eskimo parents caution their children to stay near their village to avoid being "carried off by the Indians" (Holderman, 1993). These superstitions are kept alive through the retelling of tales, and when things are missing from an Eskimo village, "the Indians" are blamed (Damas, 1984; Hall, 1975; Holderman, 1960; Morris, 1985).

CULTURE AND HERITAGE OF THE ESKIMOS

The word "Eskimo" is from the French *esquimau(x)*, possibly from *eskimot*, an Algonquian word meaning 'eater of raw flesh', but this word has now been found to have been first applied to the Algonquian Micmacs of Gaspé Peninsula because it meant 'speaking the language of a foreign land' (Mailhot, 1978) or possibly 'snowshoe-netter' (Random House, 1987). Some Eskimos believe the "eaters of raw flesh" attribution puts them in a poor light with modern audiences and so use other terms for themselves.

"Inuit," the most widely used of these terms, refers specifically to Eskimos of the eastern Canadian Arctic. The Eskimos of the Bering Sea region prefer, instead, to be called "Yupik," whereas North Slope Alaska Eskimos prefer "Inupiat," and Mackenzie Delta Eskimos prefer "Inuvialuit" (Damas, 1984).

Some people believe that the Eskimos once numbered about 100,000 and that this number dramatically decreased with contact with the White man in the nineteenth and twentieth centuries, which brought exposure to disease (Morris, 1985). Epidemics of smallpox, influenza, hepatitis, and measles have been credited with killing thousands.

The Eskimo people, more than any other native Alaskans, have managed to preserve artifacts as well as many interesting and unique native customs. Artifacts of the Eskimo can be found in various museums such as a museum outside Ketchikan at the White Salmon Falls Resort. The public can see a 1300-piece collection that includes Native basketry, Native trade beads, ivory, miniature kayaks, moccasins, 3-foot canoes, masks, furs, totems, a Chilkat blanket from the early 1800s, and more (Saari, 1997). However, the traditional way of life is changing for the Eskimo as they become assimilated into the dominant culture, take on mechanical trades, and move away from reliance on the land. Young Eskimos are leaving the villages to go away to school and are returning with new knowledge of the outside world. Some do not return.

The Eskimo people have lived in the harsh and frigid regions of western and southwestern Alaska. To survive in this frozen, non–crop producing region, the Eskimos have hunted, fished, trapped, and gathered food on the tundra. Thus the dietary mainstay of the people traditionally consisted mainly of wild meat, such as caribou, and seafood, such as seal, fish, and whale. A century ago the government brought reindeer to Alaska from Russia and Scandinavia in an effort to improve the meat supply. Only the Eskimos were allowed to own reindeer, and it proved a successful addition to the local diet (Loshbaugh, 1996). However, commercial ranching has remained small. Today, there are only eight reindeer herders and a couple of Native corporations that own herds (Loshbaugh, 1996). These foods were supplemented by berries fermented in sealskin with fat, as well as wild greens, such as sour dock.

Traditionally, dog teams were used for traveling, but this is no longer common. When dog teams were used, they had to be chained to reduce the risk of catching rabies from Arctic foxes. One tradition that remains from dogsled days is the annual Iditarod Trail sled dog race across Alaska to None. However, this is one tradition of the Natives that has almost entirely been taken over by non-Natives who can afford to pay the high cost of competition, estimated to be at least $30,000 (Rosen, 1997). Although animal rights activists annually oppose the race, it is a special event for many Alaskans and is promoted around the world as a tourist attraction (Rosen, 1997; Giblin, 1997). Today, many Eskimos use "snow machines," a motorized toboggan. Dogs are slower than snow machines, but they run on cheap fish rather than expensive gasoline and in a crisis an Eskimo could eat a dog. Dogs will always get you there; snow machines break down. On the other hand, snow machines travel up to 40 miles per hour and need no driving license. Unfortunately, when children drive snow machines, accidents often occur (Holderman, 1993).

Traditionally, kayaking served an important source for water transportation, and whaling was an important component of the economy for most Eskimos who lived near the ocean (Newberg, 1997; Lubbock, 1937; Stefansson, 1921). Today, whaling can still be found along the northern coast lines (Lefever, 1993). Some Yupik Eskimos in the Delta region subsist on salmon, seal, migratory birds, and eggs. The popular Eskimo "blanket toss game" originated from the lofting of a member of the tribe as high as possible above flat terrain to look seaward to spot whales. When a whale was spotted, open sealskin boats called "umiaks" were outfitted with paddles, bailers, and harpoons and were launched from the shore. Great knowledge and skill were required to harpoon a whale and tow it back to shore, where the entire village participated in butchering the beast. Today umiaks are replaced with outboard motorboats. Life jackets are not used because the sea temperature is near freezing and causes rapid death by fibrillation. The benefit of wearing a life jacket is

that it assists in finding the body later. Eskimos usually do not know how to swim because the water is too cold for learning purposes (Holderman, 1993).

Eskimos traditionally have been noted for their honesty. For example, if a piece of driftwood were turned in a position in which it would not have washed ashore, others would know it had been claimed and would not take it (Holderman, 1993). The concept of sharing is deeply ingrained among Native Americans who hold it in greater esteem than the White American ethic of saving (Lange, 1988; Lewis & Ho, 1975). In the Northwest culture area, primarily among Indians, the potlatch, a festive gathering of friends and neighbors, would involve not only sharing food but also blankets and other useful items (Jilek-Aall, 1981).

It is a popular misconception that most Eskimos live in dome-shaped ice-block shelters called "igloos." In fact, these shelters were used primarily as emergency bivouacs by the Canadian Eskimos. The early Alaskan Eskimos lived in dwellings that were partially underground and covered with sod. Both the ice igloo and the sod huts had long, dipped tunnels as entrances so that the cold air, which is heavier, was caught in a natural trap, thus permitting the interior of the hut to be heated more easily. Today, houses are constructed of wood frames in small modern villages that are scattered widely along the coast and major river systems (Pollick, 1997). These wooden buildings usually have central heating, running water, and sewage storage tanks. Originally "honeybuckets," black polyethylene bags, were used for sewage disposal. Honeybuckets were tied when full and thrown outside the door for collection to be taken to a dump outside the village (Morris, 1985). Many small villages had a boat that took honeybuckets out into the bay and dumped them. The beaches became polluted with old plastic bags from "honeybuckets" that washed up on shore in the summer. Today, because of government projects, many of the larger villages have a sewage treatment plant that includes a piping system where central water tanks supply water to houses by plastic pipe and raw sewage is piped out to sewage holding and treatment areas. Some houses even have "flush" toilets. However, winter temperatures play havoc with this system because of frozen lines, even though some villages have above-ground insulated pipes to avoid permafrost. Consequently, during the winter months the old honeybucket system may still be found. In the Yukon Delta regions, where it is extremely cold, the honeybucket collection is still an important part of village life. Permanent villages range in population from 20 persons to 1000, with an average of 400 persons. Most of these villages share community water supplies, electricity, churches, stores, and irregular mail service by airplane.

The social disorganization and cultural conflict that has accompanied the rapid changes among Eskimos has contributed to increased health risks for all ages of Eskimos just as living in remote areas, severe climate, harsh terrain, subsistence, and primitive life-style have (Taylor, 1988). According to the Alaska vital statistics records for 1993, the three leading causes of death in Alaska were accidents (20.2%), cancer (19.8%), and heart disease (19.4%). Nationally, accidents accounted for only 4.6% of deaths, whereas heart disease (37.45%) and cerebrovascular accidents (7.6%) were the two leading causes of death. From 1987 to 1993 approximately 7950 deaths and more than 73,000 hospitalizations of American Indians and Alaska Natives resulted from accidental injuries (National Center for Health Statistics, 1998).

Nationwide, one of three children has had a serious injury. The average figure for Alaska is higher than this. Injuries are the major cause of hospitalization within the Alaska Area Native Health Services Unit (Taylor, 1988). Alaska Native elders constitute a major risk group for poor health, chronic disease, high medical expenditures, and institutionalization (National Center for Health Statistics, 1993). Death by violence has increased significantly among Alaska Natives, who have a suicide rate, frequently related to alcohol and self-inflicted gunshot wounds, three times that of the general United States population (Kost-Grant, 1983; National Center for Health Statistics, 1998; U.S. Department of Health and Human Services, Indian Health Services, 1991b). American Indian–Alaska Native adolescents produce reports of high rates of health-compromising behaviors and risk factors related to unintentional injury, substance

use, poor self-assessed health status, and emotional distress (Blum, 1992). Even infants have an unusually high death rate in Alaska. Rates of sudden infant death syndrome, accidents and injuries, fetal alcohol syndrome, and infectious disease exceed those for the United States (Fleshman, 1992.)

Over the years the Indian Health Service has targeted specific health problems, such as the high rate of maternal and child health problems, with specific programs. In 1984, Alaska was one of 10 states to receive a Child and Adolescent Service System Program to improve state services for troubled youth (VanDenberg & Minton, 1987). An Indian Health Service work group on aging was established in 1991 to plan strategies for helping aging Alaskan Natives through the year 2000 (National Center for Health Statistics, 1993). The Indian Health Service has endeavored to bring general health services to the small villages. For many years, because of the remoteness of the villages, the Indian Health Service Bureau has sponsored regular clinics in each village, which are staffed by a community health nurse who travels to the villages by air or dogsled. In 1991, 172 Alaskan village health clinics were identified as well as an increasing number of dental services (U.S. Department of Health and Human Services, Indian Health Services, 1991b). Areas not served by clinics with on-site staff have field nurses who make rounds by airplane and have replaced the former system. In some places, teachers from the lower 49 states and native, trained health aides were the only health service available to give antibiotics, pull teeth, deliver babies, and handle both major and minor medical emergencies (Holderman, 1962, 1993; Lancaster, 1990; Ross, 1989; U.S. Department of Health and Human Services, Indian Health Services, 1992b).

The following excerpts are from letters written by a teacher's assistant living in Deering, Alaska (Holderman, 1962):

The great variety of work and the fascinating Eskimo people make life in the Arctic very interesting for this farm girl from Johnstown, Pennsylvania. As special assistant to the teacher (my husband), I find my role also includes caring for the sick (there is no doctor within 100 miles), and my LPN training comes in very handy. I also help teach, prepare the school lunch, fill out applications for villagers who know little English for OAA and ADC checks from the Territory, help pull teeth and immunize the children, conduct women's meetings, write letters and reports for the Eskimo natives, and help the Eskimos place orders from the Sears Roebuck catalogue.

They caught me as I was coming out of church and told me about a sick baby with a temperature of 105.1. This baby is always sick, and because the mother has had 8 that died, I fear for the safety of this one. The mother was shaking her when I got to the sod hut where they live to try to get her to stop crying. Eskimos can't bear to hear their children cry. I told her to put her down and keep her very quiet, and I gave her a shot of penicillin. I wanted my husband to make this visit, but when Eskimo women come to the door and he answers it, they just grunt and won't tell him. In the Eskimo culture women have their place, and men have theirs. When I got home, another mother came in with her two year old who had a temperature of 104.1. We are so lucky we haven't had a death this year. It is so depressing when we have to add another name to the death book. We are working very hard to help the Eskimos learn how to take better care of themselves and their babies, and with constant teaching we can see less sickness. We are glad it will soon be winter because without the mosquitoes and flies and less spoiled food there will be fewer fevers and sickness.

When we first came and I went through the dispensary supplies in the dispensary between our house and the school, I came across this little black doctor's bag and thought, "How quaint!" I wondered if there was any real occasion to use it. Now the little bag has lost its quaintness. There have been many occasions to carry it. When I start out at 20 below across town to see a client, I am always worried about what I'll find. I did a minor operation this week. This lady had a dreadful swollen shoulder and finally the mass came to a head the size of a fist and the doctor 100 miles away ordered me to lance it deep and wide. I went with my boiled instruments and went to work in the dimly lit cabin. One Eskimo held a flashlight and handed me what I needed. I was sure the blood would gush out, but instead the pus poured forth, several cupfuls I am sure. Later, I stopped to redo the dressing and give her more penicillin, and she is much better. She was very grateful and insisted I accept new fur mittens she had made out of reindeer skin as a token of her appreciation.

Last Saturday I was worried about Martha who had not been in to school for a few days. I had fixed her face up with salve on Monday, but it had looked pretty bad. The old grandma she lives with had sent word on Friday she couldn't come to school because "The medicine never helped." The sod house was terribly dirty, and there was no one there to care for her and keep her clean. The bugs had apparently eaten at her until the scabs spread all over. My husband and I both went and, when we saw her, knew we had to get her out of there if she was to get better. We sent for an interpreter and told the old grandma we would have to take her. The Native pastor helped, and the men just picked up the girl and carried her out to the infirmary on the porch of our house. We started with her head and gave her a general overhauling in our own portable tub. We spent hours soaking, bathing her face, and applying salve. Days later we got the scabs off, and the healing process began. The infection had spread up her nose and smelled horrible. I think it was the first time in her whole life that she had to do anything she did not want to do. Eskimo children are rarely corrected. I'm sure she never had so much washing in her whole life. I made her a clean new dress and kept rewashing her clothes to get rid of the germs. Yesterday we sent her home after a week without a trace of illness or even a scar.

Recently, health care in the villages has been provided by the Indian Health Service, which funds the Alaska Native–run health corporations, such as the Yukon-Kuskokwim Health Corporation. In addition, state and federal block grants have provided funds for regional centers. Bethel, Nome, Kotzebue, Barrow, Fairbanks, and a few subregional centers have had professional staff, including physician assistants and public health nurses. The Bethel service has provided care for 50 villages. Each village has had a clinic staffed with health aides supported and trained by Yukon-Kuskokwim Health Corporation from Bethel. Daily telephone contact has been made with physicians in Bethel. Public health nurses have visited every 2 to 3 months, and the physician visits every 2 years. The health aides have had high school diplomas and five or six training sessions every 6 weeks. Their level of expertise has varied but has increased over time as they have assessed clients and discussed with the physician or physician assistant by phone what should be the choice of treatment or plan. Standard drugs have been kept in the clinic, and the health aides have given them as directed. Public health nurses have done well-child care and immunizations. The major health care provider in most villages has been the community health aide (Lefever, 1997). Medical students and residents have also been used extensively as additional health care providers. This has been an important recruitment technique to provide future physicians (Bartline, 1997). Today, the major health reform affecting the United States in the 1990s is also affecting health care delivered by the Indian Health Service (IHS). The implications of the state health care reforms have unknown implications for Alaskan Natives. It is feared by some that the lack of funding sources will result in the loss of the generalist public health nurses (Nord, 1995). Dr. Trujillo, director of IHS in 1996, indicated that the health care system must be prepared to perform in a new era of health care delivery in Alaska. One of the director's strategies has been to involve the key stakeholders including the Natives in the design of the delivery system (Wiggins, 1996). One major problem that must continue to be addressed regardless of the health care system is the fact that for a variety of reasons Alaska Natives die younger and at higher rates proportionately than members of the general United States population (Andrew & Krouse, 1995).

COMMUNICATION
Language

Although some authorities have related the language of persons native to the Arctic to the Athapaskan or Algonquian language groups (Szathmary, 1984), others have found the Eskimo language or Eskimoan to be a unique language. Eskimoan is a difficult language because one word is often used to express a whole sentence. Originally the Eskimo language had no written forms; thus the recounting of events in story form and in dance provided the only record of Eskimo life. Today a phonetically written form of the Eskimo language that was developed by missionaries exists. The early missionaries and educators demanded that the Eskimo people learn English, which has now become the primary language of the younger generation of Eskimos. A few school systems have initiated bilingual study programs as a direct result of the desire of Eskimos to preserve the Eskimo heritage.

In the oral language spoken by Eskimos, present-time oriented actions are communicated with the Eskimos referring to themselves, as well as others, in the third person. For example, when referring to himself or herself, an Eskimo person would say, "Someone is going hunting," or "Someone is hungry." There is no terminology recognizing the future or vocabulary to discuss abstract concepts; language is used to describe action occurring in the present (Vaudrin, no date). Unlike children learning English who learn the passive structure of the language later, children learning Inuktitut (one dialect of the Eskimo language) learn a simple and complex form of passive vocabulary very early in language development (Allen & Crago, 1996). In the past, each person in the Eskimo culture had a defined role in the group; therefore, the anticipation of each person's action required little verbal communication. With the desire to be accepted by incoming Westerners, the Eskimo people learned to speak simple English. Idioms, abstract ideas, and double-meaning phrases were not understood in early acculturation (Vaudrin, no date). However, with English as a primary language of the young people and with the exposure to the world by means of satellite television and education, idioms and abstract ideas have begun to have meaning. Still, the nurse who cares for Eskimo clients from the bush or remote areas should avoid the extensive use of idioms, such as "a bull in a china shop," "out in left field," or "robbing Peter to pay Paul," because such idioms may lack meaning to these people who may have little or no background in urban living where such things as baseball fields are commonplace.

The language of the Eskimo people reflects their dominant concerns and interests. Certain words take on a more significant meaning than other words do. Because Alaska for the most part is a land of snow and ice, these words take on a more significant meaning. For example, there are three different words for snow for which there are no single-word equivalents in the English language. Different words are used for falling snow, soft snow on the ground, and drifting snow. Another important word for the Eskimo is ice. Again, different words describe freshwater ice, saltwater ice, and icebergs because ice also serves different and important purposes in this culture (Armstrong, Roberts, & Swithinbank, 1973; Holderman, 1993).

For the older generation, English is the second language. Thus, when one is speaking to an older person, comprehension can be facilitated by speaking slowly and in literal terms. Children who know only English may have trouble communicating with their grandparents who know only Eskimo (Taylor, 1988). Translators may be helpful, but it is important to remember that the Eskimo language has no translation for the future or for abstract ideas. When providing care to an Eskimo client, the nurse should provide an explanation about specific therapeutic interventions both in English and, if a translator is available, in Eskimo (Glassetter, 1989).

Use of silence

Eskimos tolerate periods of silence more easily than people in Western society do (Kleinfeld, 1971). In fact, it is considered rude to fill silences with chatter because such chatter only prevents one from having the space to express viewpoints. The perceived Western intolerance of silence serves to increase the Eskimo's feelings of being dominated and inferior (Kleinfeld, 1971; Vaudrin, no date). Traditionally in Eskimo culture, each adult is given the opportunity to express a viewpoint without a time limit. For example, an Eskimo may go see a White person for some reason and just sit in silence for many minutes before saying why he or she has come (Holderman, 1993). However, individuals in Western society may be insensitive to this mode of communication and interpret silence as nonparticipation or passive acceptance. Generally, Eskimos are a polite people and are unlikely to criticize other people's opinions and actions unless such actions cause a threat to the social group. There appears to be a prescription against verbal expression of negative effect (Kost-Grant, 1983). In dealing with people in Western society, the younger generation of Eskimos have for the most part adapted Western ways, which includes becoming more verbal.

Touch

There is a wide range of acceptable open demonstration of affection displayed in public among various subgroups in the Eskimo culture. However, the handshake is considered universally acceptable and a mandatory politeness. Hugging is an acceptable greeting between family members and between women friends. Eskimo men are more reserved in their expressions of affection, using a handshake with only one movement, not up and down, as a common way to greet friends and family (Glassetter, 1989). Traditional Eskimos are very modest about exposing the body, and it is often difficult to persuade older Eskimo people to undergo complete physical examinations, particularly for diagnostic purposes. The nurse who cares for Eskimo clients needs to establish a trust relationship before diagnostic examinations will be allowed. In the presence of pain and illness, however, there is less resistance to physical examinations (Schaefer, 1973).

The late Eskimo healer Della Keats supposedly healed many people through the use of touch and love (Keats, 1985). According to Keats, she inherited the skill of her hands and learned the use of herbs for healing from her mother and other Eskimo elders. Through love, touch, and a combination of old and new medicines, Keats reportedly healed her people (Pender, 1987). The older Eskimo people give credence to the power of touch as a direct result of a shaman's healing powers (Glassetter, 1989). Shamanism, a belief that a person holds supernatural powers, is a doctrine held by some primitive societies and some Eskimos.

Kinesics

Eskimos use nonverbal communication extensively through body posture and facial expression (Albert, 1988; Boas, 1938). Years of watching animal behavior for survival needs have made the Eskimo people experts in the interpretation of nonverbal language. The nurse who understands the Eskimo culture will look for nonverbal clues, such as watching the face for raised eyebrows (indicating "yes") or a wrinkled nose (indicating "no"). Eskimos seldom disagree publicly with others. Although smiles and head nods in the Western culture may indicate agreement, in the Eskimo culture they may simply acknowledge the other person's words. Among Eskimos, actual agreement is determined by action. Insincerity and deceptiveness are quickly perceived through body talk and lead to distrust and eventually to social ostracism. Thus others are evaluated by body language, and this evaluation is nonverbally communicated back by inclusion or exclusion of the person in future activities. The nurse who lives and works among the Eskimo people will eventually understand the nonverbal language of Eskimos and its significance. The old adage is true for the Eskimo that one must listen with both the eyes and the heart to hear what the people have to say about themselves and others (Glassetter, 1989; Keats, 1985).

Implications for nursing care

For effective communication to occur, the nurse must develop a trust relationship with the client that in time will give rise to acceptance of the nurse. When the nurse works in an Alaskan village, the villagers may appraise the nurse not on skills but on the nurse's endorsement of the community. Some villagers may perceive acceptance in terms of the nurse's willingness to visit in homes, to take time to have a cup of coffee, and to participate in village activities. It is important for the nurse to recognize that some Eskimos have a need to know they are accepted as individuals and as a community. Thus insincerity and discrepancy between nonverbal and verbal language will cause mistrust and block communication. When dealing with Eskimo clients, whether in villages or in an integrated mainland United States society, the nurse should be assertive but not aggressive and use a suggestive rather than a direct approach.

Some Eskimos respect the right of personal choice and self-determination as long as these actions do not affect the welfare of the family or community. Above all, the nurse must avoid direct orders because they tend to be viewed as being "bossy." When working with some Eskimo clients, it is best for the nurse to approach the situation in a roundabout way. For example, a public health nurse, while making a home visit, may notice a baby's bottle rolling around on a dirty floor. Later the nurse may see the toddler pick the bottle up, take a few sips, and throw it back on the floor. If the nurse corrects the mother about failure to protect the child from the dangers of unrefrigerated milk and bottle-mouth syndrome, that mother may not come

to the clinic or allow the nurse in the house again. However, the advice may be more readily accepted if the nurse waits until the mother brings the child in for health care, where teaching can be implemented and emphasis placed on the importance of refrigerated milk and the prevention of bottle-mouth syndrome.

Eskimos are very sensitive to the power of the dominant culture and will withdraw from any form of judgment implied by health care providers. For example, it is of little value to lecture about alcohol use, chewing tobacco, or dipping or pinching snuff. (Yupik women may "chew" up to 6 to 10 times daily.) The development of trust and acceptance is the best form of demonstrating support for the community. This approach will allow the village community to educate itself and seek to change unhealthy life-styles of community members. Health care providers should not fall into the trap of thinking that they alone can effect change, which is a collaborative interaction of support and nonjudgment between providers and the community.

When providing health teaching for a client who lacks English language skills, the nurse must use educational material that can be understood. Many educational materials available for children in English do not address the specific kinds of accidents encountered. The Emergency Medical Services program at the Yukon-Kuskokwim Health Corporation has developed four educational curricula with specific focus on safety and first-aid issues appropriate for the Alaskan Eskimos. Two sets of books were created, one written in English and the other in Eskimo, thus making culturally and linguistically appropriate materials available (Taylor, 1988).

It is also important for the nurse to be aware that some Eskimos have been found to have chronic otitis media, which has impaired their ability to learn. Services are being developed to assist with providing hearing aids for students and to develop audiological services to the Eskimos (Baxter, 1980; Baxter, Katsarkas, Ling, & Carson, 1979; Ling, 1976; Crago & Tremblay, 1991; Goodbody & Stubbing, 1991). Problems in service have often been the product of two very different cultures coming together, and they include attitudes toward hearing-aid service, noise exposure, and adequate audiovisual materials (Ilecki & Baxter, 1981).

SPACE

In the Eskimo culture individual space is often shared with family members (Lange, 1988; Roberts & Ross, 1979). What is perceived as crowded living conditions by individuals in the Western society may be viewed by the Eskimo as living in the warmth and security of the family group. The Western cultural need to be territorial, that is, owning private space, traditionally was not a value of the Eskimo people. Instead, the Eskimo people valued sharing and perceived it as an acceptable norm. Acculturation has weakened this particular value system, but family rights still take precedence over individual rights. For example, if a family member desires the privacy of a room for a few hours, this request may be accepted as a personal need. However, if this same individual demands such privacy continuously in a two-room house with five members, ridicule and accusations of selfishness may result. As the need for individual space arises, individual family members may go on hunting, fishing, or camping trips to meet privacy needs as well as to return to nature.

A handshake distance between two people is considered the acceptable space for socialization on a daily basis. Closer approaches without permission are perceived as threatening, whereas greater distances are perceived as rude. An outsider who desires input from the Eskimos in a public meeting must recognize the decision-making process of the people and the effect that spatial requirements have on the decision-making process. The public zone for communication incorporates an intimate physical space where people sit in a circle, without a leader dominating the group. Some Eskimos view Westerners as masters of the savior attitude, which can serve to block communication with an impenetrable wall (Damas, 1984).

Implications for nursing care

The nurse who cares for Eskimo clients must remember that certain requirements for spatial distances must be observed. Requirements for space must take into account that the client may have unique beliefs about space and may be disturbed when a nurse ventures into personal space to do such routine procedures as give a bed bath or provide oral care. The nurse must determine how much self-care can be implemented by the client and how much must be implemented by the nurse. When self-care is threatened, clients who are protective of space may become withdrawn, overly aggressive, or overly passive. The nurse must be careful to allow the client to make decisions about care, and thorough explanations should be given when the nurse must venture into the intimate or personal zone.

SOCIAL ORGANIZATION
Family

The extended family is the primary social unit; however, polyandry was common in traditional Eskimo society. Polyandry (the practice of a woman having more than one husband), though a cultural rarity, is believed to have existed in the Eskimo culture because of extensive female infanticide and because of the inability of some women to survive the long harsh winters (Carpenter, 1973; Holderman, 1993). The practice of female infanticide and the suicide of elderly people in the Eskimo culture may be understood in light of the harsh and frigid geography (Seltzer, 1983; Travis, 1983). In many instances there simply was not enough food, and hence the killing of female babies (who were primarily consumers rather than procurers of food) was a kind of protection for the society as a whole. Similarly, when men got beyond the age when they were able to be active hunters and women were no longer able to chew the hides and thus prepare them, they were usually expected to commit suicide or to induce their friends or relatives to kill them. Although this may seem inhumane, it was a purposeful way of preserving the culture (Nida, 1954; Seltzer, 1983). In a study of the attitudes toward the elderly in the Aleutian Islands today, Seefeldt (1984) reports that Eskimos still place more value on youth. Suicide by elders and female infanticide is no longer part of the culture. Many Eskimos who have been raised by Christians are embarrassed by this heritage. Care must be used in referring to these practices. Westerners have an intolerance for such concepts, and this intolerance can be interpreted by the Eskimo as judgmental. The elders who may remember talk by grandparents have a different understanding of such behavior. This behavior was seen as completely normal and good for the community in that the community was honored over the individual. This concept clashes with the Western concept of individual rights and is one of the main causes of friction between the emerging modern Eskimo culture and the old ways.

Among some early Eskimos, wife exchange had no negative connotations and was considered the mark of a good host (Holderman, 1993; Nida, 1954). Rules of hospitality indicated that a host should offer his wife to an unrelated visitor, with an understanding that the favor should be reciprocated.

The family unit, with its kinship ties, was paramount to survival in the harsh Arctic environment. The ideal Eskimo family group size has traditionally been considered to be four members (Holderman, 1993). Although the Eskimo society has become a distinctively individualistic society, with primary reliance on the individual and with the individual relatively free to work out problems, the survival of the group traditionally was considered more important than the survival of the individual members. Several family units would band together in a migrating social group. These social groups were not permanent because families could disband and join other groups during a lifetime. However, the roles for individuals and for families within a social group were clearly delineated, so that the groups were not weakened by the shifting of members (Nida, 1954). In fact, this shifting may have strengthened the culture by extending kinships. Extended families consisted of parents, their children (from a current or previous marriage or from adoption), grandparents, and single blood relatives. The husband was the head of the family, but the responsibility of bonding the family into a strong unit belonged to the mother. Thus, if the family was unsuccessful, the blame was placed on the woman. The woman's role for family bonding was continued into the modern cultural adaptation. However, the role is continued despite lack of male support. The male members of the Eskimo society find themselves at a loss with the depletion of the role of hunter and subsistence gatherer. Because of the intrusion of the dominant society, inactivity

and lack of jobs has led to alcoholism and family dysfunction.

Kinships were vital social relationships when Eskimos lived in isolated areas. Kinship boundaries extended beyond blood relations through such practices as wife sharing, hunting partnerships, and the adoption of children. The code of behavior between kin was as binding as that between blood relatives. These extensive kinship relationships were partially responsible for the cultural similarities in Eskimos that spread across the vast Arctic regions (Williamson, 1974). History has recorded incidences of lost Eskimo hunters who crossed paths with another Eskimo band and were killed if the lost person could not prove kinship to a member of the new group (Williamson, 1974).

In Eskimo culture today, the extended family plays a very important role. Survival no longer depends on kinships, but these relationships are far from dead. There still is a linking of families, which is evidenced by the sharing of native foods or the formation of business partnerships. These ties go beyond simple friendship considerations. Eskimos feel "to be really poor is to be without relatives" (Holderman, 1993). The extended family involves the easy adoption of babies between families. If someone finds it impossible to care for a baby, adoption is an accepted practice. Adoptions are frequently carried out with little or no litigation. An adopted child is fully incorporated into the extended family. Because of close family ties, the child is often related to the adoptive parents.

The rapid entry of the Eskimo into the American cash economy and value system has led to the restructuring of the Eskimo social and economic system. The nurse who interacts with persons from this culture must recognize that partially accepted Western values may be superimposed over Eskimo values that may still be practiced. The new elite class in Eskimo society is based on the ability to earn money without regard for old, established kinships and extended families, and a disregard for and severance of family and kinship ties underlie conflicts that may be found in villages today (Klausner & Foulks, 1982).

Individual freedom within the family or group
The culture maintains its respect for individual thought and personal freedom for behavior and de-

cisions. Perhaps there is even more freedom for individual choices than in other traditional cultures because survival of the group is less affected by personal preferences. At times, this individual freedom appears extreme because others in the society take on a noninterference attitude. For example, a husband may beat his wife without anyone lifting a finger to stop the beating, or a person may drink to oblivion day after day, and no one will take the bottle away (Roberts & Ross, 1979). The value of individual choice of behavior is honored so long as the integrity of the group is not in jeopardy. However, the Yupik Eskimos have decided as a group that alcoholism is destroying the fabric of their culture. A sobriety movement headed by an Eskimo urges the natives to become sober.

Social status within the family structure Formerly, social status was attained by successful hunters who could provide food and skins not only for their own families, but also for others. Successful hunters soon were recognized as leaders in the social group by the members. The opinions of successful hunters were given precedence over the opinions of others. A woman's status was secondary to her husband's and was gained through her own skills in keeping her family well fed and clothed. Each family member had an expected role to play. Grandparents were the primary educators of the children and imparted knowledge and skills required for survival. Children learned skills through play activities that also contributed to family needs, such as finding bird's nests for the eggs or challenging a playmate in picking the most berries (Holderman, 1993).

Some Eskimo parents do not punish or even correct their small children because tradition says that the spirits of a deceased relative guide each youngster. In the Eskimo culture the spirit of the deceased relative was considered so paramount to the survival of the young child that while a women was in labor an old woman was brought to the bedside to recite the names of the child's dead relatives. The name that was uttered at the time the child became visible was regarded as the appropriate name, and thereafter that deceased ancestor was believed to become the guardian spirit of the child (Holderman, 1993; Nida, 1954; Polk, 1987). Although this is not practiced today, many Eskimos still believe that the es-

sence of a dead relative is found in children born around the time of the death of a relative. For this reason many new babies may have the same name of a recently deceased family member.

For the Eskimo child, praise from parents and grandparents provides a positive learning experience and a strong self-concept (Polk, 1987). In Eskimo culture undesirable behavior traditionally was ignored, and if the behavior continued, the child was shamed through teasing and ridicule. Social controls within the community followed a similar pattern. There were no rigid rules. If a social standard was broken, it was assumed that the individual had a valid reason for the breach of conduct. Behavior was kept in control through teasing, gossip, and ridicule. If the behavior threatened group survival, the person was ostracized. To be isolated from the group meant certain death because an individual could not survive for long in the Arctic. The traditional Eskimo society is an example of a society that bases status on sharing and contributing to the well-being of the group and can thus establish a positive feedback system to control its members (Gove, 1982; Williamson, 1974).

Traditional Eskimos did not have any formal recognition of puberty (Polk, 1987). This was in strong contrast to other primitive societies wherein formal rituals frequently marked the coming of age. Boys are recognized by a feast at the first kill and share with all the family. In traditional Yupik Eskimo culture, girls were recognized when they danced with the older women for the first time.

For the nurse to give culturally appropriate nursing care to the client whose cultural makeup encompasses traditional values regarding social status, it is necessary for the nurse to appreciate traditional family roles. In most cases, it is also necessary to involve both nuclear and extended family members in the planning, implementation, and evaluation of nursing care.

Political structure

The political development of Eskimos has evolved out of the development of councils, native corporations, and health care corporations. The Native Land Claims Act of 1971 spurred a political development pattern similar to the political system in other states. Where once each community had an informal social structure that revolved around family and kin, now most villages have a decision-making council headed by an elected spokesperson (U.S. Department of Health and Human Services, Indian Health Services, 1991a).

Implications for nursing care

Extended family ties can be used to pressure non-compliant clients into following recommended therapy. These ties can also be used to find reasons for noncompliance because the client may not feel free to contradict the nurse. In Eskimo culture it is considered impolite to openly disagree with others. Cooperation, patience, and nonaggression are important values. Attempts to persuade or counsel another person, even to keep that person from doing something dangerous or foolish, are considered rude and are not tolerated. When health care staff attempt to "help" through advising and counseling, they are seen as "meddling" and will encounter interference (Lange, 1988). The nurse may need to resolve a difficult situation by asking other family members for guidance. The traditional view of health as a way of life becomes cloudy with the squelching of shamanism and with the miracles that modern medicine provided during the devastating infectious disease era. Some Eskimos have become dependent on Western medicine. Thus the nurse must remember that some Eskimo clients may still put blind faith in the physician's decision regarding their treatment. The fatalistic acceptance of illness may also contribute to this dependency. With the increased educational levels of the younger people and with the help of the nurse as an advocate, some Eskimos are beginning to assume more autonomy to question medical therapy and social programs. It is essential that the nurse encourage the Eskimo client to take personal responsibility for health or illness. The nurse should directly involve the client in planning health care and in activities that pursue solutions to health needs.

There is a mixture of childrearing practices in the Eskimo culture today (MacDonald-Clark & Boffman, 1995). Eskimo parents tend to use more positive reinforcements, praising desired behavior and ignoring undesired actions. Children are considered individuals as soon as they learn to express themselves. What this means for the nurse is that a child is given the right to refuse or accept health-related care. Some parents will not force a child to do something that the child refuses to do. For example, a parent may make a statement such as, "I tell Sam to brush his teeth, but he won't do it" or "JoJo won't let me put drops in her ear." The parent may tease, shame, or ridicule the child in an attempt to persuade the child, but the parent will seldom demand the appropriate behavior. The nurse needs to emphasize that certain health care behaviors or techniques such as brushing teeth or appropriately using medications are important because they may prevent more overriding problems such as dental cavities and otitis media.

It is also important for the nurse to be aware that according to a 1991 IHS survey of dental patients over 75% of Alaska Native children experienced dental decay in their primary teeth. This is commonly caused by giving a child a bottle containing carbohydrates at nap or bedtime and bottle-feeding past the age of 12 months. This high prevalence of dental caries results in increased cost of treatment and requires community-based intervention (Bruerd, 1997).

TIME

The Arctic Circle marks the point at which there is no sunrise on December 21, which is considered the winter solstice (or the shortest day of the year), and no sunset on June 21, the summer solstice (or the longest day of the year). This factor gives rise to a unique phenomenon that occurs in the northernmost part of North America. When the sun rises on May 10 in Barrow, Alaska, which is North America's northernmost city, it does not set again until August 2. As a result, there are 84 days of continuous sunlight. When the sun sets on November 18 in Barrow, it does not rise again until January 24. Therefore Barrow residents have 67 days of continuous semi-darkness. There is daylight even though the sun does not rise over the horizon. However, the daylight is very short, for example from 3 to 5 hours.

The extended periods of daylight and darkness give rise to seasonal, geographically related behavior.

For example, it is not uncommon to see small children playing outside in the summer at 2 o'clock in the morning (Gottberg, 1988). Also during the summer months, the extended hours of daylight are used for fishing. Likewise, because of the extended periods of darkness in the winter, northerners tend to sleep late. Although most northerners have rearranged their lives in recent times to synchronize themselves with the Western day-night rhythm, some Eskimos remain on "Eskimo time," which is a result of both the unusual daylight pattern and a present-time orientation. Rather than being structured by the clock, time is cyclical, based on naturally recurring phenomena: sunrise, sunset, days, nights, moons (months), and seasons (Lewis & Ho, 1975). Use of "Eskimo time" may prompt Eskimo families to keep their children out of school and in fish camp several weeks after school officially opens. Some Eskimos believe that fish camp, a present-oriented activity, is a time to be enjoyed, whereas school, a future-oriented activity, prepares children for future goals. Committing to year-round jobs on a 9-to-5 schedule is difficult for some Eskimos because of the strong urge to spend summer and fall in fish camps.

The present-time orientation of this culture is sometimes reflected in the ways in which money is spent. There is an emphasis on consumable things that give immediate benefit. Budgeting and investing for the future may not be motivating concepts. Some Eskimos who have been away from the village and have earned a large sum of money during a season may come home and "blow" it in one spending spree for the family. This action exemplifies two values: sharing what you have with others and living for today because tomorrow will take care of itself.

Use of "Eskimo time" requires readjustment by the nurse for such things as scheduling appointments for health care because some Eskimos prefer to come in when they feel like it. Consequently, a nurse who works in a remote area of Alaska should seldom schedule a clinic appointment before 9 or 10 AM and should be prepared to work late into the evening. A visiting nurse may be on a tight schedule and insist that the villagers accept a Western time frame. This insistence causes such comments as "You

are always rushed," or "You must not like our village because you are always in a hurry to leave."

Implications for nursing care

It is important for the nurse to remember that a village may practice "Eskimo time," which is quite different from city time. For example, some people may stay up late and sleep late, which may cause stress for teachers because the children may come to school half asleep and without breakfast. In the summer, when it is daylight most of the time, villagers may sleep only when they are tired and children may stay up very late. This may present real challenges for the nurse, whether in a clinic or in a hospital setting, because the lack of a definitive schedule interferes with the nurse's obtaining medical histories and the client's keeping appointments and taking medications on time and correctly. The public health nurse learns to take medical histories by village events and seasons. On the other hand, the hospital nurse must emphasize in simple terms the necessity for the medical history. In either case it is important to know a little about the client's daily routine if nursing care is to be implemented and effective. Because schedules are flexible and time is relative, the nurse needs to inquire about daily schedules before requiring medication to be taken at a certain time. Many families do not eat meals together. Therefore telling a client to take a pill at mealtime may have no meaning.

ENVIRONMENTAL CONTROL

The early Eskimos believed that the individual had three parts: body, soul, and name. All of these were considered of equal importance and combined to make the whole person. Early Eskimos also believed that everything, such as earth, wind, flowers, animals, and birds, had a spirit. An extensive "taboo" system guided the Eskimo in harmonious living with the spirits (Holderman, 1960). Each family inherited a specific taboo system, and each person had a guiding spirit to help him or her during his or her lifetime. When a girl married, she had to abide by both families' taboos (Gove, 1982). The spiritual leader, called a "shaman," had the vital role of keeping the group healthy by persuading the spiritual world to continue smiling on the people. When famine struck or illness occurred, the shaman communicated with the spiritual world during trances to learn what taboo had been broken and who needed to appease the spirits. Appeasement often meant that the guilty person confessed to breaking the taboo and suffered humiliation. It is interesting to understand that the shaman was not blamed if the shaman failed to find the cause for negative events. The people accepted their situation as a matter of fate (Blodgett, 1978; Lantis, 1960; Mitchell & Patch, 1986). Famine, bad luck, and failure in hunting meant the spirits were displeased with the Eskimo people, whereas successful hunting and times of plenty meant the spirits were pleased. Consequently, each Eskimo perceived his or her relationship with nature as being in harmony or out of harmony with the spiritual world. Today shamanism has been largely replaced by Christianity except for various remote areas of Alaska (Blodgett, 1978).

Today it is common for Eskimos to be Christian, equally divided between Catholics and Anglicans. Death is accepted as a part of life, which makes an enormous difference in attitudes about suffering, stress, and even acculturation. In the past, Eskimos were buried in wooden boxes above the ground because of the difficulty in digging graves; people are now buried in graves dug with jackhammers. Whereas wood was once at a premium and one cross contained many names, imported wood is now readily available (Lefever, 1993; Morris, 1985).

Illness and wellness behaviors

Early Eskimos believed that each person had a spiritual healer who could be offended by the person breaking a taboo. A broken taboo was manifested by the person becoming ill. Possession by harmful spirits was recognized as a cause of illness. For example, it was considered taboo to eat polar bear liver, and any Eskimo who offended the bear spirit in this manner became ill or died. Studies in the 1940s indicated that vitamin A toxicity, rather than the ill effects of the broken taboo, was the cause of illnesses associated with eating polar bear liver (Rodahl, 1964).

Written information on shamanism is limited because of the squelching of this religion by early missionaries. Folklore indicates that the shaman had

predicted the coming of the strangers who would cause the death of the Eskimo; thus, when nearly one half of the Eskimos died of diseases brought by the early traders, whalers, and missionaries, the prophecy was fulfilled. Unfortunately, while the Westerners brought medicine, they also brought new diseases to which the Eskimo people were not immune. With the influx of Westerners, the life-style of the Eskimos changed as they moved into permanent settlements to take advantage of schools, churches, and medical care. The spread of communicable disease became rampant among these people, who now lived in crowded, permanent houses. Before the influx of Westerners, the constant moving of living sites prevented the hygiene problems that were now incurred by permanent villages. Over the years the Eskimos have learned about the physical causes of illness and the appropriate techniques necessary to prevent the spread of disease. However, it has taken many years to increase the Eskimo population.

Shamanism lost face with the people as they turned to the magic of medicine brought by the Westerners to cure the devastating infectious diseases. Many of the medical people were missionaries, who implied that illness was related to the people's sinfulness and that the cure depended partly on their confession and acceptance of Western religion. The early Eskimos did not oppose the switch to the new religion because it seemed similar to shamanism. Medical treatment by Westerners was often restricted to the Eskimos whose names appeared on the church roster.

In the Eskimo culture there is a generation gap in health and illness concepts. An older person may have a more holistic view of health and believe that a happy person is less likely to develop physical ills, whereas a younger person may assign illness to direct physical causes. For example, in the case of suicidal behavior, a young person may blame alcohol, stating that if the person did not drink he or she would not commit suicide. Therefore the treatment for the prevention of suicide is to take the alcohol away. On the other hand, older Eskimos may see suicidal behavior as an illness of the spirit that creates a disharmony leading to the choice of drinking. The cure is to heal the spirit; then the need for alcohol will disappear.

Implications for nursing care

When giving culturally appropriate nursing care to Eskimo clients, whether in remote areas of Alaska or in the mainland United States, the nurse must realize that an individual's feelings of environmental control are an important factor in the nursing assessment of client status. Illness and wellness behaviors among some Eskimo clients may be attributable to past belief systems and a belief in supernatural powers. The nurse may need to combat some superstitious beliefs, such as a pain in the head will be cured by wrapping a red yarn around the head (in this case the nurse must teach the client that the continued wrapping of a red yarn to treat head pain may delay needed medical treatment).

Because some Eskimos tend to view nature as an entity that can be in equilibrium or disequilibrium, the nurse can build on this concept and teach the client that certain conditions in the body can also be in equilibrium or disequilibrium. Coupling the theory of equilibrium or disequilibrium with supernatural beliefs, the nurse may explain that certain conditions such as edema of the lower extremities may be perceived as a disequilibrium in the body. Therefore the client who attempts self-treatment with a red yarn around the leg to stop the rise of disequilibrium (edema) may actually be augmenting the chance for further disequilibrium in the body.

BIOLOGICAL VARIATIONS
Body size and structure

Ancestors of the Indians and Eskimos originated from the Mongoloid race (Banks, 1956; Zegura, 1985). Anthropologists believe that there was a land bridge between Asia and Alaska that was crossed by the early native people. Genetic studies have related the origin of Eskimos to a population of Asiatic Beringia (Szathmary, 1984). The Mongolian racial traits seen in the Eskimos include a short muscular body, large oblong skull with a definite occipital protuberance, well-developed lower jaw and maxillary bone, epicanthal folds, little or no body hair, dark-pigmented skin, and lumbar mongolian spots (Banks, 1956; Chance, 1966; Mann & Scott, 1962). The head shape and jaw structure have been attributed to the evolutionary process from prehistoric man and have little significance in the Eskimo culture today (Carpenter, 1973; Chance, 1966).

Early medical research noted the short stature and heavier weight per height of Eskimos, which was greatly different from that of Europeans and other circumpolar people, such as Icelanders and Finns (Milan, 1980). Three theories were proposed to explain this difference: (1) a genetic inheritance, (2) a combination of genetic and environmental adaptation, and (3) a condition of long-term nutritional deficiency. Part of this weight difference was attributed to the Eskimo's thicker bony skeleton and muscular chest and arms (Hrdlicka, 1930, 1941; Milan, 1980). Researchers demonstrated by the use of triceps and body skin-fold measurements that the extra weight was not caused by an extra layer of fat, negating the adaptation theory that Eskimos carried extra fat to protect the body from the cold (Hrdlicka, 1941). Muscular development resulting from an active life-style and genetic inheritance contributed to the early Eskimo's body structure.

The birth weights and heights of today's Eskimos are statistically similar to those of their White counterparts (Heller, 1947; Johnston, Laughlin, Harper, & Ensroth, 1982; Mann & Scott, 1962; U.S. Department of Health and Human Services, Indian Health Services, 1991). By 11 months of age, Eskimo infants fall within the 5% range for height on Faulkner's growth charts, whereas their weight is in the 50% range. By 18 months of age, Eskimo children are consistently heavier than their White counterparts. This pattern of growth continues until 6 years of age, when Eskimo children become lighter in terms of weight than White children. The average height of Eskimo children remains shorter throughout life. This pattern may be a genetic trait, though in the past 3 decades the Eskimos have had a growth (height) increase pattern of greater than 1 cm per decade (Milan, 1980). Some researchers believe that the growth increase is indirectly related to a decrease in hibernation. However, in 1972 Schaefer presented some convincing data directly linking the growth rate to sugar consumption. The pattern seen in Eskimos discredits the supposition that growth increase is a result of a high-protein diet. Since the Eskimo diet changed from an almost total protein intake to the current high-sugar, high-carbohydrate diet, their growth pattern has increased (Bells, Draper, & Bergan, 1973). Unfortunately, obesity is now a problem.

When using the Faulkner growth chart in health assessments of Eskimo children, the nurse must remember that the chart is based on White averages. Sequential growth patterns are needed in health and nutrition assessment. For example, it is easy to identify Eskimo children born with fetal alcohol syndrome by following the sequential growth pattern on the standard growth charts.

Skin color

Eskimos have a "tanned" complexion that becomes deep brown to black with continuous exposure to the sun. This pigmentation is part of their Mongoloid heritage. However, evolutionary selection may also explain this feature. Skin cancer research indicates that deeply pigmented skin has some natural protection from the ultraviolet rays of the sun. Therefore the evolutionary conclusion is that Eskimos are more protected from skin cancer because of their deep skin pigmentation (Young, 1986).

Other visible physical characteristics

Mongoloid heritage among Alaskan Eskimos is reflected in the lumbar pigmented spots and the epicanthal eye folds. However, neither of these characteristics gives rise to significant health problems. The nurse who cares for Eskimo children needs to be able to distinguish between mongolian spots and those bruises that might be associated with child abuse. Child abuse may be reported to health care providers by well-meaning Westerners who notice "bruises" on an infant's arms and buttocks when these are only mongolian spots. However, during physical assessment it is important for the nurse to remember to document unusual placement of mongolian spots on areas such as the wrist, legs, and chest.

Enzymatic variations

Enzyme deficiencies in lactase and sucrose have been documented in Eskimos. When given a lactose load equivalent to 3 to 4 cups of milk, 80% of Eskimo adults and 70% of Eskimo children demonstrated intolerance symptoms of flatulence and diarrhea (Bells, Draper, & Bergan, 1973; Duncan & Scott, 1972). However, most of them could tolerate a daily glass of milk without symptoms. In the past, Eskimos had no dietary source of milk after being weaned from the breast, and nutritional analysis of traditional foods indicates that the diet of adult Eskimos remains quite low in calcium. Research is needed to determine if there is a genetic protective factor for calcium metabolism or if this population is at risk for osteoporosis from calcium-deficient diets. It is essential for the nurse who works with Eskimo clients to encourage using alternative forms of milk such as cheese, yogurt, and powdered milk. The nurse should note that Eskimos rarely like milk products; however, cheese is an exception. The nurse must also remember that another source of calcium that is readily available to Eskimos is found in fish bones that are canned with the flesh. Berman, Hanson, and Hellman (1972) noted that breast feeding of both Indian and Eskimo women tended to decrease the rate of conception independent of the climate of the areas.

A small portion of Alaskan (approximately 5%) and Greenland Eskimos (approximately 10%) is intolerant of sucrose. Some classic research studies indicate that a can of soda or a piece of cake can cause debilitating diarrhea in some Eskimos (Bells, Draper, & Bergan, 1973; Shephard, 1974).

Friedrich and Ferrell (1985) found that the alpha-keto acid reductase locus is monomorphic in most cultural groups, despite earlier studies that suggested its existence as a genetic polymorphism. Thus the Eskimo population is no more prone to having an alpha-keto acid reductase locus than any other cultural group.

Susceptibility to disease

The isolation of Eskimos from outsiders caused them to be more susceptible to the devastating effects of infection. Eskimos who lacked exposure to certain diseases failed to develop antibodies to these diseases. It has been documented that Eskimos develop antibodies to antigens as well as their Western counterparts do. Thus the rapid spread of disease among Eskimos is believed to have occurred because of a lack of knowledge about hygiene techniques necessary to stop the spread of communicable disease, not because of failure to develop antibodies to antigens (Young, 1986).

Today, increased incidences of communicable diseases are still being reported among some populations of Eskimos. For example, in an epidemiological study of streptococcal disease that affected 706 Alaskan Eskimo children, throat cultures were obtained during a long-term surveillance program (Brant, Bender, & Marnell, 1982). In this study a binary-variable, multiple-regression model was used to study the association between streptococcal colonization of the children and the following six potential risk factors: age, sex, number of children in the household, region, health aide rating, and colonization rate for the child from the previous year. According to the study's findings, the factors significantly associated with streptococcal colonization among the Eskimo children included age, past colonization, competence of the local health aide in providing care, and region in which the care was provided. The study also found that the number of children in overcrowded homes and the child's sex were not apparently important to the incidence of streptococcal colonization (Brant, Bender, & Marnell, 1982).

In some remote villages in Alaska, hygiene techniques remain a nursing priority. When working with Eskimos, the nurse must implement teaching programs emphasizing hygienic practices and medical asepsis. Because some modern villages are extremely crowded, susceptibility to disease is augmented; thus the nurse must also emphasize hygienic practices with these individuals. A study by Lum, Knutson, Hall, et al. (1986) reports the significant effect that improved immunization programs, prenatal care, and improved health care have had on infant mortality. Deaths from infectious diseases, measles, and pertussis were dramatically reduced as health care was improved among southwestern Alaskan Eskimos between 1960 and 1980. Still another problem for Eskimo infants is increased exposure to *Haemophilus influenzae* type b (Hib) disease (Hall, Lum, Knutson, et al., 1987). Alaskan Eskimos have

the greatest known endemic risk for this disease, which seems to have genetic factors that contribute to susceptibility (Petersen, Silimperi, Rotter, et al., 1987; Ward, Lum, Hall, et al., 1986). In 1990 effective Hib vaccines were licensed for infants, and over the next year infants in the Delta and Bristol Bay areas of Alaska were immunized. By 1992 there had been a complete year with no Hib infections in children or adults in contrast to the approximately 18 cases per year between 1980 and 1989 (Singleton, 1992).

Tuberculosis Tuberculosis was formerly considered an illness for which Alaska Natives had inherited susceptibility (Stevenson, 1984). Today this is no longer considered true, but it is still an illness that is five times more prevalent among Alaska Natives than in the general U.S. population. In the 1970s certain regions of Alaska experienced an incidence rate of 1200 per 100,000 population, compared with 14 per 100,000 in the rest of the U.S. population. However, rather than inherited susceptibility, this incidence is related to environmental and socioeconomic issues, such as very cramped houses because of the cold temperature and poor availability of clean water (Stevenson, 1984). Effective intervention includes both prevention and curtailment of possible spread once a case is present. Health education is essential and must include not only direct information on tuberculosis, but also information on predisposing factors such as hygiene, overcrowding, alcohol abuse, and nutrition. Many rural health care providers have suggested that a general improvement in the standard of living is needed for this problem to be fully addressed (Stevenson, 1984). In a 1987 study of tuberculosis in minorities, 32 cases were reported in Alaska Natives (Centers for Disease Control and Prevention, 1989). Causes for these cases that were identified as preventable were noncompliance, intravenous drug use, HIV infection, and tuberculosis in correctional institutions (Snider, Salinas, & Kelly, 1989). Outbreaks of tuberculosis continue to occur in remote Alaskan villages (TB Monitor, 1996).

HIV and AIDS Sexually transmitted diseases have unusually high prevalence among Alaska Natives. From 1984 through 1988, Alaskan Natives had five times the reported gonorrhea and syphilis morbidity as compared with non-Native Alaskans (Toomey, Oberschelp, & Greenspan, 1989). In Canada, data from Manitoba in the early 1980s indicated that Natives were affected three times more often than non-Natives (Lee, Brunham, Sherman, & Harding, 1987). From 1982, when the first Native with AIDS was reported, until the end of 1991, 322 cases of AIDS were reported, for a cumulative incidence of 16 cases of AIDS per 100,000, as compared with 84 cases per 100,000 for all other groups in the United States (Conway, 1992). Alaska Natives are at greater risk for AIDS because of alcohol and drug use, effects of long-term unemployment and poverty, and lack of prevention activities. In the first 6 months of 1993, 42 cases of AIDS were reported, which represents a 525% increase for the same period in 1992. Although study of race exhibits no new trends, the number of cases of AIDS has doubled from 1991 to 1992 (Middaugh, 1993). However, in Canada, of the 5000 cases of AIDS reported up until 1991, fewer than 30 were in people of Native ethnic origin. In the United States the rate of AIDS cases among Native Americans for 1990 was 4 per 100,000 compared to 43 per 100,000 for blacks, 32 per 100,000 among Hispanics, and 12 per 100,000 among whites. These data would indicate that the problem is low among Native Americans despite the increases that have been reported (Metler, Conway, & Stehr-Green, 1991). Surveys among Greenland Eskimos have found a higher number of lifetime sexual partners. Over 50 percent of Native AIDS cases have been reported among homosexuals and bisexuals. Thus the pattern by some Natives with limited sexual partners may be suggestive of a reason for a lower rate and has strong implications for nursing education (Young, 1994; Hankins, Hum, Tran, et al., 1997).

Chlamydiosis, which is nonreportable, has a very high incidence rate. The symptoms caused by *Chlamydia* bacteria allow for a possible entrance for HIV. Thus there is concern that such a possibility is high among teenagers whose *Chlamydia* rate is higher than that of the general individual.

Glaucoma Eskimos are susceptible to primary narrow-angle glaucoma. Persons who have primary narrow-angle glaucoma have eyes that have a shallow chamber angle and a thicker lens, both of which

are factors that contribute to glaucoma. It is believed that the sex and increasing age of the person, particularly in the case of women, are associated factors as well. Both genetic and environmental components appear to play a major role in the development of primary narrow-angle glaucoma (Schaefer, 1973; Van Rens, Arkell, Charlton, & Doesburg, 1988).

Diabetes mellitus Although Alaskan Eskimos have been known to have low rates of diabetes mellitus, more recent studies have found that the incidence of diabetes mellitus appears to be increasing among these people (Schraer, Lanier, Boyko, et al., 1988). Although some classic research studies are suggestive that a normal glucose response is found among Eskimos (Mouratoff, Carrol, & Scott, 1967; Scott & Griffin, 1956), with each passing decade there is an increasing number of glucose-intolerant Eskimos. There are many Eskimos of mixed heritage who are listed as being full-blooded Eskimos, and this could be a factor in the discrepancy.

The risk factors for diabetes are yet to be completely understood, but there is strong evidence that obesity and high sugar intake are contributory factors among Eskimos. Over the past decade, obesity among Eskimos has increased, and it is not uncommon for Eskimos (particularly women) to be as much as 50 to 100 pounds over their ideal weight. In Canada, Schaefer (1970) noted that the incidence of diabetes was higher in the Arctic, where Eskimos have had a longer contact with a high-sugar diet. In this classic study, Schaefer concluded that the increase in known diabetes incidence among Alaskan Eskimos follows Campbell's rule, which states that diabetes morbidity generally trails 20 to 30 years behind the introduction of a Western diet. Although Eskimos are not reported to have an increased incidence of glucose intolerance, it is essential for the nurse to keep in mind that some Eskimos have a prevalence for obesity and a high sugar intake, both of which can be contributory factors in the development of diabetes mellitus. In light of this fact, the nurse must implement teaching techniques that emphasize the importance of exercise and eating right. In addition, the nurse must remember that, if Campbell's rule is correct, an increase in glucose intolerance will be evident among the Eskimo people. The key to control of glucose intolerance is prevention.

Cardiovascular disease In Alaska the incidence of cardiovascular disease among Eskimos is low in comparison with the rest of the general population in the United States. For example, Dyerberg and Bang (1978) first reported a lower incidence of coronary disease in the Greenland Eskimos. This finding was attributed to their diet, which was rich in fat from whale, fish, and seals. Further analysis revealed that the Eskimos had lower levels of plasma cholesterol and triglyceride and high plasma concentrations of certain polyunsaturated fatty acids (Sipperly, 1989). It remains unclear whether genetic factors protect this population from a high incidence of cardiac disease. However, the nurse must remember that the diet and life-style of the Eskimo people have changed dramatically in the last few decades, and those factors will certainly have a profound effect on their cardiovascular health (Young, 1986). The Western world has done extensive research on arteriosclerosis and heart disease in a search for preventive clues. As a result, Americans are encouraged to eat foods that are low in fat (less than 30% of daily caloric intake), limit their red meat and egg yolk intake, and do aerobic exercises. Traditionally, the Eskimo people subsisted on a diet that was 44% protein (sea and land animals, fish, and birds), 47% fat (polyunsaturated), and 8% carbohydrates (berries, beach greens, and roots). In a recent analysis of the dietary intake of Eskimos, protein intake was 26%, fat intake was 37%, and carbohydrate intake was 37% (Mann & Scott, 1962). Although protein and fat intake decreased significantly, carbohydrate intake increased significantly. For some Eskimos the significant increase in carbohydrates is attributable to high intakes of sugar.

In certain seasons the early Eskimos ate foods that were high in cholesterol. In other seasons their diet was devoid of cholesterol. Some studies suggest that the body uses stored cholesterol when there is no cholesterol intake (Feldman, Ho, Lewis, et al., 1972). If this is correct, seasonal food variations among Eskimos have provided a protection against heart and blood vessel disease. Today, Eskimos continue to follow a seasonal pattern of dietary habits. Regardless of whether the body uses stored cholesterol, the nurse needs to caution against excessive cholesterol intake.

Although medical knowledge regarding cardiovascular disease in the pre–Western contact Eskimo is limited, arteriosclerotic plaquing was noted in the blood vessels of mummified bodies that were dated back to 1460. The oldest body had significantly greater evidence of vascular changes (Zimmerman & Aufderheide, 1984).

In a study involving a Bering Strait Eskimo population, similar heart rates and heart-rate rhythmicity and almost identical acrophases were found in the Eskimo, the Aymara Indian, and the French populations. The study also found that Alaskan Eskimos had heart-rate means that varied by approximately 15 beats per minute (Rode & Shephard, 1984). This variation can have serious implications for the nurse who is monitoring the rhythmicity of the heart because of the variation in beats. When monitoring the pulse rate of an Eskimo client, the nurse should, when possible, take an apical rather than a radial pulse and should count the heart rate for 1 full minute.

Anemia Anemia, especially in infants and children, seems to be a direct result of a nutritional deficiency resulting from iron-poor food choices. Hereditary predisposition was eliminated as a possibility for anemia in one epidemiological study (Nobmann, 1984). For the Eskimos who live along the Kuskokwim and Yukon rivers, there is a tendency to have a diet high in fish and to store items that are relatively iron poor. A typical meal for these people includes fish soup, "pilot" bread (so named because it was originally brought in by pilots) with shortening, and black, sugared tea. Even preschoolers drink black tea in these areas, and it is believed that the tannic acid in tea interferes with iron absorption (Nobmann, 1984). Thus the diet is considered to be iron poor and additionally has an agent (tannic acid) that prohibits absorption. Sea mammals are an excellent iron source, but with the decrease in subsistence living and the easy access to store-bought foods, even the coastal people succumb to anemia.

It is believed that anemia is one of the factors that contributes to morbidity in infants and children under 3 years of age (Nobmann, 1984). Lactating mothers should be taught nutritional education by the nurse who works in infant programs and should be given vitamin and iron supplements. Infant iron-fortified formulas can now be found even in remote areas in Alaska and should be used instead of canned milk when a mother does not breastfeed. Women, Infants, and Children (WIC) and Aid to Families with Dependent Children (AFDC) programs have been established in areas throughout Alaska and provide money to purchase high-cost formula. Studies done by WIC suggest that its programs have caused a decrease in anemia (Nobmann, 1984).

Cancer The incidence of cancer in Eskimos is not significantly different from that of the rest of the American population. However, the pattern of cancer is unique. Among Eskimo men, lung, colorectal, nasopharynx, stomach, and liver cancers are the most common. In fact, lung cancer is the most rapidly increasing cancer among Alaska Native people and other indigenous populations in the Arctic (Lanier, Bulkow, Novotny, et al., 1990). High rates of cigarette use occur among Alaska Native children as well as adults. Within Alaska, the prevalence of smoking is higher among Alaska Natives (39% to 50%) than among non-Natives (25%) (Behavioral Risk Factor Surveillance, 1991, 1992). Among Eskimo women, colorectal, breast, lung, and gallbladder cancers are more common (Young, 1986). Data on 239 verified cases of malignant disease in the western and central Canadian Arctic were studied by Hildes and Schaefer (1984), who found Eskimos to be less prone to developing cancer of the skin, prostate, pancreas, and stomach. Cervical cancer is on the increase, but the cause for the rise is unclear (Toomey, Rafferty, & Stamm, 1987). Apart from risk factors such as smoking and diet, there is considerable interest in the role that infectious agents play as carcinogens. For example, hepatitis B virus (HBV) is the causative agent for hepatocellular carcinoma (McMahon, Heyward, Templin, et al., 1989). Children infected at an earlier age are at a greater risk for becoming HBV carriers, and once a carrier, a child has a 40% chance of developing liver cancer by 40 years of age (Lanier et al., 1980).

The Epstein-Barr virus has been implicated in the development of nasopharyngeal cancers. It has been found in over 90% of cases of Burkitt's lymphoma in endemic regions, though only 15% of cases in nonendemic regions show evidence of infection (Gaffey & Weiss, 1990). It is suspected that the transmission of viral agents may require a susceptible genotype or other promotional events (Lynch, Schuelke, & O'Hara, 1984). It has been reported that Greenland Eskimos have the highest documented Epstein-Barr virus titers in the world (Young, 1986). Other risk factors associated with this type of cancer include the widespread life-style habits of smoking, alcohol, and chewing tobacco. Alaska Native hospitals have reported a significant rise in nasopharyngeal cancer among teenagers and young adults (Young, 1986), and epidemiologists have attributed this increase in nasopharyngeal cancer to tobacco habits (snuff and cigarettes) that begin in pre–school aged groups rather than to the Epstein-Barr virus.

Dietary habits such as the consumption of heavily smoked fish and fermented, salted foods may also add some carcinogenic risks. Insufficient data currently exist to determine whether genetic factors contribute to the cancer patterns of the Eskimo people.

Blood variations

Eskimos as an ethnic group have a distinctive blood group variation; specifically, Rh-negative blood is absent in Eskimos (Overfield, 1977, 1995). The occasional Rh-negative factor turns up in some Eskimos of mixed race. The nurse who counsels a woman during a spontaneous abortion must be alert to her Rh factor. Complacency to importance of preventable measures can have dire consequences. As the number of mixed-race Eskimos rises, so does this risk.

Nutritional and life-style preferences

After the control of infectious diseases among Alaskan Eskimos, the health-illness pattern shifted to reflect an increase in chronic disease. This increase in chronic disease may be attributable to the fact that the Eskimo diet and life-style changed as these people assimilated many of the Western culture's bad habits, such as a sedentary life-style and a diet high in sugar, salt, and fat. Many Eskimos now use some form of locomotion to get around villages that are less than a mile long or wide, minimizing needed exercise.

Clean water is sometimes a difficult commodity to obtain in Alaska. In some villages on the ocean, drinking water must be brought in as ice from several miles up the river. In the process of being brought to the village, the chunks of ice are often handled by many people and must then be melted, boiled, and cooled.

Psychological characteristics

"The suicide epidemic in Bush Alaska continues . . ." is a headline frequently seen in Alaskan newspapers. The mental health status of Eskimos is complicated by the pressures created by traditional cultural demands, attempts at assimilation of Western values, and the harsh geographic region. Alcohol and drug abuse are the major causes of injury, accidents, and death among Alaskan Eskimos. Suicide is associated with alcohol abuse, which in turn is a symptom of a people attempting to assimilate in a rapidly changing society (Albert, 1988; Travis, 1983; VanDenberg & Minton, 1987).

The suicidal behavior in Eskimo populations is believed to have changed in pattern and quantity over the last decade. The rate of attempted suicide among Eskimos has more than quadrupled, and the incidence of completed suicides among young people has increased. In a study of Greenland Eskimos, it was found that almost 2 per 1000 of the adult population committed suicide yearly, and attempts at suicide were five times more frequent than previously. The reasons for the suicides were found to be poor childhood home background and the effects of emotional conflicts with close contacts, alcohol affliction, criminality, and instability at work (Grove & Lynge, 1979). To understand the psychological makeup and characteristics of the Eskimo people, the nurse needs to have an awareness of their history, its relationship to self-destructive behavior as evidenced among some Eskimos, and their present stress of acculturation.

For many Eskimos the rapid breakdown of organized traditional values, religion, life-style, and social relationships has led to an inability to find a meaningful role in the modern world (Albert, 1988). For example, a young Eskimo villager who is a student in a modern school, works on computers, and studies about world events may become disillu-

sioned at home where old roles may still exist. In this situation the parents may feel inadequate because they are unable to relate to the child as a result of the knowledge that the child has acquired at school. On the other hand, the child may see little importance in subsistence living skills, such as fishing or hunting, which are areas where the parents excel. After high school, the student may leave the village to attend college or trade school. However, the student may be unable to tolerate living away from the village or family and thus may return to the village after several months or years. Inadequate education and village schools do not prepare Eskimo children for the modern world. When the adolescent returns to the village, there is a difficult reacceptance of village life. The village's subsistence activities give rise to disillusionment, depression, and self-destructive behavior. Because they find that their own views and values have changed as a result of the outside experience, village life becomes stifling for many of these young people. Also, the trade or occupation learned while at school (such as computer science) often has little relevance to life in the village. The result of all of this is that the village now has a frustrated, angry individual who has not readapted to village life and who does not have the emotional ability to survive away from home and family. These contributory factors may lead to depression and hence to alcohol and drug use (Albert, 1988; Chance, 1966; Seltzer, 1980).

There is a high incidence of suicide among Eskimo males. Many Eskimo women attach meaning and purpose to life through the possibility of motherhood. Thus, Eskimo women are less likely than their male counterparts to become severely depressed. However, for Eskimo men, life is perceived as purposeless because of their detachment from the family. In many instances, Eskimo women exist primarily for their children (Albert, 1988).

In a study that compared 567 Alaska Native criminal offenders referred to mental health professionals with 939 White offenders, it was found that alcohol abuse, which is the dominant social problem for some Alaska Natives, is not clearly associated with the degree of sociocultural change. Living in larger communities and higher educational achievement are associated with greater psychosocial maladjustment than the incidence of alcohol abuse is. The region of residence has a stronger influence on the rate and type of maladjustment than the ethnic group (that is, Eskimo, Indian, or Aleut) or the ethnic density of the community of residence (that is, the proportion of Alaska Natives in the population) does (Phillips & Inui, 1986).

For some Eskimos alcohol use has become an acceptable way to escape. Binge drinking has been related to the stress of acculturation (Mala, 1984) and is characteristic for some Alaska Natives (Albert, 1988). Because binge drinking is directly related to morbidity and mortality in Alaska, programs have been set up to deal with this problem. However, programs such as Alcoholics Anonymous have been relatively unsuccessful in Eskimo treatment, just as other forms of treatment designed for and by White people have (Lange, 1988). Culturally relevant programs have proved to be much more effective and frequently involve resolution of the conflicts created by Westernization (Albert, 1988).

Some reports have identified the biological predisposition of some Canadian Eskimos to be more susceptible to the deleterious effects of alcohol (Seltzer & Langford, 1984). Canadian Eskimos are extremely rapid acetylators as tested with isoniazid (Schaefer, 1986). Eskimos also tend to clear phenytoin rapidly, as proved in Greenland Eskimos and supported by clinical observations in Canadian Eskimos. Schaefer (1986) also found that metabolism is significantly slower in Canadian Eskimos than in Whites. Although the work with biological predisposition and alcohol metabolism has been done with Canadian Eskimos, these data can easily be generalized to the Alaskan Eskimos in a more westerly area of the Arctic.

Implications for nursing care

Seltzer (1983) has reported three interesting cases of Eskimos who claimed to be possessed by spirits. The spirits appeared to represent culture-bound defense mechanisms and attempts at problem solving in Eskimos who had unresolved cultural conflicts. Although reports of spiritual possession are uncommon among mental health professionals in Alaska, Seltzer's report does emphasize the importance of knowledge of myths and customs, as well as culturally significant methods of healing, on the part of health care providers.

Understanding cultural differences will allow the nurse to relate in a positive way to persons from varied cultural backgrounds. If nursing interventions are to be successful, they must not oppose a particular cultural practice. On the other hand, if the cultural practice is detrimental to the health status of the people, the nurse must devise a teaching plan and alternative strategies to combat the negative practice. If the nurse is to use time and energy efficiently, nursing care measures must be planned and implemented cooperatively with the client and family so that it is perceived as being culturally relevant (Overfield, 1995). Community efforts are also important. For example, the Alaska Native Community Suicide Prevention Center is an example of a community-based program that has shown promising results in reducing suicides among young and young adults (DeBruyn, Wilkins, Stetter-Burns, & Nelson, 1997).

The nurse who works with Eskimo clients must know certain biological concepts that are germane to the Eskimo people to give not only adequate care, but also nonharmful care. As the Western culture influences Eskimo people, behaviors have changed. For example, Eskimos are consuming large quantities of carbohydrates, bottle-feeding instead of breast-feeding their infants, consuming large quantities of alcohol, increasing their tobacco use, and assuming a more sedentary life-style. As behaviors and health care needs of these individuals change, the nurse must modify approaches to client care accordingly.

SUMMARY

Despite the apparent Westernization of Eskimos, they have retained many of their traditional perceptions and responses to life situations. Whether in an Alaskan village or in a clinic or hospital in the mainland United States, the nurse who encounters an Eskimo client must incorporate a theoretical framework that encompasses knowledge of communication, spatial requirements, social organization, time, environmental control, and biological variations to enhance quality nursing care.

Case Study

This case study focuses on a 6-year-old Eskimo girl with chronic otitis media, anemia, poor dietary habits, noncompliance with prescribed medication, and low self-esteem resulting in failure to adjust to school. The mother brings the child to the village clinic for treatment. When taking the history from the mother, the nurse notes that the child has six siblings and comes from a home where the father is frequently absent and when present is often drunk. The nurse observes that the mother provides inconsistent direction and resorts to threats and ridicule when attempting to correct or change the child's behavior. For example, when the child does not sit still, the mother states, "You be good, or the nurse will give you a shot." The nurse notes that both ears have a gluelike discharge, which the mother states is being treated with ear drops given at the clinic 2 weeks earlier. However, the mother also states that the child refuses to allow the ear drops to be instilled because they "hurt" her ears. The nurse notes that only a small amount of the bottle has been used.

This is the second clinic visit. At the first visit, when asked about what the child ate, the mother responded that most food items came from hunting or fishing or the village store and that they usually had fish soup, pilot bread with shortening, and black, sugared tea. With a hemoglobinometer, the nurse now determines that the child's hemoglobin remains at the same low level as at the previous visit. The iron-supplement tablets given at the last visit have not been taken. When questioned about whether she eats the school lunch provided by the public lunch program, the child replies that no one likes her and that the other children take her food, and so she does not get much.

On examination of the child, the nurse finds a pale mucous membrane and poor muscle tone with decreased muscle activity. The child's temperature is 102° F, pulse is 75, blood pressure is 100/66, and respirations are 22. The nurse notes that the child complains of a sharp, constant pain in both ears and frequently pulls or tugs at both ears, seemingly in an attempt to gain relief. On examination of the ears, the nurse notes that the external canal is free of wax and that the mastoid process behind the ear is not tender to touch. However, the tympanic membrane appears inflamed.

CARE PLAN

 Nursing Diagnosis   Nutrition, altered, less than body requirements

Client Outcomes

1. Client will have increased iron level.
2. Mother will understand safety measures.
3. Parental knowledge of illness will be increased.
4. Client will have adequate dietary intake.

Nursing Interventions

1. Educate mother and client about iron-rich foods.
2. Teach mother to recognize signs of pica as being iron related.
3. Do a 24-hour recall dietary history.
4. Obtain height and weight measurements and plot on a standard chart that has been normed for Eskimo children.
5. Involve mother in designing a medication reminder sheet.
6. Reinforce with mother and client the need for taking appropriate dose of iron supplements.
7. Teach mother and client about the need to eat a nutritionally balanced diet.
8. Instruct mother to be certain to put iron supplements in a safe place so that other children cannot take the medication indiscriminately, thus avoiding iron toxicity

Nursing Diagnosis   Body temperature, altered
Health maintenance, altered
Potential infection
Pain

Client Outcomes

1. Client will have increased comfort.
2. Levels of microorganisms will be reduced.
3. Measures will be taken to prevent recurrence.
4. Parental knowledge about condition will be increased.
5. Measures will be taken to prevent the possibility of a tympanic membrane rupture.

Nursing Interventions

1. Observe for symptoms of ear discomfort such as tugging or holding ears.
2. Assess for hearing impairment or loss.
3. Examine external auditory canal for erythema.
4. Examine tympanic membrane for erythema, mobility, and bulging.
5. Teach mother and client signs and symptoms of tympanic membrane rupture, which include sudden relief of pain.
6. Teach mother and client the value of soft and liquid foods when chewing is extremely painful because of movement of the eustachian tube.

 Nursing Diagnosis   Nutrition, altered, less than body requirements.

Client Outcomes

1. Mother and client will describe causative factors related to inadequate nutrition.
2. Client will experience adequate nutrition through oral intake.

Nursing Interventions

1. Teach mother about importance of good nutrition for a child.
2. Encourage a caloric intake of at least 80 calories/kg and 1.2 g of protein/kg of body weight.
3. Encourage mother to seek additional assistance for dietary supplements such as the WIC program.
4. Encourage mother to talk with teachers about lunchtime intake.

 Nursing Diagnosis   Parental role conflict
Parenting, altered
Noncompliance with prescribed regimen

Client Outcomes

1. Client will describe experiences that cause her to alter prescribed behavior.
2. Mother will develop an appropriate alternative for previous plan for medication administration.

Nursing Interventions

1. Assess causative or contributing factors for noncompliance with prescribed therapy.
2. Assess client's rationale for noncompliance with medication.
3. Initiate health teaching for mother and client.
4. Teach mother and client importance of adhering to prescribed regimen.
5. Teach mother and client what to expect from drug regimen, including side effects.

 Nursing Diagnosis   Self-esteem disturbance

Client Outcomes

1. Client will verbalize positive feelings about self.
2. Client will take part in activities with other children in a confident manner.
3. Client will achieve grade-level objectives of school age.

Nursing Interventions

1. Encourage client to express both positive and negative feelings.
2. Encourage mother to set limits on problematic behavior, such as poor hygiene, noncompliance with medication, and other negative behaviors.
3. Accept silence of client but let her know that the nurse is there for support.

Nursing Diagnosis   Infection, risk for

Client Outcomes	Nursing Interventions

Client Outcomes

1. Mother and client will learn value of washing hands and not placing foreign bodies into the ear.
2. Mother and client will learn value of taking prescribed antibiotic for the full amount of time.

Nursing Interventions

1. Teach mother or client to administer or take prescribed antibiotic.
2. Develop a medication reminder chart.
3. Teach mother and client to seek early medical care for pharyngitis to prevent spread of infection through eustachian tube to middle ear.
4. Teach mother and client to use ear plugs for swimming, showering, and hair washing if these are available.

STUDY QUESTIONS

1. Identify why otitis media may be a common illness among Eskimo children.
2. Identify cultural factors that affect the treatment of otitis media in Eskimo children.
3. List factors that predispose Eskimos to risk as a direct result of regular consumption of tea.
4. List factors that predispose Eskimos to risk as a result of consumption of large quantities of sugar.
5. Using Campbell's rule, can you distinguish if this cultural group is at risk for glucose intolerance?
6. List several contributing factors related to alcoholism among Alaskan Eskimos.
7. Formerly tuberculosis was a disease condition to which Eskimos were believed to have inherited susceptibility. Today, however, this is considered untrue. List two factors cited that do have contributing significance for this disease.

References

Albert, D. (1988). *Impact of acculturation of Alaskan natives.* Paper presented at the Ob-Gyn Update 1988 Conference, Anchorage, Alaska.

Allen, E., & Crago, M. (1996, Feb.). Early passive acquisition in Inuktitut. *Journal of Child Language, 23*(1), 129-155.

Andrew, M., & Krouse, S. (1995, Winter). Research on excess deaths among American Indians and Alaska Natives: a critical review. *Journal of Cultural Diversity, 2*(1), 8-15.

Armstrong, T., Roberts, B., & Swithinbank, C. (Eds.). (1973). *Illustrated glossary of snow and ice.* Cambridge, England: Scott Polar Research Institute.

Banks, T. (1956). *Birthplace of the wind.* New York: T.Y. Crowell.

Bartline, K. (1997, Feb.). Medical student and resident experience in Alaska: a question of value. *The IHS Primary Care Provider, 22*(2), 23-24.

Baxter, J. (1980). My experience with the Canadian Inuit. *Journal of Otolaryngology, 9*(1), 63-66.

Baxter, J., Katsarkas, A., Ling, D., & Carson, R. (1979, June). The Nakasuk project: the conservative treatment of chronic otitis media in Inuit elementary school children. *Journal of Otolaryngology, 8*(3), 201-209.

Behavioral Risk Factor Surveillance, 1991, 1992. Fairbanks, Alaska: Office of Health Promotion, Alaska Division of Public Health.

Bells, R., Draper, H., & Bergan, J. (1973). Sucrose, lactose, and glucose tolerance in northern Alaskan Eskimos. *American Journal of Clinical Nutrition, 26,* 1185-1190.

Berman, M., Hanson, K., & Hellman, I. (1972). Effect of breast-feeding on postpartum menstruation, ovulation, and pregnancy in Alaskan Eskimo. *American Journal of Obstetrics and Gynecology, 114,* 524-534.

Blodgett, J. (1978). *The coming and going of shaman: eskimo shamanism and art.* Winnipeg, Canada: Winnipeg Art Gallery.

Blum, R. (1992, August). American Indians and Alaska Native youths. *The IHS Primary Care Provider, 17*(8), 137-145.

Boas, F. (1938). *The mind of primitive man.* New York: Macmillan.

Brant, L.J., Bender, T.R., & Marnell, R.W. (1982). Factors affecting streptococcal colonization among children in selected areas of Alaska. *Public Health Reports, 97*(5), 460-464.

Brown, S. (1997, July 27). Alaskan oil. *Tulsa World,* E1.

Bruerd, B. (1997, March). Preventing baby bottle tooth decay and early childhood caries among AI/AN infants and children. *The IHS Primary Care Provider, 22*(3), 37-39.

Carpenter, E. (1973). *Eskimo realities.* New York: Holt, Rinehart, & Winston.

Centers for Disease Control and Prevention (1989, August). *Tuberculosis statistics in the United States* (DHHS Publication No. [CDC] 89-8322). Atlanta, Ga.: the centers.

Chance, N. (1966). *The Eskimo of north Alaska.* New York: Holt, Rinehart, & Winston.

Conway, G. (1992). Prevalence of HIV and AIDS in American Indians and Alaska Natives. *IHS Primary Care Providers, 17*(5), 1-6.

Crago, M. & Tremblay, C. (1991). Obstacles, challenges, and solutions: evolution in audiological service delivery to the hearing-impaired Inuit of northern Quebec. *Arctic Medical Research,* Suppl., 633-638.

Damas, D. (1984). *Arctic: Handbook of North American Indians* (vol. 5). Washington, D.C.: Smithsonian Institution.

DeBruyn, L., Wilkins, B., Stetter-Burns, M., & Nelson, S. (1997). Violence and violence prevention. *The IHS Primary Care Provider, 22*(4), 58-60.

Dunbar, M. (1968). *Ecological development in polar regions: a study in evolution.* Englewood Cliffs, N.J.: Prentice Hall.

Duncan, I., & Scott, E. (1972). Lactose intolerance in Alaska Indian and Eskimo. *American Journal of Clinical Nutrition, 25,* 867-868.

Dyerberg, J., & Bang, H. (1978). Eicosapentaenoic acid and prevention of thrombosis and atherosclerosis. *Lancet, 2,* 117-119.

Feldman, S.A., Ho, K.J., Lewis, L.A., et al. (1972, July). Lipid and cholesterol metabolism in Alaskan Eskimos. *Arctic Pathology, 94*(1), 42-58.

Fleshman, C. (1992, Oct.). Injury and deaths among American Indians and Alaska Native infants. *The IHS Primary Care Provider, 17*(10), 186-190.

Friedrich, C.A., & Ferrell, R.E. (1985, May). A population study of alpha-keto acid reductase. *Annuals of Human Genetics, 49*(Pt. 2), 111-114.

Gaffey, M.J., & Weiss, L.M. (1990, Nov.). Viral oncogenesis: Epstein-Barr virus. *American Journal of Otolaryngology, 11*(6), 375-381.

Galens, J., Sheets, A., & Young, R. (1995). *Gale encyclopedia of multicultural America.* New York: Gale Research Inc.

Giblin, P. (1997). Cooler than cactus. *The Dallas Morning News,* 1A.

Glassetter, M. (1989, Feb. 8). Personal interview with Dolly Lefever concerning Inupiat values.

Goodbody, M., & Stubbing, P. (1991). A study on cost effectiveness of audiology services, Baffin region, N.W.T. *Arctic Medical Research,* Suppl., 646-647.

Gottberg, J. (1988). *Frommer's dollarwise guide to Alaska.* Englewood Cliffs, N.J.: Prentice Hall.

Gove, C. (1982). *The conflict between cultural persistence and acculturation as it affects individual behavior of northwestern Alaskan Eskimo.* Dissertation presented to graduate faculty of the School of Human Behavior, U.S. International University, San Diego, California.

Grove, O., & Lynge, J. (1979). Suicide and attempted suicide in Greenland: a controlled study. *Acta Psychiatrica Scandinavica, 60*(4), 375-391.

Hall, D.B., Lum, M.K., Knutson, L.R., et al. (1987). Pharyngeal carriage and acquisition of anticapsular antibody to *Haemophilus influenzae* type b in a high risk population in southwestern Alaska. *American Journal of Epidemiology, 126*(6), 1190-1197.

Hall, E. (1975). *The Eskimo storyteller: folktales from Noatak, Alaska.* Knoxville, Tenn.: University of Tennessee Press.

Hankins, C, Hum, L., Tran, T., et al. (1997, June). Low HIV prevalence among childbearing women of aboriginal origin [Letter]. *AIDS, 11*(7), 945-947.

Heller, C.A. (1947). *Alaska nutrition survey report.* Juneau, Alaska: Territorial Department of Health.

Hildes, J.A., & Schaefer, O. (1984). The changing picture of neoplastic disease in the western and central Canadian Arctic. *Canadian Medical Association Journal, 130*(1), 25- 32.

Holderman, N. (1960, March). The little men. *Alaska Call,* p. 16.

Holderman, N. (1962). Personal correspondence about life as an Alaska Native Service teacher's wife.

Holderman, R. (1993, May 15). Personal correspondence regarding Alaska Native Service teaching experiences in the 1950s and 1960s in Deering and Shungnak, Alaska.

Hollmann, F. (1993). *Current Population Reports.* Washington, D.C.: U.S. Department of Commerce.

Hrdlicka, A. (1930). *Anthropological survey in Alaska* (46th annual report). Washington D.C.: U.S. Department of Commerce, Bureau of Ethnology.

Hrdlicka, A. (1941). Height and weight of Eskimo children. *American Journal of Physical Anthropology, 28,* 331.

Ilecki, H.J., & Baxter, J.D. (1981). Arctic audiology: trials, tribulations, and occasional successes. *Journal of Otolaryngology, 10*(4), 294-298.

Jilek-Aall, L. (1981). Acculturation, alcoholism, and Indian-style Alcoholics Anonymous. *Journal of Studies on Alcohol, 9,* 143-158.

Johnston, F.E., Laughlin, W.S., Harper, A.B., & Ensroth, A.E. (1982). Physical growth of St. Lawrence Island Eskimos: body size, proportion, and composition. *American Journal of Physical Anthropology, 58*(4), 397-401.

Keats, D. (1985). *Della Keats: Eskimo healer* (Video). Kotzebue, Alaska: Manillnaq.

Kimble, G., & Good, D. (1955). *Geography of the northlands* (Special Publication No. 32). New York: American Geographical Society.

Klausner, A., & Foulks, E.F. (1982). *Eskimo capitalists: oil, politics, and alcohol.* Englewood Cliffs, N.J.: Prentice Hall.

Kleinfeld, J.S. (1971). *Some instructional strategies for the cross-cultural classroom.* Juneau, Alaska: Alaska Department of Education.

Kost-Grant, B. (1983). Self-inflicted gunshot wounds among Alaska Natives. *Public Health Reports, 98*(1), 72-78.

Lancaster, M. (1990). Botulism: north to Alaska. *American Journal of Nursing, 90*(1), 60-62.

Lange, B. (1988). Ethnographic interview: an occupational therapy needs assessment tool for American Indian and Alaska Native Alcoholics. *Occupational Therapy in Mental Health, 8*(2), 61-80.

Lanier, A., Bender, T., Talbert, M., et al. (1980). Nasopharyngeal carcinoma in Alaskan Eskimos, Indians, and Aleuts: a review of cases and study of Epstein-Barr virus, HLA, and environmental risk factors. *Cancer, 46*(9), 2100-2106.

Lanier, A.P., Bulkow, L.R., Novotny, T.E., et al. (1990). Tobacco use and its consequences in northern populations. *Arctic Medical Research, 49*(suppl. 2), 17-22.

Lantis, M. (1960). *Eskimo childhood and interpersonal relationships.* Seattle: University of Washington Press.

Lee, C, Brunham, R., Sherman, E., & Harding, G. (1987). Epidemiology of an outbreak of infectious syphilis in Manitoba. *American Journal of Epidemiology, 125,* 277-83.

Lefever, D. (1997, November 27). Personal communication.

Lewis, D., & Ho, M. (1975). Social work with Native Americans. *Social Work, 20,* 379-382.

Ling, D. (1976, July 6). Audiological problems of the Eskimo population in the Baffin zone. In Shepherd, R.J., & Itoh, S. (Eds.), *Circumpolar Health* (pp. 409-412). Toronto: University of Toronto Press.

López, B. (1986). *Arctic dreams: imagination and desire in a northern landscape.* New York: Charles Scribner's Sons.

Loshbaugh, D. (1996, Dec. 23). Rudolph's secret. *Peninsula Clarion,* Kenai, Alaska.

Loshbaugh, D. (1997, March 28). Kenai Natives sign land deal. *Peninsula Clarion,* Kenai, Alaska.

Lubbock, B. (1937). *The Arctic whalers.* Glasgow, Scotland: Brown, Son & Ferguson.

Lum, M.K., Knutson, L.R., Hall, D.B., et al. (1986). Decline in infant mortality of Alaskan Yupik Eskimos from 1960 to 1980. *Public Health Reports, 101*(3), 309-314.

Lynch, H., Schuelke, G., & O'Hara, M. (1984, June). Is cancer communicable? *Medical Hypotheses, 14*(2), 181-198.

MacDonald-Clark, N., & Boffman, J., (1995, June). Mother-child interaction among the Alaskan Eskimos. *Journal of Obstetric Gynecologic and Neonatal Nursing, 24*(5), 450-457.

Mailhot, J. (1978). L'étymologie de «Esquimau» revue et corrigée. *Études Inuit—Inuit Studies, 2,* 59-69.

Mala, A. (1984). Circumpolar health, 1984: an Alaskan perspective. *Alaska Medicine, 26*(4), 108-111.

Mann, G.V., & Scott, E. (1962, July). The health and nutritional status of Alaskan Eskimos. *American Journal of Clinical Nutrition, 2,* 31-76.

McMahon, B.J., Heyward, W.K., Templin, D.W., et al. (1989). Hepatitis B–associated polyarteritis nodosa in Alaska: clinical and epidemiologic features and long-term follow-up. *Hepatology, 9*(1), 97-101.

Metler, R., Conway, G., & Stehr-Green, J. (1991). AIDS surveillance among American Indian and Alaska Natives. *American Journal of Public health, 81,* 1469-1471.

Middaugh, J. (1993, July 27). AIDS case definition changes: the impact in Alaska. *The State of Alaska Epidemiology Bulletin, 27,* 1.

Milan, F.A. (Ed.) (1980). *The human biology of circumpolar populations.* Cambridge, Mass.: Cambridge University Press.

Mitchell, W., & Patch, K. (1986). Religion, spiritualism, and the recovery of Native American Alcoholics. *The IHS Primary Care Provider, 11,* 129.

Morris, J. (1985). Caribou and ketchup—health implications. *Nursing Practice, 1*(2), 98-101.

Mouratoff, G., Carrol, N., & Scott, E. (1967). Diabetes mellitus in Eskimos. *Journal of the American Medical Association, 199*(13), 107-122.

Murphy, K. (1997, July 10). Alaska's delicate Arctic awaits new push for crude. *Los Angeles Times,* A-1.

National Center for Health Statistics, Healthy People 2000 Review (1993). *Health, United States 1992.* Hyattsville, Md.: Public Health Service.

National Center for Health Statistics (1998). *Health United States, 1998, with socioeconomic status and health chartbook.* Hyattsville, Md.: Public Health Service.

Newberg, J. (1997, April 10). Paddle power on the water. *The Arizona Republic,* OT1.

Nida, E. (1954). *Customs and cultures.* New York: Harper & Brothers.

Nobmann, E. (1984). *Dietary factors and iron deficiency.* Anchorage, Alaska: Alaska Native Medical Center.

Nord, E. (1995, Aug.) Evolution of a public health nursing program, Yukon Kuskokwim Delta, Alaska, 1893-1993. *Public Health Nursing, 12*(4), 249-255.

Overfield, T. (1977). Biological variations. *Nursing Clinics of North America, 12*(1), 19-27.

Overfield, T. (1995). *Biologic variation in health and illness* (ed. 2). Reading, Mass.: Addison-Wesley.

Pender, J. (1987, March). Little Pinch: memoir of a healer. *Anchorage Daily News Magazine,* p. 3.

Petersen, G.M., Silimperi, D.R., Rotter, J.I., et al. (1987). Genetic factors in *Haemophilus influenzae* type b disease susceptibility and antibody acquisition. *Journal of Pediatrics, 110*(2), 228-233.

Phillips, M.R., & Inui, T.S. (1986). The interaction of mental illness, criminal behavior and culture: Native Alaskan mentally ill criminal offenders. *Culture, Medicine, and Psychiatry, 10*(2), 123-149.

Polk, S. (1987, Sept.-Oct.). Helping our children. *Children Today,* pp. 19-20.

Pollick, S. (1997, June 16). Inuit life harsh, often brutal. *The Blade,* Toledo Ohio.

The Random House dictionary of the English language (1987). New York: Random House, Inc.

Roberts, L., & Ross, C. (1979). Nursing north of sixty. *Canadian Nurse, 75*(5), 26-29.

Rodahl, K. (1964). *Between two worlds.* London: Heinemann.

Rode, A., & Shephard, R.J. (1984). Ten years of "civilization": fitness of Canadian Inuit. *Journal of Physiology, 56*(6), 1472-1477.

Rosen, Y. (1997, Feb. 28). Iditarod trail leads to more pros, fewer native racers. *Christian Science Monitor,* 1.

Ross, D. (1989). Nursing up north. *Canadian Nurse, 85*(1), 22-24.

Saari, M. (1997, June 7). Native art unearthed for all. *Ketchikan Daily News,* 1.

Schaefer, O. (1970). Pre- and postnatal growth acceleration and increased sugar consumption in Canadian Eskimos. *Canadian Medical Association Journal, 103*(10), 1059-1068.

Schaefer, O. (1971). When the Eskimo comes to town. *Nutrition Today, 6,* 8-16.

Schaefer, O. (1973). The changing health picture in the Canadian north. *Canadian Journal of Ophthalmology, 8,* 196-204.

Schaefer, O. (1986). Adverse reactions to drugs and metabolic problems perceived in northern Canadian Indians and Eskimos. *Progress in Clinical and Biological Research, 214,* 77-83.

Schraer, C.D., Lanier, A.P., Boyko, E.J., et al. (1988). Prevalence of diabetes mellitus in Alaskan Eskimos, Indians, and Aleuts. *Diabetes Care, 11*(9), 693-700.

Scott, E.M., & Griffin, I. (1956). *Diabetes mellitus in Eskimos.* Anchorage, Alaska: Arctic Research Center.

Seefeldt, C. (1984). Children's attitude toward the elderly: a cross-cultural comparison. *International Journal of Aging and Human Development, 19*(4), 319-329.

Seltzer, A. (1980). Acculturation and mental disorders in the Inuit. *Canadian Journal of Psychiatry, 25*(2), 173-181.

Seltzer, A. (1983). Psychodynamics of spirit possession among the Inuit. *Canadian Journal of Psychiatry, 28*(1), 52-56.

Seltzer, A., & Langford, J.A. (1984). Forensic psychiatric assessments in the Northwest Territories. *Canadian Journal of Psychiatry, 29*(8), 665-668.

Shephard, R.J. (Ed.) (1974). Circumpolar health: 3rd international symposium. Yellow Knife, Northwest Territory, Canada.

Singleton, R. (1992). *Haemophilus influenzae* type B infections in the Yukon Kuskokwim Delta and Bristol Bay area of Alaska. *The IHS Primary Care Provider, 17*(8), 123.

Sipperly, M. (1989). Marine lipids and coronary angioplasty: benefit. *Progress in Cardiovascular Nursing, 4*(4), 119-123.

Snider, D., Salinas, L., & Kelly, G. (1989). Tuberculosis: an increasing problem among minorities in the United States. *Public Health Reports, 104*(6), 646-653.

Statistical Reports (1991). Washington, D.C.: U.S. Department of Commerce, Bureau of the Census.

Stefansson, V. (1921). *The friendly Arctic.* New York: Macmillan.

Stevenson, M. (1984). Tuberculosis in the North: a lifestyle issue. *Canadian Nurse, 80*(1), 41-43.

Szathmary, E.J. (1984). Peopling of northern North America: clues from genetic studies. *Acta Anthropogenetica, 8*(1-2), 79-109.

Taylor, C. (1988). Trauma prevention in rural Alaska. *Journal of Emergency Nursing, 14*(5), 36A-39A.

TB Monitor (1996, April). Village TB outbreaks threaten Arctic zone. *TB Monitor, 3*(4), 42-46.

Toomey, K.E., Oberschelp, A.G., & Greenspan, J.R. (1989). Sexually transmitted diseases and Native Americans: trends in reported gonorrhea and syphilis morbidity, 1984-1988. *Public Health Reports, 104*(6), 566-572.

Toomey, K.E., Rafferty, M.P., & Stamm, W.E. (1987). Unrecognized high prevalence of *Chlamydia trachomatis* cervical infection in an isolated Alaskan Eskimo population. *Journal of the American Medical Association, 258*(1), 53-56.

Travis, R. (1983). Suicide in northwest Alaska. *White Cloud Journal, 3*(1), 23-30.

U.S. Department of Commerce, Bureau of the Census (1993). *Population profile of the United States, 1993* (Publication No. 23-185). Washington, D.C.: Government Printing Office.

U.S. Department of Health and Human Services, Indian Health Services (1991a). *Alaska Child Health Administration program description.* Washington, D.C.: Government Printing Office.

U.S. Department of Health and Human Services, Indian Health Services (1991b). *Trends in Indian Health 1991.* Washington, D.C.: Government Printing Office.

U.S. Department of Health and Human Services, Indian Health Services (1992b). Injury deaths among American Indian and Alaska Native infants. *The IHS Primary Care Provider, 17*(10), 186-190.

U.S. Department of Health and Human Services, Indian Health Services (1992c). *Trends in Indian health.* Washington, D.C.: Government Printing Office.

VanDenberg, J., & Minton, B. (1987). Alaska native youth. *Children Today, 16*(5), 15-18.

Van Rens, G.H., Arkell, S.M., Charlton, W., & Doesburg, W. (1988). Primary angle-closure glaucoma among Alaskan Eskimos. *Documenta Ophthalmologica, 70*(2-3), 265-276.

Vaudrin, B. (no date). *Native/nonnative communication.* Unpublished manuscript Anchorage, Alaska.

Ward, J.I., Lum, M.K., Hall, D.B., et al. (1986). Invasive *Haemophilus influenzae* type b disease in Alaska: background epidemiology for a vaccine efficacy trial. *Journal of Infectious Diseases, 153*(1), 17-26.

Wiggins, C. (1996, June). A business plan for the IHS. *The IHB Primary Care Provider, 21*(6), 1-4.

Williamson, R. (1974). *Eskimo underground social-cultural change in the Canadian Central Arctic. Occasional Papers* (vol. 2). Uppsala, Sweden: Institutet för Allmän och Jämförande, Etnografi, Uppsala University.

World Almanac (1997). Mahwah, N.J.: World Almanac Books.

Young, T.K. (1986). Epidemiology and control of chronic disease in circumpolar Eskimos/Inuit populations. *Arctic Medical Research, 42,* 25-47.

Young, T. (1994). *The health of Native Americans.* New York: Oxford University Press.

Zegura, S.L. (1985). The initial peopling of the Americas: an overview from the perspective of physical anthropology. *Acta Anthropogenetica, 8*(1-2), 1-21.

Zimmerman, M.R., & Aufderheide, A.C. (1984). Frozen family of Utqiaġvik: autopsy findings. *Arctic Anthropology, 21*(1), 531-564.

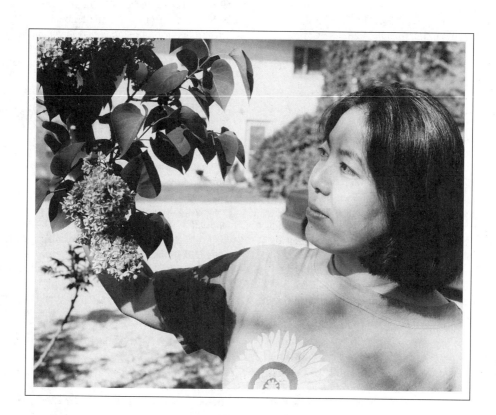

CHAPTER 13 Japanese Americans

Dianne Ishida and Jillian Inouye

BEHAVIORAL OBJECTIVES

After reading this chapter, the nurse will be able to do the following:

1. Describe the influence of acculturation on Japanese Americans.
2. Develop a sensitivity and an understanding for the communication styles within and across the Japanese-American culture to avoid stereotyping and to provide culturally appropriate care.
3. Describe the time orientation of some Japanese-American people and its influence on wellness and illness behavior.
4. Discuss the spatial needs and implications for culturally appropriate care for the Japanese American client.
5. Discuss the influence of family and social organization on behavior.
6. Explain the health care beliefs, folk beliefs, and folk practices of Japanese Americans and the influence on health-seeking behaviors.
7. Recognize physical, biological, and psychological variances that exist within and across the Japanese American culture to provide culturally appropriate care.

OVERVIEW OF JAPAN

Japan is a chain of islands that stretches in an arc more than 1860 miles (2995 km) long from the twenty-fourth parallel, off Taiwan, north to the forty-fifth parallel, just below Sakhalin Island (Information Please Almanac, 1998). Japan lies just east of the Asian mainland. The Ryukyu chain, which lies southwest, was once United States–occupied territory. Similarly, the Kuriles, which are northwest, are Russian occupied. The Tsushima Strait separates Japan from Korea.

Japan is composed of four large closely grouped islands—Hokkaido, Honshu, Shikoku, Kyu-shu—and 4000 smaller islands. In land mass, Japan is 145,874 square miles. The four main islands constitute approximately 98% of the total land mass of the country. By comparison, Japan is just slightly smaller than California (Information Please Almanac, 1998; World Almanac, 1997). The habitable and uninhabitable terrain of Japan roughly composes 0.3% of the world's total land mass, yet the population of this country accounts for 3% of the world's population. In 1997, Japan had the seventh largest population in the world with 125,716,637 people (Information Please Almanac, 1998; World Almanac, 1997). This number is expected to reach 131 million people by the year 2000. Of the number of people residing in Japan, three fourths live in cities (Information Please Almanac, 1998; World Almanac, 1997). Because the Japanese landscape is mountainous with angled slopes, only 15% of the total land area is habitable (Sargent, 1993), which accounts for the density of the population in certain regions of the country. In fact, the population of Japan is so dense that there are 861.8 people per square mile (320 sq km). If the uninhabitable areas of Japan were excluded from this equation, a more realistic figure of 3885 people for every 1500 yards (1760 yards equals a mile) would emerge (Information Please Almanac, 1998; World Alamanc, 1997).

The population explosion of Japan is attributed to industrialization and reached 65 million by 1930. After World War II, the Japanese government initiated a population policy to lower the rate of increase. Since the mid-1950s, the population growth rate corresponds to those in other Western European countries (Storry, 1993). In 1996, the birth rate for Japan was reported to be 10 per 1000; the infant mortality, 4 per 1000 live births. In 1996, the average life expecancy at birth was 77 for males and 83 for females (World Almanac, 1997).

Hokkaido is the least populated island in Japan. Although it was once a haven for outcasts, it is now an industrial site where agriculture, leisure activities, and brew-making dominate the economy.

Honshu is the island on which approximately 80% of the Japanese people reside, with the majority concentrated in the plains of Kanto (Tokyo) and Kansai (Kyoto-Osaka). Honshu is known for its distinctive business culture, major ports, and multiple airports (The Economist's Business Traveller's Guides, 1987).

Shikoku is a comparative backwater devoted primarily to agriculture. Shikoku is not a major attraction for foreign visitors. It is a subtropical island, and the people are reputedly the most outgoing of all Japanese. There is bullet train service to Hakata, which is near Fukuoka, which has a major airport.

The Ryukyu chain of islands was occupied by the United States from World II until 1972 and is perhaps the poorest of all the regions in Japan. These islands are noted for their hybrid population. Several of the islands in the Ryukyus are uninhabited. Okinawa is one of the major islands in the Ryukyus and is a major staging base for the U.S. Air Force and Army (The Economist Business Traveller's Guides, 1987).

The capital of Japan is Tokyo and, when combined with Yokohama, is the second largest city in the world. The population of Tokyo-Yokohama is approximately 14,900,000 (Basch, 1990). It is pro-

jected that the population of Tokyo-Yokohama will grow to approximately 17 million by the year 2000, making it the third largest populated city in the world (Information Please Almanac, 1998; World Almanac, 1997; Basch, 1990). Although Tokyo-Yokohama is a densely populated city, it sprawls over only 800 square miles (2000 sq km) (The Economist Business Traveller's Guides, 1987; Information Please Almanac, 1998). Tokyo is largely industrial and is the home of the Tokyo Stock Exchange (the counterpart to the New York Stock Exchange), which is the barometer for the economic climate throughout the world.

In Japan, there are approximately 60 active volcanoes. Climatic conditions are favorable with sufficient warmth and humidity in the summer for cultivation. Winters are cool and dry, unlike the subtropical and tropical winters of the rest of Asia. Significant seasonal changes vary with the direction of the prevailing wind, like much of monsoon Asia (Sargent, 1993).

Although over 67% of the total land area of Japan is forested, not all forests have commercial value because soil erosion is a problem. The sea provides the major portion of protein in the Japanese diet. Both the Japan Sea and the Pacific Ocean are rich fishing grounds. Japan's fishing catch has been the world's largest since 1972. Japan has few mineral resources and depends on imports of raw materials and fuel (Sargent, 1993).

Historically, Japan has primarily had an agriculture-based economy. The economy has changed rapidly since the late nineteenth century with industrialization, especially after World War II. Today, Japan is considered the most urbanized country in Asia.

The Ainu (hairy aboriginals whose ethnicon means 'man') are known to be the original inhabitants of Japan. Although they once occupied the whole country (Storry, 1993), it is believed that today only 15,000 Ainu remain on the islands of Sakhalin and Hokkaido (Webster's Dictionary, 1991). The ancestors of the Japanese are believed to have come from mainland Asia, crossing over from Korea. These early settlers moved eastward from Kyushu and settled in the Kansai Plain (Kyoto-Osaka regions). Eventually, they established an ordered society under chieftains who were dedicated to the cult of the sun. Buddhism was later introduced in the sixth century of our era. The ethics of Confucianism were added to the practice of sun worship and animism *(Shintō)* (Storry, 1993). Today, the Ainu maintain a culture and language that are distinctively different from the rest of the Japanese; however, the Ainu language is now almost extinct. Except for the Ainu, however, the Japanese population is ethnically and linguistically homogeneous (Sargent, 1993).

IMMIGRATION

Today the ability of Japanese Americans to identify with Japanese culture depends largely on when they arrived or whether they were born in the United States, where they live, and how much acculturation and assimilation have occurred. Before the 1890s a few Japanese scholars and businessmen came to the United States and settled along the East Coast. Because of their small numbers and desire to be acculturated and assimilated into the mainstream society in the United States, they were more readily accepted than later ones.

The large influx of Japanese immigrants between 1890 and 1924 settled primarily along the West Coast and in Hawaii. Because of the prejudice they experienced, their lack of knowledge about the new country, and the language barrier, they kept to themselves and formed relatively self-sufficient communities where they were able to retain familiar cultural values. Second-generation Japanese Americans were largely influenced by the values and norms of their parents. However, third- and fourth-generation Japanese Americans may be unfamiliar with the Japanese language and customs. In addition, 50% of the Japanese in the United States have married outside the Japanese ethnic group, promoting further assimilation into the mainstream American culture (Kikumura & Kitano, 1973).

The Japanese-American people are the only immigrant group to identify themselves by the generation in which they were born, and these generation groups are distinguishable by the individual's age, experience, language, and values. The generation groups are the *issei*, the first generation to live in the United States; the *nisei*, the second generation; the *sansei*, the third generation; the *yonsei*, the fourth generation; the *gosei*, the fifth generation; and the *rokusei*, the sixth generation (Hashizume & Takano, 1993).

These generational categories provide a framework for understanding family-related cultural values. For the *issei*, the family provided the anchor for the values and traditions of Japan. Today the family remains one of the most important factors in the lives of the Japanese people. The *issei* withstood extreme hardships and made personal sacrifices for the benefit of their children.

Before the 1890s the majority of the Japanese persons who immigrated to the United States were men. Generally speaking, it often took many years before a Japanese man was able to afford a wife or family. These men might have been 30 or 40 years of age before they looked back to Japan to find their brides through the exchange of photographs and letters. Thus these Japanese women were often 10 to 20 years younger than their husbands, and even today elderly Japanese men often have much younger wives. For the *issei* descendants there was a strong, stable family support system. The exclusion law of 1924 prevented some of the early Japanese male immigrants from finding a spouse, which resulted in a group of single elderly men who continue to reside in the United States without the support of a family. In 1965, with the lifting of the immigration restrictions based on race, creed, and nationality, Japanese immigrants were able to reestablish the continuity of family life (Kobata, 1979). The general pattern of the Japanese family is the vertical family structure, with the father and other male members in the topmost position. Many of the activities in the Japanese family occur in both the nuclear family and the extended family. Problems are handled within the structure, and the achievement or accomplishment of the individual member is a reflection on the entire family (Kitano, 1976).

Today intergenerational relations are close among most Japanese Americans. There continues to be a flow of goods, money, and services between the generations. The younger generation continues to be willing to assist and give more than what is requested and expected by the older generation

(Osaka, 1979). The *issei* descendants continue to emphasize the importance of caring for their elderly parents; however, it is important to remember that the *issei* generation never experienced caring for their own parents because they left them in Japan. Today the tradition of caring for aged parents is seen in the *issei* descendants wherein aged parents continue to maintain separate but close residences, receive contributions from all their children, and spend blocks of time with each child. Generally one child, often the oldest son or an unmarried child, assumes full responsibility for the care of elderly parents (Kobata, 1979). As indicated, family contacts are frequent among the elderly. In a study done in Chicago, researchers found that 65% of the elderly Japanese Americans surveyed indicated that they had at least daily contact with at least one child, 30% had contact once a week, and the remaining 3% lived with their children (Osaka, 1979). Similar studies have been conducted that support these findings (Kiefer, 1974; Modell, 1968). Seemingly, reliance on the family structure has resulted in less dependence on outside individual agencies and organizations.

For both the *issei* and the *nisei,* parent-child relationships tended to be intense with open expressions of emotion displayed. For these generational groups there was much tolerance and permissiveness for the child until 5 or 6 years of age, at which time parents began to place emphasis on having the child learn emotional reserve and control. On the other hand, the *sansei* group tended to adopt the child-rearing practices and attitudes of contemporary and middle-class Americans and showed much less traditionalism than the earlier generations (Strazar & Fisher, 1996; Kiefer, 1974).

The *nisei* were born in the United States during the pre–World War II period. Although this generation had a higher educational level and was more fluent in English than their parents, they still faced intense racial discrimination in housing and employment (Sato & Takano, 1983). Hostile feelings on the part of many U.S. citizens intensified in 1942 with the declaration of the war with Japan. This sentiment climaxed with the evacuation and internment of Japanese Americans when President Roosevelt signed executive orders 9066 and 9102.

Although restrictions applied to Japanese, German, and Italian aliens on the West Coast, only the Japanese, both alien and United States born, were removed from their homes in California, Washington, Oregon, Arizona, and Hawaii and forcibly placed in internment camps (Daniels, Taylor, & Kitano, 1991; Strazar & Fisher, 1996). More than 120,000 persons were imprisoned. The experiences of those who survived are well documented (Daniels, Taylor, & Kitano, 1991; Houston & Houston, 1973; Reid, 1993; Tateishi, 1984; Yoshida, 1972). What is missing, however, are the accounts by those who did not survive or whose lives were broken and warped by this experience. During the internment, 6485 Japanese Americans were born in camps. Unfortunately, 1990 Japanese Americans died in internment camps (Daniels, Taylor, & Kitano, 1991).

The evacuation and internment of the Japanese in U.S. camps have been described as the most dehumanizing experience for Japanese Americans since their immigration to the United States. It not only disrupted their families and way of life, but also had enormous financial implications that were largely created from the loss of their homes and businesses. To prove their loyalty as Americans and combat the racism that confronted them, an overwhelming number of *nisei* volunteered for the all-*nisei* 100th Infantry Battalion and its larger unit of Japanese Americans, the 442nd Regimental Combat Team (Kakesako, 1993; Yoshishige, 1993). These volunteers, who came from Hawaii and mainland internment camps, emerged as the most decorated unit for its size and duration of service (Chang, 1993).

After the war, the employment and cultural expectations of Japanese Americans from the *nisei* became more aligned with their American background. As this new generation became more acculturated, they began to rely less on the economic sanction of their *issei* fathers. These individuals sought a better way of life and upward mobility. The GI Bill offered many veterans a chance at a first-class education. Japanese Americans have been extremely successful in the assimilation process, particularly in certain states. In Hawaii, successful inroads have been made particularly in the political arena (Burris, 1993). Succeeding generations of Japanese Americans have benefited tremendously from the efforts of these earlier immigrants. Recognition of Japanese-American rights and political power occurred when U.S. Congress passed the Civil Liberties Act of 1988 to make redress payments of $20,000 to each survivor who had been incarcerated during World War II (Daniels, 1991).

Life in the United States

According to 1998 Census data, there are 1,004,645 Japanese Americans residing in the United States (U.S. Department of Commerce, Bureau of the Census, 1998; Information Please Almanac, 1998). This number represents a 0.3% increase in the population of Japanese Americans since the 1980 census. Overall, Japanese Americans represent 12.3% of the total Asian-American population. Of the number of Japanese Americans residing in the United States, 75.9% live in the West, 7.9% live in the South, 7.5% live in the Midwest, and 10.2% live in the Northeast. By states, the largest populations of Japanese Americans are found in California (312,989), Hawaii (247,486), New York (35,861), and Washington (43,799) (U.S. Department of Commerce, Bureau of the Census, 1993a; 1993b).

The median age of Japanese Americans is 36.3 years. In the United States, Japanese Americans are the oldest group of Asians by median age. In fact, even when compared with the national median age for all ethnic and racial groups (33 years), Japanese Americans have a higher median age. Of the number of Japanese Americans residing in the United States between 1980 and 1990, 20% were foreign born, compared to 12.4% of Japanese Americans living in the United States before 1975. These data are suggestive that immigration has played a major role in the increase in numbers of Japanese Americans in the United States (U.S. Department of Commerce, Bureau of the Census, 1993b).

Asian Americans tend to have larger families, compared with other ethnic and racial groups. Japanese Americans may be the exception to this statistical fact. Japanese Americans, on the average, have 3.1 persons per family, compared with the national average of 3.2 persons per family. This number is in stark contrast to other Asian groups. At the higher end of the spectrum are Hmongs with 6.6 persons per family, Cambodians with 5.0 persons per family, Laotians with 5.0 persons per family, and Vietnamese with 4.4 persons per family (U.S. Department of Commerce, Bureau of the Census, 1993b).

COMMUNICATION
Communication and culture

The official language in Japan, which is spoken by some 90 million inhabitants, is Japanese. There are two systems that are used concurrently to communicate in writing in Japanese. In the Japanese language, one system includes the *kanji,* or *honji,* ideographic characters which are borrowed from the Chinese and used to express chief meanings of words such as substantive and root meanings of verbs and adjectives (Webster's Dictionary, 1991). The other system includes two sets of *kana* symbols, which are phonetic. To represent items that have grammatical function in Japanese, the *hiragana* are used. In addition, to translate foreign words, the *katakana* are used. The *katakana* are also used in official documents and advertisements. In many ways, the Japanese language shows a remarkable resemblance to the Korean language (Webster's Dictionary, 1991). Of the number of Japanese Americans residing in the United States, 42.8% speak an Asian or a Pacific Islander language at home, 57.7% do not speak English well, and 33.0% are linguistically isolated (U.S. Department of Commerce, Bureau of the Census, 1993b).

Style Japanese characteristics in language and behavior reflect characteristics of some of the values inherent in this ethnic group. The Japanese culture is known as the "culture of anticipatory perception" or "culture of consideration" because of the importance of sympathizing with the speaker (Lebra, 1976). A concept central to the issue of communication is "empathic identification." The speaker identifies with and views the listener from the listener's point of view. The expectation is that the listener will also empathize with the speaker. Thus, verbal (that is, oral) communication can be held to a minimum. For some Japanese Americans, constant verbal communication is seen as unnecessary. For these individuals, it is more important to communicate through attitude, action, and feeling than through words (Lebra, 1976). A talkative person is considered a "show-off" or insincere (Rogers & Izutsu, 1980).

When communication occurs with someone who is not Japanese, many Japanese people do not expect to have a personal position understood without strong assertions. During these times, it may be necessary for some Japanese Americans to establish their viewpoints before the listener has appropriately comprehended the message.

Behavior and communication are defined by role expectancy and status and by an attempt to preassess the listener's feelings or wishes. According to Schon and Ja (1982), the content of communication depends on the characteristics of the persons involved. Factors such as age, sex, education, social status, family background, and marital status often influence specific behaviors. Behaviors that may be seen as negative or resistive in Western culture may, in fact, be reflective of proper upbringing for some Japanese Americans. Openness may be construed as a sign of immaturity or lack of self-control, which may bring shame to the family.

Context In a high-context culture such as the Japanese, implicit nonverbal messages are of central importance; in multiethnic low-context cultures explicit verbal messages are emphasized (Hall, 1976). Behaviors of individuals in a high-context culture reflect the value of thinking before speaking, of modesty in acts and speech. In this sense, context is also viewed as intuitive. Purpose is attached to implicit, nonverbal, intuitive communication over explicit, verbal, rational communication. This concept is related to the context of empathy with its value on sensitivity and responsiveness. It is essential for the speaker to avoid superficiality and poor subtleties of speech if intuitive understanding is to occur (Lebra, 1976). In addition, in a high-context culture, esthetic refinement and sophistication are evident in nonverbal, indirect, implicit, subtle messages. Thus it is not surprising that some Japanese Americans may be threatened by or avoid ambiguous situations (Matsumoto, 1989).

Linguistics The grammatical structure of a language frequently reflects the major theme of a culture (Johnson, Marsella, & Johnson, 1974). Four

themes relating to verbal behaviors in Japanese Americans govern interactions: (1) a strong sense of gender differences, (2) a concern for hierarchy and status that manifests itself as deference toward authority, (3) an emphasis on self-effacement, and (4) a focus on nonverbal communication. These themes can be seen in the primacy of hierarchical status in the Japanese culture, where themes of the Meiji-era (post-1868) Japan and Confucian doctrines still dominate social behavior among many Japanese Americans.

Oral language According to Lebra (1976), the Japanese culture stresses nonverbal communication, and for many Japanese Americans there is a general mistrust of spoken words. Lebra attributes this characteristic to a belief held by some Japanese Americans that indicates that the *ma-gokoro* ('true-heart', thus the innermost self) is incapable of being adequately or sincerely expressed through the outer part of the body such as the mouth, which is inclined toward deception. Directly related to the *ma-gokoro* is the importance of personal self as the monitor of self-identity. Again, words are perceived as a poor substitute for the adequate expression of sincere feelings.

Self-abasement, modesty, and apology used by Japanese Americans when communicating are viewed by some health care professionals as self-effacing behaviors. Many health care professionals believe that this type of behavior is open to misunderstanding. The complex meanings behind these attitudes and behaviors can be understood by the concept of *enryo*, which directs Japanese Americans to be modest, to defer to others, to play down personal accomplishments and achievements, and to direct attention away from oneself (Johnson, Marsella, & Johnson, 1974). Likewise, for some Japanese Americans, self-praise or the acceptance of praise is considered poor manners, resulting in denying, ignoring, or negating another trait or behavior. To many Westerners, this behavior may be interpreted as lack of self-esteem or belittling (Chang, 1981).

The concept of hierarchy and status also dictates communication patterns. For some Japanese Americans, it is considered impolite to disagree publicly with a person of higher status for fear of making this individual lose face. In traditional Japanese society, gender differences are reflected by males tending to be more economical in speech, particularly in public situations, and more direct in delivery of opinions or ideas than their female counterparts (Johnson, Marsella, & Johnson, 1974). Some Japanese-American males tend not to give an opinion, especially on mundane matters. Japanese-American women are relatively soft spoken and are more loquacious than their male counterparts. Japanese-American women are viewed as pleasant individuals who not only are cooperative, but also have less assertive, aggressive, or loud verbal behaviors (Johnson, Marsella, & Johnson, 1974). Overt conflict is minimized both inside and outside the home for both Japanese-American women and men.

Oral expression is focused on increasing harmony and avoiding conflict (Fisher, 1996; Chang, 1981). Therefore, answering "yes" to questions may be a way of avoiding embarrassment or shame and does not necessarily imply that communication is agreed with, clear, or understood (Fisher, 1996).

In studying communication apprehension among individuals in Japan, Korea, and the United States, Klopf, Cambra, and Ishii (1981) found that the Japanese frequently expressed feelings of nervousness and anxiousness. These feelings were particularly augmented in social situations that made them generally awkward and unsociable when communicating with strangers and particularly persons from different cultures.

Voice quality. Vocal qualifiers include intensity, volume, pitch, and rate or speed (Ishii, 1987). In general, Japanese speak in a high-pitched voice, which may relate to the love of traditional folk songs *(minyō)* and sentimental nostalgic songs *(enka),* which call for high-pitched voices. Gender differences are also manifested in the manner in which women are expected to speak.

Nonverbal communication. The Japanese culture is a relatively non–eye contact culture, which is seen both in public speaking and in the communication process (Ishii, 1987). Most Asian Americans consider it disrespectful to look someone directly in the eyes, especially if that person is in a superior position (Galanti, 1991). In nonverbal communication, integral

quality and explicitness of feelings are involved in the process itself and are communicated paraverbally rather than directly. High awareness of nonverbal gestures and facial mimetic nuances exist among Japanese Americans (Johnson, Marsella, & Johnson, 1974). Matsumoto and Ekman (1989) found that Japanese-American perception of emotional intensity is consistent with cultural differences noted in two separate cultures. They also noted differences in the perception of emotional intensity. For these Japanese Americans there were strong, consistent cultural differences for all emotions except disgust. They concluded that disgust may be a reaction without interpersonal context. For some Japanese Americans, emotional expression of anger is unusual and a stoic reaction is often manifested as a response to pain.

Matsumoto (1989) found that the Japanese culture strongly advocated expressions of "uncertainty avoidance" and masculinity. For some Japanese Americans, uncertainty avoidance reflects the way in which an individual perceives a threat or is threatened by an ambiguous situation. In these situations, some Japanese Americans create a belief concept to avoid uncertain encounters with others. In contrast to uncertainty avoidance is the concept of masculinity. Masculinity reflects the degree to which cultures delineate sex roles, with masculine cultures making distinct differentiations between the sexes. Women are considered the subordinate gender in the Japanese culture. Matsumoto (1989) further concluded that cultures high in power distance and low in individualism tend to emphasize the need for hierarchy and group cohesion, whereas the need for individuality is devalued. In these cultures, the communication of negative emotions threatens group solidarity and interpersonal social structure. Thus, stoicism is the usual reaction to pain and uncertain situations.

Kinesics Mehrabian (1968) estimates that, for Japanese Americans, communication of feelings and attitudes is 5% verbal, 38% vocal, and 55% facial expression. Thus, facial expression plays a crucial role in communicating emotions and attitudes. Some Westerners have noted the inscrutability of the Japanese face. It is essential to remember, however, that the traditional behavior of some Japanese Americans is to control emotions, especially in formal and public situations. This value is believed to have originated in *heijō-shin* ('ordinary state of mind') in Zen Buddhism, which advocates controlling emotions and maintaining a neutral presence. An inappropriate smile may sometimes be seen as an unconscious and reflective attempt to avoid troubling others by showing one's true feelings.

Touch Japanese culture is viewed as a nontouch culture. There is close contact with infants but less touch or physical contact among adults (Ishii, 1987). Barnlund (1989) found that Japanese Americans touch family members less frequently than people in other cultures do.

Silence Findings from several studies are suggestive that Japanese adults spend only half as much time in conversation per weekday compared with their U.S. counterparts (Klopf & Ishii, 1976; Ishii, 1987). The data further suggested that Japanese couples, especially those who had been married for some time and were happy in the relationship, usually remained silent with each other because they had developed *sasshi* ('guesswork', or 'intuitive sensitivity'). In other words, they understand each other without speaking. *Sasshi* is also highly appreciated in other situations. The ideal and ultimate pattern of communication in Japanese society is silent communication. Some Japanese Americans do not appreciate aggressive or spoken forms of communication.

Implications for nursing care

Information and explanations regarding treatments and schedules should be given by the nurse or physician. Visitors in hospitals should be welcome because family participation is expected in illness. When a child is in the hospital, the parents' feelings of responsibility and guilt may need to be addressed.

Because it is impolite to think of personal needs, some Japanese Americans, when asked if they want something to eat or drink, are likely to respond negatively. In such instances, if the nurse does not try to persuade the client to eat or drink, the nurse may be perceived as insensitive.

The nurse can learn to anticipate needs and accurately assess discomforts by relying on astute interpretation of the meaning of nonverbal expressions

and behaviors. It is essential to remember that subtle facial expressions and gestures are expected to be understood. Japanese American clients may wait silently rather than ask questions because they believe health care providers know best and will meet their needs without being asked (Sato & Takano, 1983).

Because direct expression of negative feelings is an unusual behavior for some Japanese Americans, indirect messages should not be mistaken for agreement. For example, rather than verbalize to the staff their discontent with the health care, the client may have the family request a unit change. Nurses who expect clients to express their feelings through direct action may be surprised when they encounter a Japanese-American client who is withdrawn and silent. For the nurse who is unfamiliar with the cultural behaviors of the Japanese American, behaviors in ambiguous, embarrassing, or anxiety-producing situations may be difficult to understand, and the client may be labeled as passive or nonresponsive. For some Japanese Americans, it is extremely important to control expressions of anger or pain. The nurse should be aware of situations that may cause discomfort such as the exclusion of the family from the plan of care. The nurse must also remember that some Japanese Americans consider it insulting to be addressed by their first names, especially the first generation, who follow strict hierarchical rules of deference and respect.

SPACE

Although there are variations in spatial requirements among individuals, Japanese Americans tend to have a higher tolerance for crowding in public spaces than other Americans (Watson, 1980). For these persons, more time and attention is given to the organization of their living space and perception by the senses (Hall, 1976). Families of several generations often reside under one roof, depending on available resources. Even in relative proximity, a personal space can be created. Privacy is generally maintained by family members by respecting the privacy of others and by limiting self-disclosure to persons in binding or trusting relationships (Baker, 1993; Embree, 1939). For some Japanese Americans, well-manicured gardens can provide a degree of tranquillity and peace that tends to expand personal spatial boundaries.

Japanese Americans, like other Asian Americans, tend to use less physical contact when interacting. They may also appear reserved and formal in new situations as they maintain their social zones. However, in times of crisis or celebration, Japanese-American families tend to support family unity.

Implications for nursing care

Nurses should not misinterpret the reserved and formal behavior manifested by some Japanese Americans as a dysfunctional sign. The nurse should remember that these clients need to establish a caring, trusting relationship before they engage in self-disclosure. Japanese Americans may feel uncomfortable with the overuse of physical contact or the invasion of personal space when interacting. When some Japanese Americans are hospitalized, the nurse can help the client by identifying territorial boundaries within the room. Identification of these territorial boundaries may reduce conflicts created from the invasion of privacy of others, particularly when more than one client shares a room.

SOCIAL ORGANIZATION
Effect of immigration on social organization

Most Japanese immigrants who remained in the United States eventually brought their families or picture brides. They experienced increased racial prejudice as their numbers increased. As a buffer, they tended to form fairly self-sufficient subcommunities that provided for their needs and offered social support. The traditional Japanese value system places emphasis on the family, group orientation, harmony, and mutual aid (Embree, 1939; Lee & Takamura, 1980). This value system has allowed the families and communities to survive. For many Japanese Americans, interdependence and dependence on each other is perceived as very important (Doi, 1973).

As increasing numbers of the *nisei* generation entered adulthood, they sought ways to overcome the personal, economic, and legal barriers that their parents endured. For example, Japanese Americans were frequently prevented from buying homes in desirable parts of town, using public swimming pools,

and entering many professions (Kitano, 1976). The *nisei*, some of them recent college graduates but most still teenagers, wanted to prove their loyalty as Americans and thus combat anti-Japanese sentiment. Citizen organizations sprang up in various West Coast cities in the early 1920s. In 1930, the Japanese-American Citizens League became a national organization (Hosokawa, 1969). Some of the political clout of these organizations can be seen in the successful enactment of an amendment to the Cable Act to permit *nisei* girls who married alien Japanese to regain their citizenship. In addition, a bill was passed to allow foreign-born Oriental men who served in the U.S. armed forces in World War I to be granted citizenship. The passage of this bill enabled 700 *issei* to become naturalized citizens (Hosokawa, 1969). More recently, Congress has passed laws that specifically address repartition and repatriation of Japanese Americans interned during World War II (Daniels, 1991).

Family systems

Padilla, Wagatsuma, and Lindholm (1985) report that the Japanese social structure is "vertical," meaning that relationships are clearly defined to those above or below a clearly determined line of social status. In contrast, social structures in the United States have been described as more "horizontal," implying a differentiation among social classes.

For some Japanese Americans, the self is viewed as part of a set of interpersonal relationships of which the family system is the central core (Fugita, Ito, Abe, & Takeuchi, 1991). In this sense, the self is subordinate to the family social unit, and consequently most Japanese Americans find it difficult to stand out publicly as individuals. This difficulty is evidenced by the reluctance of some Japanese Americans to give speeches, talk about themselves in casual conversations, or engage in self-serving behaviors.

The Japanese emphasize collectivity, as evidenced by cooperative family effectiveness rather than by intrafamily lineal authority or filial piety (Caudill & Scarr, 1962). Fostering of *amae*, or 'interdependency', is also seen as a method of enhancing group solidarity and social relationships. This concept is also based on preservation of harmony and the suppression of conflict (Fugita, Ito, Abe, & Takeuchi, 1991). *Amae* (passive love), as defined by Doi (1962), means 'to depend and presume upon the benevolence of others' and is often associated with the Japanese word for 'sweet' *(amai)*. This relationship may also exist between two people. Some data indicate that this concept is significant for Japanese-American families living in the United States but not for African Americans, Hispanics, or White Americans (Kobayashi-Winata & Powers, 1989). In traditional U.S. society, assertiveness is seen by Americans as a characteristic of well-behaved children. For some Japanese-American parents, assertiveness is a characteristic of the poorly behaved child (Kobayashi-Winata & Powers, 1989).

The family is one of the most important factors in the lives of most Japanese Americans. The phrase *kodomo no tame ni* ('for the sake of the children') reflects the sacrifices and hardships families would endure to ensure the success of the next generation. Intergenerational relations are close as evidenced by the flow of food, money, help, and goods between generations. In Japanese-American families, contact with other family members occurs frequently.

On (a sense of obligation within the Japanese hierarchy) forms the basis of reciprocal relationships among peers and within social networks (Fugita, Ito, Abe, & Takeuchi, 1991). Intervention and assistance are taken for granted within the family, but casual help from strangers is usually avoided because of the concern of becoming entwined in reciprocal relationships with outsiders. The reluctance to receive help from social service agencies may reflect this value. Within the Japanese-American family, *on* is seen as a sacrifice of individual needs and personal goals for the sake of others in the family. Examples of this sacrifice are when a child cares for a parent or other elderly relative to the point of sacrificing financial security, career, or social stability and when the eldest child foregoes school to work in order to send the younger children to college.

According to Kitano (1969), Japanese families traditionally value authoritarian styles of leadership where the father makes unilateral family decisions. Sue (1983) described the family life-style of Chinese and Japanese Americans as patriarchal with authority and communication exercised from the top down. Sue (1983) also noted that within these families there is a need for interdependent roles, strict adherence to traditional norms, and minimization of conflict by suppression of overt emotion. The concepts or values related to guilt and shame may be used to control family members. For some Japanese-American families, family obligations take precedence over individual desires. Problems are generally handled within the family, and negative behaviors such as delinquency, school failure, unemployment, or mental illness are considered family failures that disrupt the desired harmony of family life and reflect badly on the family. Japanese-American individuals exhibit close contact among the generations. The care of the elderly is generally the responsibility of the oldest son or an unmarried child.

Active discouragement of verbal communication, avoidance of discussion of personal problems, and limited expression of emotion have also been noted as common patterns in the traditional Japanese family (McDermott, Tseng, & Maretzki, 1973). However, recent studies (Kobayashi-Winata & Powers, 1989; Morris, 1990) have found that a process of cultural change in family norms is becoming more prevalent across generations of Japanese Americans. Today, there is a tendency to adopt more Euro-American family norms and behaviors.

Parent-child interaction Methods of childcare are inextricably linked not only to tradition and customs of a culture but also to its systems of values. These methods appear to persist from generation to generation despite the acculturation process. Parent-child relationships in Japanese-American families tend to be intense, with open expressions of emotions displayed with the mother. There is much tolerance and permissiveness for the child until 5 or 6 years of age, at which time considerable emphasis is placed on the child learning emotional reserve and control. However, third-generation Japanese Americans have tended to adopt childrearing practices and attitudes of the contemporary American middle class (Kiefer, 1974: Strazar & Fisher, 1996).

In a classic study, Caudill and Frost (1974) compared the maternal and childcare habits of Japanese Americans with those of Japanese nationals to determine the effect on infant behavior. Findings from the study suggest that Japanese-American mothers have a closer behavioral style to Americans than to their Japanese national counterparts. The data also indicate that certain patterns of behavior from their Japanese cultural heritage were nevertheless retained by these Japanese Americans, who played with their babies for longer times, held their babies more often, and sang to their babies more often than their Japanese national counterparts did (Caudill & Frost, 1974).

In interviews conducted with Japanese Americans in California, Connor (1974) found that the *sansei* were more deferential, abrasive, and associative; were less dominant and less aggressive; had less need for heterosexuality; and had greater need for succor and order compared with Whites. These individuals also value the importance of family and the preservation of the *ie*, which, translated literally, means 'household'. However, it can also imply a continuum from past to future members (including the present generation, the dead, and the unborn, with a hierarchical structure with the father as head). Higa (1974) found that Japanese-American mothers who were born in the United States were more restrictive in childrearing behaviors than immigrant Japanese Americans were. In addition, Japanese American–born individuals tended to want their children to be obedient to authority rather than be independent and aggressive.

Johnson (1972) noted that for *nisei* and *sansei* Japanese Americans, specific cultural features of the family and ethnic community served to maintain boundaries of the group even over three generations and after 80 years of residency in Hawaii. Findings from this study were also suggestive that Japanese-American fathers were somewhat emotionally detached, aloof, and quiet in the home with prolonged periods of silence between father and child. Some evidence exists that *sansei* Japanese-American fathers are less authoritative than the *issei* fathers (Smith, 1976).

Notable differences were found in childrearing practices between Japanese and American parents (Kobayashi-Winata & Powers, 1989). The respondents in the study were Japanese businessmen who lived in Houston. Findings from the study were suggestive that Japanese parents were less likely than their American counterparts to report the use of external types of punishment, such as time-out or physically and socially punishing the child. A plausible explanation for these differences is the assimilation of American cultural values that place emphasis on independence and individuality. It is believed that insistence on individuality makes it necessary to use powerful, external techniques to ensure compliance in some situations (Kobayashi-Winata & Powers, 1989).

Strazar and Fisher (1996) note that, among Japanese Americans, abortion is not generally condoned but may not be uncommon for numerous reasons. First, some Japanese believe that an unwed mother brings great shame to the family. Second, in Japan there is a great emphasis on population control, and this value has been carried over into the Japanese-American culture. Third, adoption has become more common in recent times, and often some Japanese Americans will adopt a boy to carry on the family name (Strazar & Fisher, 1996).

Family role in education attainment

The model-minority thesis surfaced in the mid-1960s because of publicity regarding high educational attainment levels, high median family incomes, low crime rates, and absence of juvenile delinquency and mental health problems among Asian Americans (Petersen, 1966). Recently, Asian Americans have been portrayed as extraordinary achievers. Based on U.S. census data, Sue and Okazaki (1990) found Asians and Pacific-Islander Americans exceeded the national average for high school and college graduates with high rates of graduation from colleges and universities.

The popular cultural view that Asian-American family values and socialization account for educational attainment is supported primarily by anecdotal and observational evidence rather than by empirical findings (Sue & Okazaki, 1990). Mordkowitz and Ginsberg (1987) found that Japanese Americans often reported that their families emphasized educational accomplishment. As a result, these students held high expectations of themselves. More importantly, they were able to control behavior because of the direct relationship between appropriate behavior and personal achievement.

Dornbusch, Ritter, Leiderman, et al. (1987) found that Asian-American students came from families who exhibited strong authoritarian behaviors and permissiveness and weak authoritative characteristics, which was directly opposite of the family environments of White students. Asian-American parents were also reported to have a lower level of parental involvement compared with White parents. Findings from the study are suggestive that authoritarianism and permissiveness were inversely related, whereas parental involvement was directly related to academic achievements. Also, Asian-American responses were not significantly different from that of other groups regarding the value of working hard, parental pressures for academic achievement, need for students to make their parents proud of them, and most importantly avoiding embarrassment to the family. Significant group differences were noted in only one area. Asian Americans were more likely to believe that success in life depends on what is studied in school, which was directly related to the grades they received in high school. According to Sue and Okazaki (1990), a plausible explanation for this behavior is the belief held by some Asian Americans that educational attainment provides opportunities for upward mobility. To the extent that upward mobility is limited in noneducational avenues, education becomes increasingly important as a means for advancement. In addition, education is perceived by some Japanese Americans as a feasible means for mobility in view of limitations for success in other areas. Sue and Okazaki (1990) concluded that the effects of culture have been confused with the consequences of society while continuing to play an important role in achievement.

Many Asian immigrants came to the United States to obtain a better education for their children. For many Asian Americans, immigration was a great sacrifice because of downward occupation mobility (Chan, 1991). Nonetheless, the sacrifice was considered necessary because many Asian Americans generally think in terms of the family and not of the individual. In this context, they are often willing to sacrifice their own socioeconomic standing in exchange for giving the next generation a better chance to "make it," or be successful in the world.

Religion

Some of the ingrained cultural values evident in Japanese Americans are derived from Zen Buddhism, Confucianism, and Shintoism. Today, these values are seemingly manifested in Japanese Americans whether they practice Catholicism, Buddhism, Protestantism, or another religion. From the earliest immigrants, who came from mostly Buddhist backgrounds, the Japanese tended to adopt the religion of the area in which they lived, which resulted in divergent religious beliefs and practices among Japanese Americans in different locales. Religion and the church have both played an important role in acculturating the Japanese within their communities (Sato & Takano, 1983).

Implications for nursing care

Because many Japanese Americans place a high value on the family system, the nurse should be aware of the significant role the family plays in providing support, interdependence, and the fulfillment of duties. Respect is also greatly valued, and the linear relationship apparent in families and in casual relationships should be maintained and supported when providing care for the Japanese-American client and family support system. Although these values are the strength of the Japanese-American family, they can create stress and disharmony not only for the client but also for the family unit. It is essential for the nurse to remember that some Japanese-American families may want to provide support to the hospitalized family member by keeping a bedside vigil, especially if the individual is elderly and doing poorly. Married men, especially *nisei* and *issei* Japanese Americans, may expect their wives to serve in the traditional caretaker role. Therefore the wife (or daughter) may be expected to be available at the bedside so that the client does not have to bother the nurses, especially with intimate care or requests for assistance. The nurse must be alert to the overextension and lack of self-care of family members in providing for the client. The nurse should make every effort to assist the family to identify resources, both financial and human, to reduce the stress created when a family member is ill. In addition, the family should be assured that they are not alone. Because family name and honor are important for this group, the nurse should be especially cognizant of the issue of confidentiality and respect. Information should not be shared with outsiders, even with extended family members who may appear close to the client. Information concerning illness is often kept within the immediate family.

Shintoism and Buddhism is suscribed to by more than 80% of the Japanese culture. Christianity is also well established in Japan. In the United States, a great number of Japanese Americans are Christians. Nonetheless, funerals for some Japanese Americans despite this Christian orientation are likely to be Buddhistic, particularly for the *issei* and the *nisei*. In addition, for some Japanese Americans, births and marriages are often colored by Shinto rituals but to a lesser extent for *yonsei* and *gosei* (Strazar & Fisher, 1996).

TIME

In a classic 1962 study, Caudill and Scarr examined Kluckhohn's value orientations in Tokyo area high schools and concluded that time orientations differed by context, with a future focus in technology and a present focus in social relations. The greatest number of generational changes in these values occurred in political considerations, whereas the smallest number occurred in the religious area. In contrast, Chang (1981) believed that this future orientation originated from a religious philosophical view of life. Buddhism teaches that death in all living things is inevitable. People are instructed not to make plans in this world without reckoning with death. According to Sato and Takano (1983), time is considered valuable and must be used wisely. The *issei* use the term "waste time" to describe inefficiency or trivial matters. Hard work in the present is seen as important for future successes.

Decisions are not necessarily made in relation to individual needs or benefits. Sato and Takano (1983) state that the *issei* perception of time was related to death, in which death is seen as continuous and suprapersonal. This view is in stark contrast to the Western view of death as personal and discontinuous. Depending on the degree of acculturation, the *nisei* also accept death more readily than the *sansei* and the *yonsei*, who are more like Americans in their attitudes toward death and time.

Implications for nursing care

Because Japanese Americans are both present and future oriented, the nurse must consider the context of the current situation. The Japanese-American client is usually prompt and adheres to fixed schedules. However, Japanese-American clients tend to be more prompt with persons they hold in high regard such as physicians than with persons not held in high regard. They generally follow directions regarding medications and treatments. Because of future orientation regarding their children, care must be taken regarding their diet and health. Japanese Americans will work hard with little regard for their health in the hope that future generations will have a better life.

ENVIRONMENTAL CONTROL
Locus of control

The value of stoicism enables some Japanese Americans to avoid embarrassing themselves through loss of control or signs of weakness or inadequacy. Padilla, Wagatsuma, and Lindholm (1985) found that *issei* Japanese-American students believe that they have an external locus of control. In contrast, *sansei* and later-generation students indicated an internal locus-of-control. *Nisei* students were in between an external and an internal locus of control. Ho (1976) noted that the external locus of control in the Japanese-American population was fatalistic, which allowed them equanimity and acceptance without question of life as it unfolds.

Illness and wellness behaviors and folk medicine

Major beliefs that have contributed to medicine in Japan influence the Japanese-American persons' view of health and illness. In the Shinto religion, people are seen as inherently good. Evil is caused by outside spirits who cause humans to succumb to temptation and harm, which can be alleviated through purification rites. Disease is believed to be caused by contact with polluting agents, such as blood, corpses, and skin diseases, which accounts for the emphasis on cleanliness (Strazar & Fisher, 1996; Sato & Takano, 1983).

Another important belief held by some Japanese Americans is based on the traditional Chinese belief of harmony and balance among oneself, society, and the universe. Some Japanese Americans believe disharmony (with society or family) or imbalance (as from lack of sleep or exercise or because of poor diet) can cause disease. Therefore restoration of balance should be the major focus of treatment. In addition, some Japanese Americans believe that illness may cause energy to slow or stop along the meridians of the body. Thus acupuncture, acupressure, massage, or moxibustion may be used to restore the flow of energy (Sato & Takano, 1983).

The *kampō* ('Chinese medicine') medical system was developed around the belief that forces of the universe affect an individual's body processes and activities. Health depends on maintaining a harmonious relationship with the universe. *Kampō* practitioners believe that dietary precautions and preventive measures help resist illness (Ishihara, 1962; Strazar & Fisher, 1996).

Certain foods have special symbolic meaning for Japanese Americans. Herbal decoctions or special foods such as soft boiled rice and *miso* soup (a soup made with fermented soybean paste) may be eaten during illness as well as to promote good health. Traditionally, on their most important holiday, New Year's Day, most Japanese Americans eat special foods that have symbolic meaning for good health, prosperity, and happiness. Such foods include *kazu-no-ko* (dried herring roe) for fertility, *mochi* (steamed rice cake) for longevity and prosperity, *soba* (buckwheat needles) served in clear broth for longevity and prosperity, and *kuromame* (black beans) for good health (Corum, 1983; Engle, 1993). Other symbolic foods include *ozoni* (a clear soup with *mochi* and vegetables) for prosperity, *gobō* (burdock) symbolic for deep family roots, and *tai* (sea bream, a large red fish served whole) for happy occasions.

Although Asian medical traditions recently have regained popularity with the holistic and preventive health movement, most Japanese Americans tend to rely on Western medicine. Some use both Oriental and Western medicine, depending on the illness and the efficacy of Western medicine. Yet for those who still subscribe to the Old-World traditional health care practices bought with them from Japan, the basis for health practices may include a mixture of traditional medical practices *(kampō)* brought to Japan from China, Shinto beliefs, and Western medical practices (Strazar & Fisher, 1996)

Implications for nursing care

Because some Japanese Americans hold traditional value orientations regarding fatalism, they often are perceived as having an external locus of control. The nurse must focus on primary prevention methods to prevent illnesses and maintain health. Health teaching and plans for a health regimen should consider the values germane to a culture that subscribes to an external locus of control. The nurse must also remember that some Japanese Americans value self-control, particularly in areas they believe may reflect weakness or inadequacy. The loss of "face" and dignity should be especially maintained in procedures and treatment.

The nurse should inquire about treatments the client is using at home and what measures are most helpful. Special foods, tea, or herbal decoctions may be important for the client to have if there are no contraindications. It is very common for family or friends to bring fruits or special Japanese food when visiting. The client and family are likely to show hospitality by offering food to the nurse and visitors. Although it is unusual for the family and the client to hold special religious ceremonies at the bedside, privacy will be needed if such ceremonies are held.

BIOLOGICAL VARIATIONS
Body size

Japanese Americans tend to be of smaller stature than their White counterparts. However, rapid westernization has brought major changes in diet and life-style. As a result, the height of the average Japanese male has increased 4 inches (with an average height of 5 feet, 8 inches). Likewise, the height of the average Japanese female has increased 2.7 inches over the last 30 years. Given this pattern of growth, it is expected that within 10 years Japanese Americans may be as tall as their American peers (Reid, 1993; Overfield, 1995).

Data from a classic study done by Roche, Roberts, and Hamill (1978) indicate that Japanese and Chinese children raised in the United States had delayed skeletal maturation rates compared with their American counterparts. Despite this finding, these children were more skeletally mature than their counterparts who lived in China and Japan. In body proportions, Japanese, like other Asian Americans, tend to have longer trunks and shorter limbs than White Americans have. They also tend to have wide hips and narrow shoulders (Overfield, 1995).

Skin color

Skin color varies among Japanese Americans. Some Japanese Americans have more yellow tone than others. One can assess jaundice by looking at the sclerae of the eyes. The amount of sun exposure can make a noticeable difference in the skin color of the same individual.

Other visible physical characteristics

Mongolian spots (bluish pigment from fetal migratory melanocytes) found generally in the lumbosacral region are present in 80% of Orientals at birth. They can often be mistaken for bruises (Jacobs & Walton, 1976; Overfield, 1995). Other areas of the skin such as nipples, areolae, scrotum, and labia majora are affected by hormones and as a result are often darker in Oriental groups than in Whites (Overfield, 1995). Keloid formation varies among Japanese Americans but is greater in this group than in White Americans. Keloid formations can be cause for concern in highly visible areas.

Enzymatic and genetic variations

Lactose intolerance occurs in a majority of the population of the world. In fact, it affects 94% of Asians, 74% of American Blacks, 79% of Native Americans, and only 17% of White Americans (Overfield, 1995; Bose & Welsh, 1973; Duncan & Scott, 1972; McCracken, 1971). The time when symptoms are first noted and the ability to consume or tolerate different amounts of milk or milk products can vary (Caskey, Payne-Bose, Welsh, et al., 1977; Lebenthal, Antonowicz, & Schwachman, 1975; Simoons, 1969).

Japanese have a higher incidence of cleft lip and cleft palate compared with the general U.S. population (Chung & Myrianthopoulos, 1968; Erickson, 1976). When the nurse provides care for a Japanese American with these anomalies, it is essential to remember that these conditions require additional attention through culturally appropriate teaching and risk-reduction strategies.

Drug interactions and metabolism

In tuberculosis therapy involving isoniazid, 85% to 90% of Asians rapidly inactivate the drug, compared with 40% of White Americans and 60% of American Blacks (Vessel, 1972). Asian clients must be carefully monitored when taking this drug to determine its efficacy.

Succinylcholine, a muscle relaxant used during surgery, is inactivated by the enzyme pseudocholinesterase. Asians are at risk for having pseudocholinesterase deficiency and thus may suffer prolonged muscle paralysis and inability to breathe after administration of the drug (Overfield, 1995; Kalow, 1972).

Genetic and physiological studies have found that Asian clients display more side effects to antipsychotic medication than their White Americans or American Black counterparts (Binder & Levy, 1981). In addition, they require significantly lower doses of antipsychotic medication to control symptoms (Lin & Finder, 1983; Yamamoto, Fung, Lo, & Reece, 1979). Another notable finding concerns flushing after ingesting alcohol (Kitano, Hatanaka, Yeung, & Sue, 1985; Wilson, McClearn, & Johnson, 1978). Evidence indicates that for some Asian Americans flushing after alcohol ingestion may not be a result of diet, experience with alcohol, or cultural values. Physiological changes noted after alcohol ingestion include faster metabolism, differences in pulse pressure, and increase in heart rate (Sue, 1987). Because of discrepancies noted in the findings relative to the influence of genetic and physiological factors on alcohol consumption, an accurate assessment of their roles cannot be determined at this time (Sue, 1987).

Susceptibility to disease

There are equal incidences of blood types A, B, and O found among Japanese Americans, with type AB found in only about 10% of Japanese Americans. Statistically, persons with type O blood are at greater risk for duodenal ulcers, whereas persons with type A blood are more likely to develop cancer of the stomach (Overfield, 1995).

Cancer of the stomach, esophagus, and liver occurs more frequently among Japanese Americans than among their White counterparts (Overfield, 1995; Rhoads, Glober, & Stemmerman, 1991; Tominaga, 1985). It is believed that eating dried salted fish is a predisposing factor for gastric cancer (Nomura, 1982; Nomura, Stemmerman, & Heilbrun, 1985). In addition, diets high in salt-cured foods and nitrites and poor in vitamin C intake have been commonly associated with greater incidence of stomach cancer. Also, drinking hot tea may contribute to the development of esophageal cancer. In recent years Japanese Americans have experienced an increased incidence of breast, prostate, and colorectal cancer (Locke & King, 1980), which has been correlated to the adoption of a Western diet and life-style.

In an age-specific comparison of hip fracture incidence among Japanese in Oahu, Hawaii, and Okinawa, Japan, and Whites in Rochester, Minnesota, hip fracture rates of Japanese in Hawaii and Japan were found to be only half that of the rate of their White counterparts. Further research is needed to pinpoint the reasons for this significant difference (Ross, Horimatsu, Davis, et al., 1991).

Kawasaki syndrome, or mucocutaneous lymph node syndrome, a disease first described in Japan and later in Hawaii, has been observed primarily in children of Japanese ancestry. This condition has been managed by medications but is often accompanied by a variety of complications of the cardiovascular system (Dean, Melish, Hicks, & Palumbo, 1982).

Pockets of high incidences of diabetes and obesity have been noted among the Japanese in Hawaii (Kawate, Miyanishi, Yamakido, & Nishimoto, 1978). These higher incidences may be a result of a combination of diet and life-style.

Longitudinal research noting the incidence of coronary heart disease has been conducted on the Japanese in Japan, in Hawaii, and on the U.S. mainland. The mortality from coronary heart disease (as well as breast and colon cancer) has been attributed to variations in diets and life-styles of Asian, Hawaiian, and mainland Japanese. Coronary artery mortality is lowest in Japan, intermediate in Hawaii, and highest on the U.S. mainland (Reed, McGee, Cohen, et al., 1982; Yano, Reed, & McGee, 1984).

Cerebrovascular disease mortality appears to be opposite that for coronary artery disease. There is a higher incidence in Japan, an intermediate incidence in Hawaii, and the lowest incidence on the U.S. mainland (Syme, Marmot, Kagun, et al., 1975; Yano, Reed, & Kagan, 1985).

Nutritional preferences and deficiencies

The Japanese place great importance on the presentation of food. For these individuals, food should be visually appealing. Color, contrast, and shapes of food are considered as important as the cooking and seasoning of a particular food. Unlike American meals that are centered around one main dish, Japanese meals usually consist of several small dishes (Corum, 1983; Giger & Davidhizar, 1990). A Japanese-American family that has been acculturated may serve a mixture of American and Japanese dishes.

Traditionally, food was cooked on a small grill by broiling, steaming, frying, or simmering. Food was cut so that it cooked quickly and evenly, preserving vitamins. Meat, which is expensive in Japan, is frequently eaten with vegetables. Traditionally, the main sources of protein were fish and soybean. *Tōfu,* a soybean product, is used extensively as a dish by itself or mixed with other dishes. The main source of carbohydrate is rice or noodles. A seasoning used extensively is soy sauce, which is high in sodium. Another flavoring, which has been losing popularity, is *aji-no-moto* (monosodium glutamate). Pickled vegetables and unsweetened green tea complete a meal. *Sake,* or rice wine, is sometimes served. Milk is often included in the diet of children but less often for adults, a finding that may be related to the high incidence of lactose intolerance in the population. The traditional diet is nutritious and low in fat but tends to be high in sodium. In Hawaii, Japanese dishes tend to be sweetened more than they are in Japan. Most Japanese Americans also consume popular American foods such as pizzas, tacos, and hamburgers.

Psychological characteristics

Cultural values related to self The concept of *enryo* emphasizes modesty, respect, and deference toward others. *Enryo* is related to *hazukashii,* the implicit fear of being ridiculed, which results in feelings of embarrassment and reticence. *Hige* is the concept of denigration of self and others (Kitano, 1970). These concepts emphasize conformity to group norms, and minimization of accomplishments (Fugita, Ito, Abe, & Takeuchi, 1991). *Gaman* refers to internalization and suppression of anger and emotion. Avoidance of confrontation and acceptances of the results of negative social interactions can be related to *gaman.*

Leong (1986) found that Asian Americans have a lower tolerance for ambiguity. Findings from this study also indicate that Asian Americans are more likely to prefer structured situations. They tend to want practical and immediate solutions to their problems (Leong, 1986). Further findings from this study are suggestive that Asian Americans are more likely to show respect for authority figures and are less likely to express their emotions. Leong (1986) concludes that Asian Americans are more likely to avoid having to express themselves verbally.

Emotional and behavioral manifestation of stress The length of residence in a new environment and generational status of an individual are important factors in determining levels of stress perceived by an ethnic group undergoing acculturation (Padilla, Wagatsuma, & Lindholm, 1985). Examining variables such as generational status, acculturation level, and personality variables, Padilla, Wagatsuma, and Lindholm (1985) found that *issei* Japanese immigrants reported the most stress and were the most externally controlled. A plausible reason for acculturation stress is the disparity noted between culture and expected individual behavior. It is interesting to note that *sansei* and later-generation students scored lower on stress, higher on self-esteem, and higher on internal locus of control. Differences in scores also indicated that *nisei* individuals may be in transition from traditional values held by their parents to values held by some Japanese Americans belonging to *sansei* or later generations.

Mental health According to Atkinson and Matsushita (1991) there is considerable evidence to indicate that Asian Americans utilize mental health services less frequently than White Americans do (President's Commission on Mental Health, 1978). Those who do use mental health services drop out at a significantly higher rate than White American clients do (Sue, 1987; Yamamoto, James, & Palley, 1968). Atkinson and Matsushita (1991) found *sansei* and *yonsei* Japanese Americans rated Japanese-American counselors as more attractive than White-American counselors when portraying a directive counseling style but less attractive when portraying a nondirective counseling style. This theory supports an earlier study (Atkinson, Maruyama, & Matsui, 1978) that found that Asian Americans demonstrated a preference for an ethnically similar counselor and a directive counseling style.

Rogers and Izutsu (1980) found that Japanese Americans had low rates of treatment from mental health services. In addition, they rarely sought hospitalization for mental disorders. Individuals who did seek professional help had more severe and advanced symptoms that required longer hospitalizations. They concluded that families probably attempted home care of these relatives as long as possible because of the shame involved in having a mentally ill family member. Mental illness is seen as a stigma and reflects poorly on the family name and honor. For some Japanese Americans, any defect, whether physical, cognitive, or emotional, is seen as deviant and nonconforming and is not generally mentioned outside the family.

Internment trauma For Japanese Americans, the imprisonment of 120,000 men, women, and children in internment camps by the United States government during World War II represents the most traumatic and salient episode of the past (Nagata, 1991).

Over 60% of those persons incarcerated were U.S. citizens. No formal charges were ever brought against them, yet they had no opportunity for a trial. In many cases, they were given less than a week's notice to move and to sell their businesses, personal property, and other personal possessions. In many instances, they were unable to sell these items or were forced to sell them for much less than their actual value, which resulted in severe economic hardship. Many were forced to move twice, first to temporary assembly centers in animal stalls at horse tracks and fairgrounds and later to internment camps in isolated areas. They lived 2 to 3 years in camps enclosed by barbed wire and armed guards. In addition, there was the psychological degradation associated with being accused of disloyalty (Nagata, 1991).

Many of these individuals believed they were victimized and rejected by their own country of citizenship (Nagata, 1991). Even today, transgenerational effects of victimization are still seen in descendants of individuals who suffered through this ordeal. Nagata (1991) found transgenerational effects of internment trauma were particularly evident in the *sansei*. Many of these individuals reported their parents maintained a silence about their experience in the camps. This lack of communication between generations about the experience further inhibited communication within some families and created secrecy about the internment. For many *sansei*, lack of knowledge created a sense of vulnerability and fear that their rights as U.S. citizens might be violated again (Nagata, 1991).

Somatization and folk traditions According to Fujii, Fukushima, and Yamamoto (1993), folk healing is often used to treat physical ailments because Asians tend to express emotional illness or distress through physical symptoms. Being "ill" is a legitimate, socially acceptable manner of receiving care. For some Japanese Americans, complaints are usually physical (Rogers & Izutsu, 1980). Kitano (1969) noted that Japanese people tend to worry needlessly about body functions and are usually obsessed about a potential problem related to their blood pressure.

Tracey, Leong, and Glidden (1986) found that Asian-American students appear to find it more ac-ceptable to react to emotional difficulties by focusing on academic and vocational concerns. When counseling was sought, Japanese-American students tended to focus more on academic difficulties than on emotional conflict.

For some Canadian Japanese, there was a stigmatism associated with mental illness. Many believed that mental illness was inherited, contagious, or incurable. These individuals viewed the psychiatrist as someone who treated only severe mental illnesses. For many of these individuals, very little interest was taken in psychotherapy and psychodynamics (Isomura, Fine, & Lin, 1987). Biological treatment methods were viewed as being more helpful than psychiatric intervention (Isomura, Fine, & Lin, 1987).

Degree of acculturation and somatization of symptoms by the Japanese was investigated by Tanaka-Matsumi and Marsella (1976). They found that among Japanese nationals, the word "headache" was associated with depression, whereas Japanese Americans and White Americans associated the word "loneliness" with depression.

Psychopharmacology Several studies have suggested that Japanese Americans do well on lower dosages of psychotropic medication for depression or mania (Yamamoto, 1982; Yamamoto, Fung, Lo, & Reece, 1979). Additionally, these individuals tend to need significantly lower maintenance dosages (Roseblat & Tang, 1987). Evidence also indicates that Japanese Americans need less maximum and stabilizing dosages for chlorpromazine. Although Japanese Americans tend to need lower dosages of psychotropic drugs, they are at risk for extrapyramidal symptoms because the drugs remain in the blood longer (Kalow, 1986; Lin, Poland, Nuccio, et al., 1989; Lin & Finder, 1983).

Alcohol use Japanese Americans appear to have lower rates of alcoholism than the rest of the U.S. population have. Some researchers believe that these lower rates may be attributed to a variety of factors such as (1) being shielded by their families, (2) seeking treatment only during the late stages of alcoholism, and (3) seeking assistance from other sources rather than state mental health facilities (Kotani, 1982). Because of these factors, it is extremely difficult to determine an accurate rate for alcoholism in this ethnic group. The untreated case method would give a better estimate of the severity of alcohol abuse in this group. This method is based on the obtainment of information on patterns of use among the general population. In a survey of untreated case methods, Sue (1987) concluded that Asian Americans are less likely than other groups to seek treatment for alcoholism. Findings from this study also indicate that although these individuals are more likely to abstain from alcohol use than other ethnic and racial groups, among those who drink heavily, Japanese American men tend to drink more than their female counterparts do (Sue, 1987).

Implications for nursing care

It is important for the nurse to teach and counsel clients about diseases common among Japanese Americans. In addition, preventive health care techniques should be emphasized. To provide culturally appropriate and competent care, the nurse must engage the support of other family members. To reduce chronicity and severity of hypertension, the nurse must stress to the client and the family the importance of limiting use of soy sauce. Because somatization is a problem among some Japanese Americans, the nurse must recognize that frequent physical ailments may be possible signs of underlying stress. Meaning must be attached to behavior if the client is to receive optimal care. It is also essential to identify previous successful strategies in order to assist the client to develop and refine coping strategies. To reduce stress, the nurse might suggest exercise because it may be perceived by the client as a nonconfrontational form of release.

It is essential for the nurse to remember that some Japanese Americans generally do not seek or delay seeking professional help for mental health problems. Of those individuals who do seek treatment, many generally do not complete treatment (Leong, 1986). Kitano (1969) speculated that the reluctance to seek treatment may be a result of several factors, including (1) strength of the family and community and the family's ability to control and hide problem behaviors, (2) different cultural styles of expressing problems, (3) inappropriateness of current therapeutic organizations, and (4) lack of relevant connections to the therapeutic community. Another factor may be related to the inability of the therapist to provide culturally responsive forms of treatment (Sue, 1987). Additionally, some Japanese Americans will look first to their families when they have emotional problems to maintain family honor (Atkinson & Matsushita, 1991; Leong, 1986). Therefore, the major goal of nursing care should be aimed at developing a trusting relationship between the nurse and the client.

SUMMARY

Japanese Americans vary in their degree of acculturation. Because of this diversification, Japanese Americans may present in the clinical setting with a variety of behaviors depending on factors such as generational, regional, and individual differences. The nurse must assess the unique needs of each individual and the extent to which the information presented applies to that person or family. The importance of establishing a trusting relationship based on respect and open communication with the client and the family cannot be underestimated.

Case Study

Mr. Robert Kiyoshi Yamamoto, a 71-year-old retired *nisei* electrician, was admitted to the hospital with complaints of nausea and difficulty keeping food down related to recurrent colon cancer with liver metastasis. For the past few weeks, Mr. Yamamoto's appetite has been steadily decreasing. His wife of 50 years states that he has been unable to keep any solid foods down but has been able to drink some fluids.

After a few days of nasogastric decompression, Mr. Yamamoto's bowel function begins to return. He is able to eat small amounts of soft foods. Because the tumor has spread despite chemotherapy,

Case Study—cont'd

Mr. Yamamoto has decided against further chemotherapy. As he becomes weaker and weaker, Mr. Yamamoto insists that his wife remain at his bedside so that he "doesn't have to bother the nurses for little things." Mrs. Yamamoto has kept a bedside vigil and rarely leaves except to go home to shower while one of three daughters stays with her father.

The nurse notices that Mrs. Yamamoto is looking tired and appears to be losing weight. Her daughters have tried to relieve their mother at night so that she can rest at home, but she insists that "Dad is restless and calls out in the night for me." Mr. Yamamoto insists that she bathe him and assist him to the bathroom. One daughter flew in from out of town to assist indefinitely if needed. All daughters take turns in keeping their mother company or relieving her when she goes home to shower or cook special foods for her husband.

Although he never says he is having pain, Mr. Yamamoto has family members constantly massaging his back and legs. He moves cautiously and winces with each movement. Mr. Yamamoto does not talk much to the staff. He lets his family talk for him. He denies pain when asked by the nurse, but tells his family otherwise. He does not sleep well.

Mr. Yamamoto's current treatment is primarily supportive care. He is constantly requesting special Japanese foods such as sushi and miso soup, which the family brings in daily. Generally, he just tastes it. The hospital staff has brought up the possibility of hospice care. A family meeting to discuss discharge plans was called by his son. Mr. Yamamoto has stated he wants to go home.

CARE PLAN

 Nursing Diagnosis Altered family processes, related to situational crisis

Client Outcomes

1. Family devises a specific rotation plan to meet each other's need for rest and support while caring for their father.
2. Family will demonstrate mutual support and cohesion.

Nursing Interventions

1. Provide empathy and support for the immediate family members who need to be at the bedside by providing family with liberal visitation, adequate space for members who stay overnight, and privacy.
2. Keep family abreast of current treatments and nature of illness to dispel any misunderstandings and to keep lines of communication open between family and staff.
3. Assess family members for signs of fatigue or overextension.
4. Explore with family members other possible extended family members or friends who would be willing and be accepted by client to keep him company or support his wife.

 Nursing Diagnosis Pain, related to cancer metastasis

Client Outcomes

1. Client will indicate to family that the pain is tolerable.
2. Client will be able to sleep 4 hours at a time at night.

Nursing Interventions

1. Observe nonverbal behaviors that indicate pain, such as wincing with movement and restlessness at night.
2. Check with family about how much pain client is having with the current treatment.
3. Give analgesic on a regular schedule without waiting for him to ask (unless refused), especially before sleep.

Nursing Diagnosis Risk for ineffective family coping, related to deteriorating course of disease of a family member

Client Outcomes

1. Family unit will use own resources and explore outside resources.
2. Family will devise realistic expectations of roles of members.
3. Open communication is maintained among family members.
4. Family members will perform care without compromising their own physical and emotional health.

Nursing Interventions

1. Develop trusting and respectful relationships with client and family.
2. Encourage the son to call family meetings as needed to discuss realistic plans and expectations of members, using health care providers as needed.
3. Assist and encourage family to explore outside resources as well as family resources to assist in dealing with the crisis.
4. Assess if basic physical and emotional needs of client and family members are being met.
5. Encourage family members to support each other, especially Mrs. Yamamoto, and devise a schedule that does not compromise their physical and emotional health.
6. Continue to monitor ability of family members to carry out treatment regimen and care.
7. Discuss management of emotional outbursts, personality changes, and mood swings with family members or those providing care.
8. Encourage realistic expectations of role performance, especially by Mrs. Yamamoto.
9. Teach coping strategies to manage tension and strain if previous techniques are no longer effective.
10. Help with identification of current stressors and strains.

STUDY QUESTIONS

1. List the important cultural values that determine health-seeking and health-practice behaviors in this cultural group.
2. Identify three interventions that incorporate these values in treating the Japanese-American client.
3. Analyze different strategies useful in communicating with the Japanese-American family.
4. Discuss the importance of understanding generational, geographical, and acculturation issues in working with the Japanese-American client.
5. Describe appropriate interventions by health care providers for clients who do not verbally express pain, discomfort, or stress.

References

Atkinson, D.R., Maruyama, M., & Matsui, S. (1978). The effects of counselor race and counseling approach on Asian Americans' perceptions of counselor credibility and utility. *Journal of Counseling Psychology, 25,* 76-83.

Atkinson, D.R., & Matsushita, Y. (1991). JapaneseAmerican acculturation, counseling style, counselor ethnicity, and perceived counselor credibility. *Journal of Counseling Psychology, 38,* 473-478.

Baker, J. (1993). *Perceptions of privacy in Japan and America.* Paper presented at the East West Center, Honolulu, Hawaii.

Barnlund, D.C. (1989). Public-private self in communication with Japan. *Business Horizons, 32,* 32-35.

Basch, P. (1990). *Textbook of international health.* New York: Oxford University Press.

Binder, R.L., & Levy, R. (1981). Extrapyramidal reactions in Asians. *American Journal of Psychiatry, 138*(9), 1243-1244.

Bose, D., & Welsh, J. (1973). Lactose malabsorption in Oklahoma Indians. *American Journal of Clinical Nutrition, 26,* 1320-1322.

Burris, J. (1993, March 21). 442nd vets "shared a tent" in battle, in politics. *The Honolulu Advertiser,* p. B-1.

Caskey, D.A., Payne-Bose, D., Welsh, J.D., et al. (1977). Effects of age on lactose malabsorption in Oklahoma Native Americans as determined by breath H_2 analysis. *American Journal of Digestive Disease, 22*(2), 113-116.

Caudill, W., & Frost, L. (1974). A comparison of maternal care and infant behavior in Japanese American, American, and Japanese families. In Lebra, W.P. (Ed.), *Youth, socialization and mental health: mental health research in Asia and the Pacific* (vol. 3). Honolulu: University of Hawaii Press.

Caudill, W., & Scarr, H.A. (1962). Japanese value orientations and culture change. *Ethnology, 1,* 53-91.

Chan, S. (1991). *Asian Americans: an interpretive history.* Boston: Twayne Publishers.

Chang, B. (1981). Asian American patient care. In Henderson, G., & Primeaux, M. (Eds.), *Transcultural health care.* Menlo Park, Calif.: Addison-Wesley.

Chang, T. (1993, March 21). A legacy of bravery: the 442nd comes home. *The Honolulu Advertiser,* 442nd Special Section, p. 4.

Chung, C.S., & Myrianthopoulos, N.C. (1968). Racial and prenatal factors in major congenital malformations. *American Journal of Human Genetics, 20,* 44-60.

Connor, J. (1974). Acculturation and family continuity in three generations of Japanese Americans. *Journal of Marriage and Family, 36,* 159-168.

Corum, A.K. (1983). *Ethnic foods of Hawaii.* Honolulu: The Bess Press.

Daniels, R. (1991). Redressed achieved, 1983-1990. In Daniels, R., Taylor, S.C., & Kitano, H.H.L. (Eds.), *Japanese Americans: from relocation to redress* (pp. 219-223). Seattle: University of Washington Press.

Daniels, R., Taylor, S.C., & Kitano, H.H.L. (Eds.) (1991). *Japanese Americans: from relocation to redress.* Seattle: University of Washington Press.

Dean, A.G., Melish, M.E., Hicks, R., & Palumbo, N.E. (1982). An epidemic of Kawasaki syndrome in Hawaii. *Journal of Pediatrics, 100*(4), 552-557.

Doi, L.T. (1962). *Amae:* a key concept for understanding Japanese personality structure. In Smith, R.J., & Beardsley, R.K. (Eds.), *Japanese culture: its development and characteristics.* Chicago: Aldine Publishing.

Doi, L.T. (1973). *The anatomy of dependence.* New York: Kodansha International Ltd.

Dornbusch, S.M., Ritter, P.L., Leiderman, P.H., et al. (1987). The relation of parenting style to adolescent school performance. *Child Development, 55,* 1244-1257.

Duncan, I., & Scott, E. (1972). Lactose intolerance in Alaskan Indians and Eskimos. *American Journal of Clinical Nutrition, 25,* 867-868.

The Economist Business Traveller's Guides (1987). *The economist publication.* New York: Prentice-Hall.

Embree, J.F. (1939). *Suye Mura, a Japanese village.* Chicago: The University of Chicago Press.

Engle, M. (1993, Jan. 4). Japanese New Year's customs demystified. *Star-Bulletin,* p. A-4.

Erickson, J.D. (1976). Racial variations in the incidence of congenital malformations. *Annals of Human Genetics, 39,* 315-320.

Fisher, N. (1996). *Cultural and ethnic diversity: a guide for genetic professionals.* Baltimore, Md.: Johns Hopkins University Press.

Fugita, S., Ito, K.L., Abe, J., & Takeuchi, D.T. (1991). Japanese Americans. In Mokuau, N. (Ed.), *Handbook for social services for Asian and Pacific Islanders* (pp. 61-77). New York: Greenwood Press.

Fujii, J., Fukushima, S., & Yamamoto, J. (1993). Psychiatric care of Japanese Americans. In Gaw, A.C. (Ed.), *Culture, ethnicity and mental illness* (pp. 305-346). Washington, D.C.: American Psychiatric Press.

Galanti, G.A. (1991). *Caring for patients from different cultures: case studies from American hospitals.* Philadelphia: University of Pennsylvania Press.

Giger, J.N., & Davidhizar, R.E. (1990). Transcultural nursing: a method for advancing nursing care and practices. *International Congress of Nursing Review, 37*(1), 199-202.

Hall, E.T. (1966). *The silent language.* Westport, Conn.: Greenwood Press.

Hall, E.T. (1976). *Beyond culture.* New York: Doubleday.

Hashizume S., & Takano, J. (1993). Nursing care of Japanese American patients. In Orque, M.S., Bloch, B., & Monrroy, L.S.A. (Eds.), *Ethnic nursing care: a multicultural approach* (pp. 219-243). St. Louis: Mosby.

Higa, M. (1974). A comparative study of 3 groups of Japanese mothers' attitudes toward childrearing. In Lebra, W.P. (Ed.), *Youth, socialization, and mental health.* Honolulu: University of Hawaii Press.

Ho, M.K. (1976). Social work with Asian Americans. *Social Casework, 57,* 195-201.

Hosokawa, G. (1969). *Nisei: the quiet Americans.* New York: William Morrow.

Houston, J.W., & Houston, J.D. (1973). *Farewell to Manzanar.* Boston, Mass.: Houghton Mifflin Co.

Information Please Almanac (1998). Boston: Houghton-Mifflin.

Ishihara, A. (1962). *Kampo:* Japan's traditional medicine. *Japan Quarterly, 9,* 429-437.

Ishii, S. (1987). *Nonverbal communication in Japan* (Orientation Seminars on Japan, No. 28). Tokyo: Office for the Japanese Studies Center.

Isomura, T., Fine, S., & Lin, T.Y. (1987). Two Japanese families: a cultural perspective. *Canadian Journal of Psychiatry, 32,* 282-286.

Jacobs, A.H., & Walton, R.G. (1976). Incidence of birthmarks in the neonate. *Pediatrics, 58,* 218-222.

Johnson, C. (1972). *The Japanese-American family and community in Honolulu: generational continuities in ethnic affiliation.* Doctoral dissertation in anthropology, Syracuse University, Syracuse, New York.

Johnson, F.A., Marsella, A.J., & Johnson, C.L. (1974). Social and psychological aspects of verbal behavior in Japanese Americans. *American Journal of Psychiatry, 131,* 580-583.

Kakesako, G.K. (1993, March 19). *Nisei* proved their loyalty on the war front. *The Honolulu Star-Bulletin,* p. A-1.

Kalow, W. (1972). Pharmacogenetics of drugs used in anesthesia. *Human Genetics, 60,* 415-427.

Kalow, W. (1986). Conjugation reactions. In Kalow, W., Goedde, H.W., & Agarwal, D.P., (Eds.), *Ethnic differences in reactions to drugs and xenobiotics.* New York: Alan R. Liss.

Kawate, R., Miyanishi, M., Yamakido, M., & Nishimoto, Y. (1978). Preliminary studies of the prevalence and mortality of diabetes mellitus in Japanese in Japan and on the island of Hawaii. *Advances in Metabolic Disorders, 9,* 201-224.

Kiefer, C.W. (1974). *Changing cultures, changing lives* (pp. 110-129). San Francisco: Jossey-Bass.

Kikumura, A., & Kitano, H.H.L. (1973). *Changing lives.* San Francisco: Josey-Bass.

Kitano, H.H.L. (1969). Japanese-American mental illness. In Plot, S.C., & Edgerton, R.B. (Eds.), *Changing perspective in mental illness.* New York: Holt, Rinehart & Winston.

Kitano, H.H.L. (1970). Mental illness in four cultures. *Journal of Social Psychology, 80,* 121-134.

Kitano, H.H.L. (1976). *Japanese Americans: the evolution of a subculture.* Englewood Cliffs, N.J.: Prentice-Hall.

Kitano, H.H.L., Hatanaka, H., Yeung, W.T., & Sue, S. (1985). Japanese-American drinking patterns. In Bennett, L.A., & Ames, G.M. (Eds.), *The American experience with alcohol.* New York: Plenum.

Klopf, D., & Ishii, S. (1976). A comparison of communication activities of Japanese and American adults. *ELEC Bulletin,* (20), 66-71.

Klopf, D., Cambra, R., & Ishii, S. (1981). A comparison of communication styles of Japanese and American college students. *Current English Studies,* (53), 22-26.

Kobata, F. (1979). The influence of culture on family relations: the Asian American experience. In Ragan, P.K. (Ed.), *Aging parents.* Los Angeles: Ethel Percy Andrus Gerontology Foundation, University of Southern California.

Kobayashi-Winata, H., & Powers, T. (1989). Child rearing and compliance: Japanese and American families in Houston. *Journal of Cross-Cultural Psychology, 20,* 333-356.

Kotani, R. (1982). AJA's and alcohol abuse. *Hawaii Herald, 3*(13), 4.

Lebenthal, E., Antonowicz, I., & Schwachman, H. (1975). Correlation of lactase activity, lactose tolerance, and milk consumption in different age groups. *American Journal of Clinical Nutrition, 28,* 595-600.

Lebra, T.S. (1976). *Japanese patterns of behavior.* Honolulu: University of Hawaii Press.

Lee, P., & Takamura, J. (1980). The Japanese Americans in Hawaii. In Palafox, N., & Warren, A. (Eds.), *Cross-cultural caring: a handbook for health care professions in Hawaii* (pp. 105-135). Honolulu: Transcultural Health Care Forum.

Leong, F.T.L. (1986). Counseling and psychotherapy with Asian Americans: review of the literature. *Journal of Counseling Psychology, 33,* 196-206.

Lin, K.M., & Finder, E. (1983). Neuroleptic dosage for Asians. *American Journal of Psychiatry, 140*(4), 490-491.

Lin, K.M., Poland, R., Nuccio, I., et al. (1989). Longitudinal assessment of haloperidol doses and serous concentrations in Asian and Caucasian schizophrenic patients. *American Journal of Psychiatry, 146*(10), 1307-1311.

Locke, B., & King, H. (1980). Cancer mortality risks among Japanese in the United States. *Journal of the National Cancer Institute, 65,* 1149-1156.

Matsumoto, D. (1989). Cultural influences on the perception of emotion. *Journal of Cross-Cultural Psychology, 20,* 92-105.

Matsumoto, D., & Ekman, P. (1989). American-Japanese cultural differences in intensity ratings of facial expressions of emotion. *Motivation and Emotion, 13,* 143-157.

McCracken, R. (1971). Lactase deficiency: an example of dietary evolution. *Current Anthropology, 12*(4-5), 479-517.

McDermott, J.F., Jr., Tseng, W.S., & Maretzki, T.W. (1973). *People and cultures of Hawaii: a psychocultural profile.* Honolulu: John A. Burns School of Medicine and the University of Hawaii Press.

Mehrabian, A. (1968). Communication without words. *Psychology Today,* p. 53.

Modell, J. (1968). The Japanese American family: a perspective for future investigations. *Pacific Historical Review, 37,* 67-81.

Mordkowitz, E.R., & Ginsberg, H.P. (1987). Early academic socialization of successful Asian American college students. *Quarterly Newsletter of the Laboratory of Comparative Human Cognition, 9,* 85-91.

Morris, T.M. (1990). Culturally sensitive family assessment: an evaluation of the family assessment device used with Hawaiian American and Japanese American families. *Family Process, 29,* 105-116.

Nagata, D. (1991). Transgenerational impact of the Japanese American internment: clinical issues in working with children of former internees. *Psychotherapy, 28,* 121-128.

Nomura, A. (1982). Stomach cancer. In Schottenfeld, D., & Fraumeni, J. (Eds.), *Cancer epidemiology and prevention* (pp. 624-637). Philadelphia: W.B. Saunders.

Nomura, A., Stemmerman, G., & Heilbrun, L. (1985). Gastric cancer among the Japanese in Hawaii: a review. *Hawaii Medical Journal, 44*(8), 301-304.

Osaka, M.N. (1979). Aging and family among Japanese Americans: the role of ethnic tradition in the adjustment to old age. *Gerontologist, 19,* 448-455.

Overfield, T. (1995). *Biologic variation in health and illness.* Menlo Park, Calif.: Addison-Wesley.

Padilla, A.M., Wagatsuma, Y., & Lindholm, K.J. (1985). Acculturation and personality as predictors of stress in Japanese and Japanese Americans. *Journal of Social Psychology, 125,* 295-305.

Petersen, W. (1966, Jan. 9). Success story, Japanese American style. *New York Times Magazine.*

President's Commission on Mental Health (1978). *Report to the president* (Vols. 1-4). Washington, D.C.: U.S. Government Printing Office.

Reed, D., McGee, D, Cohen, J., et al. (1982). Acculturation and coronary heart disease among Japanese men in Hawaii. *American Journal of Epidemiology, 115*(6), 894-905.

Reid, T.R. (1993, Feb. 7). Japanese growing taller. *The Sunday Star-Bulletin & Advertiser,* p. A-32.

Rhoads, G.G., Glober, G.A., & Stemmerman, G.N. (1991). A review of some tumors of interest for demographic study in Hawaii. *Hawaii Medical Journal, 50*(9), 326-333.

Roche, A., Roberts J., & Hamill, P.V. (1978). Skeletal maturity of youths 12-17 years: racial, geographic, and socioeconomic differentials. *Vital Health Statistics, 11*(167), 1-98.

Rogers, T., & Izutsu, S. (1980). The Japanese. In McDermott, J.F. Jr., Tseng, W.S., & Maretzki, T.W. (Eds.), *People and cultures of Hawaii: a psychocultural profile.* Honolulu: University of Hawaii Press.

Roseblat, R., & Tang, S.W. (1987). Do Oriental psychiatric patients receive different dosages of psychotropic medication when compared with Occidentals? *Canadian Journal of Psychiatry, 32,* 270-274.

Ross, P.D., Horimatsu, H., Davis, J., et al. (1991). A comparison of hip fracture incidence among native Japanese, Japanese Americans, and American Caucasians. *American Journal of Epidemiology, 133*(8), 801-809.

Sargent, J. (1993). Japan—physical and social geography. In *The Far East and Australasia 1993* (ed. 24) (pp. 371-372). London: Europa Publishers Ltd.

Sato, H., & Takano, J. (1983). Nursing care of Japanese American patients. In Orque, M.S., Bloch, B., & Monrroy, L.S.A. (Eds.), *Ethnic nursing care: a multicultural approach* (pp. 219-243). St. Louis: Mosby.

Schon, S.P., & Ja, D.A. (1982). Asian families. In McGoldrick, M., Pearce, J.K., & Giordano, J. (Eds.), *Ethnicity and family therapy.* New York: Guilford Press.

Simoons, F. (1969). Primary adult lactose intolerance and the milking habit: a problem in biological and cultural interrelations. *American Journal of Digestive Diseases, 14*(12), 819-836.

Smith, M.D. (1976). Perceptions of parental authority and adolescent independence responses from students from two ethnic groups. Unpublished master's thesis, University of Hawaii, Honolulu, Hawaii.

Storry, R. (1993). Japan—history up to 1952. In *The Far East and Australasia 1993* (ed. 24) (pp. 372-375). London: Europa Publishers Ltd.

Strazar, M., & Fisher, N. (1996). Traditional Japanese culture. In Fisher, N. (Ed.), *Cultural and ethnic diversity: a guide for genetic professionals.* Baltimore, Md.: The Johns Hopkins University Press.

Sue, D.W. (1983). Ethnic identity: the impact of two cultures on the psychological development of Asians in America. In Atkinson, D.R., Morton, G., & Sue, D.W. (Eds.), *Counseling American minorities: a cross cultural perspective* (pp. 85-96). Dubuque, Iowa: WC Brown.

Sue, D.W. (1987). Use and abuse of alcohol by Asian Americans. *Journal of Psychoactive Drugs, 19,* 57-66.

Sue, S., & Okazaki, S. (1990). Asian American educational achievement. *American Psychologist, 45,* 913-920.

Syme, S., Marmot, M., Kagun, A., et al. (1975). Epidemiologic studies of coronary heart disease and stroke in Japanese men living in Japan, Hawaii, and California: an introduction. *The American Journal of Epidemiology, 102*(6), 477-480.

Tanaka-Matsumi, M., & Marsella, A.J. (1976). Cross-cultural variations in phenomenological experience of depression, I: word association studies. *Journal of Cross-Cultural Psychology, 7,* 379-396.

Tateishi, J. (1984). *And justice for all: an oral history of Japanese American detention camps.* New York: Random House.

Tominaga, S. (1985). Cancer incidence in Japanese in Japan, Hawaii, and Western United States. *National Cancer Institute Monographs, 69,* 83-92.

Tracey, T.J., Leong, F.T.L., & Glidden, C. (1986). Help seeking and problem perception among Asian Americans. *Journal of Counseling Psychology, 33,* 331-336.

U.S. Department of Commerce, Bureau of the Census (1993a). *Population profiles of the United States: 1993* (Economic and Statistics Administration, Publication No. P23-185). Washington, D.C.: Government Printing Office.

U.S. Department of Commerce, Bureau of the Census (1993b). *We the American . . . Asians* (Economic and Statistics Administration, Publication No. WE-3). Washington, D.C.: Government Printing Office.

U.S. Department of Commerce, Bureau of the Census (1998). *Population profiles of the United States,* Internet release, June 1998.

Vessell, E. (1972). Therapy—pharmacogenetics. *New England Journal of Medicine, 287*(18), 904-909.

Watson, O.M. (1980). *Proxemic behavior: a cross-cultural study.* The Hague, The Netherlands: Mouton.

Webster's dictionary (1991). *The new lexicon Webster's dictionary.* New York: Lexicon Publication.

Wilson, J.R., McClearn, G.E., & Johnson, R.C. (1978). Ethnic variation in use and effects of alcohol. *Drug and Alcohol Dependence, 3*(2), 147-151.

World almanac (1997). Mahwah, N.J.: World Almanac Books.

Yamamoto, J. (1982). Japanese Americans. In Gaw, A. (Ed.), *Cross-cultural psychiatry.* Littleton, Mass.: John Wright–PSG Publishing.

Yamamoto, J., Fung, D., Lo, S., & Reece, S. (1979). Psychopharmacology for Asian Americans and Pacific Islanders. *Psychopharmacology Bulletin, 15*(4), 29-34.

Yamamoto, J., James, E.C., & Palley, N. (1968). Cultural problems in psychiatry therapy. *Archives of General Psychiatry, 19,* 46-49.

Yano, K., Reed, D., & Kagan, A. (1985). Coronary heart disease, hypertension and stroke among Japanese American men in Hawaii: the Honolulu Heart Program. *Hawaii Medical Journal, 44*(8), 297-325.

Yano, K., Reed, D., & McGee, D. (1984). Ten year incidence of coronary heart disease in the Honolulu Heart Program: relationship to biologic and lifestyle characteristics. *American Journal of Epidemiology, 119*(5), 653-666.

Yoshida, J. (1972). *The two worlds of Jim Yoshida.* New York: William Morrow & Co., Inc.

Yoshishige, J. (1993, March 21). Wartime heroics: a *nisei* history. *The Honolulu Advertiser,* 442nd Special Section, p. 5.

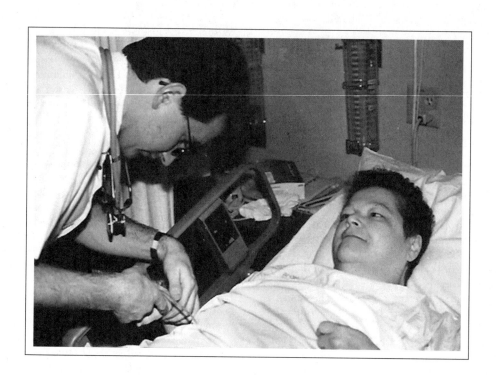

CHAPTER 14

Irish Americans

Cheryl Martin

BEHAVIORAL OBJECTIVES

After reading this chapter, the nurse will be able to:

1. Recognize cultural factors that affect the health-seeking behaviors of Irish Americans.
2. Identify specific communication approaches for Irish Americans that influence health and wellness behaviors
3. Explain the distance and intimacy behaviors of Irish Americans and how health and wellness behaviors are influenced.
4. Identify the Irish-American orientation to time and its influence on social and psychological behaviors.
5. Recognize physical and biological variances that exist within and across Irish-American groups to provide culturally appropriate nursing care.

OVERVIEW OF IRELAND

The Republic of Ireland covers approximately 85% of the island that is known as Ireland. The Republic of Ireland comprises 26 counties that became the Irish Free State in 1921. The capital of Ireland is Dublin. In 1937 the Irish Free State was given the Gaelic name *Eire* by the constitution. Ireland is bordered on the northeast by Northern Ireland (Ulster), which today remains a part of the United Kingdom, and by the Atlantic Ocean to the west and south. St. George's Channel, the Irish Sea, and the North Channel separate Ireland from Great Britain by distances averaging at least 50 miles, or 80 kilometers.

The Republic of Ireland is primarily an agricultural country and is noted for the Irish potato. Industry is flourishing, and mining has become increasingly important because of recent discoveries of lead, silver, zinc, and copper deposits. Most of the countryside in Ireland is low land, is situated less than 500 feet above sea level, and is underlain by limestone rock. Most of the surface is covered by glacial drifts that are a legacy of the Pleistocene Ice Age. In some places in Ireland the drifts have been shaped into distinctive landforms that form a continuous belt across the island.

Most of Ireland has a cool, maritime climate. For example, in July temperatures vary from 61° F in the south to 57° F in the north. Winters are extremely mild, with January temperatures varying from 44° F in the Valentia to 40° F in the northeast.

Ireland was colonized by settlers from Europe. For at least 5000 years there were successive waves of settlers who arrived from the island of Great Britain. Each group of settlers contributed to the heritage of the modern Irish nation. Even today, the Celtic influence remains dominant in Ireland. However, the eastern portion of Ireland has been particularly influenced by the Anglo-Normans, whose initial invasion in 1170 was followed by the subsequent immigration of settlers from England, Wales, and Scotland. The population of Ireland rapidly expanded during the eighteenth and early nineteenth centuries and reached a peak of 8.1 million people in 1841. However, the Great Potato Famine, which began in 1845, brought a reversal of the population trend as a result of the many deaths and massive migration to the United States and Great Britain. This exodus continued over the next 100 years, and by 1921 the population of Ireland numbered little more than half of the original 1845 figure.

In the early 1900s the Irish revolted against Britain in a battle for home rule. At the Easter Rebellion in Dublin in 1916 Irish nationalists unsuccessfully attempted to throw off British rule. In 1919 the rebels proclaimed Ireland as a republic. Unfortunately this was followed by guerrilla warfare against the British until 1921, when a peace was negotiated by General Michael Collins (Zimmermann, 1997). In 1922, the Irish Free State was established as a dominion and one of six northern counties constituting the United Kingdom. In 1948, Eamon de Valera, American-born leader of Sinn Fein ('our own', pronounced /shin fayn/), who had won establishment of the Free State in 1921 in negotiations with Britain's David Lloyd George, was defeated by John Costello, who demanded final independence from Britain. The Republic of Ireland was proclaimed on April 18, 1949. It withdrew from the British Commonwealth (Information Please Almanac, 1997).

Throughout the 1960s, two antagonistic currents dominated Irish politics. One sought to bind the wounds of the rebellion and civil war. The other was the effort of the outlawed extremist Irish Republican Army (IRA) to bring Northern Ireland into the republic (Information Please Almanac, 1997).

In the elections of 1981, FitzGerald, leader of the Fine Gael ('tribe of Irishmen', pronounced /finnuh gail/), was elected prime minister. However he resigned within a year for failure of support, and former Prime Minister Haughey was reinstated. The 1990 elections were won by Mary Robinson, who was supported by the Labour Party and the Workers Party and who became the first non-Fianna Fáil president since 1945. Amid allegations of scandal Prime Minister Haughey resigned in early 1992. Albert Reynolds was chosen by a majority of his Fianna Fáil ('army of Tara stone [= Ireland]', pronounced /feenah faw-il/) party to become the next

prime minister. However, Reynolds government fell in January of 1995 over a scandal involving the handling of the extradition of a priest convicted of child molestation in the North. In 1995 a referendum on divorce, which hitherto had been constitutionally forbidden, under certain conditions was held in November and narrowly passed (Information Please Almanac, 1997). Reynolds was replaced as prime minister by John Bruton. In a historic move, the British government invited the IRA's political wing Sinn Fein, to participate in multiparty peace talks set to resume Sept. 15, 1997. Northern Ireland secretary Dr. Marjorie ("Mo") Mowlam said that the self-imposed ceasefire the IRA declared in August was "unequivocal," which allowed the new Labour Party government to follow through on its promise to include Sinn Fein in the talks for the first time (Wallace, 1997; Clarity, 1997). United States President Clinton has expressed his approval of this process and his support of winning a peace in Northern Ireland (Elliott, 1997). In September 1997 Mary Robinson announced she would step down as president in light of the recent conviction of a Catholic priest for child molestation.

Although discrimination is illegal in Britain, the ongoing conflict with the Irish has affected Irish who are working in Britain (Dolan, 1997). Snell (1997) notes that racial discrimination and prejudice against Irish nurses can be found in British health care facilities. This is not without deleterious effects. For example, it has been noted that there is a higher incidence of mental illness among Irish-born women in Britain (Corduff, 1997). On the other hand, Irish nurses are credited with making an important contribution in Calcutta (Saidler, 1995).

Over the years music has played an important role in Irish history. In the 1990s Irish music including spiritual music, Irish Catholic hymns, Irish songwriter and singer Mary Coughlan, the Irish céilí (ceilidh, 'evening entertainment visit') bands, and the Irish band Junkster is receiving national recognition (Verna, 1997; Bhushan & Kwaku, 1997; Duffy, 1997; Sexton, 1997; Perlah, 1997).

Research concerning health care problems is evident in the Irish health care literature. For example, there has been a dramatic increase in the percentage of infants born to unmarried mothers in Ireland over the last decade. For the first 50 years of the century 2% of all registered births were to single mothers. In 1975 the figure had risen slightly to 3.7%. Within 10 years it had risen to 8.5%, and in 1990 the figure stood at 14%. It has been concluded that increased rates of sexual activity among unmarried couples resulted from the lack of information on family planning and the unavailability of artificial birth control (Nugent, 1994). Nugent (1994) notes that, although there has been a general cultural rejection of unwed mothers and babies, recently this has been replaced by a general cultural acceptance.

Another recent health problem in Ireland is a dramatically increasing suicide rate. Particularly male suicide rates by violent methods has increased in 15-24, 25-34, and 55-64 age ranges (McLaughlin & Whittington, 1996). In contrast, the undetermined death rate has fallen off. This has implications both for improving measurement procedures and for suicide prevention (Kelleher, Corcoran, Keeley, et al., 1996; Connolly & Cullen, 1995). Interestingly, there is little information in the Irish medical literature on smoking. The lack of information provides little help in the government's focus on establishing smoking cessation programs (Howell, 1996). Another health problem noted in the Irish medical literature relates to incontinence in the elderly. It was noted that only 33% of general practitioners studied were aware of the incontinence status of their clients over 75 years of age. This study suggested that general practitioners should have a high index of suspicion for incontinence in persons over 75 years of age and should assess this as a possible health problem (Prosser & Dobbs, 1997). Research in Ireland has also suggested that self-neglect in later life, or Diogenes syndrome, may be a significant problem (Johnson & Adams, 1996). Finally, work by Manning, Curran, Kirby, et al. (1997) indicates that there may be a prevalence of teenage asthma with associated allergic conditions in Ireland.

Against a background of fundamental change in the Irish health care environment, MacDougall and Doran (1995) conducted a survey to determine the information needs of all health care practitioners. This survey revealed serious deficiencies in access, awareness, and availability of information for both staff and clients and recommended a comprehensive national health information strategy to coordinate the future development of health sciences information services. In general, nursing is less institutionalized in Ireland because of the rural society with "country" traditions. Even in Dublin, which contains more than one third of the population, many of the people have relatives who live in the country, and therefore there is a mass exodus on weekends to the countryside. Nursing is considered a desirable career, and families are proud to claim a nurse "in the family" (Slack, 1982). Medicine is considered a respected profession. In 1997 the fact that some physicians who had AIDS were practicing came to light. An act was passed that allows prosecution of doctors with AIDS who continue to practice because it was believed that this put clients at risk and involved negligence (Birchard, 1997).

Today the population of Ireland is approximately 3,562,902 (1996 estimate) and is of mixed origin (Information Please Almanac, 1997). Immigration to the United States continues to be an attractive alternative for many who are distressed by the political unrest that has so long prevailed in Ireland.

IMMIGRATION TO THE UNITED STATES

The large number of Catholic Irish immigrants of the famine years were not the first Irish people to immigrate to the United States. The famine immigrants were preceded by their Irish countrymen in the seventeenth and eighteenth centuries though in smaller numbers (Fallows, 1979). Many of the earlier immigrants, particularly during the seventeenth and eighteenth centuries, were Protestants from the northern county of Ulster and thus came to the United States under less dramatic circumstances than the later immigrants did. The early Ulster immigrants arrived in the United States just in time to help the Americans win independence from England. At that time many Irish-American immigrants regarded themselves as members of the Anglo-American society. This distinction was not made to deny their Irish origin but to embrace their new heritage. By the mid-1800s Irish organizations were established in the major cities of the United

States, but even today Irish descendants regard their Irish extraction more as a point of historical interest than as an identification with social relevance for their lives. According to Greeley and McCready (1975), Irish Americans, in the process of adapting to American life, began to think and behave like their American counterparts, a fact reiterated in a study by Cornacchia and Nelson (1992). Irish Americans have become so assimilated into the mainstream of American society that today they are more likely to be professionals or managers and less likely to be laborers, service workers, or factory workers (Blessing, 1980).

There are approximately 39 million people of Irish descent who reside in the United States, or approximately 16% of the U.S. population (U.S. Department of Commerce, Bureau of the Census, 1995; Information Please Almanac, 1998). The Irish immigrant population has been steadily increasing since the early 1970s and increased dramatically in 1994 with 14.1 million between 1971 and 1980, 32.8 million from 1981 to 1990, 20.6 million from 1991 to 1993, and 17.3 million immigrants in 1994 alone (Statistical Abstract of the United States, 1996). In addition, it was estimated that in 1992 36,000 Irish immigrants were undocumented (Statistical Abstract of the United States, 1996). Irish ranks as the second largest ancestry group in the United States and is outranked only by Germans. Irish is the largest ancestry group in five states in the Northwest and ranks third (after German and African American) for having the largest ancestry group in a state (U.S. Department of Commerce, Bureau of the Census, 1995).

COMMUNICATION

The official language of Ireland is Irish (Irish Gaelic). However, English is recognized as the second official language. English is universally spoken throughout Ireland, and approximately 27% of the population know both Irish and English. Irish is more widely used in the west and is the first language of people in remote areas of Ireland.

To understand the development of language in Ireland, it is essential to understand the historical significance of the Celtic (usually pronounced /kel-tic/) language. Because the Celts (/kelts/) devel-

oped a written language quite late, the people were forced to rely heavily on the oral transmission of laws, customs, religions, and philosophy, and poetry became a useful mnemonic device for transmitting tradition. According to legend, the ancient heroes of the mythological cycle, which included Finn Mac-Cool and Cuchulain, were clearly in love with the sound of their own voices. Modern-day Irish people are much like the ancient Celts; the Irish politician and the Irish priest have the same love for using many words (Greeley, 1981). Greeley (1981) suggested that, for Irish people, playing with the language not only provided a means of communication, but also a portion of their enjoyment and pleasure. It should be noted that languages throughout the world that have survived from an earlier period have not only elaborate language structures, but also more extensive vocabularies. It has been suggested that the reason for this is that spoken language needs to be more flexible and descriptive than written language.

For people in the western part of Ireland, the vocabulary is about one half as extensive as the vocabulary of the well-educated English speaker in London. It has also been noted that people who live in the *Gaeltacht* (/gail-tahht/), or the Irish-speaking regions in the west, tend to have an extensive English-speaking vocabulary. According to Greeley (1981), modern-day Irish people delight in ridicule, scatology (elaborate obscenity), limericks, puns, and riddles. Although a modern-day Irish language exists, the Irish language for all practical purposes was almost destroyed during the second half of the nineteenth century with the onslaught of the English language.

Because many Irish persons arrived in the United States with knowledge of English, assimilation into the predominant culture was enhanced. However, despite the use of English words, some words have different meanings for the Irish. For example, the word "homely," which is commonly used in the United States to describe someone who is plain and not attractive, is used by some Irish people as an endearing word to describe hospitality. An Irish guest after a dinner may hug the host or hostess and say, "Thank you for being so homely." In Ireland it is considered inappropriate to ask for a "ride" from a cab driver. Instead the word "lift" or "drive" is used.

Nonverbal actions have special significance for the Irish. For example, holding up two fingers with the palm facing one's face is a hand gesture meant to be obscene (Lasky, 1996). In business or professional relationships it is not considered proper to give gifts. Instead, tokens of appreciation with special significance, such as Vermont maple syrup or California wine, are appreciated (Lasky, 1996).

The Irish tend to dress up rather than dress casually for business or professional events. The nurse should not be surprised if a newly immigrated Irish client comes to a health care agency very well dressed.

Implications for nursing care

It is important for the nurse to understand that some Irish Americans who may be encountered in the health care system may not have an extensive vocabulary, but the words they use may be used with exaggeration. Because language is a form of entertainment and power for some Irish people, the client may attempt to communicate needs through flowery and sometimes exaggerated words. On the other hand, some Irish tend to ignore pain and to provide no words of complaint (Zborowski, 1952, 1969). Therefore it is essential for the nurse to carefully evaluate physical signs and symptoms of pain in addition to oral descriptions to assist in an accurate assessment of the need for nursing intervention. Because of this variety of responses, it is particularly important for the nurse to be careful to not stereotype Irish-American clients relative to pain response (Spector, 1996a, 1996b). The astute nurse must keep in mind that the Irish-American client may tend to be overly verbose in descriptions of conditions, but this does not imply that the client is being objective or accurately descriptive about the nature of the condition. The nurse should use a combination of open-ended and closed questions to solicit specific information from which culturally appropriate nursing care can be planned. When assessing the client, the nurse should be aware that some Irish Americans tend to avoid saying the word "no." Instead phrases such as "I'll let you know" or "we'll see" or "perhaps" are used. It is important for the nurse to try to ana-

lyze context and demeanor to determine if the response is really negative (Lasky, 1996).

Zola (1966) compared Italian Americans and Irish Americans and their descriptive methods of presenting complaints. The findings of the study indicated that when Italian Americans and Irish Americans were asked, "Where does it hurt?" Irish American respondents were more likely to locate chief problems in the eyes, ears, nose, or throat. In a similar question the respondents were asked to identify the most important areas of the body. Again, for the Irish American respondents, the emphasis was on the eyes, ears, nose, and throat. Another finding of the study was that the Irish Americans more often than the Italian Americans denied that pain was a part of their illness. When Irish-American respondents were asked about the presence of pain, some of them hedged their replies with qualifications such as "It is more a throbbing than a pain," "It is not really a pain; it feels more like sand in my eye," or "It feels more like a pinprick than a pain." The conclusion of the study was that Irish Americans, through such comments, were reflecting something more than an objective reaction to their physical condition. Irish Americans were found to describe their chief problems in terms of specific dysfunctions. What appeared to emerge from the study was that Irish people limit and understate their physical difficulties, whereas Italians spread and generalize theirs.

With the increasing numbers of Irish clients it is helpful to have health care materials translated into Irish. However, translating client-teaching materials and various assessment materials to Irish has not always been completely successful. For example, Aroian, Patsdaughter, Levin, and Gianan (1995) attempted to utilize the Brief Symptoms Inventory to assess psychological distress among Polish, Filipino, and Irish immigrants by translating the form into the respective languages. It was found that the scale in its translated form was able to measure psychological distress with all three immigrant groups. However, problems with the psychoticism subscale occurred across all three immigrant groups, and such occurrence indicated that this subscale should be interpreted with caution when used with immigrants. Thus, although English translation to another language on written assessment materials is sometimes helpful, it cannot generally be assumed to be accurate.

SPACE

Space is an essential component in a cultural framework of nursing because from the beginning of modern time, philosophers, mathematicians, psychologists, and ethnologists have studied the phenomenon of space. Territoriality, proximity, and personal space are all terms that have been used to describe space. The word "territoriality" was initially used to describe the physical area that animals claim as their own and defend from predators, but in modern times the term has been extended to describe human behavior as well (Hall, 1959). Hall (1963) coined the term "proxemics" to describe the use of space as an elaboration of a culture. According to Hall (1966), individuals by virtue of their culture have four ways of perceiving distance: as intimate distance (from 6 to 8 inches), as personal distance (from 6 inches to 4 feet), as social distance (from 4 to 12 feet), and as public distance (from 12 to 25 feet). Hall (1966) concluded that the use of space explains communication in various cultures.

Space is a cultural phenomenon that is infrequently noted in the literature about the Irish. Greeley (1981) has noted, however, that Irish-American students often require more time to become articulate and self-confident in a high-powered academic environment and that this can be seen in the student's spatial relationships with others. The Irish-American student is more likely to sit off in a corner for several semesters, only to be "discovered" later as having produced brilliant work, for the most part in solitude (Greeley, 1981). Some authors (Fallows, 1979; Greeley, 1981) have also noted that Irish individuals are less likely to be physically affectionate in both their interpersonal and their family relationships.

Implications for nursing care

The use of space, in its simplest terms, is a means of nonverbal communication (Stillman, 1978). How individuals feel about their own personal space determines how much intrusion by others is considered acceptable. Because health care often occurs in what is described as an intimate zone, spatial issues have important implications for the nurse.

Because Irish Americans are perceived as having a past-oriented culture that relies heavily on extended family ties, the personal space of some Irish Americans is extremely limited (Fallows, 1979). In other words, because some Irish-American clients may be accustomed to having family members close by, they may have a need for proximity of family members during illness; however, according to Greeley (1981), despite the closeness of the family unit, Irish-American families have a tendency to collapse the personal space inward, more so than in other cultures. One difficulty that has been noted in Irish-American families is difficulty expressing love and affection. Some have more difficulty in expression with close family members than with more distant persons, creating an isolated and greatly expanded personal space. Others express feelings somewhat readily with a close group of intimates but not with persons more distant. The nurse should be cognizant of the possible effects of attitudes and values about space that may affect individuals from different cultures. By assessing the client on an individual basis, the nurse can provide culturally appropriate care. One major objective for the nurse may be to assist the family in recognizing the need to convey warmth, feelings, and attitudes in order to create a supportive and nurturing spatial environment for the client that will promote recovery.

SOCIAL ORGANIZATION
Family

The famine years had a profound effect on the structure of the Irish-American family. As the famine progressed, the resulting experiences dramatically altered the family system in Ireland. The immigrants brought this altered family structure to the United States and formed their own ethnic societies. Most of those who immigrated to the United States from Ireland were between 15 and 35 years of age because it was these able-bodied individuals who were most able to leave (Kennedy, 1973; McKay, Hall, & Buckler, 1989).

Ireland stands alone in losing such a large proportion of its population to emigration. Even in modern times, more Irish people live outside Ireland than in it, and most Irish families have at least some members living in the United States (Fallows, 1979). A wide range of disparity has been noted regarding the link between Irish Americans and the family in the homeland. For some Irish Americans there appears to be an almost mystical link between the family in the United States and the roots in Ireland. These roots often lead to a particular farm that may still be inhabited by a remnant of that particular clan. For other Irish Americans there is almost no link remaining except the knowledge that an ancestor originated in Ireland. The family values and ethnic traits are often transmitted to the next generation unconsciously by imitation of the parental model.

Before the famine years, families in the southern and western parts of Ireland were traditionally Irish speaking, Catholic, and subsistence farmers. The typical couple married early, had many children, and on the father's death subdivided the land among the sons. The agricultural pattern of the prefamine years no doubt was instrumental in creating the almost total reliance of the Irish on the potato crop. However, this pattern of continuous subdividing of the land among family members also contributed to the close family bonds, which were evidenced by parental demands for respectful attention and by obedience to marriages arranged by the parents to ensure appropriate bonds between families and clans. These family bonds continued even after immigration to the United States, as evidenced by the fact that it was the responsibility of many immigrants to send money back to Ireland to pay the passage for another family member to come to the United States (Kennedy, 1973).

Marriage

In the past there was intense social pressure among Irish Americans regarding mate selection; marriage within the Irish Catholic community was considered preferable. Therefore the Irish neighborhoods in the United States often served as the social context for the meeting and pairing off of the young immigrants (Wessel, 1931). For the early Irish settlers, marriage with non-Irish Catholics was a permissive alternative. However, these marriages generally followed a preferential hierarchy in which the early-arriving English or German Catholics were considered more suitable than the later-arriving Irish Catholics (Abramson, 1973; Alba, 1976). By the time of the third generation of immigrants, a tendency was noted for the socially aspiring Irish Catholic to marry a Protestant or even convert to Protestantism. These practices were generally disapproved of by other Irish-American Catholics. Even today in stable communities in the United States, intermarriage between Irish families remains one of the clearest distinctions of social acceptance and social equality in the Irish-American community.

Many studies have portrayed marriage among the Irish as an uneasy practical alliance that provided little affection or intimacy between partners. Sex and procreation were reported to be duties rather than joys or expressive activities in some of the marriages reported in the studies by Ablon and Cunningham (1981).

Bachelorhood and spinsterhood are infrequent among Irish Americans, with only 14% of men and 12% of women not married, according to a study by Greeley (1981). The typical Irish-American Catholic woman marries at 22 years of age, and the typical Irish-American Catholic man marries at 24.5 years of age. Although this is a bit older than the American average, the practice in ancient Ireland was to delay marriage until the early 30s. Greeley (1977) has noted that Irish-American Catholics are less likely than Irish-American Protestants to marry before 21 years of age. Greeley (1977) has also noted that Irish-American Catholics are less likely to become divorced and are more likely to have three or more children. The mean number of children for Irish-American families is 2.6, compared with the national mean of 2.4. As family planning becomes more progressive among Irish-American Catholics, the number of children is decreasing.

Role of women One traditional view of Irish women was that they were controlling matriarchs on whom sons and husbands were dependent (Messenger, 1969). A contrasting view held that male dominance began as a pattern in Ireland after the mass emigrations. According to Fallows (1979), the women were expected to be subservient in every way and assist their husbands with what was considered "men's work" in addition to completing their own, traditionally female tasks.

Greeley (1972) has noted that some Irish women find it hard to resist the temptation to become stiff, if not non sexually responsive, when sexual advances are made by a mate. According to Greeley (1972), sexual relations have been viewed as a matter of duty by some Irish women, whereas others are able to be warm and loving with their mate. Also, according to Greeley (1972), some Irish-American Catholic women have reported feeling obligated to admit any failures regarding sexual performance at the next confession, and some Irish-American women have felt such an obligation to the "duty" of marital sexual relations that this obligation has continued for periods of 20 or 30 years of marriage, even if no pleasure is experienced.

A representative study of female college graduates by Greeley and McCready (1975) found that Irish-American women are more likely than their Anglo-American counterparts to view the wife-mother role as the dominant one in marriage. The findings are also suggestive that Irish-American women view the mother's working as detrimental to children and see the role of the wife as a helper to her husband. The data are further suggestive that Irish-American women are less likely to stress the importance of security or of keeping up family contacts or relationships with parents or in-laws or to view their daughters' independence as important. A final conclusion of the study was that Irish-American women are less likely to report tense relationships with their mothers; however, they are more likely to report tense relationships with their fathers.

Role of men Greeley (1972) has noted that, although Irish men, particularly when intoxicated, may spin tall tales and recite romantic poetry about their true love, in intimate relationships they often become awkward and tongue tied and may become clumsy, if not rough, in any attempts at intimacy. The male dominance that began in Ireland as a result of the change in family structure between 1840 and 1940 is paralleled even today among Irish Americans (Fallows, 1979).

Adolescent Irish Americans

Porteous (1985) conducted a study of adolescents in England and Ireland to determine if problems experienced by adolescents varied systematically with age, sex, and culture. The data from this study indicate that in both countries boys may be less mature than girls in problem experience and at the same time are more concerned with authority, self-image, and behavioral problems, whereas girls appear to have more worries in personal and emotional areas. The data are also suggestive that in both countries both boys and girls are more concerned with feelings of inadequacy, which increase with age, whereas the concerns expressed by both boys and girls in other areas seemingly decrease with age. The data are further suggestive that Irish adolescents have a less mature problem pattern than their English counterparts; however, Irish adolescents in the study admitted to having more worries. The conclusion of the study was that cultural differences are specifically reflected in adolescent problem experiences.

Religion

In Ireland and in the United States the primary cultural force and national unifier of Irish culture has been the Catholic Church. In fact, the parish rather than the neighborhood has traditionally defined the family's social context (Campinha-Bacote, 1997). The Church of Ireland is an independent Anglican church found in both the Republic of Ireland and Northern Ireland. The church traces its Episcopal succession from the pre-Reformation Church in Ireland. Christianity is believed to have existed in Ireland before the missionary activities of Patrick, the Patron Saint of Ireland, in the late fifth century. The early church in Ireland was monastic, without parochial or diocesan divisions or central government. If there was authority within the structure of the church, it rested with the abbot and the bishops.

As church members in the United States, both Irish-American Protestants and Irish-American Catholics have had a significant effect on the development of hospitals, schools, colleges, and churches, not only in the growing cities on the East Coast, but also in towns and cities across the country (Shannon, 1981).

In Ireland the Catholic Church has been faced with a dilemma because of the desire to preserve the Catholic moral tone. In this regard the Catholic Church has found it necessary to relegate the prevention of AIDS through the promotion of condoms and safe sexual practices to the government as its official responsibility. Most Catholic churches advocate abstinence before marriage and avoidance of sexual behavior by some high-risk groups, such as homosexuals.

Political influences

Immigrants from Ireland have significantly contributed to the development of the United States from its inception (Griffin, 1981). In fact, eight Irish individuals signed the Declaration of Independence, and five died in the Boston Massacre. About one third of the people in the United States can trace all or part of their lineage to Irish ancestry. It has been reported that three presidents, including Andrew Jackson, James Buchanan, and Chester Arthur, were sons of Irish immigrants. Irish individuals have been active in all walks of American life, including the formation and growth of trade unions and active service on police forces across the country, and have served admirably in the army and in the navy (Griffin, 1981).

Irish Americans have enjoyed a significant and spectacular rise in the political arena in this country, in part because of the block voting of these individuals in large cities, where they generally were the largest single group. The fact that this voting practice assured the Irish of political influence was evident by the 1800s, particularly in Boston, where the first Irish-American mayors were elected. During this same period in New York, the Irish controlled many political machines. Among the most noted Irish-American political bosses were John F. Fitzgerald, Richard J. Daley, "Big Tim" Sullivan, and James Michael Curley. The success of the Irish resulted partially from their strong sense of group solidarity, their fluency with the spoken word, and their personal charm. Historically the Irish were known as

the most successful enhancers of corrupt politics. Today, the voting patterns for Irish Americans remain about the same as that for other Americans. In addition, with the election of the first Irish Catholic president in 1960 (John F. Kennedy), the issue of an Irish Catholic president was resolved.

Implications for nursing care

The nurse must keep in mind that the one reemerging theme among Irish Americans is the significance of the family and family structure. It is difficult for people from other cultures to perceive the importance of the family structure to some cultural groups such as the Irish Americans. Because Irish Americans are viewed as having a relational orientation that is lineal in nature, nursing interventions are likely to be successful only if family involvement in the care and treatment of the client is maximized.

Kluckhohn and Strodtbeck (1961) viewed relational orientation in families as having three subdivisions: lateral (collateral), lineal, and individualistic. For families with a lateral (collateral) mode of orientation, the goals and welfare of laterally extended groups, including siblings and peers, take on paramount importance. This type of family assumes responsibility for all of its members. Therefore the goals of the individual family members become subordinate to those of the family group. When the lineal mode is present as the major focus in family groups, the goals and welfare of the group may also have primary importance because the family members view culture and kinship bonds as the primary basis for maintaining lineage.

A contrasting mode that is held by some families is the individualistic mode of orientation. For families with this orientation, individual goals are viewed as being more important than specific lateral or lineal goals. In this type of family each individual member is held responsible for personal behavior and is therefore judged according to personal accomplishments (Campinha-Bacote, 1997).

Because Irish Americans are perceived as having a lineal relationship, it is important for the nurse to seek the family's advice and opinions on treatment for the client. In addition, because the family is perceived as being a source of anxiety and tension because of restricted family roles, it is important for the nurse to assist the family in identifying the boundaries of each role and the characteristics of the roles. If the family determines that the boundaries are restricted and do not overlap, the nurse must accept this fact and recognize and appreciate that such families function with a hierarchical ranking of family roles. Therefore lack of recognition on the part of a nurse may foster feelings of anxiety and tension on the part of those persons who are considered to be at the top of the hierarchical ranking, such as the father or the mother.

Because Irish Americans tend to delineate roles and behaviors within the family structure based on gender, it is important for the nurse not to minimize the significance of ranked ordering of behavior. For example, some Irish-American women may view their role as primary caretaker of the family. Therefore, when they are ill, their role function is greatly compromised. In this case the client must be assisted in developing strategies to help the family meet its needs in the absence of the primary caretaker.

It is also important for the nurse to remember that for some Irish Americans religion and religious views take on paramount importance in maintaining the social integrity of the individual. The astute nurse should solicit information on religious practices that are deemed essential to the optimal functioning of the Irish-American client. Lack of recognition of the significance of religious beliefs may serve to augment problems and difficulties encountered with illness.

TIME

According to Kluckhohn and Strodtbeck (1961), the cultural interpretation of time has a three-point range of variability that includes past, present, and future orientations. Based on this model Irish Americans are viewed as having a past-oriented culture. Kluckhohn and Strodtbeck have noted that all cultures must deal with all three time orientations. Cultures differ regarding time perspective in the preferential ordering of the orientations, and a great deal about a society can be learned and predicted from this preferential ordering. For example, Irish

Americans are perceived as members of a first-ordered, past-oriented society because some Irish Americans have a strong allegiance to the past, worship their ancestors, and have a strong family tradition. In addition, persons from cultures with past-oriented time perspectives may have the attitude that nothing new ever happens in the present or will ever happen in the future because it all happened in the far-distant past. For example, an Irish American who is shown a new invention may remark, "Our ancestors were making something similar to this 100 years ago." Persons in the dominant culture may find it difficult to understand the respect that Irish Americans have for tradition, and at the same time some Irish Americans do not appreciate the typical American disregard for tradition.

On the other hand, many Irish of today are present and future oriented in terms of working hard to achieve a future objective. The Irish tend to maintain a hard work ethnic and to have difficulty tearing themselves from a long day at the office to indulge in a social function (Lasky, 1996). Timing for business functions is considered very important. However, the opposite is true of social gatherings. Fun-filled functions usually begin 20 to 30 minutes after the designated time. Nevertheless, once a party has started, Irish Americans tend to indulge in light-hearted events hardily and often late into the night. Some Irish are offended when individuals attempt to leave a social event early (Lasky, 1996).

Implications for nursing care

Because some past-oriented people are perceived as lacking an understanding of rhythmicity and periodicity, it is likely that they may also be perceived as being noncompliant regarding scheduled medical and therapeutic interventions. Because some individuals with a past time orientation view man as being subjugated to nature, there may be a tendency for a fatalistic orientation that affects the time orientation. In other words, some people with a past time orientation believe that time and nature will alleviate the problem and tend to wait until the last possible moment to seek medical intervention for acute or chronic medical problems.

The astute nurse must recognize that noncompliance is not necessarily an inherent quality of the personality but may be related to a lack of understanding regarding the time perspective. For example, individuals with a past-oriented perspective view time as being elastic, and therefore a moment in time has the possibility of being recaptured (Mbiti, 1970). The nurse should plan activities that encourage the client to adhere to the necessary aspects of the time perspective, as in the case of time-released insulin or heart medication. The client should be encouraged to relate adherence to a medical regimen to a business schedule that tends to require adherence to a fixed schedule (Lasky, 1996).

ENVIRONMENTAL CONTROL
Locus of control

Kluckhohn and Strodtbeck (1961) developed a five-concept value-orientation framework that includes (1) perceptions of human nature, (2) relationship of man with nature, (3) time orientation, (4) activity orientation, and (5) relational orientation. In this model, Irish Americans are viewed as being a past-oriented culture because some Irish Americans believe that man is basically evil and subjugated to nature, and so their family and social relationships are lineal in nature. Also, they tend to cling to a past-oriented value orientation regarding the family and family relationships and tend to consider past values and traditions to be of paramount importance to future growth and development. Greeley and McCready (1975) found in a national sample of Anglo-American Protestant males and Irish-American Catholic males that Irish Americans were more fatalistic, less authoritarian, less anxious, and more trusting than their Anglo-American counterparts. Because Irish Americans hold a value orientation that views man as being subjugated to nature, some Irish Americans are viewed as having an external locus of control.

Perception of illness

According to Zola (1966), every individual has an orientation to problems that corresponds with the way this person handles problems. For Irish Americans the world view of life is expressed through fasts, which are symbolic of prior deprivations in their lives. Some Irish Americans have life patterns that have alternated between overindulgence and self-deprivation (Zola, 1966). Many psychologists believe that the expected and limited nature of these irregular, extreme cycles is correlated with alcohol use and that for some Irish Americans continued use of defense mechanisms to ignore or dispel previous conditions or symptoms is the norm rather than the exception. Some Irish Americans have a view of life that states that "life is black and long suffering and therefore the less said about life the better" (Zola, 1966). It is this statement that best reflects the way in which some Irish Americans handle the concept of illness.

Although in some cultural groups ignoring bodily complaints is not normative, for some Irish Americans this appears to be a culturally prescribed and supported defense mechanism. For some Irish Americans the use of defense mechanisms (ignoring and denying) appears to be the typical way of coping with psychological and physiological needs. For example, some Irish Americans will say, regarding an illness, "I ignore it as I do most other things." This point reemphasizes the fact that for some Irish Americans there is a tendency to understand the implications of the illness but, at the same time, to refrain from expressing illness-related complaints.

Illness and wellness behaviors

The consistency of the Irish illness behavior can also be perceived in two other contexts. First, for some Irish Americans illness or the perception of illness helps perpetuate a self-fulfilling prophecy. Some people believe that the way in which Irish Americans communicate complaints, but do very little to make treatment easy, has assured them of continued suffering (Zola, 1966). Second, for some Irish Americans illness behavior can be linked to sin and guilt ideology, which seems to pervade a major portion of Irish-American society today. This is evidenced by the fact that in the Irish-American culture there is great restraint, which opens the door for constant temptation, which must be denied. The perception held by some Irish Americans is that the flesh is weak and the individual is very likely to sin. This theme is reinforced even in the way in which symptoms are localized. According to Zola (1966), Irish Americans localize complaints in the eyes, ears, or throat, which might be a symbolic reflection of the more immediate source of sin and guilt. For example, it might be said that these three localized areas of complaints are congruent with what should have been seen, what should have been heard, or what should have been said.

Folk medicine

Some Irish Americans subscribe to folk medicine beliefs that can be perceived as neutral health practices (neither having benefit nor producing harm), such as the "blessing of the throat" and the wearing of holy medals to prevent illnesses. Additional folk medicine beliefs that are considered neutral include the practices of tying a bag of camphor around the neck to prevent flu during the flu season, never looking in a mirror at night, closing closet doors to prevent evil spirits from entering the body, and finally and above all maintaining a strong family with lots of love to prevent illnesses. Irish methods to prevent illness and protect health include not going to bed with wet hair, drinking nettle soup to clear the blood, and eating porridge at night before going to bed. Irish methods to restore health that are likely to have little effect include tying onions to wrists or dirty socks around the neck to cure a fever, curing a cold by eating a whole raw onion and having a shot of whiskey, curing flatulence by placing one's rear end toward the fire, and wrapping hot bread, sugar, and soap in a linen cloth and placing it on an infection to cure boils and cuts (Spector, 1996b).

Other folk medicine beliefs practiced by some Irish Americans may be perceived as harmful, such as eating a lot of oily foods, cleansing the bowels every 8 days with senna, and seeing a doctor only in an emergency. For some Irish Americans the first level of intervention is often home treatment because of the belief that a doctor should be seen only in an emergency, and this practice may create a reactive

rather than a preventive model of treatment. For example, for the treatment of a throat condition, the first level of intervention may be home treatment with such things as iodine or kerosene to paint the throat or honey and lemon to soothe the throat. Another example of a practice that might be perceived as harmful is the home treatment of nausea and other stomach ailments that might have serious implications with such remedies as drinking hot tea, taking castor oil, or eating potatoes or gruel.

Some Irish Americans subscribe to folk medicine practices that may be perceived as beneficial, such as getting lots of rest and going to bed early, enjoying fresh air and sunshine, exercising outdoors, dressing warmly, and keeping the feet warm. Many also believe that one must eat good food, take vitamins, and balance the diet. In addition, there seems to be an overriding belief that to stay healthy one must be goal oriented and nurture a strong religious faith. The combination of positive thinking along with healthful practices such as exercise and adequate rest can contribute to optimal wellness (Spector, 1996).

Implications for nursing care

Because some Irish Americans are perceived as having an external locus of control, the astute nurse must devise a teaching plan that emphasizes the importance of preventive techniques to maintain optimal wellness and prevent illness. The nurse should recognize the importance of assisting the client in developing a sensitivity and an understanding about wellness that will alleviate fatalistic beliefs about life in general and illness in particular. It is important for the nurse to understand that compliance with a health regimen is much more complex than the mere recognition and prescription of such a plan. The nurse must keep in mind that philosophical beliefs and attitudes play a major role not only in the perception of health and wellness, but also in compliance behavior.

Because the first level of treatment for an illness for some Irish Americans may be home treatment, it is important for the nurse to ascertain for the client which of these practices are neutral or beneficial and thus may be retained and incorporated into the plan of care and which of these practices are harmful. The nurse must devise teaching strategies that assist the client in developing an understanding about harmful folk medical practices in order for such practices to be eliminated from the typical health care regimen of the client. The nurse must realize that complete avoidance of harmful practices is initially difficult and that a reduction in such behaviors should be considered significant.

BIOLOGICAL VARIATIONS

It has been found that certain Irish people have genetic susceptibility to certain biological variations. Byrne, Cama, Vigliarolo and Levato (1997) suggested that neural tube defects (NTDs) may result from a genetic susceptibility interacting with environmental exposures occurring early in pregnancy. A high-rate area of Ireland was compared to a low-rate area of Italy. The results of their study support the notion that geographic differences in occurrence of NTDs are attributable at least in part to differing prevalences of genetic susceptibility factors.

A study on bimaxillary dental protrusion was conducted with a sample of 20 Northern Irish people. On average, tooth size for the overall maxillary and mandibular dentition was 5.7% larger in the bimaxillary sample than in the control sample (McCann & Burden, 1996).

When mutations of chromosomes were studied in Northern Irish persons with cystic fibrosis, it was determined that three major cystic fibrosis mutations are delta F508, G551D, and R117H (Hughes, Hill, Macek, et al., 1996). Mutation G551D of exon 11 of the cystic fibrosis transmembrane conductance regulator gene is one of the most common mutations in clients of European origin (Cashman, Patino, Martínez, et al., 1995).

Siblings of Irish persons with abdominal aortic aneurysm have been studied in the Irish population. It was determined that there is a high incidence of abdominal aortic aneurysm among brothers of clients diagnosed with this illness. This study highlights the need to counsel siblings on their risk of aneurysm (Fitzgerald, Ramsbottom, Burks, et al., 1995).

Lipton and Marbach (1984) conducted a study to examine interethnic differences and similarities in reported pain experiences among African-Americans, Irish persons, Italians, Jewish persons, and Puerto Ricans and found that responses, attitudes, and descriptions of pain were relatively similar after controlling for variables shown by previous studies to influence reported pain experiences. These variables included symptom history; signs elicited on physical, radiographic, and laboratory examination; and social, cultural, and psychological data. No significant intraethnic differences were noted regarding the clients' emotionality (that is, stoicism versus expressiveness) in regard to pain and the overall interference in daily functioning attributed to pain. The data are suggestive that the pain experiences reported by African-American, Italian, and Jewish clients were almost identical, whereas the pain experiences of Irish and Puerto Rican clients appeared to be relatively distinctive from those of the other groups and from those of each other. The variable that most influenced differences for Irish clients was social assimilation. The conclusion of the study was that intraethnic homogeneity is present for most aspects of the pain experience; however, intraethnic heterogeneity also exists for factors that influence the experience of pain.

AIDS risk

Of the number of reported cases of AIDS in the United States among Irish Americans, there is a low incidence reported for homosexuals (Lewis, 1988). The number of reported cases of AIDS among Irish Americans appears to be predominantly related to intravenous drug use. This has been further substantiated in a study by Walsh (1987), in which 11,640 persons in Ireland were tested for antibodies to the AIDS (human immunodeficiency) virus. Of this number, 626 were found to have antibodies to the virus, and 412 of these were identified as being intravenous drug users, including 28 infants born to mothers who were intravenous drug users (Lewis, 1988). The data would indicate that Irish people subscribe, in part or in full, to the doctrines of the Catholic Church, which include monogamous relationships, no premarital relationships, and no homosexual relationships. On the other hand, lack of sexual enhancement, failure to relieve aggressive tendencies, and characteristics of a dominant family life-style may be related to the incidence of AIDS among Irish persons who are intravenous drug users (Lewis, 1988). MacHale and Newell (1997) studied the level of knowledge regarding sex education. Although the level of knowledge was found it to be generally high one third of sexually active respondent Irish school-going teenagers were involved in high-risk behavior. For students who were sexually active only 67% used condoms all the time, whereas 33% used them sometimes or never.

Marsh, Hone, White, et al. (1996) studied nosocomial infection rates and pneumonia rates in Ireland and across Europe. Very little difference was found between the Irish groups and Europe-wide rates.

Psychological characteristics

Alcoholism Among American ethnic groups, Irish Americans have been ranked the highest or near highest in terms of heavy alcohol intake, loss of control, and untoward social consequences (Estes & Heinemann, 1986; Walsh, 1968, 1969; Walsh & Walsh, 1973; Butler, 1996). Pubs are a popular and common venue for revelry in Ireland. Beer without ice or beer mixed with lemonade (a shandy) and served warm are favorite Irish drinks (Lasky, 1996). The Irish in Ireland have ranked among the highest groups internationally for the prevalence of alcohol-related problems (Walsh, 1969). When compared to men in England and Wales, men in Ireland are more likely to drink at high-risk levels and are more likely to experience drinking problems than their counterparts (Harrison, Carr-Hill, Sutton, 1993). Stivers (1976) concluded that heavy drinking among Irish men is directly related to the patterns and characteristics of the familial, social, and economic systems. It has been further suggested that membership in the hard-drinking Irish peer group was traditionally legitimized because of the status of the sons who did not inherit land (Ablon & Cunningham, 1981).

Greeley (1972) concluded that the Irish often drink for reassurance, to escape from intolerable psychological burdens, and to repress sexuality and aggressiveness. Greeley (1972) has further characterized the domination of the Irish-American mother as a causative factor in male alcoholism because she rules her family by strong will or by subtly manipulating the sympathies of her husband and children. Ablon and Cunningham (1981) have substantiated the possibility of female domination as an etiological factor in the development of alcoholism among Irish men. They found that problem drinking was positively linked most closely to the Irish and that, in cases where a man's parents were both Irish, a serious alcohol problem was likely to be present. They also found that in cases where a man had an Irish mother but a father from another ethnic group, if that father was characterized as a heavy drinker, even if not an alcoholic, the subject was likely to have a drinking problem. Farren and Dinan (1996) also noted that a significantly higher percentage of alcoholics studied had a positive family history of alcoholism. Farren and Dinan (1996) concluded that there is validity in an alcohol typology theory among the Irish and that age of onset is a useful defining criterion

Adolescents and drinking behavior O'Conner (1978) noted that an expectation for enhanced sociability was directly related to drinking among Irish young adults. The respondents in this study had a prominent wish for a reduction in anxiety. Very little information is available regarding the drinking behavior of Irish adolescents. More information about adolescent Irish drinking would be helpful in addressing Irish adult drinking behavior.

Christiansen and Teahan (1987) conducted a study that examined the drinking behavior of Irish adolescents in two stages. The first stage compared the drinking behavior of Irish adolescents with the drinking behavior of American adolescents. During the second stage the adolescents' expectations regarding the effects of alcohol were measured. In the study it was believed that adolescent expectancies might initially arise from social learning processes, including acculturation from parents who drink or are alcoholics. However, the data from the study are suggestive that Irish adolescents drink less and experience fewer alcohol-related problems than their American counterparts across all ethnic adolescent groups, including Irish Americans. The findings of Christiansen and Teahan are not surprising because approximately 95% of the population in Ireland is Roman Catholic, and adolescents are prohibited from drinking as a religious decree at the time of confirmation and are expected to pledge abstinence until 21 years of age. However, although Irish adolescents did not report as many alcohol-related problems as their American counterparts, when social drinking occurred among these adolescents, drinking-related problems were noted. A conclusion was that Irish adolescents had a lower expectation for sexual enhancement; however, they believed that alcohol would result in increased arousal and release of aggression.

The problems identified in Irish adolescents, such as lack of sexual enhancement and lack of ability to release aggression, have also been noted among adult Irish alcoholics. Although Irish adolescents are noted to drink less than American peers and experience fewer alcohol-related problems, Ireland has one of the highest rates of alcoholism among the adult population.

Schizophrenia Straub, MacLean, O'Neill, et al. (1997) have presented some support for a possible schizophrenia vulnerability locus in region 5q22-31 in Irish families. This was the result of a genome scan for schizophrenia genes in 265 Irish individuals. It has been noted that allelic variation at the DRD2 locus or other genes in the surrounding chromosomal region do not account for the genetic susceptibility (Su, Burke, O'Neill, et al., 1993). However, it has been noted in the British literature that Irish-born people in Britian have the highest rates of first and subsequent admissions to psychiatric hospitals of any immigrant group since 1971 (Doolin, 1994). They are three times more likely to be admitted to a mental institution than White British-born people and twice as likely to be admitted as a person of Afro-Caribbean origin, which is the next highest group (Cochrane, 1989). Doolin (1994) suggests that the fact that Irish men are more likely to be diagnosed as alcoholic than schizophrenic in Britain is

suggestive of a stereotypical and racist view of Irish people being drunks. Stopes-Roe and Cochrane (1980) also noted that ethnic group membership has been shown in England to be one of the sociodemographic variables that is related to overt or diagnosed level of psychopathology.

Implications for nursing care

The nurse should remember that for Irish Americans alcoholism is influenced by a variety of factors, including patterns and characteristics of the family, social and economic conditions, and psychological orientation, rather than a biological variation per se. Because some Irish-American adults and adolescents drink for reassurance and to escape what is perceived as an intolerable burden, the nurse must develop strategies to teach such individuals more positive ways to alleviate stress and tension. Such individuals should be taught to verbally communicate feelings and anxiety rather than repressing or denying such feelings. The client must be taught the value of verbal expression to communicate needs. In addition, it is important to assist these clients in developing positive outlooks on life that may be perceived as positive coping strategies. The nurse also must remember the value of working not only with the client, but also with the family because some Irish Americans perceive family relationships as being paramount to a healthful existence.

The nurse might devise a family systems strategy that identifies perceived and actual roles within the family structure. After the roles are delineated, the nurse should assist the family in identifying undesirable behaviors manifested by persons in the particular roles. Changing behaviors that negatively affect the entire family system cannot be accomplished overnight. Such interventions will likely need repeated reinforcement. However, the nurse must remember that because some Irish Americans report that their drinking behavior is a result of their situation in life, it is important to consider the family's social and economic variables as a realistic beginning point in the initial intervention and treatment of such clients.

SUMMARY

Irish Americans have enjoyed extraordinary success in the United States. Although once faced with religious bigotry and economic hardship, they managed to cope with these problems and frequently turned them to their advantage.

Nurses should develop a sensitivity and understanding of individuals from a transcultural perspective to provide culturally appropriate nursing care. Nursing schools throughout the United States should incorporate transcultural courses and transcultural concepts into the nursing curriculum to foster the development of a transcultural understanding. One such institution that has developed a course to facilitate transcultural understanding is Vanderbilt University, which has a course titled

"International Perspectives of Nursing and Health Care." This course was designed to offer graduate and undergraduate students an experiential learning opportunity for the development of a theoretical base in nursing and health care in countries other than the United States. During this experience students spend time in Dublin, Edinburgh, and London. Macy and Morgan (1988) described the experiences of students in this course; for example, while in Dublin, students noted that 90% of the deliveries were attended by midwives, who were usually assisted by student midwives. During this experience students were able to compare the differences in nursing and medical techniques found in other countries and to assess the need to modify care based on transcultural concepts.

Case Study

Mr. Jonathon McMartin, a 46-year-old Catholic Irish American, is admitted to an in-house alcoholic treatment center at a local hospital. Mr. McMartin came to the United States 10 years ago with his wife and his five children, who now range from 11 to 23 years of age. Of the five children, four still live at home. In addition, Mr. McMartin's mother and father live within five blocks of him. Mr. McMartin also has seven siblings; three of these siblings still reside in Ireland, and four live in the same city as Mr. McMartin. Mr. McMartin reports to the nurse therapist who admits him to the unit that his problem occurred because he feels isolated from his immediate family. He states that his wife is very cold and unaffectionate and appears to mobilize the children to her way of thinking. Mr. McMartin says his children appear very distant from him and closer to their mother. He also reports that as a child growing up he felt the same way about his mother and father: he felt close to his mother and very distant from his father. Mr. McMartin reveals to the nurse that he believes he can stop drinking any time he desires.

CARE PLAN

 Nursing Diagnosis   Health maintenance, altered, related to use and abuse of alcohol

Client Outcomes

1. Client and family will verbalize a desire to learn more about alcoholism and appropriate techniques to reduce symptoms.
2. Client and family will verbalize a willingness to comply with psychiatric therapeutic regimen.
3. Client and family will verbalize an understanding of the need to comply with routine, scheduled follow-up visits to maintain an alcohol-free environment.

Nursing Interventions

1. Identify with client and family sociocultural factors that influence health-seeking behaviors.
2. Determine with client and family their knowledge level about alcoholism and the severity of this illness.
3. Determine with client and family their willingness to adapt to an alternative life-style free of alcohol.

Nursing Diagnosis   Parenting, altered, risk for, related to perceived emotional distance in family

Client Outcomes

1. Parents will develop an adequate base for effective parenting.
2. Parents will develop realistic expectations of self, spouse, and children within the family system.

Nursing Interventions

1. Assist parents in identifying present expectations of self, spouse, and children within the family system.
2. Assist family in developing and creating a positive learning environment for family growth.
3. Identify with family perceived areas of failure to meet expectations.
4. Provide family with opportunities to express feelings about unmet expectations.
5. Assist family in identifying major components within role identity that may create conflict within family system.
6. Encourage family to engage in closeness-related behavior such as touching to develop a more cohesive family system.

 Nursing Diagnosis   Communication, impaired, related to sociocultural variables creating interpersonal distance in family

Client Outcomes

1. Family will be able to communicate with health care personnel about personal and family-related needs.
2. Family will be able to communicate feelings about interpersonal relationships and effects of alcohol on the family system.
3. Each family member will be able to send precise, understandable messages to one another through appropriate verbal and nonverbal communication.

Nursing Interventions

1. Assist family in developing adequate communication techniques to communicate feelings and anxieties to one another.
2. Assist family in developing the ability to determine discrepancies in communicated verbal and nonverbal behavior.
3. Assist family in developing appropriate language skills and nonverbal perception to decrease the possibility of faulty perception.

 Nursing Diagnosis   Family processes, altered, related to an alcoholic family member

Client Outcomes

1. Family will participate in care and maintenance of the alcoholic family member.
2. Family will assist nurse in assisting client to return to a high level of wellness.
3. Family will verbalize difficulties encountered in seeking appropriate external resources.

Nursing Interventions

1. Determine family's understanding of client's condition.
2. Determine support systems available to family from external resources.
3. Determine with family supportive networks of friends and extended family members.
4. Involve family in care and management of client.
5. Encourage family to verbalize fears and anxieties.

 Nursing Diagnosis   Self-esteem disturbance related to emotional distancing of significant others

Client Outcomes

1. Client and family will verbalize positive and realistic feelings about self and the family system.
2. Client and family will make positive statements about self and the family system and display appropriate behavior accordingly.
3. Client and family will set realistic goals for self and the family system and implement a plan to follow through on activities to achieve these goals.
4. Client and family will perceive self and family in a positive manner.

Nursing Interventions

1. Design and implement client and family education to clarify values and beliefs that are perceived as negative influences.
2. Encourage client and family to engage in family therapy.
3. Assist family in developing an understanding about the need for the client to engage in psychotherapy, whether as an individual or in a group.
4. Encourage family to seek and attend appropriate self-help groups.

STUDY QUESTIONS

1. List appropriate nursing interventions that can be implemented to facilitate communication within this family system.

2. Describe the family structure of some Irish-American families and the effect the family organization may have on health-seeking behaviors and explain how this may affect nursing interventions when providing care for Mr. McMartin.

3. Identify how Mr. McMartin's behavior may be affected by time and space variables.

4. List at least two etiological reasons for the development of alcoholism within an Irish-American family.

5. Identify sociocultural variables within an Irish-American family that may facilitate perceived emotional distance.

References

Ablon, J., & Cunningham, W. (1981). Implications of cultural patterning for the delivery of alcoholism services. *Journal of Studies on Alcohol, 42*(Suppl. 9), 185-206.

Abramson, H. (1973). *Ethnic diversity in Catholic America.* New York: John Wiley & Sons.

Alba, R. (1976). Social assimilation among American Catholic national-origin groups. *American Sociological Review, 41,* 1030-1046.

Aroian, K., Patsdaughter, C., Levin, A., & Gianan, M. (1995, Spring). *International Journal of Social Psychiatry, 41*(1), 31-46.

Bhushan, N., & Kwaku, E. (1997, Aug. 30). Musicians: sound recording industry. *Billboard, 109*(35), 59.

Birchard, K. (1997, Aug. 9). Ireland brings in tough negligence law. *Lancet, 350*(9075), 421.

Blessing, P. (1980). Irish. In Thernstrom, S. (Ed.), *Harvard encyclopedia of American ethnic groups.* Cambridge, Mass.: Belknap Press.

Butler, S. (1996, July). Substance misuse and the social work ethos. *Journal of Substance Misuse for Nursing Health and Social Care, 1*(3), 149-154.

Byrne, J., Cama, A., Vigliarolo, M., & Levato, L. (1997, Jan.-Feb.). Patterns of inheritance in Irish and Italian families with neural tube defects: comparison between high and low rate areas. *Irish Medical Journal, 90*(1), 32-34.

Campinha-Bacote, J. (1997). Understanding the influence of culture. In Haber, J., Krainovich-Miller, B., Leach McMahon, A., & Price-Hoskins, P. (Eds.) *Comprehensive psychiatric nursing.* New York: McGraw-Hill.

Cashman, S.M., Patino, A., Martínez, A., et al. (1995, Jan.-Feb.). Identical intragenic microsatellite haplotype found in cystic fibrosis chromosomes bearing mutation G551D in Irish, English, Scottish, Breton and Czech patients. *Human Heredity, 45*(1), 6-12.

Christiansen, B., & Teahan, J. (1987). Cross-cultural comparisons of Irish and American adolescent drinking practices and beliefs. *Journal of Studies on Alcohol, 48*(6), 558-562.

Clarity, J. (1997, Sept. 10). With new promise for peace, talks resume in Ulster. *New York Times, 146*(50911), p. A1.

Cochrane, R. (1989). Mental hospital admission rates of immigrants to England: a comparison of 1971 and 1981. *Social Psychology, 24,* 2-11.

Connolly, J., & Cullen, A. (1995). Under-reporting of suicide in an Irish county. *Crisis, 16,* 34-38.

Corduff, E. (1997, March 12-16). Invisible exports. *Nursing Times, 93*(11), 28-31.

Cornacchia, E.J., & Nelson, D.C. (1992). Historical differences in the political experiences of American Blacks and White ethnics: revisiting an unresolved controversy. *Ethnic and Racial Studies, 15*(1),102-124.

Dolan, B. (1997, March 12-18). No Irish, no blacks. *Nursing Times, 93*(11), 28-29.

Doolin, N. (1994, Aug.) The luck of the Irish? *Nursing Standard, 8*(46), 40-41.

Duffy, T. (1997, Aug. 16). Shadows bring music to Matt Molloy to light. *Billboard, 109*(33), 48.

Elliott, M. (1997, Aug. 18). Looking for a legacy? *Newsweek, 130*(7), 47.

Estes, N., & Heinemann, M.E. (1986). *Alcoholism.* St. Louis: Mosby.

Fallows, M. (1979). *Irish Americans.* Englewood Cliffs, N.J.: Prentice Hall.

Farren, C.K., & Dinan, T.G. (1996, May). Alcoholism and typology: findings in an Irish private hospital population. *Journal of Studies in Alcohol, 57*(3), 249-252.

Fitzgerald, P., Ramsbottom, D., Burks, P., et al. (1995, April). Abdominal aortic aneurysm in the Irish population: a familial screening study. *British Journal of Surgery, 82*(4), 483-486.

Greeley, A. (1972). *That most distressful nation: the taming of the American Irish.* Chicago: Quadrangle Books.

Greeley, A. (1977). *The American Catholic: a social portrait.* New York: Basic Books.

Greeley, A. (1981). *The Irish Americans.* New York: Harper & Row.

Greeley, A., & McCready, W. (1975). The transmission of cultural heritages: the case of the Irish and Italians. In Glazer N., & Moynihan, D.P. (Eds.), *Ethnicity: theory and experience.* Cambridge, Mass.: Harvard University Press.

Griffin, W. (1981). *A portrait of the Irish in America.* New York: Charles Scribner's Sons.

Hall, E.T. (1959). *The silent language.* New York: Fawcett.

Hall, E.T. (1963). A system for the notation of proxemic behavior. *American Anthropologist, 65*(5), 1003-1026.

Hall, E.T. (1966). *The hidden dimension.* New York: Doubleday.

Harrison, L., Carr-Hill, R., & Sutton, M. (1993, Nov.). Consumption and harm: drinking patterns of the Irish, the English, and the Irish in England. *Alcohol, 28*(6), 715-726.

Howell, F. (1996, Jan.-Feb.). Smoking in Irish journals: a content analysis 1960-1994. *Irish Medical Journal, 89*(1), 18-20.

Hughes, D., Hill, A., Macek, M., et al. (1996). Mutation characterization of CFTR gene in 206 Northern Irish CF families: thirty mutations, including two novel, account for approximately 94% of CF chromosomes. *Human Mutations, 8,* 340-347.

Information please almanac (1997). Boston: Houghton Mifflin Company.

Johnson, J., & Adams, J. (1996, July). Self-neglect in later life. *Health and social care in the community, 4*(4), 226-33.

Kelleher, M., Corcoran, P., Keeley, H., et al. (1996, Jan.-Feb.). Improving procedures for recording suicide statistics. *Irish Medical Journal, 89*(1), 14-15.

Kennedy, R. (1973). *The Irish: emigration, marriage, and fertility.* Berkeley: University of California Press.

Kluckhohn, F., & Strodtbeck, F. (1961). *Variations in value orientation.* Evanston, Ill.: Row, Peterson.

Lasky, J. (1996). Ireland: culture bytes. *Chronicle Features.* Internet, Nov. 22, 1997.

Lewis, C. (1988). AIDS in Ireland. *Canadian Medical Association Journal, 138,* 553-555.

Lipton, J.A., & Marbach, J.J. (1984). Ethnicity and the pain experience. *Social Science and Medicine, 19*(12), 1279-1298.

MacDougall, J., & Doran, B. (1995, Nov.). Health care information services in Ireland. *Topics in Health Care Information Management, 16*(2), 1-9.

MacHale, E., & Newell, J. (1997, March). Sexual behaviour and sex education in Irish school-going teenagers. *International Journal of Studies in AIDS, 8,* 196-200.

Macy, J., & Morgan, S. (1988). Learning on the road: nursing in the British Isles and Ireland. *Nursing Outlook, 36*(1), 40-41.

Manning, P., Curran, K., Kirby, B., et al. (1997, April-May). Asthma, hay fever and eczema in Irish teenagers (ISAAC protocol). *Irish Medical Journal, 90,* 110-112.

Marsh, B., Hone, R., White, M., et al. (1996, May-June). European nosocomial infection survey: analysis of Irish data. Irish Intensive Care Pneumonia Survey Group. *Irish Medical Journal, 89*(3), 96-98.

Mbiti, K. (1970). *African religions and philosophies.* New York: Anchor Books.

McCann, J., & Burden, D. (1996, Dec.). An investigation of tooth size in Northern Irish people with bimaxillary dental protrusion. *Europe Journal of Orthodontics, 18*(6), 617-621.

McKay, J., Hall, B., & Buckler, J. (1989). *A history of world societies.* Boston: Houghton Mifflin Co.

McLaughlin, C., & Whittington, D. (1996). Suicide in Northern Ireland: a comparison of two quinquennia (1982-1986 and 1987-1991). *Journal of Psychiatric and Mental Health Nursing, 3*(1), 13-20.

Messenger, J. (1969). *Inis Beag: Isle of Ireland.* New York: Holt, Rinehart & Winston.

Nugent, J. (1994, Nov.). Cross-cultural studies of child development. *Zero to Three, 15*(2), 1-5.

O'Conner, J. (1978). *The young drinkers: a cross-national study of social and cultural influences.* London: Tavistock Publications.

Perlah, J. (1997, Aug. 23). In print. *Billboard, l09*(34), 93.

Porteous, M.A. (1985). Developmental aspects of adolescent problem disclosure in England and Ireland. *Journal of Child Psychology and Psychiatary, 26*(3), 465-478.

Prosser, S., & Dobbs, F. (1997, Aug.). Case-finding incontinence in the over-75. *British Journal of General Practice, 47*(421), 498-500.

Saidler, S. (1995, May-June). Nursing overseas. Irish nurses to the rescue in Calcutta, *World of Irish Nursing, 3*(2), 17-8.

Sexton, P. (1997, Aug. 30). RCE sees a multi-genre 'Slide' to success for Irish act Junkster. *Billboard, 109*(35), 14.

Shannon, W. (1981). Foreword. In Griffin, W.D. (Ed.), *A portrait of the Irish in America.* New York: Charles Scribner's Sons.

Slack, P. (1982). Nursing in southern Ireland. *Nursing Times, 78*(4), 138-141.

Snell, J. (1997, March 12-18). Joke over. *Nursing Times, 93*(11), 16-18.

Spector, R. (1996a). *Cultural diversity in health and illness, guide to heritage assessment and health traditions.* East Norwalk, Conn.: Appleton-Century-Crofts.

Spector, R (1996b). *Guide to heritage assessment and health traditions.* Stamford, Conn.: Appleton & Lange.

Statistical Abstract of the United States (1996). U.S. Department of Commerce, Bureau of the Census. Washington, D.C.: Government Printing Office.

Stillman, M. (1978). Territoriality and personal space. *American Journal of Nursing, 78,* 1671- 1672.

Stivers, R. (1976). *A hair of the dog: Irish drinking and American stereotype.* University Park, Pa.: Pennsylvania State University Press.

Stopes-Roe, M., & Cochrane, R. (1980). Mental health and integration: a comparison of Indian, Pakistani and Irish immigrants to England. *Ethnic and Racial Studies, 3,* 316-341.

Straub, R., MacLean, D., O'Neill, F., et al. (1997, March). Support for a possible schizophrenia vulnerability locus in region 5q22-31 in Irish families. *Molecular Psychiatry, 2,* 148-155.

Su, Y., Burke, J., O'Neill, F., et al. (1993, March). Exclusion of linkage between schizophrenia and the D_2 dopamine receptor gene region of chromosome 11q in 112 multiplex families. *Archives of General Psychiatry, 50*(3), 205-211.

U.S. Department of Commerce, Bureau of the Census. (1995). *We asked . . . . You told us ancestry. Economics and Statistics Administration.* Washington, D.C.: Government Printing Office.

Verna, P. (1997, Aug. 23). Albums: Spotlight. *Billboard, 109*(34), 91.

Wallace, B. (1997, Aug. 4). Stilling the guns. *Maclean's, 110*(31), 34.

Walsh, B.M., & Walsh, D. (1973). Validity of indices of alcoholism: a comment from Irish experience. *British Journal of Preventive Social Medicine, 27,* 18-26.

Walsh, D. (1968). Alcoholism in Dublin. *Journal of the Irish Medical Association, 61*(371), 153- 156.

Walsh, D. (1969). Alcoholism in the Republic of Ireland. *British Journal of Psychiatry, 115,* 1021-1025.

Walsh, J. (1987, Sept. 8). AIDS. *The Irish Times, 8.*

Wessel, B. (1931). *An ethnic survey of Woonsocket, Rhode Island.* Chicago: University of Chicago Press.

Zborowski, M. (1952). Cultural components in response to pain. *Journal of Social Issues, 8,* 16-30.

Zborowsky, M. (1969). *People in pain.* San Francisco: Jossey-Bass.

Zimmermann, T. (1997, Sept. 8). Recalling Ireland's pragmatic hero. *US News and World Report, 123*(9), 14.

Zola, I. (1966). Culture and symptoms: an analysis of patients' presenting complaints. *American Sociological Review, 31,* 615-930.

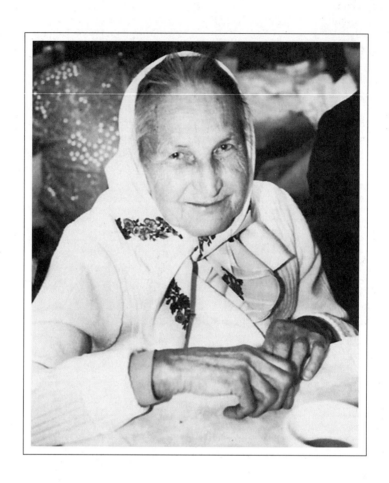

CHAPTER 15 Russian Americans

Linda S. Smith

BEHAVIORAL OBJECTIVES

After reading this chapter, the nurse will be able to:

1. Describe how health care practices in Russia have affected the health of Russian Americans.
2. Identify at least two health problems unique to Russian Americans.
3. Explain how Russian-American people use space and gestures as a part of communication.
4. List at least two future-oriented values for Russian Americans.
5. Identify the importance of family to Russian Americans.
6. Describe specific characteristics of the Russian language.

OVERVIEW OF RUSSIA

Russia (The Russian Federation) is the largest of the 15 republics once known as the Soviet Union and the largest republic of the Commonwealth of Independent States (CIS). Before the collapse of the Soviet Union, Russia was known as the Russian Soviet Federal Socialist Republic. Russia stretches from the Baltic Sea across the northern Eurasian land mass to the Bering Strait, where a Russian island lies only 3 miles from an island that is part of Alaska.

Russia occupies 6,592,800 square miles with both European and Asian components. This Russian land mass totals roughly 77% of the land once known as the Soviet Union and is almost twice the size of the United States. Of the number of people in Russia, 147,987,000 people are 81.5% Russian, 3% Ukrainian, 3.8% Tatar, and 11.7% other, to total over 40 nationalities (Brunner, 1997). It is important to un-

This chapter was written with special consultation of two Russian health care professionals who have now immigrated to the United States: Olga Messinova, M.D., Ph.D., former surgical nurse during and after World War II, and Mara Lisnyanskaya, former Medical Sister with over 15 years of nursing experience.

derstand that non-Russians living inside and outside of Russia insist on their separate identities.

Russia's enormous land area is divided by the Urals (a mountain system constituting the traditional boundary between Europe and Asia) into two land localities—European Russia and Siberia. European Russia is smaller in size but includes the greatest number of people as well as Russia's two largest cities, St. Petersburg (named "Leningrad" until September 1991) and Moscow, Russia's capital.

Russia is the largest country in the world and comprises 21 republics. Russian land includes Eastern Europe and stretches across northern Asia and onto the Pacific Ocean. On Russia's western borders, neighbors include Finland, Poland, Norway, Estonia, Belarus, and Ukraine. To the south, Russia is bordered by Azerbaijan, Georgia, Kazakhstan, China, Mongolia, and North Korea. Because of its geographic massiveness, Russia's climate is extremely varied with all types of weather conditions except tropical. Therefore Russian land can be plain and grassy, wooded, mountainous, frigid, and marshy and includes northern tundra and southern desert regions (Brunner, 1997; Hoffman, 1992).

Russian territory spans 11 time zones and includes 30% of the world's gas reserves, 20% of the world's coal reserves, 20% of the world's gold, and 6% of the world's oil. Other natural resources include uranium, diamonds, copper, lead, and silver. Russia has at least 40 billion barrels in proved oil reserves.

However, despite the richness of the country, Russia's gross national product (GNP) has dropped 19.6% since 1985, and personal income dropped 19.7% from 1991 to 1992 (Green beats red, 1993; Hofheinz, 1993). The 1995 World Bank Gross Domestic Product purchasing power parity estimate was $5300 per person with an average per month inflation rate of 7% (Brunner, 1997). Although millions of Russian workers have not been paid their salaries in months, a "shadow economy" has surfaced whereby Russians conceal part of their incomes and may actually have a higher living standard than figures represent because of their propensity for tax avoidance. In 1998, Russia showed the first fragile signs of economic growth in over 10 years. However, 25% of Russians remain classified as poor (Caryl, 1998a). Russians are well educated. Approximately one sixth of the world's scientists work in Russia, most Russians have at least a high school education, and there is a 95% literacy rate. However, the average Russian enjoys few luxuries.

Moscow is Russia's largest city (nearly 9 million people) and also its capital. St. Petersburg, to the north and west of Moscow, has 4.9 million people. Russia is highly industrialized. In addition to its defense industry, Russia is known for steel, metal work, appliance manufacturing, forestry, nuclear power, iron, cement, and chemicals. Russia's chief crops are grain, cotton, sugar beets, potatoes, and sunflowers. Nearly three fourths of Russia's mineral wealth is located in the Siberian regions. Some 10 million Russians are farmers. However, farming remains mostly collective, with Russians currently producing only half of the needed grain, meat, and dairy products needed for the Russian population (Information Please Almanac, 1998).

After the fall of the Soviet Union on December 21, 1991, Russia and 10 other former Soviet republics joined in a Commonwealth of Independent States (Johnson, 1992). In early 1992, Russia made radical changes that had enormous implications for Rus-

sians, including privatization programs and lifting of price freezing, which had stifled free enterprise for decades. Russia became a constitutional republic and a United Nations member and adopted a constitution that includes a multiparty system and scheduled elections. This new constitution, adopted late in 1993, gave the president ruling powers independent of the Russian Parliament (Brunner, 1997).

Life today in Russia

Today, in Russia, life continues to be extremely difficult and frustrating. Anti-Semitism continues. Railroad stations are crowded with homeless people because of unemployment Public transportation, once the pride of the country, has decayed as a result of poor maintenance and lack of repair parts. (Hofheinz, 1993; Stanglin & Pope, 1992). An estimated one million children are homeless in Russia. These children represent the offspring of the unpaid or unemployed. They have been forced into the streets by cruelty, alcoholism and neglect. They are beggars, glue or gas sniffers, and prostitutes (Carpenter, 1997). Because of an international fall in oil prices, Russia's major export, state revenues were cut, and wages owed to public servants, from teachers to soldiers, have grown to 7.6 billion rubles a month (Caryl, 1998b). Crime has also escalated. After the dissolution of the Soviet Union, few if any controls enforced law and order within the country. What did remain, however, was a tradition of abusing power and innovative officials who had learned how to exploit the system. Thus, crime exploded. Theft and gang rings have proliferated, along with weapons and explosives (Kunstel & Albright, 1996).

Russia's economy has experienced numerous serious problems in the past few years. Russia's gross domestic product (GDP) has dropped every year since 1989, with the exception of a less than 1% increase in 1997. After the 4.6% drop in 1998, an additional decline of 5% to 6% was expected in 1999. In 1997, the Russian government collected 10.8% of the GDP in taxes and spent 18.3% (Aron, 1998). The annual inflation rate is 30%; the rate of inflation in 1998 was 84.4%. These high inflation rates have caused financial disaster for Russians. Unemployment has increased to 11.5% of Russia's workforce, and this rate is expected to increase as the crisis worsens (Iams, 1998). In February of 1999, the currency exchange rate was about 23 rubles to the dollar (Bush, 1999), meaning it takes the equivalent of 80 rubles to simply buy a four dollar meal at Mc-Donalds.

As a result of the changing economy in Russia, vital statistics and general health have been greatly affected. For example, according to 1998 estimates, the death rate was 15/1000 persons. The infant mortality rate was 23.26/10000 live births, and life expectancy at birth was 58.6 years for men and 71.6 years for women (Factbook: Russia 1999). Tuberculosis has been a major concern, killing over 100,000 people in the last few years. In that time, over two million Russians have been exposed to tuberculosis. Medications are terribly expensive and hard to find. Only a few pharmaceutical firms exist following the August 1998 financial collapse. One brand of antihypertensive medication costs 350 rubles for just 20 pills.

Although agriculture remains primarily collectivized, independent farmers, with only 3% of the land, continue to produce 30% to 40% of Russia's fruits and vegetables. Even so, during the first 6 months of 1992, milk production declined by 30% and meat production by 25% in at least one Russian region (Dobbs, 1992). Millions of small farmers sell produce from small yard or kitchen plots and gardens (Caryl, 1998a). During the week of May 25, 1998, Moody's Investor Services (an influential financial agency that evaluates credit ratings) lowered Russia's credit rating for the second time in 2 months. Bailout plans for Russia's desperately poor economy are not moving fast enough to facilitate the payment of Russia's debts. Therefore the great fear is that Russia may be forced to devalue or print more rubles. Both of these options would further jeopardize Russia's fragile economic and social environments (Saffron, 1998).

Russian economic problems have translated into a declining health status for its people. Data from the World Health Organization (WHO) are startling. Russian men now live an average of 57.7 years as compared with 65 years in 1987. In the United States, men expect to live 72 years and women nearly 79 years (Barr & Field, 1996; Health care collapse, 1997). In just 1 year, between 1992 and 1993, male

life expectancy at birth declined 3 years. In Russia, parasitic infestations and respiratory infections account for almost half of all infant deaths. In the United States, these disorders represent less than 10%. In adults, Russia's leading causes of premature deaths are trauma, poisoning, respiratory diseases, and childbirth and pregnancy complications. Infant mortality is 25 per 1000 births (Barr & Field, 1996; Brunner, 1997). The chance of a woman dying from complications of pregnancy, childbirth, or unsafe abortions during her lifetime rose to 1 in about 1000 in Russia (Birth and Death, 1995).

Hospitals and clinics are poorly managed, equipped, and maintained. Most physicians have inadequate training and are paid dreadfully low salaries. Furthermore, hospitals and clinics lack adequate plumbing and heating and can often supply only 10% to 20% of the needed pharmaceuticals (Barr & Field, 1996). Even meager allocations to health care are misspent by local authorities. As further evidence of a decaying health care system, Russian children are sicker now than before the collapse of the USSR, perhaps because of a more open social climate. Sexually transmitted diseases, suicide, drug and alcohol abuse, and teen pregnancies have escalated. The number of abortions for girls 17 years of age or less has doubled in the last 5 years (Abortions among teens, 1995). Syphilis cases among the 15- to 17-year-old age group increased 73 times when compared with 1990 data (Study: Russian kids, 1998).

The psychological implications of the hardships in Russia are great. The proportion of Russians reporting depression is 70%; agitation and anxiety, 61%; and meaninglessness, 42% (Gloom in the time, 1992). It is easy to see why more than twice as many suicide attempts were made in 1991, compared with 1990 (Stanglin & Pope, 1992).

History

Historically, Slavic tribes began migrating into Russia around the fifth century of our era, and the first Russian state was established in the ninth century by Scandinavians. Mongols overran the country until 1480, and Ivan the Terrible became the first tsar in 1547. Peter the Great (1682-1725) tried to westernize Russia, but the pace was slow. Russia had no universities until 1755. In 1917, after Tsar Nicholas II abdicated (and during the October Revolution), Lenin and the Bolsheviks overthrew the government. Between 1918 and 1924 the tsar and his family were murdered, the Bolsheviks declared ideological war on Europe, Joseph Stalin (Josif V. Dzhugashvili) became general secretary, and the United Soviet Socialist Republic (USSR) was established.

Recent political change in Russia has been dramatic and historic. The current political situation began on March 11, 1985, when the former USSR KGB chief, Secretary Konstantin Chernenko, died and was replaced by Mikhail Gorbachëv.

Between 1985 and 1990, the Gorbachev-Shevardnadze team created a new human rights movement within the USSR. Gorbachev reforms, identified as *perestroika* ('restructuring') and *glasnost'* ('openness'), swept the Russian Republic with promises of democracy and freedom. However, Gorbachev inherited a sad and decaying empire (Anderson, 1992). Gorbachev believed that free enterprise and a carefully controlled form of democracy could be the overhaul needed for communism. To help him with this plan, he heralded a known reformer, Boris Yeltsin.

Yeltsin proved to be forceful, authoritarian, proud, chaotic, and critical of Gorbachev's leadership. Therefore, in a powerful move of control, Gorbachev publicly humiliated and fired his former protégé. This embarrassing termination triggered Yeltsin to campaign against the Communist Party and to run as a candidate for a parliamentary seat as the people's deputy from Moscow. Yeltsin achieved enormous popularity among the people, 90% of the vote, and became leader of a growing group of people who opposed communism (Anderson, 1992).

In February 1990, the USSR's Central Committee eliminated a constitutional clause that guaranteed the leading role of the Communist Party. On December 25, 1991, the Russian Federation became an independent republic (Billy, 1993). Yeltsin left the Communist Party in 1990. After confrontations with the Baltic republics, Gorbachev began discussions that would lead toward the creation of a "voluntary" union of the Republics.

In May 1991, all Soviet citizens were given the right to emigrate. The law titled "On the Procedure for the Exit from the USSR and Entry into the USSR of Citizens of the USSR" came into full effect in January 1993. This law was heralded as one of the most significant steps toward an open Russian society and marked the end of communist-enforced isolation (Burlatsky, 1991). This law restored the rights of the Russian people to live, work, and travel anywhere in the world.

In a historic move the citizens of the Russian Republic elected Yeltsin as president by democratic vote (Kostikov, 1991). However, shortly thereafter Gorbachev was overpowered in a dramatic conspiracy coup. Since that time, there have been ongoing struggles over rulership of this land as power has passed back and forth between Yeltsin and coup forces. Yeltsin had great power but failed to use this power to make immediate and necessary reforms. Yeltsin's popularity declined dramatically as a result of internal fighting among the 1033-member parliament (also called Congress of People's Deputies).

The Congress (or *Duma*), Russia's highest legislative body, is dominated by an anti-Yeltsin majority of ex-communists (Yeltsin rival backs down, 1993). His economic policies have received much criticism, and by the spring of 1993, eight attempts on his life were reported (Eight attempts reported, 1993). However, Yeltsin has continued to push for democratic reform (Witt, 1993), including opening classified Soviet archives, allowing Russians the right to own property and business, and attempting to stabilize the unit of Russian currency, the ruble. Other reforms include increasing social care for the needy, formalizing a system of granting benefits and privileges (Yeltsin: Main points, 1993), enforcing public disclosure of environmental accidents, dismantling state economic controls, and cutting the military by one half, including dramatic nuclear arms cuts, to invest energy in other areas.

In December 1994, Yeltsin drew criticism for sending Russian troops into the southern republic of Chechnya after their drive for independence from Russian control. Fighting was fierce and resistance costly. However, just before presidential elections in June 1996, Yeltsin agreed to a cease-fire. Soon after Yeltsin won the 1996 elections, he underwent bypass surgery. The Chechnyan war formally ended in May 1997. (Brunner, 1997).

IMMIGRATION TO THE UNITED STATES

As Russia has undergone rapid changes over the years, life in Russia has been increasingly unbearable to some, and immigration to the United States has dramatically increased. Thus the likelihood has significantly increased that a nurse in the United States may care for Russian clients and their families.

The first wave of Russian immigration to the United States occurred after the Revolution (1917) in the 1920s. These immigrants were highly intelligent and generally well educated. The second wave of Russian immigrants occurred after World War II. In this wave, Russian immigrants had a mixture of backgrounds. Russian Jews were and are well educated with approximately 13.5 years of education. Most entered the United States as refugees because of emerging and ever-increasing anti-Semitism. For many Russian Jews, the Jewish communities in which they settle provide tremendous social and economic support. For most Russian immigrants to the United States, their sphere of family and friends rests primarily with other Russian Americans, caused in part by U.S. immigration laws, unchanged since 1952, that offer the right to U.S. immigration based on family preference. Therefore the majority of new Russian Americans are related to earlier Russian immigrants.

For the past 20 years, the United States encouraged the USSR to allow free immigration, particularly for the 2 million Soviet Jews residing in that country. A wave of Soviet Jews immigrated to the United States in 1973 as a direct result of a law passed by Congress to facilitate Jewish immigration. Because of this law, more than 66,480 Soviet Jews immigrated to the United States between 1975 and 1980 (Schiff, 1979).

Historically, from 1971 to 1991, approximately 181,000 Russian Jews entered the United States. In 1991, of the number of Russians entering the United States, almost two thirds were Jewish. (In the red, 1992). Historically, Soviet Jews were the most oppressed ethnic group in the USSR (Azarian, Boland, & Skripchenko, 1996). Additionally, policies of the former USSR encouraged, even mandated, the immigration of the family as a unit. Therefore, when younger family members wished to leave Russia, older parents also had to leave. Over half the immigrants to Chicago (62%) stated that leaving Russia was not their decision (Brod & Heurtin-Roberts, 1992; Kohn, Flaherty, & Levav, 1989).

In 1988, in the United States, there were 406,022 persons who were listed as Russian immigrants (U.S. Department of Commerce, Bureau of the Census, 1988). For the most part, those who immigrate to the United States are well educated and courageous people who are voracious readers and passionately devoted to the arts. Despite years of hardship, Russian immigrants are proud people. Russian immigrants come to a specific location because they have relatives or other contacts in these locations, which means that pocket populations of Russian Americans have emerged in various regions of the United States.

Recent immigrants did not endure the long delays and confusion that earlier immigrants endured. Some recent immigrants were processed and arrived in the United States within a year or less. In some cases, resentment has surfaced among earlier immigrants, who often endured 10 or more years of waiting and turmoil.

In 1991, 57,000 people born in the former Soviet Union were granted permanent resident (immigrant) status. With this statistic in mind, the Soviet Union, in its final year as a nation, provided more U.S. immigrants than any other nation of the world. These numbers reflect a dramatic change in Soviet policy. Before 1989, fewer than 3000 Soviet citizens per year were allowed to emigrate. However, in 1988, restrictions on emigration eased. In 1989, the U.S. Department of Justice Immigration and Naturalization Service reported 11,000 Soviet immigrants and more than 25,000 in 1990. Starting in 1992, Russian immigration was reported separately. However, demographic data based on reported city of birth were compiled for Soviet Union immigrants, and whenever possible, the republic of birth origin was identified. From these data, the following Russian immigration data were listed and reported. The number of Russian immigrants in 1989 was 2167; in 1990, 4766; and in 1991, 10,652. In 1989, most Russian immigrants settled in California. In 1991, most Russian immigrants settled in one of five states: New York (34.2%), California (25.3%), Massachusetts

(5.4%), Illinois (4.9%), and Pennsylvania (4.4%). In 1990, Russian immigrants settled in urban settings, primarily in Boston, Chicago, New York, and Philadelphia. In 1991, Portland, Sacramento, Los Angeles, and San Francisco received immigrants (U.S. Department of Justice, 1992). The current Russian population in San Francisco is approximately 80,000 (Fish, 1992).

Currently, immigration of Russian Jews is down from 36,000 per year in the early 1990s to 21,000 per year in 1995 and 1996. Employment opportunities and welfare cuts were named as possible reasons for the change. However, 60,000 Jews are waiting in Moscow for U.S. immigration interviews (Ups and downs, 1996). Immigration also includes a seldom-reported yet growing number of U.S.-adopted Russian children. Since 1992, Russia, with its limited resources to care for orphaned children, has become the number one source of foreign children adopted by U.S. citizens, with a total of 3,816 children adopted by American adults in 1997 and 2454 in 1996. This number is expected to grow. These children are Russian-speaking and usually have special educational and health needs (Azarian, Boland, & Skripchenko, 1996; Russia may tighten, 1997). There are estimated 2,952,987 of Russian descent currently residing in the United States (Information Please Almanac, 1998).

Life today for Russians in the United States

Russian Americans report new freedoms in the United States. For example, Russian-American Jews are often able to fully practice their faith for the first time, arriving in the United States, and Russian parents commend the skills their children learn in schools. They especially appreciate skills of thinking, analysis, and discussion (generally unheard of in their country). Russian-Jewish women are familiar with working outside the home in good paying professions. As refugees, Russian-American Jews are entitled to resettlement services, training programs, financial help, and permanent resident status in the United States. (A *refugee* comes to the United States because of declared political problems, such as anti-Semitism and because they seek political safety; an *immigrant* is identified as someone who simply

wishes to live in another country.) However, over half of the newly arriving Russian Jews are over 50 years of age and therefore have difficulty in adapting to a new culture.

The recession in the United States has made the transition more difficult for new Russian-American immigrants. However, Russian immigrant communities often provide supportive services such as career guidance, networking, training programs, classes in English as a second language (Hill, 1992), and free health care.

Americans should understand that in Russia preventive care and medical treatment, though limited, are free. Education, including postsecondary university and professional studies, is also free though teachers are poorly paid and less qualified than before 1991. Therefore, many Russian immigrants have had some form of technical training or advanced education. Nevertheless, Russian immigrants have difficulty in understanding the concepts of insurance, private pay, malpractice, and diagnostic related groups. Concepts such as "credit" are entirely new.

COMMUNICATION
Dialect, style, and volume

The official language of Russia is Russian. This language consists of a 33-character Cyrillic alphabet named after the ninth-century apostle to the Slavs, St. Cyril. St. Cyril created the alphabet so that the Bible could be translated to be used for liturgy in the Slavic countries (Moore, 1988). In the tenth century, the Cyrillic alphabet was adopted by Russians simultaneously with Christianity. The old Cyrillic alphabet was renovated twice, once by Peter the Great and again in 1918. Russian is the most important of all the Slavic languages and belongs to the eastern branch of the Slavic linguistic family. Approximately one sixth of the world's population speaks Russian.

For most Russians, English is the most popular language of all the Western languages. This new-found popularity of English on the part of the Russian people is related to media broadcasts, movies, rock video television programs, and Western business opportunities. In addition, professional literature (including health and medicine) is often in

English, and medical students are frequently required to read English medical journals.

Russian is sometimes referred to as a "house green" language because articles (such as "the") and verbs (such as "is") are often unnecessary. The Russian language is a flexible, beautifully rich language. Paralanguage qualities such as tone, inflection, speed, and verbal pauses contribute to the variety and meaning of Russian words and sounds. Russians freely use paralanguage and other nonverbal indicators to denote the value being placed on what is said. The spirit of the Russian people, their warmth and love, comes through clearly in this dialect (Binyon, 1983). Just as in the United States, the Russian language carries geographic variances.

Some Russian-American people may have studied English in Russia. However, the English they learned is British English, which often is significantly different in sound, spelling, and pronunciation from American English, making language comprehension difficult. Additionally, American geographical accents can cause problems.

Although many well-educated Russians studied English at some point in their education, English proficiency is not always easy, especially for older Russian-American immigrants. In the United States, Russian speakers rank fifteenth of total speakers. Of the 241,798 recently immigrated Russian Americans, 14,939 do not speak any English and 50,356 speak English poorly (U.S. Department of Commerce, Bureau of the Census, 1997). Importantly, younger immigrants have made the adjustment to English with less difficulty. For younger Russian immigrants, the first priority on arrival in the United States is to learn conversational English; the second priority is to enroll children in school; and the third priority is to find employment.

Using interpreters is important because of potential language barriers. Family, especially younger family members, may be embarrassed and anxious during the crisis of an illness or problem. In a study of Russian immigrants in Virginia, Duncan and Simmons (1996) found that in half of the households, no one could read English. Interpreters translate more than words. They must also convey nonverbal and subtle meanings. Therefore, attention must be paid to the issues of confidentiality (Azarian, Boland, & Skripchenko, 1996).

Many elderly Jewish immigrants speak Yiddish. For these people, the practice of speaking Yiddish was greatly discouraged by Russian (and Soviet) authorities as being an "antistate" activity. Younger Jewish immigrants seldom speak Yiddish (Gennis, 1989; Smith, 1989).

Fortunately, many medical, chemical, and scientific terms are cognates, and although the written appearance of the word is different between Russian and English, the sound is similar. A few medical cognates are: organ(ism), appetite, function, pulse, doctor, hospital, physical, diagnosis, normal, and problem.

The volume of speech used by Russian Americans is not significantly different from that used by some Irish-American people. In Russia, because loud demands were often necessary to receive medical care, some Russians became loud when attempting to be understood or get attention. Thus even normal conversation may seem loud and boisterous.

Touch

Russians often use touch freely with intimate and close friends. It is not unusual to see Russian women embracing and kissing other women and Russian men embracing and kissing other men. Friends who have been separated often greet each other, in public or in private, in this fashion. The technique of kissing each cheek three times seems to be a cultural trait adopted from the Middle East. The gentle kiss of a man on a woman's hand is a gesture of respect and admiration. Also, a handshake of agreement from a Russian is often more binding than a signed document.

Russian people are commonly perceived as being kind, caring, and generous. When trust has been established, they express these feelings willingly and publicly. They are by nature and experience, however, cautious. Some Russians evaluate situations and people with great care. Emotions are also freely expressed. Russians have a quick appreciation for jokes and satire, often venting their feelings in this form of expression. It has been said that Russian people cry and laugh easily

(R. Feldman, personal communication, April 28, 1998; Smith, 1991).

Context

Russian people who learned English in Russian schools may have learned from a nonnative speaker. Therefore the sound of English will be different. Tourists traveling in Russia are often approached by native Russians who are eager to practice conversational English with a native English speaker. However, for most new Russian immigrants, conversational English is likely to be unrecognizable.

Russian people have learned through years of communist rule to look and act neutrally. With strangers and in crowded places, eye contact is avoided, affect is flat, posture is not erect, and eyes are diverted. Upon arriving in the United States, Russian Americans often express great wonder at the freedom with which Americans make nonverbal connections with strangers. However, Americans tend to be cooler with close friends and family than Russians are. In Russia, it is common to visit friends without warning, whereas in the United States this practice is uncommon (Gottlieb, 1990).

Kinesics

Until trust and comfort have been established, Russian Americans will use few gestures. They do, however, feel free to maintain eye contact, and they do allow and expect nurses to use touch and gestures freely during the implementation of nursing procedures. Older Russian Americans who are immigrants are more entrenched in social amenities, often preferring to express themselves verbally. "Please" and "thank you" are integral to their speech, and they use these words at every possible opportunity. Nodding one's head is a gesture of approval; outstretching one's hand is a gesture of salute. When compliments are given, they are sincere. Flowers are presented during important meetings as a gesture of tribute. The person seated first in a room is the one with the most authority or prestige.

Implications for nursing care

Russian Americans expect the nurse to be warm and caring, to "feel" for them, and to help them cope with physical and emotional problems. The most often expressed expectation of the nurse by the Russian American is that the nurse be friendly. This expectation is demonstrated by an "inviting" open posture, a smile, and a low and calm voice. Touch, when appropriate, is considered a sign of friendliness and caring (Brod & Heurtin-Roberts, 1992). Russian Americans do not appreciate a light, "chatty" approach to health care, and they want to be certain that the nurse understands them. Russian Americans can easily become very shy, especially recent immigrants. Because their English may be tenuous, Russian Americans may be hesitant to ask for clarification.

Russian Americans, therefore, expect the nurse to speak slowly and clearly and to choose simple words when needed. Russian Americans also tend to be poor listeners and may be unable to represent themselves accurately (Barnathan, 1991). However, gestures and demonstrations, to clarify and promote understanding, are expected and appreciated. "Look at my eyes," explained one Russian American. "My eyes will tell you that I do not understand because I will have a stupid expression!"

In most instances, Russian Americans will comply with medical directives and teachings if they believe that the nurse is trustworthy, sincere, and competent. Nurses will not be believed or trusted by Russian Americans if they are perceived to be masklike, robotic, or phony in their caring behaviors. Nurses should address Russian-American clients by "Mr." or "Mrs." followed by the family name. However, use of the first name, followed by the patronymic (their father's first name plus a feminine or masculine ending depending on the person's sex) may be an acceptable alternative. Well-educated and professional Russian-American women often retain their maiden name. Using this formal method of address will convey the nurse's respect. To address a Russian by his or her first name only is improper and presents a grave social error. Russians also object strongly to terms of endearment, such as "dear," "hon," "sweety," and "hi, guy," when used by health care workers (Smith, 1996). As explained by Russian-American R. Feldman (personal communication April 28, 1998), "I want you to believe me when I tell you I have a problem. Here the nurses are perfect. We will respect them and listen to them. They know their job, and they know what they are supposed to do."

Russian Americans tend to speak freely regarding physical problems. Once language is no longer an issue or problem, the nurse will find that clients respond warmly. However, Russian Americans may be uncomfortable using gestures when speaking to the nurse. The nurse must be aware that although younger Russian immigrants adapt well to English older Russian immigrants may not. Often, elderly Russian immigrants choose to associate only with Russian-speaking friends and relatives, which presents a difficult problem if an interpreter is unavailable. To add to this difficulty, Russian Americans may allow only Russian to be spoken at home. Because many Russian Americans are multilingual (Yiddish, German, French, Polish, Latin, and so on), it is an advantage if the nurse understands another language familiar to the client. (However, only 14% of Russian Jews consider Yiddish their mother tongue.) One way to convey respect and an understanding of the culture is to provide avenues for client teaching through Russian literature. Health literature written in Russian may prove to be a better client teaching aid than video films. Additionally, cognate words, relatives, and interpreters should be used whenever possible.

The challenge is for nurses to expand their own culture to care effectively for members of the Russian-American ethnic group. These skills can strengthen the nurse as a person and as a health care professional.

SPACE

The Russian culture exists on two very different levels. To strangers and new acquaintances, a Russian will remain aloof, preferring to speak and work in the social or public zone. However, once friendship and familiarity have been established Russian people are comfortable within a personal zone. The intimate zone is reserved for spouse or children except for health care workers performing within a professional capacity. When hospitalized, Russians are extremely compliant and are able to tolerate the loss of privacy.

Individuals are perceived according to the boundaries they maintain, which include the degree of permeability and flexibility. Permeability is generally defined as the degree to which a boundary is open or closed; for the most part, permeability varies from closed to open. When an individual has closed boundaries, very little exchange occurs between this person's internal and external environments, and the person may be perceived as being quiet, withdrawn, and set in his or her ways. On the other hand, if boundaries are open, much exchange occurs between the person's internal and external environments, and this individual may be perceived as being talkative, social, and one who enjoys taking risks. Russian Americans may be very superstitious. Do not speak of death or potentially negative events in the abstract.

Flexibility is defined as the ability of a person to move along a permeability continuum. A person who is sometimes closed and sometimes open and who thereby uses the entire permeability continuum is considered flexible. On the other hand, a person who always gravitates toward the closed end of the continuum, which is indicative of a low degree of flexibility, is described as a rigid, closed person. A person who is always open and never closed is described as an open individual. People who are perceived as rigid and closed may be quiet and withdrawn and seldom if ever share intimate secrets, dreams, or thoughts, even with best friends or a spouse (Scott, 1988).

Some Russian persons are perceived as rigid and closed because they remain aloof and distant. However, the word "friend" is not a casual term to Russians. It appears that friendship is taken more seriously by Russian Americans. Close Russian friends may embrace, but mere acquaintances will probably not even shake hands. Russians may prefer to greet and meet acquaintances on a verbal level only.

Implications for nursing care

The nurse who cares for the Russian-American client will generally find that health-assessment procedures done in the intimate zone are accepted without argument or problem provided that adequate information and justification have been given before the procedure and permission from the client has been requested and provided. For the most part, the nurse should be aware that Russians prefer to remain at a social distance rather than an intimate distance with caregivers. If personal distance must be invaded to provide therapeutic assistance, the nurse should provide careful explanation before the intervention to alleviate stress and anxiety created by the violation of space. As with all aspects of care, it is important for the nurse to modify approaches based on an evaluation of the individual client and family.

SOCIAL ORGANIZATION
Family

Russian-American people are very family oriented, and family relations and roles have a significant influence on them. Both in Russia and the United States, extended family members often live together, relying on each other for financial and emotional support, child care, and completion of household tasks.

For the Russia-American immigrant, who may have left children, siblings, and parents to come to the United States, family members in the United States become even more significant. Therefore, Russian Americans are a very closely knit group. Within a few years after immigrating to the United States, Russian children tend to become rapidly assimilated into the American culture, leave home, and may even leave the geographic area. Remaining family members are often elderly and without job or language skills. Frequently they isolate themselves from American contacts (Smith, 1996).

One Russian American explained that her children were also her best friends. Because she had so few other contacts, her son had become enormously important to her. In Russia, even in one- or two-room apartments, parents often live with married children and grandchildren, which may be one reason that the number of children in a Russian family is usually two or less. Another relationship to family size in Russia is the very large number of abortions performed each year. In 1989, 6.5 million Soviet women had abortions resulting from economic chaos and an acute shortage of contraceptives (Family & Health, 1989).

Within the Russian family structure, the father tends to have the greatest influence. Children, especially male children, look up to the father and absorb his values and beliefs. Additionally, the husband of the household makes decisions on behalf of the family, though he does consult with his wife, especially when the wife is well educated. Children primarily are cared for by women. Family violence is uncommon in Russian households, though arguing and dishthrowing may occur during family disagreements.

Education, family, and cultural activities are values that begin when children are infants. During social gatherings, children are often seen dancing with their parents. Fathers will often walk arm and arm with a child through an art museum in an effort to instill an appreciation of history and culture. Children as young as 5 years of age learn to read classic literature and attend the ballet, opera, and concerts. Girls and boys are encouraged to achieve good grades in school and go on to college. Some Russians fear that in the absence of state funding, the development of the arts, including ballet, theater, music, and painting, will deteriorate (Buttweiler, 1992).

Most Russians come to the United States with few possessions, but they come full of the joy of life, which contributes to their success (Smith, 1991). Another factor contributing to success is that they have made immigration to the United States a family project. Russian Americans complain of feeling stifled and desperate in Russia. A "group" identity has been reinforced by the Russian problems they were forced to endure. Therefore a strong bond develops in Russian-American communities because of similar backgrounds, culture, language, life-styles, educational levels, and geographical core. Despite the ethnic bond found in many Russian-American communities, Russian Jews have historically felt isolated from dominant Russian life and culture, and this heritage has helped to maintain a strong ethnic identity. Russian Americans rely on person-to-person networks and referrals.

The life of the elderly Russian immigrant is a difficult one. In Russia, elders found important roles helping support their children with child care and household duties, and, in return, Russian adult children cared for their parents. Once here in the United States, parents and children may withdraw from each other. Elders may represent the "old" country, the culture that no longer applies, and parents may lose their authority and family status (Smith, 1996). For the elderly, fears may increase because of concerns over the acculturation of their children and grandchildren and the real fear of being alone and without resources during illness and death. Because of language barriers and age, they may be unwilling and unable to begin their careers over.

One Russian American explained, "In Russia, we gathered together many, many people at my house. We could talk endlessly about politics. Russians love to come together with friends and neighbors, forming a very close connection with each person we live and work with. But in the United States, everyone is very busy. They drive in separate cars, have separate houses, and separate neighborhoods. Americans watch television at home rather than go out to the theater or see friends. Here in America I am less social and my friends are few."

Individualism

Russian Americans are hard working and have very little tolerance for people who do not have the wish to work. They are self-reliant and independent. Russian Americans who become ill will use home care, hospitalization, or both, as much as possible rather than become a burden to their family. They have a strong desire to stay in their own homes and will remain independent until the last possible moment.

This strong individualism would appear to contradict former Russian social structure, in which individual achievements were seen in terms of their value to the group. Strong individualism has been a common Russian-American response to the forced Soviet collectivism endured in Russia. Being anticommunists, Russian Americans tend to vote Republican (Gold, 1991). However, being a product of a society in which the individual was not valued, Russian Americans may resist committing anything to writing, fear taking responsibility for their actions (Barnathan, 1991), and find themselves underprepared for a way of life that depends on initiative, creativity, and responsibility (Brod & Heurtin-Roberts, 1992). Problems occur when the nurse or physician expects the Russian American to make independent decisions regarding self-care and self-help. Many look to the health care establishment to give them this advice (Duncan & Simmons, 1996).

Position of women in the family and in society

Russian-American women, who are almost completely liberated on the job and in professional circles, are not liberated at home. Although both husband and wife have full-time employment outside the home, most Russian men prefer to have their wives do the cooking, shopping, and housework. Without the modern conveniences of time-saving electrical appliances such as microwave ovens, washers, dryers, and vacuum cleaners, Russian woman would spend at least an additional 40 hours per week on household chores (Binyon, 1983; Ross & Searing, 1992).

In Russia, although jobs for women are considered equal, salary and authority are not (Ross & Searing, 1992). On average, Russian women earn 30% less than their male counterparts. Although these statistics were "Soviet" in origin, it is interesting to note that in 1989, 50.8% of all Soviet workers were women, and women accounted for 67% of physicians, 87% of economists, 58% of engineers, and 89% of bookkeepers (Koval, 1989). Of all working-age Soviet women, 92% either worked or went to school, and one out of three marriages failed (Binyon, 1983). Although Russian women can retire at 55 years of age, the size of their pensions is very small.

Burdens of food shortages, long waiting lines, and inadequate child care are problems for the working Russian woman. Unfortunately, with the fall of communism, the percentage of women in government has decreased dramatically (as a result of the change in government-forced quotas). Besides unequal wages for Russian women, sex discrimination permeates Russian society. Hence, most Russian women need to learn assertiveness, positive self-esteem, and a new vision of their important societal role. It is interesting to note that the Russian language has no phrase for sexual harassment (Ross & Searing, 1992; Smith, 1997).

The issue of poor self-esteem for women is one reason for the rapid increase in prostitution among women in Russia. Many escort agencies and personal massage services for men opened within the first 6 months of 1992. With the relaxing of puritanical communist mores, beautiful obedient women have become status symbols for Russian men, and the Moscow newspapers are full of advertisements for these kinds of services (Sloane, 1992). Not only within Russia are Russian women seemingly exploited, numerous web sites promote Russian brides and escorts. Tens of thousands of women from the former Soviet Union are trafficked yearly all over the world. They are attractive, well educated, and desperate to leave a desperate country. Profit margins are high and without passports or money, these women are easily victimized (Pope, 1997). Russian women are beautiful and keenly interested in fashion.

Spirituality and religious beliefs

Religion in Russia is mainly Eastern Orthodoxy. Until the eighteenth and nineteenth centuries in Russia, literacy was traditionally associated with the Russian Orthodox Church. Historically, the church was highly regarded by the people, mostly uneducated peasants, as a source of guidance and power. This undoubtedly contributed to the manner in which the people bowed to authority (Billy, 1993).

In Russia, the nonreligious constitute 60% of the population. The next largest group at 25% is Russian Orthodox. The remaining religions include Tatar Muslims and Jews. One Russian American explained, "We were not raised with God; we made fun of the religious" (R. Feldman, personal communication, April 28, 1998).

In Russia, traditionally, Russian Jews could not own property or land, which may explain why many became merchants. As a result of this role, other Russian ethnic groups developed resentment and anti-Semitic feelings. With the relaxation of censorship and a new emphasis on Russian nationalism, there has been a resurgence of anti-Semitism.

Russian Jews immigrated to the United States and other countries in a greater percentage than non-Jewish Russian people. The more Jewish oppression and anti-Semitism in Russia, the greater was the rate of immigration. The immigration has led to further discrimination. New freedoms of speech and expression have brought out old, otherwise buried, prejudices. In this newfound climate, Russian Jews feel persecuted and often fear for their children.

Although religious expression in Russia had major social roadblocks since the 1917 Bolshevik revolution, Russian people take religion very seriously. However, recent *perestroika* and *glasnost'* changes, along with the dramatic fall of communism in Russia, witnessed a resurgence of religious freedoms. Christianity has had a remarkable revival.

The Russian Orthodox Church requires followers to observe fast days as well as a "no-meat" rule on Wednesdays and Fridays. During Lent all animal products, including dairy products and butter, are forbidden. Fasting also occurs during Advent. It is believed that God is served in a more powerful way during periods of fasting. However, even if fasting is strictly observed, special allowances are made for illness and pregnancy. Fear, sin, and punishment have been major themes for the Russian Orthodox Church.

After more than 70 years of war against religion, most Russians hope that the Orthodox Church will be able to positively influence the people's family, moral, and social values and consequently decrease the rate of divorce. As the Russian Orthodox Church attempts to reclaim state-confiscated churches and land, more and more Russians are returning to their once-hidden faith. Before *perestroika* and *glasnost'*, religious expressions were prohibited in Russia. However, some churches did remain open. As a result some people believed that Russian Orthodox Church leaders were obliged to report to the Secret Service and confessions were not confidential. In addition, the training of Russian Orthodox priests was poor because of the general absence of good academic education programs. Today in Russia the church holds the power of hope for the many people who attend services. This hope is brief, strong, and desperate because of the hardship of Russian life, especially for the elderly.

Implications for nursing care

In all human societies, actions that are done for survival, such as eating, elimination, sex, and health practices, though physical, take on cultural and social regulations. Cultural functions and norms dictate behavior patterns in a profound way. It is essential for nurses to understand the role culture plays to provide safe, compassionate, and effective nursing care.

Despite persecution and hardships, Russian-American people have maintained a significant degree of individualism. Russian-American parents have taught their children an appreciation for land and country. One Russian immigrant explained,

"Whether good or bad, it is still mine. I still love my homeland." Another Russian American said it this way: "I miss everything—my home, my language, my friends. Here, I am another personality. I am not me. I cannot say what I want because I don't know the right words. This makes me tired and frustrated. I want so much to visit Russia, my country." It is important for the nurse to understand that strong feelings of national pride are only experienced by some Russian immigrants.

Because Russian Americans have strong family ties and values, the nurse must remember to involve the entire family, including extended family members, in the planning and intervention of care. Because the father is perceived as having a paramount role and function in the Russian family, the astute nurse will solicit the opinions and advice of the father before presenting a treatment and intervention plan to the rest of the family. In this instance, if the father's opinions and advice are solicited before the presentation to the rest of the family, the father may be of particular assistance in getting the family's cooperation and support. Because the entire Russian family becomes the client, time, respect, and information must be presented to the entire family. Goals of health and health care need to be presented as family goals and family benefits (Azarian, Boland, & Skripchenko, 1996).

Some Russian Americans hold particular beliefs in regard to religion, death, and dying. Therefore it is important for the nurse to respect these beliefs and practices and incorporate them into a therapeutic plan of care that will assist the client in returning to a high level of wellness. Because of a belief that the human body is sacred, Russian Americans will be reluctant to donate organs. More importantly, the nurse needs to keep imminent death topics away from the terminally ill. Tell the head of the family first. "We choose to give mercy to the person; that person must not know that he or she will soon die. We don't need time to prepare a will because we have so few possessions to write wills about," replied one Russian woman.

Russian Americans tend to feel displaced and isolated. Nurses need to be extremely thorough in gathering data in the psychosocial and physical assessment. The nurse must also remember to be tolerant of visitors to Russian-American clients. Russian Americans are accustomed to long discussions with friends, which they find socially and spiritually rewarding. Therefore, unless visitors become potentially harmful toward client outcomes, they should generally be permitted and supported.

TIME

Some Russian Americans hold a perspective of time that is past, present, and future oriented. For these people, there is a future within the present and a present within the past. On the other hand, some Russian Americans, particularly the well educated, hold only a future orientation. One example of this cultural attitude is seen in immigration.

Although the study of history and heritage is important to Russian Americans, most look to the future more than to the past, a characteristic related to socialism and Marxism. "Not now," such ideology preaches, "the future!" "Work hard now and have patience; suffer now so that the future will be better." Because living conditions in Russia for most immigrants were desperate, now they feel hope.

Another important example of future orientation is seen in the Russian people's almost universal belief in education for themselves and their children. Education begins early and is reinforced in the home. For Russian Americans who espouse a belief in future orientation, education is viewed as an awakening or a light. Lack of education is viewed as a void or darkness. Self-learning and lifelong learning are valued and practiced. On immigration to the United States, Russian children are encouraged to attend school immediately, even before they have any knowledge of English. In fact, Russian children learn English very easily. It is obvious that present efforts are vehicles for future achievements.

Implications for nursing care

For the Russian American, the United States offers opportunities for goal establishment and attainment impossible in Russia. However, one main obstacle faced by nurses caring for Russian Americans is that they may be content to continue to live poorly and not take advantage of health care opportunities (Dobbs, 1992).

For some Russian immigrants who hold time orientation that is a combination of past, present, and future beliefs, it is important for the nurse to remember that such an individual may be reluctant to seek preventive therapeutic interventions. The nurse must design and implement teaching strategies that will assist the client in developing an understanding about the implications of past and present behavior on future wellness and quality of life.

On the other hand, Russian immigrants who hold a future orientation value preventive therapeutic techniques that have long-range future benefits on wellness and wellness behavior. Because these individuals have a future orientation, the nurse will find it easier to encourage preventive screening techniques than with past-oriented individuals. In fact, the client may even request information on preventive techniques and their benefits. However, routine health mammograms and cholesterol checks were not performed by Russian Americans in the Duncan and Simmons study (1996).

To a Russian American, punctuality is important and arriving late for an appointment is considered rude. Therefore the nurse must remember to keep appointments and be punctual because this will help build rapport and trust with the Russian-American client. One Russian explained that to have been late for work under the former Soviet regime meant death; tardiness was considered a sabotage of social goals.

ENVIRONMENTAL CONTROL
Locus of control and effect on wellness and illness behaviors

The Russian culture instills in its members a belief that man has little control over nature. This control is especially apparent in health care activities, which in Russia are free for everyone. Spiritually, however, Russian Americans with Russian Orthodox beliefs may have difficulty with current self-help practices. These beliefs center around ideas of Christ's teachings. It is believed that Christ will give as much help as is deserved in relation to the strength of the beliefs, which means that an ill person who is not re-

covering may somehow not have had enough faith. Illness in this sense is perceived as a punishment. Russian Americans who espouse these beliefs have an external locus of control.

In contrast, some Russian Americans believe that one can control both internal and external forces in the environment, thereby creating opportunities for high levels of wellness. This perception is regarded as an internal locus of control. When Russian Americans have an internal locus-of-control orientation, they are likely to have a unique self-care approach to illness and hospitalization.

Russian methods of health treatment

In Russia, *fel'dsher*s deliver a great deal of primary health care. The *fel'dsher* is a medical aide with 3 years of training (Vlassov, 1989). After 3 years of medical school, the *fel'dsher* is trained in basic preventive medicine, with a special focus on mothers and preschool children, in suturing, and in emergency care techniques. *Fel'dsher* centers generally serve collective farms and therefore are in the center of each village. Because of their proximity to the population, *fel'dsher* centers become the first point of referral for clients. *Fel'dsher* centers are organized by regions, with approximately four *fel'dsher* centers to every hospital (Brown, 1979). When Russians are ill, they are expected to stay in bed and call the clinic. The physician or *fel'dsher* often makes a house call that same day, determines the severity of the problem, and makes a recommendation. Once or twice each year industrial and chemical workers are required to have a complete physical examination.

Other Russian health care alternatives sometimes used are charm men and barbershops. In the past, barbershops were equipped to do a procedure called "cupping," which was used primarily for the treatment of respiratory tract disorders. In this procedure, approximately 15 cups are heated, placed up and down the back, and left in place for about 10 minutes. Believed to extract evil humors from the body, the cups leave ecchymosis-like marks that may last for days (Carr, 1983). Cupping is a technique currently taught to Russian nursing students and is still practiced in some Russian-American communities.

Currently, the Russian health care system is suffering greatly as a result of the plummeting Russian economy. In 1990, the Soviet health minister agreed that over half of all rural hospitals and clinics had no sewage-drainage systems, 80% had no hot water, and 17% had no running water. Severe shortages have been reported for such things as suture material, catheters, bandages, diagnostic equipment, sterilization units and autoclaves, medications, syringes, needles, and gloves (Feshback & Friendly, 1992). Unsterile needles have been blamed for the dramatic increase in the number of AIDS cases, especially among children. Tragically, hundreds of Russians have contracted AIDS in hospitals as a result of sloppy sterilization procedures and a chronic needle shortage (Edwards, 1993). Even when immunizations are available, parents, fearful of contaminated needles, are refusing to have their children vaccinated.

According to Corwin (1990), a 950-bed Russian hospital received 1 needle plus per day for the first half of 1990. As a necessary response to this shortage, the medical ministry sent out a report explaining how to sterilize and reuse disposable needles. As a result of the shortage, Russian people found themselves without medical resources and have consequently turned to home remedies and faith healers.

In Russia, approximately 75% of all deaths are related to cardiovascular disease, cancer, and trauma (trauma on the roads, in the homes, and in the work place) (13,000 die, 1992). Additionally, during 1991, incidence rates in Russia for dysentery and other enterically transmitted diseases increased substantially. In the Tom river basin in Siberia between 1990 and 1991, the number of cases of diphtheria, pertussis, and measles increased by 54.7%, 25.1%, and 12.2% respectively. Measles vaccine was unavailable. Polluted water is blamed for the increase in gastrointestinal disturbances (82%), hepatitis A (47%), and dysentery (22%) over national incidence rates (Monisov, 1992). To compound matters, working conditions have worsened, and salaries for doctors and nurses have plummeted, causing many health professionals to go on strike or leave their professions (Russian nurses, 1992). Russians may now have to pay for the once-free health services (Androshin, 1990; Russian doctors, 1992).

Russian labor and delivery practices are often brutally traditional, without Lamaze techniques, and abortion is practically the only form of birth control. It is possible that a 37-year-old woman could have had as many as 10 abortions. Contraceptives are of poor quality and difficult to obtain, and all types of hormones taken for any reason are popular.

In Russian hospitals, clients necessarily take care of each other. Giving bedpans, feeding clients, performing client-teaching functions, and even bathing clients are tasks that are more often performed by other clients than by nursing staff. Therefore clients assume a major role in their own care and are discharged after lengthy hospital stays (Dennis, 1989). Despite this, Russian clients report their love and admiration for the wonderful dedicated nurses who care for them. "I couldn't have made it without my nurses," one cardiac client explained (Smith, 1989).

Although the Russian health care system may lag behind that of the United States, preventive health care is practiced. Russian people believe that physical screening is the answer to good health care and is widely accepted among Russian immigrants. Female Russian Americans are quite familiar with frequent and routine pelvic and Pap screenings, gastric acid tests, sedimentation rates, and prothrombin times. In contrast, however, they are unfamiliar or unaccepting of mammograms, routine breast examinations, and cholesterol screenings and state that the cholesterol findings are inconclusive and of little or no value.

One concern Russian Americans have is that the United States medicine system lacks a powerful emphasis on prevention. One Russian American responded:

Too many pills. Pills for everything without a clear reason. In Russia, physicians make house calls. If I have a fever, I will stay home, and the doctor will come. This is why United States doctors consider Russians as crying too much and complaining too much. We are used to less intensive medicine. Here, I need to call for an appointment, and it's 1 month away. In Russia we have more alternative medical therapies—the whole cleansing of the body of toxins, massages, acupressure, and acupuncture. In our hospitals, we have prescribed massages. Here, the doctors don't even consider alternative medicine or any Oriental medical practice.

Folk medicine

Russian immigrants, especially the elderly, may still practice some homeopathic or folk medicine. For example, one client had an amber necklace from Riga and refused to allow treatment for a thyroid condition. The client stated, "Those pills make me sick. My necklace will cure everything with my thyroid except cancer." However, when laboratory work indicated her condition was worsening, she accepted medication (Ruby, 1989). Amber is ground into a powder and added to hot water and is used as a kind of medicinal potion.

Other home remedies include herbs, which are prepared as drinks or enemas, and charcoal in water, which is ingested for the treatment of stomach acidity. Hot steam baths are considered healthful for pneumonia and upper respiratory tract infections. Mineral water and plasters are also used. Because of their belief in the healing qualities of mineral water, emerging Russian health care providers are using products that are rich in curative properties.

Russian Americans strongly believe in the usefulness of massage. This philosophy seems to stem from a kind of chiropractic idealism related to the spine and back (Avakyan, 1990). In addition, orthopedic shoes for foot or leg pain are commonly used.

Some Russian Americans use dry heat for the treatment of back pain. Others use a raw dough of dark rye flour and honey that is placed on the spinal column. Another back remedy is a loosely knit or compacted pad made of rough, coarse wool or animal hair, which is placed directly on the bare skin in the lower back region.

Headaches are often treated with a strong ointment placed behind the ears and temples and along the back of the neck. For the treatment of rhinitis, Russian Americans may extract raw onion juice and place several drops in each nares with a medicine dropper. A cold may be treated by immersion of both legs in hot water containing strong salts. Sore throats are said to be relieved by a salt and baking soda gargle. Leech therapy is still widely taught and practiced in Russia. Leeches are particularly useful because of the anesthetic, vasodilatation, and anticoagulant properties of leech saliva (Truax, 1991).

Health is seen as the greatest of all gifts and goals. Russians will define health as a mental, physical, and spiritual harmony, the greatest of which is spiritual. Body systems are blended and functioning as God created them to be with each part doing its job in perfect interrelatedness. When the mind is troubled, the body will respond negatively. Holistic medicine is a way of life for Russians, through the use of cosmic energy work. Spirituality carries a very important place in Russian medicine. Illness, in contrast, is defined as disharmony among body systems.

Practices at the time of death

Russian families with members who have recently died often keep vigil over the coffin for hours. The family members must wear black. The deceased person is washed, dressed, and placed in the coffin before the wake and funeral. A black wreath is placed on the door of the deceased person's home. At the funeral, a priest (if the family is Catholic or Russian Orthodox) places holy oil on the forehead while making the sign of the cross. A paper band is placed on the forehead with this prayer: "Oh God, Father, be merciful to thy servant (name) and accept into thy fold (name)." A piece of paper is placed on the dead person's chest, symbolic of a ticket into heaven. Each member of the grieving family places a few symbolic grains of soil onto the coffin.

Implications for nursing care

The nurse should be aware that the Russian-American client will find the way in which health professionals relate somewhat different from that to which they are accustomed. Traditionally, American physicians and nurses have been taught to have a nondirective, listening approach to client interactions. This approach is unsatisfactory for Russian immigrants, who seem to need almost immediate information and answers. Subjective symptoms may be difficult to assess because of lack of information presented by the client.

Russian Americans are nearly 100% compliant with follow-up medical appointments. Generally, Russian Americans are respectful and admire their physicians and nurses. They ask appropriate questions and accept what they are told. Russian Americans do not, however, often use walk-in or emergency services. Usually, Russian Americans will call the physician and wait until he or she is available, a practice that is based on their medical experiences in Russia.

Russian Americans tend to comply with most medical directives, doing whatever is needed to get well and stay independent. However, some Russian Americans may stop taking medications with any sign of a side effect, even if the side effect is unrelated. This is particularly noted with psychotropic drugs. The nurse may also notice that a kind of cancer phobia exists among elderly Russian immigrants, who seem to have an "if it isn't broken, don't fix it" philosophy in relation to screenings for stool guaiac tests, sigmoidoscopies, and mammograms. Diagnostic tests are often refused, resulting in lack of early detection (Ruby, 1989). Russian families may further complicate care by forbidding health care professionals from disclosing a cancer diagnosis to loved ones. However, the concept of "do not resuscitate" can be a significant problem for the Russian family who is unable to understand not doing everything possible for a loved one.

Many traditional Russian medications are available and frequently purchased through the Internet and used. Several large pharmaceutical firms in New York cater to Russian clients.

BIOLOGICAL VARIATIONS
Body size

Obesity is especially common among elderly Russian women. This problem is attributed to the lack of fresh fruits and vegetables in Russia. Many culturally preferred foods are high in saturated fats and salts. Many Russian people retain their traditional dietary preferences, and as a result, the problem of overuse of saturated fats and salts often continues after immigration to the United States. Russian physicians estimate that as much as 50% of their population is overweight (Blackman, 1989) but undernourished (Monisov, 1992). Duncan and Simmons (1996) found that 65% of their study population was obese. Stature and color among Russian Americans are quite similar to that of other White American clients seen by the health care provider because most Russians are White.

Enzymatic variations

Russian Americans do not have problems with hypervitaminosis or hypovitaminosis, and, biochemically, laboratory parameters are the same (Gennis, 1989). The one exception is that the cholesterol levels of Russian Americans are generally well above normal.

Susceptibility to disease

Hypertension Blood pressure screening is routine in Russia, and Russian Americans are keenly aware of the causes and effects of hypertension and will identify themselves as either hypertensive or borderline hypertensive. Although Russian Americans are often very hypertensive, they may not have been treated for the disorder because of the lack of antihypertensive drugs in Russia (Health care, 1988). Diet is also likely to be a contributing factor to hypertension.

The death rate from coronary heart disease for Russian men is five to six times higher than that in Western countries, with 53% of deaths caused by heart disease (Russian health, 1998).

Tuberculosis Tuberculosis (TB) exposure has also been noted in greater incidence among Russian Americans than in the general populace. TB is again spreading across Russia because of a debilitated health system, political instability, and an indifference to end it by the medical establishment (TB epidemic, 1998). The population in Russia is routinely immunized 2 days after birth with bacillus Calmette-Guérin (BCG), which is an effective treatment when a high prevalence of tuberculosis exists. The problem, however, is that this type of immunization causes tuberculin reactions to read positive and makes purified protein derivative (PPD) readings unclear. BCG immunization cannot be assumed. After abnormal PPD readings, many clients have radiographs that indicate signs of old cases of tuberculosis (Brinton & Ladyzhensky, 1992; Gennis, 1989).

Cancer After studying the differences in somatic mutation, based on an analysis of peripheral blood lymphocytes, Jones, Thomas, and Tucker (1995) found that, because of chronic exposure to environmental toxins including smoking, DDT-like pesticides, and the Chernobyl nuclear power plant accident, the mutant frequency of Russians was higher and the risk of health consequences was higher for Russians because of accumulated genetic damage. The population of adult Russians accumulated genetic damage at a 250% higher rate than that of Americans.

Dental needs

Most Russian Americans tend to value dental care because traditionally they have had easy and free access to dental care and often have bridges and removable plates. Recently, Russian dentists traveling abroad claimed that the dentistry they practice is 50 years behind that of the United States. Toothbrushes and toothpaste are difficult to obtain in Russia, and many Russian people lack these essential oral hygiene products (Update on visiting, 1992). Dental health was identified as a major priority by Russians in Virginia with over 75% as self-identifying as having dental problems (Duncan & Simmons, 1996).

Eye care needs

Because eye care and eye surgery have received a great deal of Russian money and attention, most Russians have had access to eye care.

Nutritional preferences and deficiencies

Recent efforts toward a national health movement in Russia have been slowed because of Russia's chronic shortage of fresh fruits and vegetables. Sausage, potatoes, and bread are standard foods for breakfast, lunch, and supper. The Russian immigrant who has come from a rural district will prefer to eat cabbage, buckwheat, millet, barley, and bread (Russian bread is a kind of heavy rye bread and can weigh as much as 12 pounds per loaf), along with sour milk and salted pork (if the person is non-Jewish). Salted meats are usually kept in a barrel and stored all winter in a kind of fruit cellar. Meat, as a delicacy, may be severely rationed. Thus, most Russians respect food and handle it with great care. Not a single morsel of food, especially meat, is wasted.

Psychological characteristics

Illness and wellness behaviors Many Russian-American people believe that American medicine is the best in the world. Russian Americans, accustomed to home visits by health care workers in Russia, would like to have United States physicians and nurses provide home care when possible. In emergency departments, some Russian Americans may become frustrated by the voluminous paperwork required to establish financial competence. In some cases, these individuals may have a difficult time understanding why so many of the emergency beds are filled with drug overdoses and shooting victims (Brokaw, 1991). Moreover, older Russian-American people consider the medical system a natural place for seeking help. For these immigrants, the clinic and its staff are viewed in a social context. Russian Americans, familiar with making loud demands to receive care in Russia, may appear pushy, manipulative, abrasive, and excessive.

Having endured a lifetime of poor medical care, poor nutrition, and continued frustration, elderly Russian Americans also have a higher number of somatic complaints compared with other groups the nurse may encounter. These complaints may be caused partially by the cultural stigma of psychiatric illness and treatment by "just talking." Russian Americans do not trust psychiatrists, psychologists, or other counseling services. Thus they may magnify aches and pains disproportionately rather than describing an emotional problem (Brod & Heurtin-Roberts, 1992). Expressing psychosocial problems, such as depression, through somatic complaints was also noted by Azarian, Boland, and Skripchenko (1996).

Complaints such as pain and paresthesia, vertigo, anorexia, and hysteria have been commonly related by the client to a disease. Unfortunately, these diseases were sometimes present but have not been adequately treated.

Russian Americans tend to perceive health care professionals as high status people. Feelings of poor self-concept are elevated when attention is received; for example, "I must have some worth if a high status person pays attention to me." Russian Americans may thus seek health care as a social exercise to increase feelings of worth.

Russian Americans generally have many important health-promoting behaviors. For example, Russian Americans usually do not smoke, drink alcohol excessively, or engage in violent crime. Having been accustomed to media portrayals of average people doing extraordinary deeds, Russian Americans long for quality newspaper and television programs that provide enthusiasm and inspiration for them. Russian Americans are familiar with hard work and difficulties, but most enjoy American freedoms and believe in the future. Gottlieb (1990) wrote of an interview with a Russian American who proclaimed, "This is land of achievable dreams. If you want something and you are willing to work hard for it, you can get it . . . . I have my pride, and I am going somewhere."

Mental health In Russia, citizens with mental disorders could expect years of prisonlike hospitalization under the influence of potent mind-numbing drugs. Psychiatric wards contained many clients who had refused military service (Langone, 1989; Pope, 1996).

Additionally, Russian citizens who tried to evangelize others or organize labor unions were labeled as insane and hospitalized in prisonlike psychiatric hospitals. This practice was scorned by the rest of the world's psychiatric community, who found the diagnosis of "sluggish schizophrenia," used in Russia to describe these persons, very objectionable. Hospitalization occurred despite Soviet law, which stated that citizens could be forcibly hospitalized only if they displayed signs of deep depression, were suicidal, or threatened the lives of others.

There are indications that such psychiatric practices changed after the mid-1980s. In 1987 the May 1 issue of *Psychiatric News* carried a report of a change in policy in the USSR regarding psychiatric treatment and treatment of the homeless, which were discussed at a meeting between the Chairman of the American Psychological Association (APA) Council on International Affairs, Harold Visotsky, M.D., and the Soviet Deputy Ambassador, Yevstafiev (APA representatives, 1987). In the meeting with the APA delegation, Yevstafiev identified a change to "maximum humanization." Apparently Soviet psychiatrists were trying to improve their tarnished image by releasing political prisoners and placing

psychiatry under the governance of the Ministry of Health rather than the Ministry of Internal Affairs (police) (Langone, 1989). Traditional Russian psychiatric therapies include hydrotherapy, physiotherapy, insulin therapy, inhalation therapy, work therapy, and drug therapy (Hess, 1971).

In the United States, when psychiatric illnesses are diagnosed in Russian Americans, the most common mental health problem is depression. This problem is identified primarily in elderly immigrants who traveled with their children to the United States. They are unfamiliar with the language and customs, have left home and family, and often can get only minimum-wage jobs because of their age. Even after a diagnosis is given, they remain reluctant to maintain compliance with taking antidepressant drugs because of a fear of such medications in general and a reluctance to experience any side effects. Because of decreased emotional, physical, and financial resources and the realities of illnesses that may accompany aging, including diabetes and heart disease, older Russian-American immigrants are at great risk for depression. Many Russian immigrants experienced a lifetime of stress including two world wars, political turmoil, religious persecution, poor health care, financial problems, and nutritional deficits. Often dependent on family or themselves for the first time in their lives, older Russian Americans may feel noncontributive, helpless, isolated, and demoralized (Azarian, Boland, & Skripchenko, 1996; Brod & Heurtin-Roberts, 1992; Kohn, Flaherty, & Levav, 1989; Smith, 1996).

Alcoholism In Russia, alcoholism is a major and growing national health problem. As an important response, the first Alcoholics Anonymous (AA) groups began emerging in Moscow (Rosenberg, 1992). Alcoholism, since the Soviet Union breakup, is worsening because of the chronic stress of obtaining needed food, unstable prices, inflation, and social upheavals. Unfortunately, two groups hit hardest by increased alcoholism are women and teenagers.

Since the collapse of the Soviet Union, Russian alcoholism is becoming as much a problem for women as for men. Between 1990 and 1992, vodka consumption for women and men was almost equal. According to Peter Balashov, director of the adolescent department of Russia's largest drug and alcohol treatment hospital, there is one female for every four male alcoholics. Balashov further reported that 60% of adult Russian drinkers abuse alcohol and that on any given day, 7% to 8% of the work force could not work because of alcoholism (Rosenberg, 1992). Through a group called American Russian Recovery Options at Work, 50 Russian alcoholism experts were trained (between 1992 and 1995) in the United States regarding AA treatment methods (Williams, 1992).

Although alcoholism is an enormous problem in Russia, it has not emerged as one of the most significant mental health problems found among Russian-American immigrants. A plausible explanation is that Russian immigrants want to survive in the United States and Russian alcoholics stay in Russia; Russian alcoholics have lost hope and vision (Williams, 1992). Another reason for the low rate of alcoholism is that it is not common for Russian-American Jews to drink excessively because of culturally imposed restrictions. In addition, Russian Americans do not generally use illegal drugs, which might lead to promiscuous sexual behavior. Perhaps the lack of these self-abuse problems is attributable to attitudes and values, high levels of education, and cohesiveness of this skewed Russian population. Unfortunately, because Russian Jews did not drink, they were often ridiculed and further ostracized by Russian society.

Radiation accidents and toxic pollution

Environmental pollution in the Commonwealth of Independent States is a growing concern for European and Asian neighbors. It has also been a major health problem for Russians as a result of polluted air, contaminated food, and contaminated water. Unfortunately, communism and an indiscriminate industrialization policy left Russia and the other republics too poor and disorganized to fix the massive pollution problems. Nearly 70 million Russians breathe polluted air at levels five times the limit allowed there. Over 130 nuclear explosions (mostly for the purpose of scientific study) have occurred in European Russia, and one out of every 10 barrels of oil

produced in Russia is spilled. A single Siberian oil spill measures 6 feet deep, seven miles long, and 4 miles wide. An estimated 30% of all food is contaminated with pesticides, and Siberian forests in Russia are disappearing at a rate of 5 million acres per year. Over 50,000 square miles of land were radioactively contaminated after the 1986 Chernobyl disaster (Prokhorov, 1990; Stanglin & Pope, 1992). Russian nuclear reactors have been called old, huge time bombs. The Chernobyl disaster, according to the U.S. Department of Energy, will cause an additional 6000 deaths in the European community over the next 50 years (Hofheinz, 1992b).

Implications for nursing care

American nurses quickly recognize that Russian Americans are very friendly, interesting, likable, and generally well educated. The nurse should be aware, however, that Russian immigrants may be very skeptical of psychiatric services because psychiatric treatment often appears similar to persecution. Education about psychiatric symptoms and the modalities of treatment available in the United States are an essential part of a psychosocial intervention strategy. The client and the family should feel that they are participants and decision makers in treatment selections and strategies.

The nurse who cares for Russian Americans must be aware of possible nutritional implications for nursing care. Because very recent immigrants may be unable to tolerate American foods, the nurse would be wise to introduce new foods slowly. Religious dietary restrictions may also be a concern. Additionally, nutritional deficits must be identified and immediately treated with dietary and medical supplements.

Although alcoholism is not a reported problem among Russian Americans, residual effects of alcoholism, whether physiological or psychological, must be looked for in individuals and families. In addition, the nurse must assist Russian-American clients in identifying coping strategies that will reduce anxiety and tension, depression, and low self-worth, thereby reducing the potential for mental health disorders.

Hypertension is reported to have a high incidence among Russian-American people. The nurse should use motivational strategies to devise teaching techniques that emphasize the benefits of dietary restraints, weight control, and adequate exercise. In addition, the Russian-American client who is hospitalized for hypertension must appreciate the need for medication adherence and timely reporting of all unusual and untoward signs and symptoms.

Although undocumented in current literature, Russian Americans may be suffering physically and psychologically from the ill effects of water, air, and land pollution. The nurse should be keenly alert to these possible effects and assess clients accordingly.

For Russian Americans, U.S. nurses and physicians represent the front-line liaison to a whole array of social and medical benefits. Russian immigrants tend to expect the health care professional to provide social and financial as well as medical services for them. If medical benefits are financially available, as in many Russian-Jewish immigrant groups, this may not be a severe problem. However, many Russian Americans arrive without the ability to access appropriate health care services. If they are underpaid or unemployed, Russian immigrants may not have any insurance coverage. The nurse must also understand that Russian Americans are very proud people, perhaps too proud to go on public assistance. One response offered by the Russian immigrant may be, "If I am sick, I'll have to go back to Russia to get care." Therefore, as a resource liaison, the nurse should identify and facilitate access to all possible health and assistance programs.

SUMMARY

As nurses transcend their own cultural mind-set, they learn to accept and use cultural uniqueness as an indicator for nursing interventions. Among experiences that are assisting nurses in gaining a transcultural perspective are transcultural educational experiences such as those offered by the United States–Russian Nurse Exchange Consortium Organization. Since 1993 this group has sponsored over 20 exchanges of health care professionals between the United States and Russia.

In addition to gaining an understanding of persons in other cultures, the nurse must increase knowledge to provide culturally appropriate care to immigrant clients. Complexity, variety, and cultural diversity contribute to the nurse's challenge and responsibility toward Russian Americans.

Case Study

Victor and Vera have immigrated to Milwaukee, Wisconsin, from St. Petersburg, the second largest city in Russia. They are Jewish and believe that the strong anti-Semitism they felt in Russia had become unbearable. Their only alternative, they decided, was to leave the country and join relatives in Milwaukee. Mt. Sinai Samaritan Medical Center offered 1 year of free health care to them when they arrived. Now, 3 years later, Victor and Vera continue to seek services at this large teaching hospital and clinic. Victor and Vera are both 58 years old, and Vera speaks very little English. Victor has found a new peer group at the brewery, his place of employment. However, Vera has been unable to find work and prefers to stay near family and friends. The Milwaukee Jewish Family Services has been minimally successful in involving Vera in social activities. Vera reads and sits in her chair most of the day. Recently, she has become more withdrawn, with an overwhelming feeling of sadness and loneliness for her native land. She regrets immigrating and has focused her bitter feelings inward.

A painful venous occlusion brings Vera to the health clinic, where the nurse examines her lower extremities and finds swelling, tenderness, edema, and a positive Homans' sign on Vera's left leg. A health history is difficult because of the language barrier, but with the help of Victor and an interpreter, the nurse learns about Vera's sedentary life-style, high-fat and high-cholesterol intake, and recent episodes of sadness. Victor is supportive but impatient for his wife to "get back on her feet again." Vera says very little.

Case Study—cont'd

On laboratory examination, Vera's plasma low-density lipoprotein level is 240 mg/dL. Left ventricular hypertrophy is noted on the electrocardiogram. Vera is obese and has a blood pressure of 180/116. Slight hemorrhages of the retinas are also noted.

Vera is presented with two medical diagnoses: symptomatic hypertension and depression. The nurse realizes that Vera's dietary instructions need to be presented with great care and attention given to cultural habits and beliefs. The nurse shows Vera an extensive list of "good" foods (written in Russian) and asks her to identify her favorites. With Vera's help and the help of the dietitian, the nurse works out a weekly menu. The nurse must also teach Vera specific techniques for controlling her hypertension. Vera is instructed to take her own weight and blood pressure every morning, record them on a graph, and bring the graphs with her for her every-other-week clinic visits. It is explained to Vera that she will need to diligently follow medication, dietary, and exercise regimens to decrease her risk of further disability. Vera is especially motivated to help herself because of her fear of losing her eyesight and thus being unable to read (her favorite pastime). Walking is encouraged after Vera's leg becomes asymptomatic.

After all instructions are repeated carefully and slowly several times, Vera is escorted into a private office. The nurse, who has known Vera for 3 years, asks her about her sadness and isolating behaviors. Vera adamantly rejects the nurse's suggestion that she see a psychiatric consultant.

A few important psychosocial questions could include:

- Who do (did) you turn to for help and hope? How is that different (the same) now that you are in the United States?
- What part in your life does religion play?
- What was life like in Russia?
- How is your life different now? What is the most significant difference?
- What do you miss (not miss) the most about Russia?
- What were the decisions that brought you to the United States?
- Help me understand what it's like to leave everything you have ever known—language, culture, friends, family—to come to the United States.
- What important information do I need to best help you help yourself?

CARE PLAN

 Nursing Diagnosis   Nutrition altered: more than body requirements (fat, salt), related to cultural food preferences and sedentary life-style.

Client Outcomes

1. Client will maintain a 1500-calorie/day, low-cholesterol diet.
2. Client will decrease her weight by 4 pounds per month.
3. Client will walk 2 miles per day (after leg has healed).
4. Client will learn to swim and will swim twice weekly at the Jewish Activity Center.

Nursing Interventions

1. Teach client about importance of exercise.
2. Teach client about menu planning in relation to avoidance of high-salt, high-fat foods.
3. Encourage and support compliance with medications, exercise, diet, and follow-up care.

 Nursing Diagnosis   Coping, ineffective, related to chronic feelings of loneliness and isolation

Client Outcomes

1. Client will attend activities at Jewish Family Services twice a week.

Nursing Interventions

1. Encourage and support social networking.

2. Client will join a social group at the local synagogue.
3. Client will enroll in English at the Milwaukee Area Technical College (MATC).

2. Introduce client to Jewish Services and involve client's family in relation to compliance.
3. Arrange for client to visit the library of Russian books and journals located at Jewish Family Services.
4. Help client make initial contacts for classes in English as a second language held at MATC.
5. Arrange transportation for client for all activities and clinic visits.

 Nursing Diagnosis   Coping, ineffective, related to lowered self-esteem and separation from previous contacts

Client Outcomes

1. Client will network with other Soviet immigrants.

Nursing Interventions

1. Show respect for client's cultural preferences.
2. Provide reading materials for client.
3. Introduce client to other Soviet immigrants outside her family and follow up with kindness, caring, and honest concern.

STUDY QUESTIONS

1. Why is it important that Vera's own list of foods be used when the nurse is making out a weekly menu?
2. How will the nurse keep Vera motivated toward self-help and self-care?
3. What role will Vera's family play in her recovery?
4. During client teaching, how much space should be between the nurse and Vera?
5. How may the nurse use Vera's spiritual values and beliefs to the best advantage?
6. What role does language play in this nurse-client relationship?
7. In addition to what is listed in the care plan, how else might the nurse increase Vera's self-esteem and decision-making potential?
8. When talking with Vera, what should the nurse be careful *not* to do?
9. How may Vera's attitudes toward self-learning and life-long learning enhance nursing-care strategies?
10. Why did Vera adamantly refuse psychiatric consultation? What should the nurse do now?

References

13,000 die on Russian roads (1992, Sept. 25). *The Journal Times*, p. 5A.

Abortion among teens on increase (1995, Oct. 24). *The Journal Times*, p. 3A.

Anderson, J. (1992, Nov. 1). Two men clashed and a nation rose. *Parade Magazine*, p. 10.

Androshin, A. (1990). Free medical services: the end of a myth. *Business in the USSR, 7*, 28-29.

APA representatives meet with Soviets to discuss abuse of psychiatry in USSR (1987, May 1). *Psychiatric News*, p. 37.

Aron, L. (1998). Russian outlook. American enterprise institute for public policy research. www.aei.org/ro/ro9464.htm.

Avakyan, G.N. (1990). Pressure and massage therapy to relieve fatigue. *Advancing Clinical Care, 5*(5), 10-11.

Azarian, A., Boland, R.J., & Skripchenko, V. (1996). Providing health care for the Russian-speaking patient. *Medicine & Health, Rhode Island, 79*(9), 323-327.

Barnathan, J. (1991, Nov. 4). The Russians aren't coming. They're here. *Business Week*, p. 100.

Barr, D.A., & Field, M.G. (1996). The current state of health care in the former Soviet Union: implications for health care policy and reform. *American Journal of Public Health, 86*(3), 307-312.

Billy, C. (1993). *Fodor's Russia and the Baltic countries.* New York: Random House, Inc.

Binyon, M. (1983). *Life in Russia.* New York: Berkley Publishing Group.

Birth and death (1995, Sept. 13). *The Journal Times* (Racine, Wisc., AP), p. 2B.

Blackman, A. (1989). Here come the trainers. *Time, 133*(15), 102.

Brinton, K., & Ladyzhensky, A. (1992). Clinical management of immigrants' immunization histories: a focus on Soviet health records and BCG. *Nurse Practitioner, 17*(4), 21-22.

Brod, M., & Heurtin-Roberts, S. (1992). Older Russian émigrés and medical care. *The Western Journal of Medicine, 157*(3), 333-336.

Brokaw, T. (1991, Nov. 10). American dreaming. *The Washington Post,* p. C7.

Brown, L. (1979). At the centre of things. *Nursing Mirror, 148*(10), 20-21.

Burlatsky, F. (1991). Coming and going in the USSR. *Soviet Life, 7*(418), 14, 45.

Bush, K. (1999, Feb. 18). *Net assessment of the Russian economy.* Center for Strategic and International Studies. www.csis.gor/ruseura/rus_econ.html.

Buttweiler, J. (1992, Nov. 21). Fall of communist rule threatens future of arts. *The Journal Times,* p. B1.

Carpenter, D. (1997, April 21). Victims of change, homeless children pose new troubles for reformed Russia. *The Greenville News,* p. 4A.

Carr, M. (1983). Kindness and consideration. *Nursing Mirror, 157*(2), 26-28.

Caryl, C. (1998a). Only a fool pays taxes in capitalist Russia: a shadow economy keeps the country going. *US News & World Report, 124*(12), 38.

Caryl, C. (1998b). Czar Boris awakes. *US News & World Report, 124*(13), 45-46.

Collee, J. (1992, Aug.). An injection of aid. MSMC Newsletter, pp. 10-15.

Dennis, L.I. (1989). Soviet hospital nursing: a model for self-care. *Journal of Nursing Education, 28*(2), 76-77.

Dobbs, M. (1992, Aug. 24-30). Russia, one year later: arguing every step of the way. *The Washington Post National Weekly Edition,* pp. 16-18.

Duncan, L., & Simmons, M. (1996). Health practices among Russian and Ukrainian immigrants. *Journal of Community Health Nursing, 13*(2), 129-137.

Edwards, M. (1993). A broken empire. *National Geographic, 183*(3), 2-20.

Eight attempts reported on Yeltsin's life (1993, Feb. 20). *The Journal Times,* p. 4A.

Factbook. (1999, March 16). Russia, people. www.od-ci.gov.cia publications/factbook/rs.html.

Family and health (1989). *Soviet Life, 3*(390).

Feshback, M., & Friendly, A. (1992, April 25). Rubbishing of a superpower: review of Ecocide in the USSR. *The Economist,* pp. 99-100.

Fish, P. (1992, Feb.). Russia in San Francisco. *Sunset Magazine,* p. 24.

Gennis, M. (1989, Sept.). Personal communication with assistant professor of medicine and program director of Internal Medicine, Sinai Samaritan Medical Center/University of Wisconsin, in charge of health care for all Soviet immigrants.

Gloom in the time of *glasnost'* (1992). *Time, 139*(19), 13.

Gold, S.J. (1991, Nov.-Dec.). Russian Jews in California. *Society,* pp. 76-80.

Gottlieb, A. (1990, March). Coming to America. *McCalls, 117,* 70-79.

Green beats red in new Russian markets (1993, March 28). *The Journal Times,* p. 8B.

Health care in communion with Hippocrates (1988). *Soviet Life, 6*(381), 30-31.

Health care collapse cuts Russian life spans (1997, Feb. 16). *The Atlanta Journal- Constitution* (AP), p. E3.

Hess, G. (1971). Impressions of mental health service delivery systems in Finland, Poland, Soviet Russia, and Czechoslovakia. *International Journal of Nursing Studies, 8*(4), 223-235.

Hill, R. (1992, March 3). Recession sours Soviet immigrants' first taste of capitalism. *The Washington Post,* p. C1, C4.

Hoffman, M.S. (Ed.) (1992). *The world almanac and book of facts.* New York: Pharos Books.

Hofheinz, P. (1992, July 27). The new Soviet threat: pollution. *Fortune,* pp. 110-114.

Hofheinz, P. (1993). Russia 1993: Europe's time bomb. *Fortune, 127*(2), 104-108.

Iams, J. (1998, September 22). Russia prints more Rubles; leaders plot jumpstart. *USA Today,* p. 6B.

In the red (1992, March 23). *New Yorker,* p. 25.

Information please almanac (1992). New York: Houghton Mifflin Company.

Information please almanac (1998). New York: Houghton Mifflin Company.

Jones, I.M., Thomas, C. B., Tucker, B., et al. (1995). Impact of age and environment on somatic mutation at the hprt gene of T hymphocytes in humans. *Mutation Research, 338*(1-6), 129-139.

Kohn, R., Flaherty, J.A., & Levav, I. (1989). Somatic symptoms among older Soviet immigrants: an exploratory study. *The International Journal of Social Psychiatry, 35*(4), 350-360.

Kostikov, V. (1991). Boris Yeltsin's political victory. *Soviet Life, 7*(418), 2-5.

Koval, V. (1989, March). Working women: common problems. *Soviet Life, 3*(390), 24-25.

Kunstel, M., & Albright, J. (1996, Nov. 17). Russian mobsters growing bolder. *The Atlanta Journal-Constitution,* p. C2.

Langone, J. (1989). A profession under stress. *Time, 133*(15), 94-95.

Miss Russia wins world crown. (1992, Dec. 13). *The Journal Times,* p. 2A.

Monisov, A.A. (1992). Public health assessment—Russian Federation. *Journal of the American Medical Association, 267*(10), 1323.

Moore, R. (Ed.). (1988). *Fodor's 89 Soviet Union.* New York: Fodor's Travel Publications.

Pope, V. (1996). Mad Russians. *US News & World Report, 121*(24), 38-43.

Pope, V. (1997). Trafficking in women. *US News & World Report, 122*(13), 38-44.

Prokhorov, D. (1990). The geography of disease. *Business in the USSR, 7,* 30-31.

Rosenberg, N.D. (1992, June 25). Russians tour treatment centers. *Milwaukee Journal,* p. B1.

Ross, J., & Searing, S.E. (1992). Women's studies take on Russian flavor. *Wingspread: The Journal, 14*(2), 1, 8-9.

Ruby, M. (1989). Sinai Samaritan to double free care for Soviets. *Jewish Chronicle,* p. 8.

Russia may tighten controls on adoptions by foreigners. (1997, Nov. 29). *The Journal Times* (Racine, Wisc., AP), p. 7A.

Russian doctors, ambulance medics strike. (1992, April 24). *The Journal Times,* p. 12C.

Russian health on life support (1998, Jan. 26). *The Journal Times* (Racine, Wisc., AP). p. 7A.

Russian nurses and physicians (1992). *American Journal of Nursing, 92*(7), 9.

Saffron, I. (1998, May 30). Russia earns IMF praise, but gets bad credit rating. *The Atlanta Journal-Constitution,* p. B-1.

Schiff, A. (1979). Language, culture and Jewish acculturation of Soviet Jewish émigrés. *Journal of Jewish Communal Service,* 44-57.

Scott, A. (1988). Human interaction and personal boundaries. *Journal of Psychosocial Nursing, 26*(8), 23-27.

Sloane, W. (1992, Nov. 25). Escort, massage services thriving in Russia. *The Journal Times,* p. 2A.

Smith, H. (1991). *The new Russians.* New York: Random House.

Smith, L.S. (1989). Soviet nursing and health care. *Advancing Clinical Care, 4*(5), 41-44.

Smith, L.S. (1996). New Russian immigrants: health problems, practices, and values. *Journal of Cultural Diversity, 3*(3), 68-73.

Stanglin, D., & Pope, V. (1992). The wreck of Russia. *US News & World Report, 113*(22), 40-49.

Study: Russian kids sicker than during USSR days (1998, March 13). *The Journal Times* (Racine, Wisc., AP), p. 10A.

TB epidemic in Europe (1998, March 25). *The Journal Times* (Racine, Wisc., AP), p. 6A.

Truax, S. (1991, March). Misunderstood and repulsive: leeches prove medical value. *Compass Readings,* pp. 68-70.

Update on visiting "The Soviet Union." (1992, Jan.-Feb.). *Traveling Healthy and Comfortably, 5*(1), 1-6.

Ups and downs (1996). *US News & World Report, 121*(8), 16.

U.S. Department of Commerce, Bureau of the Census (1988). *Current population reports, divisions and states.* Washington, D.C.: Government Printing Office.

U.S. Department of Commerce, Bureau of the Census (1997, modified March 6). *Russian* [On-line], Available at census.gov/population/socdemo/language/table 5.txt

U.S. Department of Justice, Immigration and Naturalization Service (1992, April). *Immigration from the former Soviet Union, 1989-1991* (Bulletin No. 10). Washington, D.C.: Government Printing Office.

Vlassov, P.V. (1989). History of paramedical training in Russia. *Advancing Clinical Care, 4*(5), 27-31.

Williams, J. (Reporter). (1992, June 26). Russian doctors visit Milwaukee (WITI Television).

Witt, H. (1993, March 24). Inside the Russian court. *Chicago Tribune,* p. 1, 13.

Yeltsin: Main points (1993, March 21). *The Journal Times,* p. 11A.

Yeltsin rival backs down (1993, March 26). The *Journal Times,* p. 3A.

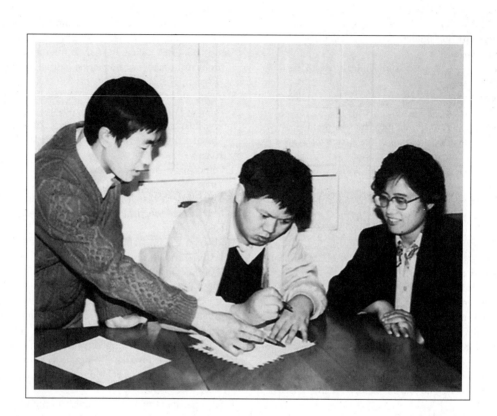

CHAPTER 16

Chinese Americans

Karen Chang

BEHAVIORAL OBJECTIVES

After reading this chapter, the nurse will be able to:

1. Describe the effect of Chinese philosophy and values on Chinese Americans.
2. Explain the ways that Chinese Americans communicate.
3. Describe the influences of the family system on Chinese Americans.
4. Explain the time concept of Chinese Americans.
5. Describe the illness behaviors of Chinese Americans.
6. Identify the biological variations of Chinese Americans.
7. Articulate the implications of providing effective nursing care for Chinese Americans.

OVERVIEW OF CHINA

China (The People's Republic of China) occupies the eastern portion of Asia and is slightly larger in area in square miles than the United States (Information Please Almanac, 1998). In fact, China occupies roughly 3,691,521 square miles (9,561,000 square kilometers). The coastline of China is roughly a semicircle. The greater part of China is mountainous; it is only in the lower portions of the Yellow and Yangtze rivers that there are any extensive low plains. The principal mountain ranges include the T'ien Shan ('Celestial Mountains') in the northwest part of the country; the K'unlun chain, which runs south of the Takla Makan and Gobi deserts; the Tangkula mountain range, which connects the K'unlun chain with the borders of China and Tibet (modified from Information Please Almanac, 1998); and the Ta Hsing-an mountain range in western Manchuria. The plains in China include Manchuria, Inner Mongolia, and Hainan. Manchuria, which is largely an undulating plain, is connected with the northern China plain by a narrow lowland corridor. Inner Mongolia contains the rich fertile southern and eastern portions of the Gobi Desert. Hainan ('sea-south'), which encompasses 13,200 square miles, is an island that lies just off the southern coast of the country.

In 1997, the estimated population of China was 1,221,591,778. The average annual rate of natural increase in the population is 0.96%. The birth rate in China is 15.52 live births per 1000 persons, compared with 16.3 per 1000 for the United States (Information Please Almanac, 1998; U.S. Department of Commerce, Bureau of the Census, 1993a). In 1997, infant mortality in China was 37.9 per 1000, compared with 9.8 per 1000 for the United States (Information Please Almanac, 1998; National Center for Health Statistics, 1998). The population of China makes it one of the densest countries in the world (331 people per square mile).

The capital city of China is Beijing ('northern-capital'; previous spelling, Peking), which has an estimated population of 12,510,000. The largest city in China is Shanghai ('on-sea'), which has an estimated population of 14,150,000. Other large cities include Tianjin (9,420,000), Canton (2,914,000) and Wuhan (3,284,200) (Information Please Almanac, 1998; World Almanac, 1997).

The principal agriculture products of China include rice, wheats, grains, and cotton. Approximately 60% of persons who participate in the labor force in China work in agriculture or forestry. The major industrial products for export include iron, steel, petroleum, textiles, oil, limestone, and a wealth of other natural and man-made resources.

The president of China is Jiang Zemin (1993-   ) and the premier is Li Peng (1987-   ). The ruling governmental authority in China is the Communist Party. The National People's Congress is the chief legislative organ. Within the governmental hierarchy, the State Council has the executive authority. It is the Congress, however, that elects the premier and the deputy premiers. In China, the ministries are under the auspices of the State Council, which is headed by the premier.

OVERVIEW OF CHINESE AMERICANS

The majority of Chinese Americans are immigrants from Taiwan, Hong Kong, and mainland China. Chinese Americans have the largest population among Asian immigrants. According to the U.S. Bureau of the Census, 1,645,472 Chinese Americans reside in the United States, representing 0.7% of the total U.S. population (U.S. Department of Commerce, Bureau of the Census, 1998; Information Please Almanac, 1998). Of the number of Chinese Americans residing in this country, 52.4% live in the West, 27.0% live in the Northeast, 12.4% live in the South, and 8.1% live in the Midwest (U.S. Department of Commerce, Bureau of the Census, 1993c). The states with the largest population of Chinese Americans are California (704,850), New York (284,144), and Hawaii (68,804). A total of 66% of Chinese Americans live in five states—California, New York, Hawaii, Illinois, and Texas (U.S. Department of Commerce, Bureau of the Census, 1993b).

Of the number of Chinese Americans residing in the United States before 1975, 18.5% were foreign born; of the number residing in the United States between 1975 and 1979, 11.4% were foreign born;

and between 1980 and 1990, 39.4% were foreign born. Immigration has definitely contributed to the growth in the Chinese-American population over the past two decades. It is interesting to note, however, that the percentage of Chinese Americans who are foreign born differs considerably across time periods. The median age of Chinese Americans residing in the United States is 32.1 years, compared with 33 years for the general U.S. population. In addition only 6% of all Asian Americans are 65 years of age or older, compared with 13% of the general U.S. population (U.S. Department of Commerce, Bureau of the Census, 1993b).

Chinese Americans are noted for maintaining high educational standards. In 1990, 77.2% of Chinese-American males and 70.2% of Chinese-American females 25 years of age or older held a high school diploma. In 1990, 46.7% of Chinese-American males and 35.0% of Chinese-American females held a bachelor's degree (U.S. Department of Commerce, Bureau of the Census, 1993c).

Of the number of Chinese Americans in the United States, 65.9% participate in the work force. Chinese Americans have lower labor-force participation rates when compared with those of Filipinos (75.4%) and Asian Indians (72.3%). Although the per capita income for most Japanese Americans is $19,375, Chinese Americans have a per capita income of only $14,876. The poverty rate for Chinese Americans is 14.0%, compared with 13.0% for the general U.S. population (U.S. Department of Commerce, Bureau of the Census, 1993b).

Before 1965 most Chinese immigrants had little or no education, and many were alone because their families were not allowed to come with them. They were forced to immigrate for political, social, or economic reasons. The majority of them came from Guangzhou (Canton) and took up occupations such as mining, railroad construction, and farming. After 1965 immigration laws eased in the United States, the better-educated professionals and specialists began to immigrate. Now families were allowed to immigrate together. These immigrants came from Taiwan, mainland China, and Hong Kong. As a result, a wide cultural and linguistic diversity exists among Chinese Americans.

A wide range of educational levels also exists among Chinese Americans. There are many college-educated professionals, yet there is a larger number of barely literate individuals working in low-paying occupations (Mangiafico, 1988; Wong, 1982; Yeung & Schwartz, 1986).

Chinese culture is dominated by Confucius's teachings, which encourage individuals to pursue filial piety, righteousness, decorum, and wisdom. A harmonious relationship with nature and other people is stressed, and a person is expected to accommodate rather than confront. If private interest conflicts with community interest, a person is expected to submit to the interest of the group rather than advocate personal concerns. Public debating of conflicting views is unacceptable. A person is expected to be sensitive to what people think and to be gracious toward others so as not to make them "lose face." Self-expression and individualism are discouraged, whereas showing filial piety to parents and loyalty to family, friends, and government is highly praised. Modesty, self-control, self-reliance, self-restraint, and face-saving are frequently taught to Chinese people. When they fail to follow these cultural practices, they feel shame or guilt. Consequently, the Chinese appear to be quiet, polite, pleasant, and unassertive and often suppress feelings such as anger or pain.

Reciprocation, or treating others as one would wish to be treated, is often used in interpersonal relationships. Interpersonal interactions have a hierarchical structure, so that older or higher-status people have authority over younger or lower-status people. A person's status is always referred to during interactions. For example, brothers address each other as "older brother" and "younger brother" in addition to the first name. Educational achievement and professional success are highly valued because pride and honor are brought to the family and the community as a result. Therefore Chinese parents willingly provide support for children to pursue higher education.

The sharp contrasts between the Chinese and the American cultures cause a high level of stress among Chinese Americans during the acculturation process. Some may hold on to traditional Chinese culture, observe holidays according to the lunar calendar, and maintain Chinese customs; some may reject all their traditional heritage; and some may assimilate both the Chinese culture and the American culture. Poorly adjusted individuals may not be able to perform tasks productively, may have low self-esteem, and may exhibit some lawless behaviors. Second- and third-generation Chinese Americans, who are already well assimilated into the Western culture, may not be influenced much by traditional Chinese culture. However, they may experience the identity problem of being culturally and linguistically American even though others perceive them as Chinese (Albert & Triandis, 1985; Becker, 1986; Chang, 1981; Chen & Yang, 1986; Encyclopedia Americana, 1983; Louie, 1985; Orque, Bloch, & Monrroy, 1983).

COMMUNICATION
Dialect

Linguistic diversity causes communication problems among Chinese people. Although the official Chinese language is Mandarin (*Pŭtonghùa*), there are many dialects spoken that are not understood by other groups of Chinese. All the dialects have the same written characters, however, which have been relatively stable for 3000 years though having undergone great changes. This stability in the language permits all literate Chinese to be able to communicate in writing. Each Chinese character (or logogram) consists of only one syllable. Each character has its own meaning, but if one character is combined with another character or more, the meaning of the combination produces words with differing concepts. There are four tones in Mandarin (as well as a neutral tone), and changes of tone produce complete changes in the meaning of a syllable or a word. The Chinese language generally does not use copulas and plurals (though both exist) and has no tenses.

Style, volume, and touch

The Chinese value silence more than Americans do and avoid disagreeing or criticizing. Disagreements are not verbalized so that harmonious relationships will be maintained, at least outwardly. To raise one's voice to make a point, a common behavior for some Americans, is viewed by some Chinese people as being associated with anger and a sign of loss of control. To avoid confrontation, the word "no" is rarely used; furthermore, the word "yes" can mean 'no' or 'perhaps'. A direct "no" is avoided because it may cause the same individual to lose face. Hesitancy, ambiguity, subtlety, and implicity are dominant in Chinese speech. Understanding nonverbal cues and contextual meanings is also necessary during communication. For example, serving someone a banana with tea indicates an unacceptable marriage arrangement. To communicate effectively, all parties involved must participate (Argyle, 1982).

Chinese people do not ordinarily touch each other during conversation. Touching someone's head indicates a serious breach of etiquette. Touching during an argument indicates shameful loss of self-control. In the same respect, putting one's feet on a desk, table, or chair is regarded as impolite and disrespectful. On the other hand, public displays of affection toward a person of the same sex are quite permissible. Public displays between the opposite sex, however, are not considered acceptable, and as a result, the Chinese are often viewed as shy, cold, polite, unassertive, or uninterested (Fisher, 1996; Chen & Yang, 1986; Watson, 1970).

Context

Communication among the Chinese is high-context communication, which is the opposite of communication among mainstream Americans in many ways. A high-context communication is one in which most of the information is either in the physical context or internalized in the person, whereas very little is in the coded, explicit, transmitted part of the message. A low-context communication is just the opposite; that is, the mass of the information is vested in the explicit code (Hall, 1976).

Chinese people perceive and value more nonverbal and contextual cues than do Americans. For example, facial expressions, tensions, movements, speed of speaking, and location of interactions are perceived during interactions and have some meaning (Anderson, 1986). Chinese people have a tendency to view what is immediately perceptible, especially visually perceptible, and seek intuitive understanding through direct perception. Intuitive understanding is valued more than logical reasoning (Gudykunst, Stewart, & Toomey, 1985).

Kinesics

Chinese people greet others by bowing. Nodding the head may indicate 'yes', whereas shaking the head may indicate 'no'. To answer a question such as "Haven't you had anything to eat?" is problematic for many Chinese Americans. They may be confused about whether to answer affirmatively or negatively: "Yes, I haven't had anything," or "No, I would like something." Many Chinese Americans experience feelings of shame and embarrassment when they cannot communicate well. Some apologize frequently for their linguistic inabilities because they think they are inconveniencing others. Even though most Chinese do not express their emotions, some may narrow their eyes to express anger and disgust (Argyle, 1982). Chinese people have less eye contact than Americans have because, in the Chinese culture, excessive eye contact may indicate rudeness (Watson, 1970).

Chinese Americans experience a great amount of stress when they are in health care facilities. The language barrier and their different cultural background often cause confusion, depression, frustration, helplessness, and powerlessness. However, they feel that they would inconvenience the health care worker by asking questions and thus are often embarrassed to ask questions when no health care workers speak their language (Smith & Ryan, 1987). These emotional experiences are often not orally expressed but may be indicated by nonverbal cues. Frequently, observing nonverbal behaviors and encouraging clients to verbalize will help identify these psychological problems.

Implications for nursing care

It is important for the nurse to remember that there are diversified Chinese dialects that are not comprehensible to other Chinese groups. If the client needs a translator in the health care setting, the nurse must first find out which dialect the client speaks and then find a translator who can speak that dialect.

Because the Chinese language is quite different from English, the nurse must remember that when

Chinese Americans communicate in English they often experience a great amount of stress. The nurse may observe these symptoms of stress and can help the client relax to lower the stress level. Because Chinese Americans tend to be quiet, polite, and unassertive and tend to suppress feelings such as anxiety, fear, depression, or pain, it is important for the nurse to recognize nonverbal cues and their cultural meanings to develop culturally appropriate nursing care plans.

Some Chinese Americans hesitate to ask questions when they do not understand; therefore, after rapport has been established, the nurse should elicit and encourage Chinese Americans to verbalize their feelings and ask questions. The nurse should avoid using negative questions to elicit responses because negative questions are comprehended differently in the Chinese language.

In addition, because some Chinese Americans do not ordinarily touch another person during conversation, it is important for the nurse to explain the necessity of touching, particularly when therapeutic assistance is needed. Showing respect, demonstrating empathy, and being nonjudgmental can help establish rapport with Chinese American patients. The nurse can communicate better with Chinese-Americans by understanding cultural practices and differing communication styles as well. Therapeutic communication techniques can be used to promote conversations to help Chinese-American patients express thoughts and feelings and to ensure mutual understanding, especially when the nurse believes that the patient is experiencing anxiety, fear, depression, or pain.

SPACE

In studying human spatial relationships, Hall (1976) divided humans into two groups: contact and noncontact. People from a contact group interact with each other by facing each other more directly, being closer, touching more, making more eye contact, and speaking more loudly than members of a noncontact group. People from a contact group may perceive people from a noncontact group as being shy, uninterested, cold, and impolite. Conversely, people from a noncontact group may view people from a

contact group as being pushy, aggressive, obnoxious, and impolite (Hall, 1963). Both Chinese Americans and most middle-class mainstream Americans are categorized as noncontact individuals. However, from the Asian person's point of view, Americans face each other more, touch more, and have more visual contact than Asians do. Chinese people feel more comfortable in a side-by-side or right-angle arrangement and may feel uncomfortable when placed in a face-to-face situation. Americans prefer to sit face to face or at right angles to each other. In the Asian culture, the person of higher status has the prerogative of sitting as proximally as desired; thus the burden of correct behavior is on the person of lesser status (Samovar & Porter, 1988; Watson, 1970).

Implications for nursing care

Because Chinese Americans are categorized as noncontact, it is important for the nurse to remember that some Chinese Americans may be erroneously perceived as being extremely shy or withdrawn. It is equally important for the nurse to remember that some Chinese Americans may view tasks that are associated with closeness, increased eye contact, and touch as being offensive or impolite. The nurse can reduce these misunderstandings by providing explanations when performing these tasks. Because some Chinese Americans feel uncomfortable with face-to-face arrangements, the nurse may seek the client's input in terms of comfortable seating arrangements.

SOCIAL ORGANIZATION
Effect of immigration on social organization

Many early Chinese immigrants came to this country as contract laborers or with money that was borrowed from various Chinese-American organizations. These organizations assumed a supervisory role for these early immigrants once they arrived in the United States. The Chinese immigrants were similar to immigrants from other ethnic and cultural groups in that most of them were unfamiliar with the language and the culture of the United States. Therefore many of the early Chinese immigrants worked as laborers in gangs. Although many of these individuals were physically smaller than those in other ethnic or cultural groups in the

United States, they were hard workers. Historically, Chinese Americans helped build the United States by constructing railroads and working at other equally taxing jobs. Early Chinese immigrants worked cheaply and saved money by living frugally. These virtues made many of the early Chinese immigrants employable, but they were feared and hated as competitors by other American workers (Lyman, 1974).

By 1851 there were 25,000 Chinese Americans living in California alone (Sung, 1967). By 1870 the number of Chinese immigrants in the United States had increased to 63,000. In 1880 approximately 6000 Chinese persons entered the United States. Nearly twice as many entered the United States in 1881, and nearly five times as many entered in 1882 (Sung, 1967). However, in 1882 an exclusionary immigration law reduced the inflow of Chinese immigrants to less than 1000 until the year 1890. Because of this law the initial Chinese immigration was almost exclusively male. The immigration of Chinese men to the United States was believed to be a tentative rather than a permanent move, and during the 1880s the number of Chinese persons leaving the United States was greater than the number entering.

In addition to the Chinese Exclusion Act of 1882, other laws that severely curtailed not only immigration, but also the possibility of a Chinese person becoming a naturalized citizen were enacted in the United States. Furthermore, some of these laws were specific enough to require citizenship as a prerequisite for entering many occupations and for owning land (Sowell, 1981). From 1854 to 1874, there were laws that prevented Chinese people from testifying in court against White men (Lyman, 1974). Some historians believe that such laws in effect made it possible to declare "open season" on Chinese Americans because many of these individuals had no legal recourse when robbed, vandalized, or assaulted. The almost total exclusion of Chinese immigration from 1882 to 1890 had devastating long-range effects on Chinese Americans that are still evident. Because the early Chinese immigrants were almost exclusively male, there was little hope for a normal social or family life. Many of these early male immigrants had wives and children in China whom they would not

see for many years, if at all. Because of the severe restrictions on economic opportunities, it was impossible to earn enough money to book passage to China.

Over the years, the few Chinese women who had managed to immigrate into the United States were able to produce a small number of first-generation children. When these children grew up, there was a slight ease in the serious shortage of women that remained characteristic of Chinese Americans from the early immigration period until World War II. In addition, an unknown number of Chinese women were smuggled into the United States for the specific purpose of prostitution (Lyman, 1974). As recently as the 1960s, many illegal aliens from China entered the United States to pursue a better life. As a result, many Chinese residents deliberately avoided census takers.

Despite the fact that economic opportunities for early Chinese immigrants were highly restricted, many Chinatown communities took care of their own indigents. This fact may explain why even during such disasters as the San Francisco earthquake in 1906 and the Great Depression of the 1930s, many Chinese Americans did not seek or receive federal aid.

In 1943 the Chinese Exclusion Act of 1882 was repealed, and that repeal did help ease the imbalance of the male-to-female ratio and permitted a more normal family life to develop among a very family-oriented people. After the repeal of the Chinese Exclusion Act of 1882, the bulk of the new Chinese immigrants were female (Sung, 1967). The labor shortages of World War II opened many new job opportunities that were not previously available to Chinese Americans. Thus many Chinese Americans abandoned traditional Chinatown occupations to move into these new jobs (Sowell, 1981).

In 1940 only 3% of Chinese Americans in California had jobs that were considered "professional," compared with 8% of the White population. By 1950 the percentage of Chinese Americans in professional fields had doubled to 6%. Over the next decade the percentage of Chinese Americans working in professional fields tripled, and for the first time passed the percentage of Whites working in professional fields. By 1970 it was reported that Chinese Americans in general had a higher income or higher occupational status than most other Americans. In 1970 at least one fourth of all employed Chinese Americans were working in scientific or professional fields (Sowell, 1981).

Family

The Chinese culture emphasizes loyalty to family and devotion to tradition and deemphasizes individual feelings (Chen & Yang, 1986). The Chinese are willing to submit their own interests to those of the family, which maintains a strong and cohesive bond. The family is expected to take care of its members, both immediate and extended. Doing so brings honor to the family; not doing so brings shame (Kim, 1988; Louie, 1985).

The Chinese family generally has a hierarchical structure. The older children have authority over younger children, and the younger children must show respect and deference to authority figures. Failure to do so causes shame for the family. The authority figures have more influence on decision making, and these decisions are made on the basis of consensus rather than majority. The individual learns to submit to the prevailing opinion rather than disagree (Anderson, 1986; Gudykunst, Stewart, & Toomey, 1985). However, the values of the Chinese-American family are eroding in the acculturation process. Many youngsters do not show respect to the elderly, and many elderly persons cannot count on their children or relatives for help. Many older Chinese Americans thus suffer mental illnesses, and some commit suicide (Tien-Hyatt, 1987).

Marital status

Because of the early Chinese Exclusion Act in the United States, there was a disproportionately large number of Chinese men compared with Chinese women. Many of the early unmarried Chinese men who came to the United States had virtually no opportunity to marry; thus in 1890 only 26.1% of the total number of Chinese-American men were married. The percentage of married Chinese-American women from 1890 to 1950 ranged from 57.4% to 69.1%. During this time there appeared to be a lower

percentage of single Chinese women who immigrated, which was partially accounted for by the Chinese tradition of females marrying at a younger age. Chinese Americans divorce less frequently than their American counterparts (Sung, 1967).

Religion

The four primary religions of China are Taoism, Buddhism, Islam, and Christianity. Of these four primary religions, Taoism has the least number of professed followers. Among Chinese and Chinese Americans, Christianity is regarded as a newcomer; nevertheless, its effects are pronounced. Christianity is viewed as being partially responsible for the introduction of the Western culture into China as well as to Chinese Americans. Today the number of Chinese Roman Catholics is increasing rapidly, particularly among foreign-born Chinese Americans (Fisher, 1996; Sowell, 1981).

Implications for nursing care

It is important for the nurse to remember that Chinese Americans are a family-oriented people who normally put family loyalties before personal interests. In addition, the Chinese-American family has traditionally had a hierarchical structure. Chinese Americans believe that they have a major responsibility in taking care of family members and relatives. Therefore family members may view the hospitalization or health care needs of a family member as a personal concern. The nurse needs to understand this sense of responsibility and be sensitive to the family's needs. Opinions and ideas of the family members should be incorporated into the plan of care. Also, it is important to provide health care education to all family members, not just the client, when procedures are to be done.

Chinese Americans vary widely in educational background and socioeconomic status, have varied cultural and religious values and practices, and have different rates of acculturation. For example, some Chinese Americans speak English very poorly, whereas others can communicate in English without any problem. Some have medical insurance, whereas others do not. Some use herbal medicine, whereas others do not. If the client has a language barrier, a translator is needed and can usually be found in the local Chinese community. Visual displays, flip charts, or exhibits can be used to facilitate the client's understanding.

Most Chinese Americans have strong family ties. By assessing the client's kinship relationship and identifying authoritative family members, the nurse can effectively use the influential family members to achieve the therapeutic goals. The nurse should help Chinese Americans with few support systems seek community resources.

Chinese women are very uncomfortable and uneasy when examined by male health professionals. Therefore a female nurse should be present and assist in the examination.

TIME

The Chinese have a different perception and experience regarding time; it is not past, present, or future oriented. Some Chinese Americans perceive time as a dynamic wheel with circular movements and the present as a reflection of the eternal. This metaphoric wheel continually turns in an unforeseeable direction, and individuals are expected to adjust to the present, which surrounds the rotating wheel, and seek a harmonious relationship with their surroundings (Kim, 1988; Yuen, 1987).

Hall (1963) has described the time concept of Asians as "polychronic" and that of Westerners as "monochronic." An individual with a polychronic time orientation adheres less rigidly to time as a distinct and linear entity, focuses on the completion of the present, and often implements more than one activity simultaneously. On the other hand, an individual with a monochronic orientation to time emphasizes schedules, promptness, standardization of activities, and synchronization with clocks.

When making decisions regarding current and future events, some Chinese people may be affected by traditions and customs. Before making decisions they may seek symbols, correlations, and intuitive understanding, as well as consider significances, consequences, future situations, and present factors. They do not make decisions according to an individual's own benefit (Gudykunst, Stewart, & Toomey, 1985).

Implications for nursing care

Because Chinese Americans are perceived as being polychronic, which more or less implies that they are present-time oriented, it is important for the nurse to remember that some Chinese Americans may not adhere to fixed schedules. Polychronic individuals may arrive late for appointments; may insist on completing a task before moving on to a new task, even though the new task may be time related; and may implement more than one task at a time. It is important for the nurse to recognize that when some Chinese Americans make decisions related to current events they may appear hesitant because of the need to consider as many variables as possible.

ENVIRONMENTAL CONTROL

Many Chinese Americans may not believe that they have control over nature because they subscribe to a belief in fatalism and may view people as adjusting to the physical world, not controlling or changing the environment (Gudykunst, Stewart, & Toomey, 1985). In traditional Chinese teaching, a harmonious relationship with nature is stressed. The concepts of *yin* and *yáng* represent the power that regulates the universe and that exists within the body and food. *Yang* represents the positive, active, or "male" force, and *yin* represents the negative, inactive, or "female" force. Body systems are categorized into *yin* and *yang* groups. For example, the liver, heart, spleen, lungs, and kidneys are *yin,* and the gallbladder, stomach, large intestine, small intestine, bladder, and lymphatic system are *yang.* The *yin* forces store the strength of life, and the *yang* forces protect the body from outside invasions. Some Chinese people believe that an imbalance between *yin* and *yang* will result in illness and a balance between *yin* and *yang* can enhance health.

Food is also grouped into *yin*/"cold" and *yang*/"hot" groups and is considered to be either the cause or the treatment of illnesses. A person with leukemia may believe that too many "cold" foods have been consumed. Diseases or conditions with excessive *yin* forces, such as cancer, postpartum psychoses, menstruation, or lactation, are treated with foods with *yang* qualities, such as beef, chicken, eggs, fried foods, spicy foods, hot foods, vinegar, and wine. Diseases or conditions with excessive *yang* forces, such as infections, fever, hypertension, sore throat, or toothache, require foods with *yin* quality, such as bean curds, honey, carrots, turnips, green vegetables, fruits, cold foods, and duck (Ludman & Newman, 1984). In addition, the Chinese often use vegetables such as bok choy, tea, honey, or prunes to treat constipation; they use chrysanthemum, crystal (preserved ginger?), ginseng, or other herbal decoctions to treat indigestion (Hess, 1986).

Fengshŭi (translated to mean 'wind [and] water'), which some Chinese Americans subscribe to, is the art of location, orientation, and design of physical structures in an effort to achieve proper harmony and balance (Fisher, 1996). Positive *fengshui* wards off evil spirits and promotes good health and prosperity. Shapes of objects, buildings, and so on take on significance for some Chinese Americans and can be correlated with either good or bad luck. For example, a triangular building is considered to be bad luck and would not usually be used by Chinese Americans for house construction. Likewise, it is believed that doors should not open directly facing traffic because this would allow evil spirits direct access to the building. Similarly, it is believed that the best location for a building is directly facing water whereas the rear of the building should face mountains in an effort to encourage prosperity and at the same time offer protection.

Some Chinese Americans hold beliefs related to colors and numbers, and such objects may take on significance in health care. For example, the number four (*sì*) is considered bad luck, whereas the number eight (*ba*) is considered good luck. The color white is considered bad luck because it is a color of mourning, whereas the color red is considered good luck. Thus a person born on 8/8/88 would be considered to be extremely lucky, whereas a person born on 4/4/44 would be considered to be extremely unlucky. It is conceivable that a Chinese American subscribing to these beliefs might have considerable difficulty going for diagnostic testing in a triangular building that was located at 444 Fourth Street where all the personnel wear white laboratory coats (Fisher, 1996).

Illness and wellness behaviors

Cultural differences and language barriers play a major role in the utilization of health services by Chinese Americans. Many Chinese Americans use both Western and Chinese medical services (predominantly herbal medicine). Typically a Chinese American will treat minor or chronic illnesses with Chinese medical services and acute or serious problems with Western medical services (Liu, 1986). Traditionally, the Chinese believe in preventive health practices. Some Chinese Americans will first seek Chinese medicines and try to manage on their own. When physiological signs indicate that conditions are getting worse, they will then seek Western medicines. This practice is especially common among Chinese-American psychiatric clients because of the emphasis the Chinese culture puts on self-control and self-sufficiency.

Many Chinese Americans tend to underutilize medical services because of low socioeconomic status. Although unemployment rates for Chinese Americans are lower than those for the general population, underemployment among Chinese Americans is much higher. Underemployment problems include a shorter work week, a mismatch between education and employment, and longer working hours for the same pay. In addition, at least 14% of Chinese Americans live at or below the poverty level. Many elderly male Chinese Americans live alone with a low income as a result of early immigration laws. Immigrant families may have no medical insurance because they may not be familiar with medical insurance, they may not believe in insuring health, or they may not be able to afford it (Fisher, 1996; Liu, 1986). In fact, Takeuchi, Chung, and Shen (1998) noted that factors such as marital status, length of residence in the United States, education, employment, and average household income were associated with health insurance coverage among Chinese Americans.

Chinese Americans may fear medical institutions because of language barriers and unfamiliarity with medical institutions or because of an inadequate understanding of illnesses and treatment modalities. As a result, some Chinese Americans may not comply with medical treatments. Many diagnostic tests, such as amniocentesis, glucose tolerance testing, ultrasonography, or drawing blood, are often perceived as being dangerous and unnecessary (Minkler, 1983).

Some Chinese Americans have a tendency to self-medicate with over-the-counter drugs, herbal remedies, tranquilizers, and antibiotics (Campbell & Chang, 1973; Gallo, Edwards, & Vessey, 1980; Hess, 1986; Louie, 1985; McLaughlin, Raymond, Murakami, & Goebert, 1987). In addition, some Chinese Americans may save part of a prescribed medicine and take it at their own discretion at a later time (Campbell & Chang, 1973). Some Chinese people respond to pain stoically because of a fear of addiction and because of the value the culture puts on self-control (Thiederman, 1989). For some Chinese people the predominant pain preparations are topical ointments and balms (Hess, 1986).

Chinese Americans use both herbal medicines and Western medicines at the same time to treat illnesses. Because some herbal and Western medicines have similar effects, using both can create problems. For example, ginseng is a tonic stimulant and an antihypertensive medicine. The client may overmedicate by taking antihypertensive drugs and ginseng at the same time.

Chinese herbal medicines are boiled in a specified amount of water over low heat until the desired concentration is reached. The medicines are then taken as a single dose. If the client does not feel better after the initial dose, the client may need to return to the herbalist. Because of this tradition, some Chinese Americans are unfamiliar with the practice of taking drugs when feeling well. In addition, the practice of taking multiple drugs in tablet or capsule form at various times and over several days or weeks can be confusing (Hess, 1986; Liu, 1986; Louie, 1985).

Folklore and folk practices

Restoring the balance of *yin* and *yang* is the fundamental concept of Chinese medical practice, which includes acupuncture, herbal medicines, moxibustion, massage, skin scraping, and cupping. Acupuncture involves the insertion of metal needles through specific body points to treat or cure illnesses with excessive *yang* forces, such as pain, stroke, or asthma. Herbal medicines are categorized according to the properties of *yin* or *yang* and their therapeutic functions and are prescribed on the basis of the *yin-yang* nature of the particular illness. Moxibustion involves heat treatment of illnesses such as mumps or convulsions. When moxibustion is used as a treatment, the ignited moxa plants are placed near specific areas of the body. After moxibustion, tiny craters about 1 cm in diameter can be observed on the skin. Massage is used to stimulate the circulation, to increase the flexibility of the joints, and to improve the body's resistance to illnesses. Massage is a useful technique to relieve tension. Skin scraping involves applying special oil to the symptomatic area and rubbing the area with the edge of a coin in a firm, downward motion. This treatment is used to treat colds, heatstroke, headache, and indigestion. Linear multiple bruises may be observed on the skin as a result of this process. Cupping is used to treat headaches, arthritis, and abdominal pain. A vacuum is created inside a cup by burning of a special material, and the cup is then placed immediately on the selected area and kept there until it is easily removed. Circular, ecchymotic, painful burn marks 2 inches in diameter can be observed on the skin after this treatment (Boyle & Andrews, 1989; Louie, 1985; Spector, 1996).

Implications for nursing care

Because Chinese Americans often believe that they do not have control over nature and maintain a fatalistic outlook on life, they may be hesitant about seeking health care treatment. In addition, because some Chinese Americans subscribe to the theory of *yin* and *yang*, which attempts to restore balance to the body, such individuals are more likely to engage in self-treatment. Therefore, the nurse must be able to distinguish between practices that could be harmful, neutral, or beneficial to the client's particular medical problem. For example, some Chinese Americans from Southeast Asia or urban areas in China may practice native healing processes in which they may tie a string around the wrist, burn incense, or make food offerings to the spirits. As long as these practices are not harmful, the nurse should respect them and allow them to continue (Gallo, Edwards, & Vessey, 1980). The nurse who observes that a Chinese-American client is taking herbal medicine in addition to the prescribed medicine should caution the client about the possibility of overmedicating.

Some Chinese Americans who subscribe to the theory of *yin* and *yang* believe that food has *yin* and *yang* qualities. Therefore the nurse must help the client select the appropriate foods according to these beliefs. Also, hospital food could be unfamiliar to some Chinese Americans. If the client wishes, the nurse may encourage the family to bring in some native foods.

BIOLOGICAL VARIATIONS

People are the product of both genetic factors and environmental influences. For example, it has been hypothesized that the epicanthic fold that gives the Chinese a slant-eyed look may have evolved as a protection against blinding blizzards of snow or sand (Bleibtreu & Downs, 1971). The "yellow" color of the Chinese skin is believed to be caused by a smaller amount of melanin in the skin compared with the skin of Black people (Race and ability, 1967). Others have theorized that Chinese people may have a thickened corneum, creating the yellowish skin color (Molnar, 1983). Most Chinese people have thick straight hair. Chinese men tend to lack facial hair.

Body size and structure

Chinese Americans tend to be shorter at all ages and tend to complete their growth earlier than other Americans (Molnar, 1983). On the standard growth charts, the mean height and weight of Chinese-American children fall in the 10th percentile, whereas the mean height and weight of mainstream American children fall in the 50th percentile (Boyle & Andrews, 1989). On the average, Asians have longer trunks and shorter limbs than Whites. Some Chinese Americans have wider hips and narrower shoulders than other Americans. The children of Chinese immigrants are generally taller than native Chinese children, but their sitting and standing height ratios do not change. Asians have smaller chest volumes than Whites. The average forced expiratory volume for Chinese Americans is 2.53 liters, compared with 3.22 liters for White Americans. The average forced vital capacity is 3.27 liters for Chinese Americans, compared with 4.30 liters for White Americans (Overfield, 1995).

Skin color

The majority of Chinese infants have mongolian spots (irregular areas of deep blue pigmentation observed primarily in the sacral and gluteal regions and occasionally in other areas of the body). Neonatal jaundice is seen in 50% of Chinese infants. The bilirubin level peaks on the fifth and sixth days of life, compared with the second and third days for other races. Bilirubin levels higher than 12 mg/dL occur in 25% to 40% of Chinese infants. In addition, blood levels higher than 15 mg/dL occur in 15% to 23% of Chinese infants. Breast-feeding elevates the bilirubin level. The physician may suggest that the mother stop breast-feeding until the baby's bilirubin levels return to normal (Boyle & Andrews, 1989; Overfield, 1985).

Enzymatic and genetic variations

A majority of Chinese Americans have a lactase deficiency and are unable to tolerate fresh milk. Lactase splits milk sugar, lactose, into simple glucose and galactose. Lactase deficiency may cause a person who drinks fresh milk to have flatus, abdominal cramps, diarrhea, or vomiting. However, the person can often eat cheese because bacteria do the work of lactase. This enzyme may also be induced by long-term consumption of fresh milk.

Chinese people have relatively high incidences of thalassemia and G-6-PD deficiency. Thalassemia is a type of hemoglobin abnormality characterized by a high rate of red blood cell destruction, necessitating frequent blood transfusions. G-6-PD deficiency is another red blood cell defect causing fragility of the red blood cells. Persons with G-6-PD deficiency are prone to anemia when exposed to certain drugs such as analgesics (aspirin, phenacetin), sulfonamides and sulfones, antimalarials (primaquine, quinacrine), antibacterials (nitrofurantoin, chloramphenicol, *para*-aminosalicylic acid), vitamin K, probenecid, and quinidine (Molnar, 1983; Overfield, 1995).

Another genetic difference is that Chinese people usually experience noticeable facial flushing and vasomotor symptoms after drinking alcohol. This may explain the low alcoholism rate among the Chinese (Overfield, 1995) (see Chapter 7).

Susceptibility to disease

Immigrants from Indochina and mainland China have common health problems, such as tuberculosis, intestinal parasites, malaria, malnutrition, anemia, and hepatitis. Most Southeast Asians received vaccinations (bacillus Calmette-Guérin, BCG) against tuberculosis in their childhood (Overfield, 1995; Gallo, Edwards, & Vessey, 1980).

Cancer Chinese people are known to be at risk for cancers of the nasopharynx, esophagus, stomach, liver, and cervix. The intake of fermented and moldy foods and nitrosamines contained in corn, bran, millet, and pickled vegetables is believed to be a possible contributing factor for esophageal and liver cancers. Recent studies have revealed a downward trend for these cancers among Chinese Americans. On the other hand, low-risk cancers for Chinese people (colon, rectum, lung, female breast, and leukemia) are gradually increasing among Chinese Americans (King & Locke, 1988; Yu, 1986; Overfield, 1995).

Mortality and leading causes of death

In 1990, mortality data revealed the four leading causes of death for Chinese Americans to be identical to those for White Americans: heart disease, cancer, cerebrovascular disease, and accidents (National Center for Health Statistics, 1993). However, the proportional mortalities are different. Chinese Americans have a lower mortality from heart disease (32%) than White Americans (39%) and a higher mortality from cancer (27%) than White Americans (21%). The fifth leading cause of death for Chinese Americans is pneumonia and influenza. Suicide ranks seventh as a cause of death for Chinese Americans compared with ranking tenth for White Americans. Chinese women have a higher suicide rate than White women. The causes of the higher suicide rate need further investigation (National Center for Health Statistics, 1993; Yu, 1986).

Psychological characteristics

Many Chinese Americans believe that psychiatric illnesses indicate an inability to solve problems or are manifested by behavior that is out of control, bringing shame to the individual and the family. Therefore the family will often attempt to manage the sick person on their own for as long as possible. As a result, hospitalized Chinese psychiatric clients appear more disturbed than other clients (Binder, 1983).

Chinese Americans experience multiple psychosocial stresses while adapting to the new culture and environment, including cultural conflicts, language difficulties, poverty, and discrimination. Many Chinese Americans experience depression and social loneliness, but few seek help until psychosomatic discomfort is experienced. Chinese Americans tend to seek help from physicians rather than psychiatrists or other mental health professionals for psychosomatic complaints (Hsu, Hailey, & Range, 1987; Kuo, 1984; Yeung & Schwartz, 1986).

Recent empirical studies have revealed that Asians require lower dosages than Whites for several psychotropic medications such as lithium, antidepressants, and neuroleptics. Asians require lower oral dosages and blood levels of lithium. The plasma levels of desipramine (an antidepressant) are higher and peak earlier for Asians than for Whites. Asians experience extrapyramidal effects at lower neuroleptic doses than Whites do. The plasma levels of diazepam at a given oral dose are higher in Asians than in Whites. Asians are reported to tolerate better the sedating effects of diphenhydramine. The causes for such differences are considered to be both genetic and environmental, an indication that further investigation is needed (Lawson, 1986; Pi, Simpson, & Cooper, 1986).

Implications for nursing care

It is important for the nurse to know that growth and development norms for Chinese Americans are different from White American standards. A standard growth chart for healthy Chinese children and adolescents is available (Whaley & Wong, 1987). However, the nurse should not rely on the growth chart alone. An assessment of general health status is necessary to identify malnutrition, anemia, or growth retardation (Gallo, Edwards, & Vessy, 1980).

The nurse should reassure the Chinese-American mother that it is normal for her newborn to exhibit more jaundice than other American babies do. Otherwise, the mother may feel guilty and believe that the jaundice is caused by something she ate. The observed mongolian spots on Chinese-American infants should not be interpreted as lesions.

When working with a Chinese-American family that has a family member with a physical or mental problem, the astute nurse will make use of general or mental health facilities easier by providing information regarding the services, encouraging the family to seek help early, and arranging for follow-up care. Rather than waiting until the symptoms are advanced, the nurse should assist the family in getting appropriate care for their family member as soon as possible.

The following case report illustrates the profound effect of the Chinese culture on a client with a medical problem and psychotic symptoms. An 83-year-old Chinese woman exhibited psychotic symptoms at home for 15 months until the family could not handle the situation any longer and admitted her to a hospital. The family members felt guilty and ashamed because they could not take care of their mother. After admission, a health history revealed that the client had had a gastrectomy about 13 years earlier, and her blood level of vitamin B_{12} was 91 mg/dL (normal is 180 to 900 mg/dL). She was treated with vitamin B_{12}, and the psychotic symptoms disappeared. Perhaps, if the family had brought the patient to the hospital earlier, they could have avoided 15 months of agony (Binder, 1983).

Client and family teaching are important in providing care for the Chinese-American client and family. Lack of knowledge related to illnesses and treatment is a common problem and causes fear and anxiety. The nurse can assess the family's understanding of illnesses and treatment and provide education accordingly. If the client takes herbal medicines, the nurse should provide education to increase the client and family's awareness of the synergistic and antagonistic effects of Western and herbal medicines taken together. Because Asians are known to require lower dosages of psychotropic medications, the nurse should provide education about these medications and observe their effects and side effects. The nurse should also emphasize the importance of taking medicines as prescribed and discourage the practice of taking medicines only when symptoms of the illness are present. In addition, the nurse should keep in mind that Chinese Americans have a relatively high incidence of G-6-PD deficiency; therefore it is essential to urge

the client to seek help early when any side effects of medication are experienced.

The need for teaching about medication is illustrated by the following example. A Chinese-American man took captopril at home as prescribed for 1 week and developed severe thirst and hyponatremia, leading to irreversible neurological damage (Al-Mufti & Arieff, 1985). He was polydipsic and drank about 7 liters daily. If he had been taught the side effects of captopril and had been encouraged to seek help when he experienced this side effect, his death could possibly have been avoided.

Although many Chinese women breast-feed their babies, recently many Chinese American women have changed to bottle-feeding in adapting to the Western culture. The nurse should provide information regarding the benefits of breast-feeding and encourage mothers to breast-feed for at least 6 weeks (Minkler, 1983). If the mother has to stop breast-feeding because of jaundice, the nurse can teach the mother to express milk to continue breast-feeding when the baby is ready to be breast-fed again.

Dietary education is also very important in providing care for the Chinese-American client and family (Kolonel, 1988). Some Chinese Americans believe in the theory of *yin* and *yang* and eat foods accordingly when they are sick. For example, post partum and after surgery, some Chinese Americans will not drink or eat anything with *yin* qualities, such as cold drinks, vegetables, salad, or cold meat; they will eat only chicken, beef, or fried foods. The nurse should help the client select foods and drinks and encourage the family to bring the desired foods from home.

Chinese foods usually are cooked with soy sauce and monosodium glutamate (MSG). The nurse must remember that many preserved foods are also high in salt content. Therefore the nurse should inform patients who require a salt-restricted diet to reduce their sodium intake gradually by reducing the use of soy sauce, monosodium glutamate, and preserved foods and should discourage the high intake of fermented and moldy foods, which are considered to contribute to the high incidence of esophageal and liver cancer. The nurse should also encourage clients to reduce their intake of foods that have no nutritional value. Because many Chinese Americans may be unable to tolerate fresh milk because of a lactase deficiency, the nurse should encourage the use of tofu (bean curd) or other protein and calcium-rich foods to replace the need for fresh milk.

SUMMARY

The number of Chinese Americans in the United States is steadily increasing. As immigration of the Chinese continues, the nurse will encounter more Chinese Americans in health care facilities. Because of the complex cultural values and beliefs, diversified acculturation, and various educational levels among Chinese Americans, the nurse needs to work with individuals to assess their unique values, communication styles, social organization, time concepts, illness behaviors, and biological variations to provide effective and individualized nursing care. The nurse should convey respect to the client, encourage pride in the Chinese culture, reduce feelings of shame, and facilitate adaptation to the Western culture.

Case Study

A 40-year-old Chinese woman is admitted to a local hospital with the diagnosis of uremia. Her blood urea nitrogen (BUN) level is 168 mg/dL (normal is 8 to 18 mg/dL). She has a history of hypertension and was previously given a prescription for hydrochlorothiazide (HCTZ), which she stopped taking because of increasing dizziness, dry mouth, and weakness. She is single, lives alone, has no immediate family nearby, has a temporary job, and has no medical insurance. Her physician prescribes peritoneal dialysis and HCTZ. The following are noted by the nurse on assessment: blood pressure, 180/100; respirations, 20 per minute; pulse, 110 per minute; height, 5 feet, 1 inch; weight, 100 pounds; dry skin with multiple scratching marks; no urine output; and complaints of blurred vision, itchiness, weakness, and insomnia. Her gait is slightly unsteady. She talks with a soft and low voice and speaks English slowly but not fluently. She sometimes asks questions that have already been discussed. Although she smiles frequently during conversation, she appears tense and restless. The nurse notices some hand tremors, shaky voice, and twisting fingers. Although she has limited information about peritoneal dialysis, the woman changes the subject as the nurse explains the procedure.

CARE PLAN

 Nursing Diagnosis   Pain related to pruritus

Client Outcomes

1. Client will verbalize discomfort to others when it exists and will relate relief with therapeutic measures.

Nursing Interventions

1. Explain pruritus will be decreased when client's BUN level is down.
2. Keep client's room cool and avoid excessive warmth from clothes or blankets because warmth will increase itchiness.
3. Apply cool lotions to dry and itchy areas.
4. Apply cool wet soaks to reduce itchiness if client desires.
5. Ask client's doctor if any medicines can be used to decrease itchiness.
6. Encourage client to engage in diversional activities.
7. Advise client to keep her fingernails short to avoid injury to her skin when she scratches.

Nursing Diagnosis   Anxiety related to peritoneal dialysis

Client Outcomes

1. Client will verbalize her understanding of peritoneal dialysis and will experience less anxiety after teaching.

Nursing Interventions

1. Assess client's understanding of peritoneal dialysis.
2. Present information to client related to peritoneal dialysis by using pamphlets and drawings.
3. Explain rationale for peritoneal dialysis.
4. Describe feelings the client may have during dialysis.
5. Contact dialysis nurse to obtain some audiovisual aids to help client understand.

 Nursing Diagnosis   Noncompliance related to side effects of HCTZ

Client Outcomes

1. Client will describe the experience that caused her to stop taking HCTZ, describe appropriate treatment of side effects, and demonstrate appropriate alternatives to the previous plan.

Nursing Interventions

1. Assess any other contributing factors for stopping HCTZ (such as cost; refer to social worker to seek any financial help).
2. Identify current effects and side effects of HCTZ on client.
3. Teach effects and side effects of HCTZ.
4. Assist client in reducing discomfort (such as dizziness—change positions slowly; dry mouth—ice chips, hard candy; weakness—get plenty of sleep and ask for help for what she is limited in doing).
5. Explain client's dizziness; weakness could be improved when her BUN level is down.
6. Ask client to verbalize what she understands.

 Nursing Diagnosis   Communication, impaired verbal, related to foreign-language barrier

Client Outcomes

1. Client will be able to communicate basic needs and relate feelings of acceptance.

Nursing Interventions

1. Talk slowly and clearly to client.
2. Write down important information.
3. Use gestures, actions, pictures, and drawings to facilitate client's understanding.
4. Encourage client to teach others some Chinese words.
5. Seek a translator to discuss important matters.

STUDY QUESTIONS

1. List at least three contributing factors for hypertension among Chinese Americans.
2. Delineate at least two things that the nurse can do to facilitate the communication process between the nurse and the Chinese American client.
3. Identify at least two factors about lack of family structure and its significance to the Chinese culture that may contribute to the difficulties of hospitalization for the Chinese-American client.
4. Describe factors regarding the time concept that may hinder health care services for a Chinese American client.
5. Describe health and illness practices that may augment problems associated with the treatment of hypertension for Chinese-American clients.

References

Albert, R.D., & Triandis, M.C. (1985). Intercultural education for multicultural societies: critical issues. In Samovar, L.A., & Porter, R.E. (Eds.), *Intercultural communication: a reader* (ed. 5) (pp. 373-385). Belmont, Calif.: Wadsworth.

Al-Mufti, H.I., & Arieff, A.I. (1985). Captopril-induced hyponatremia with irreversible neurologic damage. *The American Journal of Medicine, 79,* 769-770.

Anderson, J.M. (1986). Ethnicity and illness experience: ideological structures and the health care delivery system. *Social Science Medicine, 22*(11), 1277-1283.

Argyle, M. (1982). Intercultural communication. In Samovar, L.A., & Porter, R.E. (Eds.), *Intercultural communication: a reader* (ed. 5) (pp. 31-44). Belmont, Calif.: Wadsworth.

Becker, C.B. (1986). Reasons for the lack of argumentation and debate in the Far East. In Samovar, L.A., & Porter, R.E. (Eds.), *Intercultural communication: a reader* (ed. 5) (pp. 243-252). Belmont, Calif.: Wadsworth.

Binder, R.L. (1983). Cultural factors complicating the treatment of psychosis caused by B_{12} deficiency. *Hospital and Community Psychiatry, 34*(1), 67-69.

Bleibtreu, H.K., & Downs, J.F. (1971). *Human variations: readings in physical anthropology.* Beverly Hills, Calif.: Glencoe Press.

Boyle, J.S., & Andrews, M.M. (1989). *Transcultural concepts on nursing care.* Glenview, Ill.: Scott, Foresman.

Campbell, T., & Chang, B. (1973). Health care of the Chinese in America. *Nursing Outlook, 21*(4), 245-249.

Chang, B. (1981). Asian-American patient care. In Henderson, G., & Primeaux, M. (Eds.), *Transcultural health care* (pp. 225-278). Reading, Mass.: Addison-Wesley.

Chen, C.L., & Yang, D.C.V. (1986). The self-image of Chinese-American adolescents: a cross-cultural comparison. *International Journal of Social Psychiatry, 32*(4), 19-26.

Encyclopedia Americana (International ed., vol. 6) (1983). Danbury, Conn.: Grolier.

Fisher, N.L. (1996). *Culture and ethnic diversity: a guide for genetic professionals.* Baltimore, Md.: Johns Hopkins University Press.

Gallo, A.M., Edwards, J., & Vessey, J. (1980). Indochina moves to main street: little refugees with big needs (Part 4). *RN, 43,* 45-48.

Gudykunst, W.B., Stewart, L.P., & Toomey, S.T. (1985). *Communication, culture, and organizational process.* Newbury Park, Calif.: Sage.

Hall, E.T. (1963). A system for the notation of proxemic behavior. *American Anthropologist, 65,* 1003-1026.

Hall, E.T. (1976). *Beyond culture.* New York: Anchor Press/Doubleday.

Hess, P. (1986). Chinese and Hispanic elders and OTC drugs. *Geriatric Nursing, 7*(6), 314-318.

Hsu, L.R., Hailey, B.J., & Range, L.M. (1987). Cultural and emotional components of loneliness and depression. *The Journal of Psychology, 121*(1), 61-70.

Information please almanac (1998). Boston: Houghton Mifflin.

Kim, Y.Y. (1988). Intercultural personhood: an integration of Eastern and Western perspectives. In Samovar, L.A., & Porter, R.E. (Eds.), *Intercultural communication: a reader* (ed. 5) (pp. 344-351). Belmont, Calif.: Wadsworth.

King, H., & Locke, F.B. (1988). The national mortality survey of China: implications for cancer control and prevention. *Cancer Detection and Prevention, 13*(3-4), 157-166.

Kolonel, L.N. (1988). Variability in diet and its relation to risk in ethnic and migrant groups. *Basic Life Science, 43,* 129-135.

Kuo, W.H. (1984). Prevalence of depression among Asian-Americans. *Journal of Nervous and Mental Disease, 172*(8), 449-457.

Lawson, W.B. (1986). Racial and ethnic factors in psychiatric research. *Hospital and Community Psychiatry, 37*(1), 50-54.

Liu, W.T. (1986). Health services for Asian elderly. *Research on Aging, 8*(1), 156-175.

Louie, K.B. (1985). Providing health care to Chinese clients. *Topics in Clinical Nursing, 7*(3), 18-25.

Ludman, E.K., & Newman, J.M. (1984). The health-related food practices of three Chinese groups. *Journal of Nutrition Education, 16,* 4.

Lyman, S. (1974). *Chinese Americans.* New York: Random House.

Mangiafico, L. (1988). *Contemporary American immigrants.* New York: Praeger.

McLaughlin, D.G., Raymond, J.S., Murakami, S.R., & Goebert, D. (1987). Drug use among Asian-Americans in Hawaii. *Journal of Psychoactive Drugs, 19*(1), 85-94.

Minkler, D.H. (1983). The role of community-based satellite clinics in the perinatal care of non–English speaking immigrants. *The Western Journal of Medicine, 139*(6), 905-909.

Molnar, S.C. (1983). *Human variation: races, types, and ethnic groups* (ed. 2). Englewood Cliffs, N.J.: Prentice Hall.

National Center for Health Statistics, Healthy People 2000 Review (1993). *Health, United States, 1992.* Hyattsville, Md.: Public Health Service.

National Center for Health Statistics (1998). *Health, United States, 1998, with socioeconomic status and chartbook.* Hyattsville, Md.: Public Health Service.

Orque, M.S., Bloch, B., & Monrroy, L.S.A. (1983). *Ethnics in nursing care: a multicultural approach.* St. Louis: Mosby.

Overfield, T. (1995). *Biological variations in health and illness.* Reading, Mass.: Addison-Wesley.

Pi, E.H., Simpson, G.H., & Cooper, T.B. (1986). Pharmacokinetics of desipramine in Caucasian and Asian volunteers. *American Journal of Psychiatry, 143*(9), 1174-1175.

Race and ability (1967, Sept. 29). *Time,* p. 46-47.

Samovar, L.A., & Porter, R.E. (1988). *Intercultural communication: a reader* (ed. 5). Belmont, Calif.: Wadsworth.

Smith, M.J., & Ryan, A.S. (1987). Chinese-American families of children with developmental disabilities: an exploratory study of reactions to service providers. *Mental Retardation, 25*(6), 345-350.

Sowell, T. (1981). *Ethnic America.* New York: Basic Books.

Spector, R.E. (1996). *Cultural diversity in health and illness* (ed. 3). East Norwalk, Conn.: Appleton-Century-Crofts.

Sung, B. (1967). *A story of Chinese in America.* New York: Collier.

Takeuchi, D.T., Chung, R.C.Y., & Shen, H.K. (1998). Health insurance coverage among Chinese Americans in Los Angeles County. *American Journal of Public Health, 88*(3), 451-453.

Thiederman, S. (1989). Stoic or shouter, the pain is real. *RN, 52*(6), 49-51.

Tien-Hyatt, J.L. (1987). Self-perceptions of aging across cultures: myth or reality? *International Journal of Aging and Human Development, 24*(2), 129-148.

U.S. Department of Commerce, Bureau of the Census (1993a, June 12). *News Release,* Commerce News.

U.S. Department of Commerce, Bureau of the Census (1993b). *Population profile of the United States, 1993* (pp. 23-185). Washington, D.C.: Government Printing Office.

U.S. Department of Commerce, Bureau of the Census (1993c, Sept.). *We the Americans . . . Asians.* Washington, D.C.: Government Printing Office.

Watson, O.M. (1970). *Proxemic behavior: a cross-cultural study.* The Hague, The Netherlands: Mouton.

Whaley, L.F., & Wong, D.L. (1987). *Nursing care of infants and children* (ed. 3). St. Louis: Mosby.Wong, B.P. (1982). *Chinatown: economic adaptation and ethnic identity of the Chinese.* New York: Holt, Rinehart, & Winston.

World almanac (1997). Mahwah, N.J.: World Almanac Books.

Yeung, W.H., & Schwartz, M.A. (1986). Emotional disturbance in Chinese obstetrical patients: a pilot study. *General Hospital Psychiatry, 8,* 258-262.

Yu, E.S.H. (1986). Health of the Chinese elderly in America. *Research on Aging, 8*(1), 84-109.

Yuen, J. (1987). Asian Americans. *Birth Defects Original Article Series, 23*(6), 164-170.

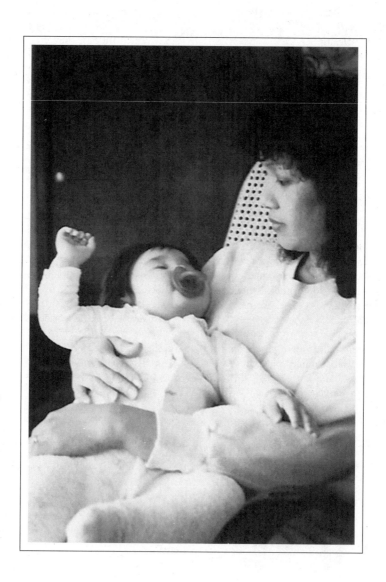

CHAPTER 17 Filipino Americans

Anna Rambharose Vance

BEHAVIORAL OBJECTIVES

After reading this chapter, the nurse will be able to:

1. Describe the problems encountered regarding communication when giving culturally appropriate nursing care to Filipino-American clients.
2. Explain the Filipino-American orientation to time and space and the relevance to culturally appropriate nursing care.
3. Describe how health care beliefs, values, behaviors, medical and folk practices, and attitudes affect health-seeking behaviors of Filipino-American clients.
4. Identify how beliefs of Filipino Americans affect the internal locus of control and subsequently the environmental control variable.
5. Develop a culturally sensitive care plan for a Filipino-American client.

OVERVIEW OF THE PHILIPPINES

The Philippine Islands constitute an independent nation located in the Pacific Ocean approximately 450 miles off the southeastern coast of China. Taiwan is the nearest neighbor and is approximately 65 miles to the north; Indonesia is 150 miles to the south.

More than 7000 islands compose the Philippine Archipelago; however, the largest islands, Luzon (40,420 square miles) and Mindanao (36,537 square miles), account for 94% of the country's total land area. All the remaining islands are less than 6000 square miles in area. Most of the Philippine Islands are hilly and mountainous, with very little level land. The principal island, Luzon, has several mountains that run from the north to the south of the island. The range, known as the Sierra Madre, runs parallel with the northeastern coast combined with the central Cordillera to form the spine of the Philippines. The highest mountain is Mount Apo (6690 feet) on

Mindanao. The islands are of volcanic origin (Information Please Almanac, 1998).

The Philippine Islands enjoy warm, even temperatures throughout the year. The average monthly temperature in the Philippines ranges from 76° F to 84° F. Cooler temperatures are found at higher altitudes; however, temperatures below 60° F are a rare occurrence. Typhoons usually strike the Philippines at least once a year. The average rainfall for most of the islands is at least 60 inches of rain per year, with some areas receiving up to 125 inches of rain.

The population of the Philippines in 1997 was estimated at 76,103,564 with a birth rate of 28.97 live births per 1000 persons; an infant mortality of 35.2 per 1000 and a population density per square mile of 657 (Information Please Almanac, 1998). Most of the people in the Philippines are of Malaysian (that is, Austronesian) descent. However, people of Chinese, American, and Spanish origin are also native to

403

the Philippines. The population is unevenly distributed, with Luzon, Cebu, Negros, Bohol, Leyte, and Panay being the most heavily populated islands (Information Please Almanac, 1998).

The economy of the Philippines is based on agriculture. One of the principal crops is rice, which occupies about half the farmed land in the Philippines. Corn and coconut are also very important crops. Other crops of some significance include root crops, fruits, nuts, sugar cane, abaca, tobacco, ramie, kapok, and rubber. Although agriculture is the principal industry, the yields per crop per acre are among the lowest in Asia (Ennis & Inaba, 1977). Causes of low productivity of agriculture in the Philippines include poor farm management, inadequate use of fertilizers, poor seeds, and lack of incentive on the part of the farmers because many are tenant farmers (Ennis & Inaba, 1977). The lack of agricultural productivity has resulted in a variety of dietary deficiencies among the people including insufficient iron and vitamins (Cheong, Kuizon, & Tajaon, 1991; Solon, Solon, Mehansho, et al., 1996). The living environment also results in the prevalence of *Ascaris lumbricoides* worm populations in Filipino children both in urban and rural areas (Monzon, 1991). Approximately 46% of the labor force depends on agriculture for its livelihood. Fishing is also a major industry in the Philippines, with the number of persons engaged in fishing being second only to those in agriculture. Because fishing is a major industry, it provides one of the primary dietary mainstays, second only to rice. The rest of the work force is divided between service (18.5%) and industry and commerce (16%). Major products include textiles, pharmaceuticals, chemicals, food processing, and electronics assembly. Natural resources include forests, crude oil, and metallic and nonmetallic minerals. The gross domestic product (1995 estimate) is $179.7 billion with $2530 per capita. The unemployment rate is 9.5% (Information Please Almanac, 1998).

More than 40% of the country is covered by forest. Resources found in the forest include Philippine mahogany and pine. Minerals mined in the Philippines include gold, copper ore, and chromite. The country continues to lack adequate supplies of mineral fuels, though coal is mined on the islands of Cebu and Mindanao.

The Philippine Islands suffered enormous destruction during World War II (McKay, Hill, & Buckler, 1988). During the war the United States extended economic aid to the Philippines because it maintained large military bases on the islands. Following through on its promise to grant independence, which was made during the war, the United States granted independence to the Philippines in 1946. From 1946 to 1965 the Philippines pursued an American-style, two-party government. However, in 1965 President Ferdinand Marcos subverted the constitution and ruled as a lifetime dictator. Marcos abolished martial law in 1981 but retained most of his own power. From 1981 to 1986 there was a growing resistance to Marcos's rule. In 1986 Corazón Aquino, whose politically involved husband was assassinated, possibly by Marcos's supporters, won a spectacular electoral victory over Marcos and forced him to flee the country (McKay, Hill, & Buckler, 1988). In the year that followed, the Aquino government survived coup attempts by Marcos supporters. Negotiations on renewal of leases for United States military bases threatened to sour relations between the two countries. However, when volcanic eruptions from Mount Pinatubo severely damaged Clark Air Base in July 1991, the United States simply abandoned the base. In 1992 General Fidel Ramos, who had the support of outgoing Corazón Aquino, won the presidency, and the opposition gained control of Congress. In September the United States Navy turned over the Subic Bay naval base to the Philippines, ending a long U.S. military presence. Elections for both houses of Congress in May 1995 gave a resounding victory to candidates backed by the president and provided him with a fresh mandate for economic reforms. After protracted negotiations the Moro National Liberation Front agreed in 1996 to a government plan leading to more political autonomy in the south (Information Please Almanac, 1998).

IMMIGRATION TO THE UNITED STATES

Three different waves of Filipino immigrants have come to the United States: the first-wave, or pioneer, group, the second-wave group, and the third-wave, or new immigrant, group (Orque, 1983). Although "Philipino American" is the correct spelling because there is no *F* in the Philipino alphabet, "Filipino

American" is the accepted English spelling (Cantos & Rivera, 1996). The feminine form "Filipina" is acceptable usage though not appearing often.

First-wave immigrants

The first-wave, or pioneer, group is diverse particularly because of the diverse times of arrival of its members in the United States and their reasons for immigrating. The first-wave Filipino immigrants were originally drafted to work on trade ships that were traveling from China to the United States (Bartlett, 1977). From 1565 to 1815 hundreds of Filipinos escaped from the trading ships and went first to Mexico and finally to Louisiana and other regions throughout the United States. In 1907 with the passage of the gentleman's agreement that restricted Japanese immigration, Filipinos were recruited to work in Hawaii on sugar plantations (Daniels & Kitano, 1970; Lasker, 1969). Many of the first-wave Filipino immigrants worked on California farms or in Alaskan canneries, and still others worked as cooks or domestic helpers. From 1907 to 1930 Filipinos provided inexpensive and unskilled labor such as housekeepers, janitors, farmhands, and cooks. Most of the first-wave immigrants were men who came from the Ilocos region, though some did come from the Bisayan and Manila areas of the Philippines (Hart, 1981; Melendy, 1977). In 1934 the United States passed what was known as the Tydings-McDuffie Act, which held Filipino immigration to an annual quota of no more than 50 persons. This act established a Philippine commonwealth and changed the legal status of Filipinos from "nationals" to "aliens" in the United States. When Filipinos were labeled "nationals," they had the rights of citizenship except the rights to vote, own property, or marry. However, with the new alien status the technical rights of limited citizenship were abolished (Parreno, 1977).

Second-wave immigrants

The second wave of immigration began after the Philippine Islands won independence from the United States in 1946, when the annual quota was raised to 100 persons. Many Filipinos who served in the U.S. Armed Forces immigrated to the United States with their families after World War II. Lott (1976) noted that during this period many of the Filipino men were physically separated from their immediate kin and denied full participation in the larger American society. Therefore many of the second-wave group, particularly the men, relied on communal arrangements as their social group.

Third-wave immigrants

The new immigration group, or the third wave of immigrants, is composed of those Filipinos who have immigrated to the United States since 1965 as a result of the liberalization of the immigration quota. In 1974, Urban Associates, Inc., reported that in the 10-year period from 1960 to 1970, the Filipino population doubled, with 343,000 Filipinos residing in the United States. From 1965 to 1990 the population of Filipino Americans almost doubled again, and according to the 1998 census there were 1,450,512 Filipinos in the United States (Information Please Almanac, 1998). This number represented a 0.6% increase in the Filipino population since the 1980 census (U.S. Department of Commerce, Bureau of the Census, 1993a). Filipino Americans represented 20.6% of the total Asian-American population (U.S. Department of Commerce, Bureau of the Census, 1993b). By geographical location, 52.4% of Filipino Americans reside in the West, 27.0% reside in the Northeast, 8.1% in the Midwest, and 12.4% in the South (U.S. Department of Commerce, Bureau of the Census, 1993c). Today, in the United States, Filipino Americans constitute the third largest group of Asians and are outnumbered in terms of population only by Chinese Americans and Japanese Americans.

Of the number of Filipino Americans residing in this country before 1975, 21.7% were foreign born. Of the number residing in this country between 1975 and 1979, 11.1% were foreign born, and between 1980 and 1990, 31.6% were foreign born. Immigration has definitely contributed to the dramatic increase in the number of Filipino Americans residing in the United States (U.S. Department of Commerce, Bureau of the Census, 1993b).

The median age of Filipino-American people residing in the United States is 31.3 years, compared with 33 years for the general U.S. population. In addition, only 6% of all Asian Americans are 65 years of age or older, compared with 13% of the general

U.S. population (U.S. Department of Commerce, Bureau of the Census, 1993b).

Among Filipino Americans, third-wave immigrants appear to be better educated than members of the first and second waves; however, some of these people still experienced discrimination. In general, Filipino Americans are noted for high educational standards. In 1990, 84.2% of Filipino-American males and 81.4% of Filipino-American females 25 years of age or older held a high school diploma, and 36.2% of males and 41.6% of females held a bachelor's degree. (U.S. Department of Commerce, Bureau of the Census, 1993c).

Of the Filipino Americans residing in the United States, 75.4% participate in the work force, compared with Chinese Americans (65.9%) and Asian Indians (72.3%). The income level of Filipino Americans has not increased consistently with educational achievement. For example, although the per capita income for most Japanese Americans is $19,373, Filipino Americans have a per capita income of $13,616. The poverty rate for Filipino Americans is 6.4%, compared with 13.0% for the rest of general U.S. population (U.S. Department of Commerce, Bureau of the Census, 1993b). Takaki (1989) reports in *Strangers from a Different Shore* that for many Filipinos, though they toil in America, they still experience an "unfinished dream" with a society unwilling to embrace its own diversity.

COMMUNICATION
Dialect and language

One of the greatest difficulties that faced Filipinos during the 1960s was the task of forming a more integrated national community. This task was made even more difficult because of sociological diversity and because more than 93 dialects were spoken in the Philippines at the time (Voegelin & Voegelin, 1977). The boundary between "language" and "dialect" in the Philippines is blurred. The most common languages are Ilocano, Cebuano, Bicolano, Pampango, and Chabacano (Cantos & Rivera, 1996). Although 86% of Filipinos speak one of eight major languages as their mother tongue, the fact remains that many diverse languages and dialects are spoken across the country. Filipinos have long recognized

the problem with dialect and language, and in 1930 a policy was adopted by the government to develop a national language based on Tagálog. In addition to Tagalog, English and Spanish were also adopted as the official languages of the Philippines. However, adoption of a national language by the people was slow, and by 1960 only 44.5% of Filipinos spoke Tagalog, 39.5% spoke English, and 2% spoke Spanish (Corpuz, 1965). At that time more than 93 Filipino languages were being spoken in the country, with 86% of the total population speaking one of the eight major languages as their mother tongue (Melendy, 1977). Although the most widely used language today is Tagalog (Orque, 1983), 85% of young and middle-aged Filipinos speak English. Although Tagalog is the official national language, English appears to be the universal language of the Philippines. In fact, the Philippine Islands make up one of the largest English-speaking nations (Zabilka, 1967).

In the United States Filipino immigrants have been willing to undergo discomfort and cultural alienation with the hope that the children might improve the economic status of the people through education. However, one tragic flaw in this scheme is the language barrier encountered by the children in the public school systems in the United States (Melendy, 1977). Even today, the public schools are not able to cope with the problem of bilingual education in languages other than Spanish and English.

Style

Shimamoto (1977) noted that the elderly Filipino man is generally concrete in thinking and pragmatic in problem solving. Shimamoto also noted that when a Filipino man acknowledges emotions in an oral manner this may be interpreted as a sign of unmanliness or weakness.

Tone

Filipino Americans tend to use tone of voice to emote or to romanticize the language (Cantos & Rivera, 1996). An individual may get loud in the presence of a group of family members or may get agitated or emotional when nervous or frightened. Typically however, Filipinos are soft spoken and will say nothing rather than disagree.

Context

There is a tendency for Filipinos to avoid direct expression of disagreement. This protects them from losing face or respect. For example, it was noted in a regional psychiatric hospital that a Filipino male physician, who was a family practitioner, would not disagree directly with a female psychiatrist. In areas of disagreement, the physician would communicate information to the psychiatrist by telling the nursing staff to relay the message (Davidhizar, 1997). In this scenario the difficulties were encountered because Filipinos are a polite people who do not like to disagree, particularly with people in authority, and because some Filipino men experience discomfort with women as authority figures.

Some Filipino people experience difficulties when discussing topics that are considered personal, including sex, tuberculosis, and socioeconomic status. The issues of sex and sex education are considered so sensitive that Filipino parents generally do not openly or deliberately discuss them with their children (Guthrie & Jacobs, 1976). Because tuberculosis is a dreaded and feared disease among Filipino people (in the Philippines the morbidity and mortality for this disease remain high as a result of unsanitary living conditions), discussion about tuberculosis may also be avoided by some Filipino people (Hooper, 1958; Orque, 1983; Wooley, 1972).

Some Filipinos have an expressed need for modesty, privacy, and confidentiality. Therefore, it is often difficult for the nurse to begin interventions immediately without a period of "small talk," which includes topics considered safe conversation, such as the weather, the condition of family members, or sports events. It is also important for the nurse to remember that Filipino-American clients may be hesitant to express feelings and emotions in a group setting. Filipinos are sensitive to the concept of shame or saving face. It may be only out of strong respect for the health care professional that personal information that is needed to plan adequately for health care will be disclosed (Orque, 1983).

Kinesics

Nonverbal language is important for Filipino persons. For example, direct eye contact in the Filipino culture between an older man and a younger woman may be indicative of either seduction or anger. Little eye contact is likely to be used with superiors and authority figures. Another situation in which a nurse may encounter nonverbal communication on the part of a Filipino-American client is in a group setting. Because some Filipino people fear losing face in public situations, the Filipino-American client may be very hesitant to express personal feelings in a group setting and may resort to remaining silent. It is important to assess the meaning of silence and to determine if it means approval or not.

Filipinos tend to be very polite and therefore tend to behave agreeably even to the extent of personal inconvenience (Cantos & Rivera, 1996). The term for this form of agreement is *pakikisama*, which means 'getting along with others at all costs'. Some Filipino nurses have difficulty giving commands to staff but rather prefer to request politely that they do an assignment. Another trait for which some Filipinos are known is *amor propio*, which is actually a Spanish term adapted to the Filipino language, meaning 'self-esteem'. Therefore, when a Filipino's *amor propio* is wounded, there is a tendency to preserve personal dignity by silence or aloofness to demonstrate self-pride. Filipinos will tend to agree even when they mistrust the physician or nurse because they do not want to risk hurting the other person's feelings. Therefore for some Filipinos a hesitant "yes" could be indicative of a positive "no" because they wish to avoid a direct, blunt "no." In the Filipino language there are hierarchical terms for "yes" and "no." The term used depends on whether one is speaking to a person of lower, equal, or superior status. When uncertain as to the status of the person with whom they are conversing, some Filipino Americans will use a silent nod to avoid giving possible offense. Also, a Filipino-American client will commonly address a physician or nurse as "Doctor" or "Mrs."; however, if the name is unknown, this same individual may only nod (DeGracia, 1979).

Touching is not uncommon, though handshakes are not commonly practiced by Filipino Americans. Elderly people are shown respect by kissing hand, forehead, or cheeks (Wilson & Billones, 1994).

Implications for nursing care

It is important for the nurse to remember that a large majority of first-wave Filipino immigrants came to this country with little or no education and may have extreme difficulty comprehending English, especially English spoken in medical jargon. Therefore the nurse should use interpretive aids such as pictures and interpreters. It is also important for the nurse to remember that if an interpreter is used the interpreter should speak the same language as well as the same dialect as the client. The nurse should be aware that many Filipinos use a nonverbal response such as a smile or a raised eyebrow as an acknowledgment to what has been said rather than giving a verbal response (Espíritu, 1995). Therefore it is important to watch the Filipino client when speaking rather than waiting for a verbal response.

Regardless of immigration-wave status, the Filipino-American client may view the nurse as an authority figure and therefore may relate to the nurse with formality and modesty. Because gender and age differences also have particular significance in the Filipino culture, it would be wise for the nurse to consider both gender and age when communicating with the client. For example because an elderly person is highly revered in the Filipino culture, it would be inappropriate as well as disrespectful for the nurse to address the elderly Filipino-American client by first name. The nurse might try using such Tagalog designations as *"opo"* or *"oho,"* which are used to show respect and honor to the person being addressed (Orque, 1983). The Tagalog designation *"po"* should be inserted when an elderly Filipino American is addressed because it conveys respect and is similar to designations in the English language such as "madam" or "sir" (Guthrie & Jacobs, 1976).

It is important for the nurse to remember that direct eye contact for Filipinos has various connotations. A young female nurse who is assigned to an elderly Filipino-American male client may encounter difficulties when communicating with this client because the client may remain aloof and reserved and may avoid eye contact altogether (Bush & Babich, 1978).

Because Filipino men, regardless of age, have great difficulty verbally acknowledging emotions,

Shimamoto (1977) recommended that the nurse assume an authority-figure role during the development of the nurse-client relationship. Because of the Filipino trait of deference toward authority figures, Filipino-American men, regardless of age, are likely to respect the nurse's position and to listen and adhere to the nurse's suggestions because of the position. It is important for the nurse to appear knowledgeable and competent when communicating with a Filipino-American client and to avoid talking down to the client. It is also important for the nurse to remember that because some Filipino men experience discomfort with women as authority figures, difficulties may arise even in nurse-physician relationships. For example, when a female nurse is communicating with a Filipino-American male doctor, the nurse should use sensitivity in offering suggestions or criticism. Some Filipino Americans encounter difficulties in group settings, particularly in situations where both men and women are present. Therefore, one-on-one encounters may be best, so that the client or professional with whom the nurse is talking feels free to express true feelings and emotions (Orque, 1983).

Because Filipino-American clients tend to be modest, it is important to offer female clients not only a gown but also a robe. Male clients should be offered pants as well as a gown (Cantos & Rivera, 1996).

SPACE

Some Filipino Americans tend to collapse their space inward and to limit the amount of personal space available. This is caused in part by the Filipinos' strong feeling for family. On immigration to the United States the personal space of Filipino Americans also collapsed inward because some of the people lived in urban ghettos, "little Manilas," that were vastly overpopulated (Burma, 1954).

Implications for nursing care

Filipino Americans are perceived as a family-oriented cultural group. Therefore it is not uncommon for a Filipino client to have the entire family, which includes nuclear and extended family members, hovering at the bedside. Even an adult who is unmarried with no relatives in the vicinity is likely to have a number of Filipino-American visitors because they are sensitive to the loneliness that illness can provoke. The astute nurse will use family members to the advantage of the client. Rather than viewing their presence as an overcrowding of space in the hospital for both the health care professionals and the client, the nurse should capitalize on these customs and traditions by involving family members in educational training programs that will assist the client in returning to an optimal level of functioning. In addition, it is important to solicit family and client input to develop shared goals.

It is also important for the nurse to remember that Filipino Americans are familiar with a limited personal space because it is always shared with other family members. Therefore the space provided in a hospital setting may appear to be overextended, thus necessitating the need for the client to collapse personal space inward even more so. While hospitalized, Filipino Americans may be reluctant to venture out of the personal space that is allocated and may be reluctant to leave their room for any reason (DeGracia, 1979).

SOCIAL ORGANIZATION
Family

Most of the first-wave immigrants who came to the United States were not allowed to immigrate with their wives. This immigration pattern was responsible for a disproportionate ratio of males to females. The male-to-female ratio in 1930 for Filipinos residing in the United States was 14 to 1, compared with 1.1 to 1 for the rest of the population (Melendy, 1977). Lott (1976) noted that because Filipino men were separated from their families, they tended to rely on communal arrangements with other Filipino immigrants who often came from the same island in the Philippines. Most of the first-wave immigrants had little or no education and because of discriminatory practices that existed throughout the United States did not receive more education or a better job.

After World War II, when the immigration policies became more relaxed in the United States, more Filipino women began to enter the country and a more normal family pattern followed. Despite the fact that more women were able to immigrate during the second and third waves, it has been noted that the age of Filipino-American husbands continues to exceed that of their wives. Because of this disproportionate age, many young Filipino-American women have been widowed early, thus leading to the establishment of the Filipino matriarchal system. In 1974 a total of 69% of Filipino-American families were matriarchal with young children and at least 23% of all Filipino-American families were extended (Urban Associates, 1974). Wagner (1973) noted that the ratio of extended families to nuclear families was at least twice that of the rest of the U.S. population. Today, however, married couples represent approximately 83.6% of all Filipino-American households, whereas female-headed households (matriarchal) make up only 11.8% of Filipino-American families (U.S. Department of Commerce, Bureau of the Census, 1993c).

In 1974, 38% of all Filipino-American families had five or more members (Urban Associates, 1974). Today, this number is decreasing somewhat, and the average Filipino-American family has 4.0 persons, compared with the national average of 3.2 (U.S. Department of Commerce, Bureau of the Census, 1993c). Pollard (1995) studied ethnic groups in relation to twinning rates in California. Numbers of Filipino twins were similar to that of Chinese and Japanese but higher than that of Koreans, Thai, and Vietnamese, an indication that twinning rates are modified by both migration and interethnic mixing.

Although the number of matrifocal families has decreased, the matriarchal system remains an integral part of Filipino cultural values. The matriarchal system may be the reason that the family has taken on paramount importance for Filipino Americans. This is evidenced even during times of illness. When a member of a Filipino-American family becomes ill, family members often keep a bedside vigil and participate in client care. Burr and Mutchler (1993) noted that Filipino-born women who are less acculturated are more likely than women from some other ethnic groups to move in with others who are more acculturated.

Family systems and the relationship to culture
The Filipino culture is a blend of various heritages, though there are some basic traits that most Filipino people manifest. Individualization is a key to understanding the Filipino culture and an individual of Filipino descent. As a result of the Chinese influence on family solidarity, Filipinos on the Philippine islands tend to socialize with people from the same region. This same clannishness is evident in the United States among the many organizations in the Filipino communities. Persons in the younger generations may have values that are in direct opposition to the traditional values held by older persons. In the Philippine Islands today, many youths resemble their Western counterparts, particularly in areas of social values, dress, and music (DeGracia, 1979). Although these same similarities exist among adolescents in the mainstream United States and Filipino-American adolescents, many Filipino-American youths still observe such traditional values as respect for elders, love of family, and preservation of self-esteem.

In the Filipino culture there is a strong feeling for family, which is a result of the Chinese influence. Today, these strong feelings for family continue and may be manifested by old-fashioned patterns imposed by the family patriarch or the equally authoritarian matriarch. The Filipino child is taught always to give deference to an elder and never to question the decision of an elder. In return for such obedience, the Filipino child receives solicitous protection from elders. In the absence of both parents, the eldest Filipino child becomes the ruling authority and must be obeyed. A study by Lantican and Corona (1989) comparing Mexican-American primigravidas in El Paso, Texas, with Filipino primigravidas in Manila found that both groups had adequate social support. The network size for the Filipinos was 5.74, compared with 5.78 for the Mexican Americans. In the case of 78% of the Filipinos studied, immediate family members provided the most support. Filipinos also reported that sisters were most likely to be the first to receive information about the pregnancy, with husbands listed third. This was in contrast to the Mexican Americans studied, who reported discussing the pregnancy first with their husbands. Lantican and Corona (1989) also noted that both

Mexican-American and Filipino-American women used their family as a major source of support during pregnancy.

Religion
Filipinos are predominantly Roman Catholic, which has been attributed to the influence of the Spanish missionaries in the Philippines as early as 1520. In 1965 82.9% of the Filipino population was Roman Catholic, 7.6% was Aglipayan, 4.1% was Muslim, 2.3% was Protestant, 0.5% was Iglesia ni Kristo, 0.2% were Buddhist, 0.5% were other religions, and 1.8% had no religion (Zabilka, 1967). By 1998 some 84% of the Filipino population were Roman Catholic, 10% are Protestant, 5% were Muslim, and 3% were Buddhist or other (Information Please Almanac, 1998).

Birth rituals
Filipino mothers are encouraged to eat well and to get plenty of sleep at night. In the last few months of pregnancy she is discouraged from staying in a dependent position such as sitting or sleeping during the day for fear of water retention. Sexual intercourse during the last 2 months of pregnancy is considered taboo. Eating prunes, sweet foods, or squid are also considered taboo for a pregnant woman (White, Linhart, & Medley, 1996; Kittler & Sucher, 1989). It is believed that such foods will respectively make the baby wrinkled, lead to a large baby and difficult delivery, and tangle the baby's cord inside the mother. If a physician is not available, a midwife may be called on to assist in the delivery. Fathers are usually not present but rather are with male friends for support while their wives deliver. A pregnant Filipino woman may walk around the room to promote dilatation. Most Filipino women will moan or grunt during labor. Others may become loud and almost hysterical (Weber, 1996). Traditionally it was an expectation of all Filipino mothers to breast-feed. This tradition is changing. In a study by Adair and Popkin (1976) Filipino women who ceased breast-feeding early or did not breast-feed were studied. It was found that a low birth weight reduced the likelihood of breast-feeding. This is significant because there are already high risks related to low birth weight and proved benefits of breast-feeding. Thus,

these researchers noted that special emphasis should be given by nurses to promoting breast-feeding. For example, a working mother may have the baby fed formula while she is at work or may have breast milk left for the baby. Traditionally male circumcision was not done at birth. Today it is more common for a male baby to be circumcised before discharge from the hospital.

Death practices

If a client has a diagnosis of terminal disease, the client should not be told without consulting the family. The family will usually want to disclose the prognosis to the client. The family will usually want the Catholic chaplain to give the Sacrament of the Sick. When a Filipino client is given a terminal diagnosis, most will prefer to die at home with dignity. A decision to not resuscitate is usually a very difficult decision and will be decided by the entire family. Death is given very high regard by Filipino Americans. Death is a spiritual event, and the client and family may ask for religious medallions, rosary beads, and other objects of spiritual significance to be near the client. The family may pray at the bedside of a dying family member. If a client dies in a hospital room, the family members will usually want to say good-bye before having the body taken out of the room and may want to wash the body. Most Filipinos will not allow organ donation and do not practice cremation (Wilson & Billones, 1994).

Implications for nursing care

In the Philippine Islands the family unit is the basic unit of social organization. Several generations of Filipinos are linked by descent and marriage. For some Filipinos, family relationships are so important that many of the kinfolk live under the same roof or as close to each other as possible. Furthermore, membership in a family union is perceived by some Filipinos as being more important than membership in a trade union (Caringer, 1977). Therefore many nursing implications are based on family structure and organization. Because Filipino-American clients are very family oriented, the nurse must remember that these clients may always have their families hovering about them. The sick Filipino child may feel lost without the mother constantly at the bedside, and when grandparents are ill, the entire family may keep vigil at the bedside out of respect for the elderly. Whenever it is possible, the nurse should arrange for family members to stay at the client's bedside during a hospital stay. Family members will want to bring food from home that is soothing for the body, such as rice soup, and in most cases clients will expect that this will occur.

It is important for the nurse to remember that the family structure of first-wave and second-wave immigrants may be significantly different from that of third-wave immigrants in that more matriarchal family structures may be found in the earlier generations. Thus the varying family structures may present the need for unique and varying approaches to health care needs. Another implication for nursing care is associated with the fact that some first-wave and second-wave immigrants have a limited education compared with third-wave immigrants, who were better educated when they came to this country. When a Filipino-American client from the first-wave or second-wave group is hospitalized, it is important that the nurse not only involve families but also recognize the need to modify educational approaches to the family's and client's level of understanding.

TIME

Filipino Americans appear to have both a past- and a present-time orientation. According to Kluckhohn and Strodtbeck (1961), human nature has a postulated range of variations, including evil, good and evil, and good. People react to these value orientations by virtue of a time frame of reference. For example, past-oriented people view human nature as being basically evil, and so control and discipline of the self are continuously required if any real good is to be achieved. On the other hand, present-oriented people view human nature as a mixture of good and evil, and so although control and effort are needed, lapses in control and effort can be understood and need not always be severely condemned. For some Filipino Americans there is a prevailing attitude that one should unquestionably accept what life and death bring because, regardless of human effort, supernatural forces are mitigating and control the world. It is this attitude that influences some Filipino Americans' time orientation.

Because Filipino Americans are both past and present oriented, they distinguish between social and business time. They tend not to become too aggravated when social functions do not start on time, and so they operate on "Filipino time." This trait results in part from their past orientation, which values human relationships and human nature over current events. However, Filipino Americans do equate success in business in Western society with a prompt observation of business time, which is perceived as being both present and future oriented (Orque, 1983). Nevertheless, for some Filipino Americans there is a prevailing attitude that time and providence will solve all (Corpuz, 1965).

Implications for nursing care

Because Filipino Americans are both past and present oriented, it is important for the nurse to remember that often a Filipino-American client may ignore health-related issues, preferring to leave these things in the hands of God *(bahala na)*. Some Filipino Americans may use the term *talaga*, which means 'destined' or 'inevitable'. When some Filipino Americans are ill, past-time orientation become obvious because of a tendency to attribute conditions to the will of God and to cope with illness by praying and hoping that whatever God's will is, it is best for the individual.

Because of their past-time orientation, there is a tendency among some Filipino Americans toward noncompliance regarding medical regimens. In addition, these same individuals may not adhere to appointments or scheduled deadlines for health-related matters.

ENVIRONMENTAL CONTROL

As indicated, Filipino Americans are perceived as being both past and present oriented and have a tendency to believe that events, particularly illnesses, are related to supernatural forces. As a result of this belief, some Filipino Americans have a value orientation that is perceived as fatalistic. Thus some Filipino Americans have an external locus of control

that is evidenced by a belief in supernatural forces and by the methods of treatment of illness.

Folk medicine

Filipinos and Filipino Americans support at least two, often competing, medical systems. A Filipino individual who becomes ill might consult both a folk healer and a Western-trained physician. Filipino Americans are like other ethnic groups in that they continue to practice folk medicine simply because it works (McKenzie & Chrisman, 1977). In some situations folk remedies may be the only treatments available for Filipino Americans, whereas in other situations some Filipino Americans will combine folk remedies with the therapy prescribed by Western health professionals. It is important for the nurse to remember that folk beliefs are an important part of some Filipino Americans' lives and therefore may significantly influence health practices.

Folk medicine has enjoyed a long history; in fact, folk medicine is believed to be older than contemporary scientific medicine. Some anthropologists believe that folk beliefs have persisted through the generations because they are so closely interwoven with other aspects of culture. Moreover, the therapeutic value of many of the health practices has been verified scientifically (McKenzie & Chrisman, 1977). The Filipino folk medicine system is based primarily on the Malaysian culture but may also be based on the Bisayan culture. The Filipino culture has been influenced by Indian, Chinese, Arabian, Spanish, Mexican, and American belief systems. It is believed that many of the elements of the health practices found in the Philippines may actually have been borrowed from these cultures.

In the Filipino culture, certain illnesses may be assigned to natural causes such as overeating, poor diet, or excessive drinking. These illnesses would normally be treated with home remedies, including such things as herbal preparations, decoctions, massage, sleep, and exercise.

Illnesses are believed to be caused by supernatural agents. Some Filipino people associate disease with the total life situation, with the result that disease can have both natural and supernatural causes. Some Filipinos believe that there are invisible spirits that replicate the life of the individual and possess supernatural powers that are generally denied to most humans (Hart, 1966; McNall, 1989).

Individuals who subscribe to supernatural causes of disease may feel protected from harmful supernatural influences by such things as talismans, amulets, prayer, and seeking advice from a folk healer. Sickness and death are believed by some Filipinos to be the result of actions of angry ancestral spirits or witches, evil eyes, or the lethal bite or power of a supernatural animal. In such cases, if the client does not recover or if the illness worsens, the client will generally seek the advice of various folk medicine specialists. The client may also seek the advice of a conventional medical practitioner if resources are available. In the Philippine Islands it is not uncommon for a physician to incorporate certain aspects of the folk medicine belief system, such as the theory of hot and cold, when implementing the treatment plan (Hart, Rajadhon, & Coughlin, 1965).

A variety of folk medicine healers exists in the Filipino culture, including shamans and curers. A shaman is a priest or priestess who practices folk remedies. A curer diagnoses illness by palpating the pulse. Many Filipino curers believe that the pulse is the best place to detect an illness because the pulse is an outlet, or a substation, of the heart. They believe that, if the pulse lies, the heart lies (Lieban, 1967). An ill person's pulse may be either "hot" or "cold," depending on the type of illness. Some Filipinos believe that a healthy person has a balance regarding hot and cold air elements in the body. However, it is believed that, if the body becomes too hot or subsequently too cold, the circulation of the blood will be increased or decreased and the person will experience a loss of appetite and fatigue that will ultimately lower the body's natural defenses against the illness. It is believed by some Filipinos that both metaphysical and real hot and cold temperatures will cause an illness if absorbed by the body in excessive amounts.

Many Filipino individuals also believe in the theory of the four humors. The body humors include phlegm or mucus, air or vapors, bile, and blood. Filipinos who subscribe to this theory accept one overriding theme that involves health in relationship to air or wind (*mal aire*). For these Filipinos there are two ways in which one can become ill. One way is related to air and includes exposure to a normal draft or breeze that results in an illness such as a cold. The other way is by absorbing excessive amounts of hot or cold air, which ultimately will cause an imbalance of these principles in the body. A Filipino mother may wrap the navel of her baby with a cloth to prevent air from entering the body through the navel cord. Some Filipinos use coconut oil to soak or rub the skin in order to prevent wind from entering the pores. Some Filipinos believe that air circulates in the veins and, if hot air is absorbed through the pores, it will be carried to the brain by the blood, resulting in mental illness (Hart, 1981). Another *mal aire* illness includes the means by which the spirits penetrate the body by magically propelling thorns, pebbles, bones, and other foreign objects into the body.

Illness and wellness behaviors

Three concepts underlie Filipino health beliefs and practices: flushing, heating, and protection. Flushing is believed to keep the body free from debris; heating is believed to maintain a balanced internal temperature; and protection is believed to guard the body from outside influences. Flushing is based on the premise that if the body is a container it can collect impurities. Heating involves the belief that hot and cold qualities must be in balance in the body. Protection involves safeguarding the natural boundaries of the body from supernatural as well as natural forces. Among Filipinos who subscribe to the theory of flushing, there is a complex system of beliefs based on the theory that flushing is a complex system of stimulating perspiration, vomiting, flatulence, or menstrual bleeding for the sole purpose of removing evil forces from the body. A common home remedy used to promote flushing is vinegar. Vinegar may be used to flush the body to cure an ailment such as a fever or a chest cold. In such cases the vinegar is mixed with items such as water, salt, or hot pepper. Drinking this mixture will stimulate perspiration and subsequently remove all the evil or bad things from the body. It must be remembered that such practices are not all that unorthodox when compared with the Western medical system (McKenzie & Chrisman, 1977).

Because Filipinos are deeply religious and a God-fearing people, they believe that many diseases and illnesses are the will of God. When a Filipino client is given a poor prognosis, the client may continue to hope for a cure despite the severity of the problem. This attitude may help to explain why some Filipino clients are uncomplaining and frequently suffer in silence.

Implications for nursing care

It is important for the nurse to remember that Filipino folk-related health practices may be beneficial, neutral, or harmful. Folk practices that are beneficial or neutral should be incorporated into the plan of care. However, the nurse should develop educational training programs that will help the client and family to identify and eliminate folk practices that are harmful.

Some Filipino Americans have an external locus of control that is based on the belief that illness may be caused by external forces, which may be either natural or supernatural. Therefore it is important for the nurse to remember that the client's noncompliance with medical regimens may be based on a fatalism-based system. It is important for the nurse to ascertain whether the client's noncompliance is based on fatalistic beliefs or a lack of understanding.

The nurse should be aware that many Filipino Americans relate health to food. For example, eating healthful food such as vegetables, meat, chicken, and fruits are related to maintaining health. Eating pigeon soup is related to protecting health or preventing illness. Eating chicken soup is related to restoring health. In addition some Filipino Americans believe actions taken relate to health. For example, praying relates to maintaining health. Soaking one's feet in salted water after working in the fields and avoiding too much sun or rain protect health and prevent illness. Taking herbal medicines and special home remedies such as pounding ginger with coconut oil and massaging painful joints are remedies that will restore health. Another home remedy is toasting uncooked rice until brown, adding water, and drinking the resulting mix for stomachache. Wounds may be treated by boiling guava leaves and drinking the fluid (Spector, 1996).

BIOLOGICAL VARIATIONS
Body size and structure

In the United States prematurity is defined as a birth weight of less than 2500 g (5 pounds, 8 ounces). When controls for income, maternal age, parity, and smoking were done, Filipino Americans tended to have a lower mean birth weight than their White counterparts have (Morton, 1977). Morton suggested that the birth-weight requirement for maturity should be lowered for some ethnic groups, including Filipino Americans, and recommended that prematurity be redefined as less than 2200 g (4 pounds, 14 ounces) for Filipino Americans and Blacks.

Filipinos are short and tend to have very small frames. Some Filipinos have short limbs in comparison with the trunk size. At 3 years of age the mean standing height is 85.7 cm (33.7 inches) for Filipino boys and 84.8 cm (33.4 inches) for Filipino girls. Thus Filipino children are considerably shorter than White children, in whom the mean standing height is 95 cm (37.4 inches) for boys and 93.9 cm (37 inches) for girls (Meredith, 1978). However, the average height and weight of Filipinos is quite similar to that of Thais and Vietnamese persons. Filipinos tend to lag behind Japanese persons in both height and weight. The height of Japanese boys and girls from birth to 1 year of age exceeds the height of Filipinos (Matawaran et al., 1966). It is believed, however, that Filipinos overcome this difference by 21 years of age and that their growth increments are quite similar to those of Japanese persons.

In a classic 1958 study, José and Salcedo observed that Filipino American women tended to be leaner and slimmer than their White counterparts. Anchacosa-Angala and Márquez-Sumabat (1964) noted that body weight for Filipino Americans increased significantly when an increase in skin-fold thickness occurred. Based on data, they concluded that skin-fold thickness could be used as an index of leanness and fatness for Filipino Americans.

Kusumoto, Suzuki, Kumakura, and Ashizawa (1996) compared foot morphology between Filipino and Japanese women and found that Filipino women showed pronounced deformity of the great toe laterally, "like a hallux valgus," without any complaints (p. 373). A pathological deformity of the hallux valgus appears to be related to the Filipino genetic structure.

Skin color

Mongolian spots are commonly found at birth on Filipino infants. Normal pigmentation among Filipinos ranges from brown to peach brown, and it is extremely difficult to detect conditions such as cyanosis in darker-pigmented skin. In addition, some darker-skinned Filipinos may also have heavy deposits of subconjunctival fat, which contains high levels of carotene in sufficient quantities to mimic conditions similar to jaundice. If the nurse is to distinguish between carotenemia and jaundice, it is necessary for the nurse to inspect the posterior portions of the hard palate of the client in an extremely good light or in bright daylight (Roach, 1977).

Other visible physical characteristics

Filipinos are classified as members of the Mongoloid race because of very common racial characteristics, including the brown skin color, almond-shaped inner eye folds, and extremely sparse body hair, particularly in men, in whom chest hair is often absent. Hair on the head is typically coarse but also tends to be either straight or wavy (Garn, 1965). In addition, male pattern baldness appears to be a rarity among Filipino Americans (Garn, 1965).

Chung and Kau (1985) noted that the tendency for cleft lip or cleft palate was highest for the Japanese, Chinese, and Filipinos, compared with Whites and Hawaiians. These researchers also noted that the high-risk groups had smaller dimensions than Whites and Hawaiians in regard to cranial-base measurement, facial height, palatal length, and mandibular length, which might be contributing factors to the higher incidence of cleft lip and cleft palate.

Enzymatic and genetic variations

Motulsky, Stransky, and Fraser (1964) found a high prevalence of glucose-6-phosphate dehydrogenase (G-6-PD) deficiency among Filipinos. It would appear that G-6-PD deficiency affects Filipinos as severely and as quantitatively as it affects persons found in the Mediterranean group. In addition, alpha-thalassemia, a form of which is known as he-moglobin H disease, is prevalent in Filipinos, Chinese persons, Thais, and Greeks (Wallerstein, 1976).

Susceptibility to disease

Cardiovascular disease Heart disease remains the leading cause of death in the United States. In this category are coronary artery and hypertensive heart diseases. Both of these diseases vary in frequency by racial group. Weisse, Abiuso, and Thind (1977) and Gordon (1976) noted that Whites and Blacks in the United States have similar age-adjusted mortalities for coronary artery disease. Gerber (1980) noted that White mortalities for coronary artery disease are higher than those of either Japanese Americans or Filipino Americans. Gerber's study also suggested that mortalities for coronary artery disease are higher in urban areas than in rural areas and that differences in mortality noted among races are probably not attributable to genetic factors but to environmental ones. This conclusion was based on the fact that when Japanese Americans or Filipino Americans moved from rural to urban areas the mortality for coronary artery disease rose, which was believed to be directly related to changes in life-style, diet, and work patterns.

Other research studies have demonstrated a connection between a high rate of coronary artery disease and sedentary life-styles. Some researchers believe that a sedentary life-style increases total cholesterol blood levels, particularly low-density lipoproteins. These conditions are believed to be conducive to coronary artery disease across races (Clarkson, Hintermister, Fillyaw, & Stylos, 1981; Hartung, Foreyt, Mitchell, et al., 1980; Anderson, 1983).

Frerichs, Chapman, and Maes (1984) conducted a study of mortalities of seven ethnic groups in Los Angeles County during 1980. The study found that, for all causes of death, age- and sex-adjusted rates were highest among Blacks, intermediate among Whites and Hispanics, and substantially lower among Asians and Pacific Islanders. The study also found that for cerebrovascular diseases the mortality among Blacks was again the highest, with Whites and Japanese being intermediate and Hispanics, Filipinos, Chinese, and Koreans being the lowest.

Gerber (1983) noted that the life expectancy at birth for both males and females is greatest for Japanese persons, followed by Filipinos and then Whites. The findings of this study are suggestive that Filipino Americans would benefit more from the elimination of variables, stressors, or both, that predispose them to coronary heart disease and cerebrovascular accidents than other ethnic groups would, with exclusion of Japanese persons because of this higher predicted life expectancy at birth.

Hypertension Stavig, Igra, and Leonard (1988) found that the prevalence of controlled and uncontrolled hypertension in the United States is lower for persons of Asian descent, except for Filipinos. In fact, the California Department of Health Services hypertension study found that Filipino Americans have one of the highest prevalences for hypertension, second only to Blacks (Requiro, 1981). The analysis of the data from the study by Stavig, Igra, and Leonard (1988) indicated that Asians and Pacific Islanders with hypertension are less likely to be aware of the condition, to seek treatment or take medication for the condition, or to control the condition through diet. In addition, these ethnic groups recorded lower frequencies of hospital stays for the condition, fewer days of bed disability, and fewer days of not feeling well as a result of hypertension than all other ethnic groups. The study concluded that because of their high levels of poverty and lack of education and the relationship of these factors to health-seeking behavior for hypertension, additional study is needed to help improve health care for Filipino Americans.

Klatsky and Armstrong (1991) reported a study in which 4211 Filipino men and women were compared with Japanese, Chinese, and other Asians for incidence of hypertension. This study noted that the Filipino men and women had the highest rate of hypertension of any of the groups.

Young, Lichton, Hamilton, et al. (1987) noted a high positive relationship between sodium intake and the prevalence of hypertensive disease. This study examined the relationship between ethnicity and blood pressure in young adults of six ethnic groups residing in Hawaii. The findings suggested that body weights and heights of Whites and Hawaiians tended to exceed those of Chinese, Filipinos, Japanese, and Koreans. The study noted that both systolic and diastolic pressures were significantly higher in men than in women across all races. The study also found no significant differences between sexes or across races regarding urinary excretion of sodium and potassium.

Stavig, Igra, Leonard, et al. (1986) conducted a study to determine the death rates in California for hypertension-related diseases for the periods 1969 to 1971 and 1979 to 1981. The data indicated that, during both periods, age-standardized rates for composite hypertension-related mortality were highest for Blacks, followed by Whites, and lowest for Asians and Pacific Islanders. Filipinos, who were noted to have high prevalence rates of hypertension, tended to have a lower rate of hypertension-related mortality. Findings from this study are suggestive that the possible reasons for the decline in hypertension-related mortality may include population awareness, level of treatment, control of hypertension, knowledge of cardiovascular risk factors, improved medical technology, and modification of behavior. A study by Klatsky and Armstrong (1991) also found that Filipino men and women had the highest prevalence of hypertension when Chinese, Japanese, other Asians, and Filipinos were studied.

Diabetes mellitus There is an increased incidence of diabetes mellitus among Filipino Americans. Sloan (1963) concluded that diabetes mellitus occurs three times more often among Filipino Americans than it does among White Americans.

Cancer Kolonel (1985) conducted a study comparing the cancer-incidence rates for Filipinos in Hawaii. The significant increases in the incidence of thyroid cancer among Filipino women in Hawaii caused this group to have the highest incidence of thyroid cancer among all ethnic groups in Hawaii. In addition, the data indicated a lack of increase in female breast cancer rates among Filipinos in Hawaii and a lower than expected increase in colon cancer rates. In contrast to this study, Goodman, Yoshizawa, and Kolonel (1988) noted that the incidence rates for thyroid cancer remained relatively stable from 1960 to 1984. However, this study also concluded that, when Filipinos in Hawaii were compared with other ethnic groups in Hawaii, Filipinos were found to have the highest reported incidence rates for thyroid cancer. The conclusion of this study was that environmental influences may be responsible for the unusually high rate of thyroid cancer among Filipinos in Hawaii.

Young, Ries, and Pollach (1984) found that the rates of gallbladder and urinary bladder cancer for women exceeded those for men among the Filipino population. The primary site of cancer having the highest survival rate for both Filipino men and women was found to be the thyroid gland. The 5-year relative survival rate for cancer of the thyroid gland was 91%, whereas the survival rate for other primary sites of cancer, including the esophagus and the pancreas, were found to be uniformly low. Rosenblatt, Weiss, and Schwartz (1996) compared the incidence of primary liver cancer among ethnic groups and found Filipino males born in the United States to be 6.5 per 100,000 compared to Whites with 3.4 per 100,000 and Filipino women none per 100,000 compared to 1.1 for Whites. The incidence of liver cancer was lower for Filipinos born in the United States than those born in the Philippines.

Gallbladder disease Yamase and McNamara (1977) examined the hospital-admission rates for gallbladder disease in Chinese, Japanese, Koreans, Filipinos, Hawaiians, Portuguese, Puerto Ricans, and Whites. This study found that although differences in admission rates among races were statistically significant they were not clinically significant.

Amyotrophic lateral sclerosis Studies have indicated that there is a prevalence for amyotrophic lateral sclerosis among Filipino Hawaiians that exceeds that found among Whites and Japanese Hawaiians (Matsumoto, Worth, Kurland, & Okazaki, 1972). However, the findings from other studies are suggestive that the excess in regard to amyotrophic lateral sclerosis found among Filipinos in Hawaii is more or less a function of population and age distribution rather than a true racial or ethnic difference (Kurtzke, 1982).

Palatal mucosal changes The habit of reverse smoking is practiced in various parts of the world including the Philippines (Ortiz, Pierce, & Wilson, 1996). In a study of reverse smokers compared to conventional smokers in Cabanatuan City in the Philippines it was found that 96.7% of reverse smokers exhibited palatal mucosal changes including leukoplakia, mucosal thickening, fissuring, pigmentation, nodularity, erythema, and ulceration, compared to only 26.7% of conventional smokers (Mercado-Ortiz, Wilson, & Jiang, 1996). This study

provides a basis for classification of the palatal mucosal changes among reverse smokers and has implications for nurses in terms of health care teaching with Filipino women.

AIDS Research by Woo, Rutherford, Payne, et al. (1988) in San Francisco indicates that the number of AIDS cases has disproportionately increased among Asians and Pacific Islanders (177%), compared with increases among Blacks, Whites, Hispanics, Native Americans, and Alaska Natives (54%). The incidence of AIDS among Filipinos was reported to be 92 per 100,000. Longitudinal studies are being done with children born to HIV-1 antibody–positive Filipino women (Manaloto, Caringal, Santiago, et al., 1996).

Nutritional preferences

Some Filipino Americans reflect their culture through the preparation and consumption of specific foods. Because some Filipino Americans subscribe to a theory of hot and cold, foods with these properties are incorporated into their dietary regimen. For example, it is customary to include both "hot" and "cold" foods in cooking, such as mixing beans, which are considered hot foods, with green vegetables, which are considered cold foods, regardless of how they are prepared (Orque, 1983). In addition, Filipino Americans who practice imitative magic may incorporate the concept of magic into the preparation and consumption of foods. For example, a pregnant Filipino woman may believe that eating dark foods such as prunes will produce a dark-complected baby (Affonso, 1978; Pimentel, 1968).

For some Filipino Americans religious or family customs also dictate foods that are prepared and consumed. For example, Filipino Catholics may abstain from eating meat during Lent, particularly on Ash Wednesday and Good Friday. Zaide (1961) concluded that Filipino beliefs and customs are so entrenched in the culture that some Filipinos may even refrain from eating meat during the burial of a relative.

The traditional foods for Filipinos include rice, fish, and vegetables. For Filipino Americans typical dishes include *adobo, pancit,* and *lupia. Adobo* is a method of preparation that includes cooking certain meats such as pork, chicken, or beef that have been marinated in vinegar, garlic, and other typical Filipino condiments. The meat is simmered slowly until it becomes tender and brown (Day, 1974). *Pancit* is a pasta made of rice or wheat noodles and is cooked with chicken, ham, shrimp, or pork in a soy and garlic-flavored sauce. *Lupia* is similar to the Chinese egg roll and is either deep fried or prepared fresh with selected vegetables (Day, 1974). Although Filipino Americans have changed their diets to reflect customs traditionally found in the United States, they also tend to retain ethnic food habits (Lewis & Glasby, 1975).

Psychological characteristics

Flaskerud (1984) conducted a study to determine whether there was a difference in perspective placed on problematic behaviors exhibited by six minority groups: African Americans, Native Americans, Chinese Americans, Mexican Americans, Filipino Americans, and Appalachians. The findings of the study indicated that there are differences in perceptions of problematic behavior and its management between mental health professionals and minority groups. Flaskerud also concluded that although these differences are related to different levels of education and expertise they are also likely to be related to cultural influences on conceptual explanations of problematic behavior and appropriate management. Cultural groups that were considered dominant viewed problematic behavior as mental illness and recommended psychiatric treatment, whereas cultural groups that were considered ethnic minority groups (including Filipino Americans, Chinese Americans, Mexican Americans, African Americans, Native Americans, and Appalachians) viewed the behavior from a broader perspective that encompassed spiritual, moral, social, economic, vocational, recreational, personal, physical, and psychological assessments. Marsella (1980), who studied depression in various cultural settings, reported that depression occurred infrequently in Filipinos. Psychological defenses vary by culture and thus result in a different configuration of depression (Rosenbaum, 1989). López (1990) noted that nurses from the Philippines who were working in America experienced conflict between being submissive and being assertive regarding client assignments and cli-

ent load. Spangler (1992) and Leininger (1991) also looked at differences in nurses who were Filipino versus White American.

Alcohol use A study by Danko, Johnson, Nagoshi, et al. (1988) found that, although Filipinos and Hawaiians have substantial alcohol usage if they drink, a large proportion of Filipino Americans are abstainers. Lubben, Chi, and Kitano (1988) found that approximately 50% of the women in a population sample of 298 Filipinos were abstainers, whereas approximately 80% of the men in the sample were drinkers, an indication that heavy drinking is almost exclusively a male activity among Filipinos. The study concluded that the only significant variable found among Filipino men and women in regard to drinking was regular participation in religious services.

Implications for nursing care

It is important for the nurse to remember that because Filipino Americans tend to have darker-pigmented skin than that of White Americans, it is essential to be able to distinguish between the norm and carotenemia, jaundice, or cyanosis. When the nurse is inspecting the skin of a Filipino American, it is important that the nurse inspect the buccal mucosa for petechiae. When looking for evidence of carotenemia, the nurse can substantiate this finding if a yellow tint is absent in the palate when the sclerae are yellow (Roach, 1977). If the nurse is unable to determine the presence of carotenemia, the client's stool may be observed to determine if it is light or clay colored and the urine may be examined to determine if it is a dark golden color.

Because some Filipino Americans have a prevalence for enzymatic conditions such as G-6-PD deficiency, lactose intolerance, or thalassemia, it is important for the nurse to encourage the client to eat meals that are high in protein and to replace whole milk with high-calcium substitutes such as buttermilk, yogurt, and sharp cheese, or add lactic aids to foods or other dairy products.

Filipino Americans are essentially very gentle and mild and have passive temperaments. It is believed that the reason for the passive temperament is the desire of Filipinos to maintain a harmonious balance between man and nature. These people generally are neither assertive nor aggressive and may often appear guarded or reticent. The nurse may often misunderstand this need for passivity and may misconstrue and mislabel this behavior as an inferiority complex. Very often Filipino Americans are erroneously labeled as passive-aggressive and as having a personality disorder with anger as the underlying cause. When angry, Filipino Americans do have a temperament that is passive-aggressive, and this anger often produces anxiety, which is usually handled through covert and passive means. Behavioral manifestations of passive-aggressive behavior are evidenced through such behavior traits as procrastination, stubbornness, intense craving for acceptance, and varying demands for attention (DeGracia, 1979).

The nurse should be cognizant that some Filipino foods are high in purine, such as *dinuguan* (from *dugu* 'blood'), which is a food prepared from the small intestines, liver, heart, kidney, and blood of pork. Because *dinuguan* is extremely high in purine, a client who is following a purine-restricted diet should be instructed to modify the diet with leaner meats than pork organs. Because Filipinos, particularly men, have been reported to be hypertensive, the nurse should instruct these clients to modify traditional high-sodium Filipino diets. Foods that are considered high in sodium include traditional Filipino condiments such as soy sauce. For the client following a diet moderately restricted in sodium, the nurse may suggest brands of soy sauce that have a lower or reduced sodium content. The client who is following a diet totally restricted in sodium can be taught to prepare certain dishes such as *adobo* by marinating the meat overnight in a mixture of lemon juice, onions, garlic, sugar, and crushed peppercorns (Orque, 1983).

The nurse should also be aware that intercultural differences in expression of depression may be the result of differences in social structure and world view. The concept of self is culture specific and must be considered in transcultural care of depressed people (Rosenbaum, 1989).

SUMMARY

The literature dealing with Filipino Americans has sometimes been confusing because Filipinos have been lumped together in the literature with Asians, Spanish-speaking people, and "other" categories (Orque, 1983); therefore the nurse must apply data carefully from the literature to Filipino-American clients who receive care. In addition, the nurse should be careful to notice the dates on research studies of Filipino Americans because many studies in the literature are old and may not reflect current needs. It is important for the nurse to assess the Filipino-American client carefully and to keep in mind what is known about the client's cultural background so that culturally appropriate care can be provided.

Case Study

Mr. Rom Recio, a 46-year-old Filipino American, is admitted to the hospital with a diagnosis of hypertension. Mr. Recio has lived in an urban area in Los Angeles, coming from the Philippines 2 years earlier. This is Mr. Recio's third admission to the hospital because his hypertension is uncontrolled. Mr. Recio has repeatedly refused to comply and take the Aldomet (methyldopa) the physician prescribed for him during the initial diagnostic hospitalization. The nurse notes on examination that Mr. Recio's blood pressure is 140/104; pulse, 88; respirations, 16; and temperature, 98.6° F.

Although Mr. Recio speaks English, occasionally he has difficulty understanding what is being communicated in English terminology. Mr. Recio has a wife and three children, ages 10, 12, and 15. Mr. Recio's wife speaks very little English; however, all the children are proficient in English. When Mr. Recio is examined by the nurse, he states that he believes the problem with his blood has occurred because of disfavor with God.

CARE PLAN

 Nursing Diagnosis   Health maintenance, altered, related to hypertension

Client Outcomes

1. Client and family will verbalize desire to learn more about condition and preventive techniques to reduce symptoms.
2. Client and family will verbalize a willingness to comply with prescribed medical regimen.
3. Client will verbalize an understanding of the need to comply with routine schedule for antihypertensive drugs.

Nursing Interventions

1. Identify with client and family sociocultural factors that influence health-seeking behavior.
2. Determine with client and family knowledge of hypertension and severity of illness.
3. Determine with client and family knowledge and level of adaptation to news about condition of hypertension.
4. Identify with client and family necessity for adherence to prescribed time limits for taking antihypertensive drugs.

 Nursing Diagnosis   Communication, impaired verbal, related to recent immigration and the use of English as a second language

Client Outcomes

1. Client and family will be able to communicate basic needs to health personnel.
2. Client will be able to communicate feelings and anxieties about present diagnosis.

Nursing Interventions

1. Use visual aids that will aid client in understanding the condition.
2. Use gestures or actions that communicate various tasks and procedures to be done.
3. Write down messages to provide visual stimulation about procedures to be accomplished.

 Nursing Diagnosis   Family processes, altered, related to an ill family member

Client Outcomes

1. Family will participate in care of the ill family member.
2. Family will assist nurse in assisting client in returning to a high level of wellness.
3. Family will verbalize difficulties encountered when seeking appropriate internal and external resources related to care and management of a family member with hypertension.

Nursing Interventions

1. Determine family's understanding of client's condition.
2. Determine support systems available to family from external resources.
3. Determine with family a supportive network with friends available.
4. Involve family in care and scheduling of client-centered activities (such as taking Aldomet on time).
5. Encourage family to verbalize difficulties.

Nursing Diagnosis   Noncompliance related to anxiety as manifested by ideology that the present condition is a result of God's disfavor

Client Outcomes	*Nursing Interventions*
1. Client will verbalize fears related to health needs. 2. Client will verbalize factors that contribute to feelings of anxiety. 3. Client will identify alternatives to present coping patterns necessary to reduce feelings of anxiety. 4. Client will verbalize understanding for compliance with taking Aldomet when scheduled.	1. Identify with client and family negative experiences with present conditions or delivery of services of the health care system. 2. Correct any misconceptions about illness, medication regimen, or both. 3. Identify health care practices that are beneficial, neutral, or harmful. 4. Give client simple and precise instructions about medication regimen. 5. Determine whether noncompliance in taking medication is a result of side effects or anxiety.

STUDY QUESTIONS

1. What factors related to culture are most likely to influence the noncompliance exhibited by Mr. Recio?
2. Explain how the Filipino-American orientation to time may influence Mr. Recio's health-seeking behavior and his adherence to specific schedules.
3. Describe the locus-of-control variable that some Filipino Americans have that may influence health-seeking behavior.
4. Describe at least three other nursing interventions that can be implemented to facilitate communication between Mr. Recio, his family, and the health care team.
5. Describe the structure of some Filipino-American families and the relationship the family may have on health-seeking behavior.

References

Adair, L.S., & Popkin, B.M. (1996, Jan.). Low birth weight reduces the likelihood of breast-feeding among Filipino infants. *Journal of Nutrition, 126*(1), 103-112.

Affonso, D. (1978). The Filipino American. In Clark, A. (Ed.), *Culture, childbearing, health professionals* (pp. 128-153). Philadelphia: F.A. Davis.

Anchacosa-Angala, S., & Márquez-Sumabat, L. (1964). Skinfold thickness as indication of leanness-fatness in some female college students. *Philippine Journal of Nutrition, 17,* 176-197.

Anderson, J. (1983). Health and illness in Pilipino immigrants. *Western Journal of Medicine, 139,* 811-819.

Bartlett, L. (1977). The Filipino "Cajuns." *Dixie,* p. 9.

Burma, J. (1954). *Spanish-speaking groups in the United States.* London: Duke University Press.

Burr, J., & Mutchler, J. (1993). Nativity, acculturation, and economic status: explanations of Asian American living arrangements in later life. *Journal of Gerontology, 48*(2), 55-63.

Bush, M., & Babich, K. (1978). Cultural variation. In Longo, D., & Williams, R. (Eds.), *Clinical practice in psychosocial nursing: assessment and intervention.* East Norwalk, Conn.: Appleton-Century-Crofts.

Cantos, A., & Rivera, E. (1996). Filipinos. In Lipson, J., Dibble, S., & Minarik, P. (Eds.), *Culture and nursing care.* University of California at San Francisco, School of Nursing: UCSF Nursing Press.

Caringer, B. (1977). Caring for the institutionalized Filipino. *Journal of Gerontological Nursing, 3*(7), 33-37.

Cheong, R., Kuizon, M., & Tajaon, R. (1991, Dec.). Menstrual blood loss and iron nutrition in Filipino women. *Southeast Asian Journal of Tropical Medicine in Public Health, 22*(12), 595-604.

Chung, C.S., & Kau, M.C. (1985). Racial differences in cephalometric measurements and incidence of cleft lip with or without cleft palate. *Journal of Craniofacial Genetic Development and Biology, 5*(4), 341-349.

Clarkson, P.M., Hintermister, R., Fillyaw, M., & Stylos, L. (1981). High density lipoprotein cholesterol in young adult weight lifters, runners, and untrained subjects. *Human Biology, 53*(2), 251-257.

Corpuz, O. (1965). *The Philippines.* Englewood Cliffs, N.J.: Prentice Hall.

Daniels, R., & Kitano, H. (1970). *American racism: exploration of the nature of prejudice.* Englewood Cliffs, N.J.: Prentice Hall.

Danko, G.P., Johnson, R.C., Nagoshi, C.T., et al. (1988). Judgments of "normal" and "problem" alcohol use as related to reported alcohol consumption. *Alcoholism, 12*(6), 760-768.

Davidhizar, R. (1997, Nov.). Personal communication about her experience as a nursing director in a psychiatric hospital.

Day, B. (1974). Philippine fare. *Gourmet,* p. 25.

DeGracia, R.T. (1979, Aug.). Cultural influences on Filipino patients. *American Journal of Nursing,* 1412-1414.

Ennis, T., & Inaba, M. (1977). Philippines. In *The volume library.* Nashville, Tenn.: Southwestern Company.

Espíritu, Y.L. (1995). *Filipino American lives.* Philadelphia: Temple University Press.

Flaskerud, J. (1984). A comparison of perceptions of problematic behavior by six minority groups and mental health professionals. *Nursing Research, 33*(4), 190-197.

Frerichs, R.R., Chapman, J.M., & Maes, E.F. (1984). Mortality due to all causes and to cardiovascular diseases among seven race-ethnic populations in Los Angeles County, 1980. *International Journal of Epidemiology, 13*(3), 291-298.

Garn, S. (1965). *Human races* (ed. 2). Springfield, Ill.: Charles C Thomas, Publisher.

Gerber, L.M. (1980). The influence of environmental factors on mortality from coronary heart disease among Filipinos in Hawaii. *Human Biology, 52*(2), 269-278.

Gerber, L.M. (1983). Gains in life expectancies if heart disease and stroke were eliminated among Caucasians, Filipinos and Japanese in Hawaii. *Social Science and Medicine, 17*(6), 349-353.

Goodman, M.T., Yoshizawa, C.N., & Kolonel, L.N. (1988). Descriptive epidemiology of thyroid cancer in Hawaii. *Cancer, 61*(6), 1272-1281.

Gordon, T. (1976). Heart disease in adults. *Vital Health Statistics, 11*(6), 1-43.

Guthrie, G., & Jacobs, P. (1976). Childbearing and personality development in the Philippines. University Park, Pa.: Pennsylvania State University Press.

Hart, D.V. (1966). The Filipino villager and his spirits. *Solidarity, 1,* 66.

Hart, D.V. (1981). Bisayan Filipino and Malayan folk medicine. In Henderson, G., & Primeaux, M. (Eds.), *Transcultural health care.* Reading, Mass.: Addison-Wesley.

Hart, D.V., Rajadhon, P.A., & Coughlin, R.J. (1965). *Southeast Asian birth customs: three studies in human reproduction.* New Haven, Conn.: Human Relations Area Files.

Hartung, G.H., Foreyt, J.P., Mitchell, R.E., et al. (1980). Relation of diet to high-density-lipoprotein cholesterol in middle-aged marathon runners, joggers, and inactive men. *New England Journal of Medicine, 302*(7), 357-361.

Hooper, H. (1958). A Filipino in California copes with anxiety. In Seward, G. (Ed.), *Clinical studies in cultural conflict.* New York: Ronald Press.

Information please almanac (1998). Boston: Houghton Mifflin.

José, F., & Salcedo, J. (1958). Subcutaneous fat distribution and body form of Filipino women. *Acta Medica Philippina, 14,* 161.

Kittler, P., & Sucher, K. (1989). *Food and culture in America.* New York: Van Nostrand Reinhold.

Klatsky, A.L., & Armstrong, M.A. (1991). Cardiovascular risk factors among Asian Americans living in northern California. *American Journal of Public Health, 81*(11), 1423-1428.

Kluckhohn, F., & Strodtbeck, F. (1961). *Variations in value orientations.* Evanston, Ill.: Row, Peterson.

Kolonel, L.N. (1985, Dec.). Cancer incidence among Filipinos in Hawaii and the Philippines. *National Cancer Institute Monogram, 69,* 93-98.

Kurtzke, J.F. (1982). Epidemiology of amyotrophic lateral sclerosis. *Advances in Neurology, 36,* 281-302.

Kusumoto, A., Suzuki, T., Kumakura, C., & Ashizawa, K. (1996, Sept.-Oct.). A comparative study of foot morphology between Filipino and Japanese women, with reference to the significance of a deformity like hallux valgus as a normal variation. *Annals of Human Biology, 23*(5), 373-385.

Lantican, L.S., & Corona, D.F. (1992, Oct.-Dec.). Comparison of the social support networks of Filipino and Mexican-American primigravidas. *Health Care of Women International, 13*(4), 329-338.

Lasker, B. (1969). *Filipino immigration.* New York: Arno Press.

Leininger, M. (1991). Culture care of Philippine and Anglo-American nurses in a hospital context. In Spangler, S. (Ed.), *Culture care diversity and universality: a theory of nursing* (pp. 119-146). New York: National League for Nursing.

Lewis, J., & Glasby, M. (1975). Food habits and nutrient intakes of Filipino women in Los Angeles. *Journal of American Dietetic Association, 67,* 122-125.

Lieban, R.W. (1967). *Cebuano sorcery: malign magic in the Philippines.* Berkeley: University of California Press.

López, N. (1990). *The acculturation of selected Filipino nurses to nursing practice in the United States.* Doctoral dissertation, University of Pennsylvania.

Lott, J. (1976). Migration of a mentality: the Filipino community. *Social Casework, 57,* 165-172.

Lubben, J.E., Chi, I., & Kitano, H.H. (1988). Exploring Filipino American drinking behavior. *Journal of Studies of Alcohol, 49*(1), 26-29.

Manaloto, C., Caringal, L., Santiago, E., et al. (1996, May-June). Longitudinal studies of children born to HIV-1 antibody positive Filipino commercial sex workers (CSW): diagnostic dilemmas. *International Journal of the Study of AIDS, 7*(3), 212-220.

Marsella, A. (1980). Depressive experience and disorder across cultures. In Triandis, H., & Draguns, J. (Eds.), *Handbook of cross-cultural psychology* (pp. 237-289). Boston: Allyn & Bacon.

Matawaran, A., et al. (1966). Preliminary report on the average heights and weights of some Filipinos. *Philippine Journal of Nutrition, 19,* 318-332.

Matsumoto, N., Worth, R.M., Kurland, L.T., & Okazaki, H. (1972). Epidemiology study of amyotrophic lateral sclerosis in Hawaii: identification of high incidence among Filipino men. *Neurology, 22,* 934-940.

McKay, J., Hill, B., & Buckler, J. (1988). *A history of world societies.* Boston: Houghton Mifflin.

McKenzie, J., & Chrisman, N. (1977). Healing herbs, gods, and magics. *Nursing Outlook, 25,* 326-328.

McNall, C. (1989). Healing we cannot explain. *American Journal of Nursing, 89*(9), 1162-1164.

Melendy, H. (1977). *Asians in America: Filipinos, Koreans, and East Indians.* Boston: Twayne.

Mercado-Ortiz, G., Wilson, D., & Jiang, D. (1996, Oct.). Reverse smoking and palatal mucosal changes in Filipino women. Epidemiological features. *Australian Dental Journal, 41*(10), 300-303.

Meredith, H. (1978). Research between 1960 and 1970 on the standing heights of young children in different parts of the world. In Reese, H., & Lipsitt, L. (Eds.), *Advances in child development and behavior* (pp. 1-59). New York: Academic Press.

Monzon, R.B. (1991, Dec.). Replacement patterns of *Ascaris lumbricoides* populations in Filipino children. *Southeast Asian Journal of Tropical Medicine in Public Health, 22*(4), 605-610.

Morton, N.E. (1977). Genetic aspects of prematurity. In Reed, D.M., & Stanley, F.J. (Eds.), *The epidemiology of prematurity.* Baltimore: Urban & Schwartzenberg.

Motulsky, A.G., Stransky, E., & Fraser, G.R. (1964). Glucose-6-phosphate dehydrogenase (G6PD) deficiency, thalassaemia, and abnormal haemoglobins in the Philippines. *Journal of Medical Genetics, 1,* 102-106.

Orque, M. (1983). Nursing care of Filipino American patients. In Orque, M.S., Bloch, B., & Monrroy, L.S.A. (Eds), *Ethnic nursing care: a multicultural approach.* St. Louis: Mosby.

Ortiz, G., Pierce, A., & Wilson, D. (1996, Sep.). Palatal changes associated with reverse smoking in Filipino women. *Oral Disease, 2* (9). 232-237.

Parreno, H. (1977). How Filipinos deal with stress. *Washington State Journal of Nursing, 49,* 3-6.

Pimentel, L. (1968). The perception of illness among the immigrant Filipinos in Sacramento Valley. Master's thesis, Sacramento State College, Sacramento, California.

Pollard, R. (1995, Dec.). Ethnic comparison of twinning rates in California. *Human Biology, 67* (6), 921-931.

Requiro, R. (1981). Filipino hypertension rate leads Asian-Pacific group. *Philippine News, 20,* 12.

Roach, L. (1977). Color changes in dark skin. *Nursing '77, 7,* 48-51.

Rosenbaum, J. (1989). Depression: viewed from a transcultural nursing theoretical perspective. *Journal of Advanced Nursing, 14,* 7-12.

Rosenblatt, K.A., Weiss, N.S., & Schwartz, S.M. (1996, May). Liver cancer in Asian migrants to the United States and their descendants. *Cancer Causes Control, 7*(3), 345-350.

Shimamoto, Y. (1977). Health care to the elderly Filipino in Hawaii: its cultural aspects. In Leininger, M., & Carbol, K. (Eds.), *Transcultural nursing care of the elderly,* Proceedings from the Second National Transcultural Nursing Conference. Salt Lake City, Utah: University of Utah College of Nursing.

Sloan, N. (1963). Ethnic distribution of diabetes mellitus in Hawaii. *Journal of the American Medical Association, 183*, 419-424.

Solon, F., Solon, M., Mehansho, H., et al. (1996, Nov.). Evaluation of the effect of vitamin A–fortified margarine on the vitamin A status of preschool Filipino children. *Europe Journal of Clinical Nutrition, 50*(11), 720-723.

Spangler, Z. (1992). Transcultural care values and nursing practices of Filipino-American nurses. *Journal of Transcultural Nursing, 4*(2), 28-37.

Spector, R. (1996). *Guide to heritage assessment and health traditions.* Stamford, Conn.: Appleton & Lange.

Stavig, G.R., Igra, A., & Leonard, A.R. (1988). Hypertension and related health issues among Asians and Pacific Islanders in California. *Public Health Reports, 103*(1), 28-37.

Stavig, G.R., Igra, A., Leonard, A.R., et al. (1986). Hypertension-related mortality in California. *Public Health Reports, 101*(1), 39-49.

Takaki, R. (1989). *Strangers from a different shore.* Boston: Little, Brown & Co.

Urban Associates, Inc. (1974). *A study of selected socioeconomic characteristics of ethnic minorities based on the 1970 census* (HEW Publication No. 5). Arlington, Va.: U.S. Department of Health, Education, and Welfare.

U.S. Department of Commerce, Bureau of the Census (1993a, June, 12). *News release,* Commerce News.

U.S. Department of Commerce, Bureau of the Census (1993b). *Population Profile of the United States,* Publication No. 23-185. Washington, D.C.: Government Printing Office.

U.S. Department of Commerce, Bureau of the Census (1993c, Sept.). *We the Americans . . . Asians.* Washington, D.C.: Government Printing Office.

Voegelin, C.F., & Voegelin, F.M. (1997). *Classification and index of the world's languages.* New York: Elsevier.

Wagner, N. (1973). Filipinos: a minority within a minority. In Stanley, S., & Wagner, N. (Eds.), *Asian-Americans: psychological perspectives.* Palo Alto, Calif.: Science & Behavior Books.

Wallerstein, R. (1976). Blood. In Krupp, M., & Chatton, M. (Eds.), *Current diagnosis and treatment.* Los Altos, Calif.: Lange Medical Publications.

Weber, S.E. (1996). Cultural aspects of pain in child-bearing women. *Journal of Obstetric, Gynecologic and Neonatal Nursing, 25*(1), 67-72.

Weisse, A., Abiuso, P, & Thind, I. (1977). Acute myocardial infarction in Newark, New Jersey: a study of racial incidence. *Archives of Internal Medicine, 137,* 1402-1405.

White, J., Linhart, J., & Medley, L. (1996, Sept.). Culture, diet, and the maternity. *Advance for Nurse Practitioners.* 26-28.

Wilson, S., & Billones, H. (1994). The Filipino elder: implications for nursing practice. *Journal of Gerontological Nursing, 20*(8), 31-36.

Woo, J.M., Rutherford, G.W., Payne, S.F., et al. (1988). The epidemiology of AIDS in Asian and Pacific Islander populations in San Francisco. *AIDS, 2*(6), 473-475.

Wooley, P. (1972). *Syncrisis: the dynamics of health—an analytic series on the interactions of health and socioeconomic development:* Vol. 4. *The Philippines.* Washington, D.C.: U.S. Department of Health, Education, and Welfare.

Yamase, H., & McNamara, J. (1977). Geographic differences in the incidence of gallbladder disease: influence of environment and ethnic background. *American Journal of Surgery, 123,* 667-670.

Young, F., Lichton, I.J., Hamilton, R.M., et al. (1987). Body weight, blood pressure, and electrolyte excretion of young adults from six ethnic groups in Hawaii. *American Journal of Clinical Nutrition, 45*(1), 126-130.

Young, J.L., Ries, L.G., & Pollach, E.S. (1984). Cancer patient survival among ethnic groups in the United States. *Journal of National Cancer Institute, 73*(2), 341-352.

Zabilka, G. (1967). *Customs and culture of the Philippines.* Rutland, Vt.: Charles E. Tuttle.

Zaide, G. (1961). *Philippine history: developing our nation.* Manila, the Philippines: Bookman.

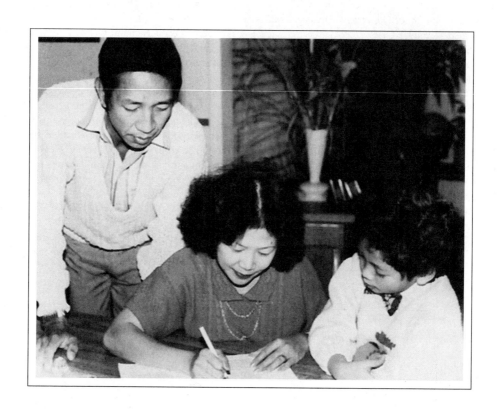

CHAPTER 18 Vietnamese Americans

*Ruth Yoder Stauffer**

BEHAVIORAL OBJECTIVES

After reading this chapter, the nurse will be able to:

1. Identify two important Vietnamese cultural values that influence all Vietnamese behavior.
2. Describe the organization of the Vietnamese family.
3. Articulate at least three explanations for the causes of illness that influence traditional Vietnamese thinking.
4. Discuss briefly the basic *yin* and *yang* theory of Chinese medicine and how it is expressed in the cause and treatment of disease.
5. Identify four barriers for Vietnamese Americans using the U.S. health care system.
6. Describe possible sources of anxiety that may be experienced by a Vietnamese American working as a translator and interpreter in a clinic serving recent refugees.
7. Articulate ways the nurse might modify "routine" procedures in a clinic or hospital to accommodate a Vietnamese-American client.

OVERVIEW OF VIETNAM

Vietnam is situated on the eastern coast of the Indochinese peninsula, bordered on the north by China, with the Gulf of Thailand surrounding the Mekong delta on the south. On the west, Vietnam is bordered by Cambodia (Kampuchea) and Laos and, on the east, by the South China Sea. The country is slightly smaller than Japan, with 127,000 square miles. Vietnam, along with Laos and Cambodia, is often referred to as "Indochina," or "Southeast Asia." These three countries are strikingly dissimilar, however, with completely different languages, unrelated

*Former Mennonite Central Committee relief worker in Vietnam; more recently worked with the Mennonite church in the Vietnamese communities in Honolulu, Hawaii, and the Washington, D.C., area.

social roots, long histories of separate development, and often strife.

The northern part of Vietnam is mountainous with deep valleys and the industrial Red River delta. The central ribbon is a long, narrow corridor with a mountain range, coastal plain, and miles of beautiful white sand beaches. The southern part of Vietnam is mostly the flat Mekong delta, the agricultural area where most of the rice for the country and for export is grown. Vietnam is considered a tropical country, though the north has four distinct seasons and the south has two seasons: rainy and dry.

The population of Vietnam is over 75,123,880 million people (1996 estimate), which includes "lowland people" (often urban and more educated), rural village people (with varying degrees of sophistication and education), and mountain people (made up of at least 30 different groups or tribes with a culture all their own). The Chinese are the largest minority, with 1 million people (based on pre-1975 figures). The mountain people number approximately 1 million (Information Please Almanac, 1998).

Vietnam has a recorded history of over 2000 years, with legends that cover an additional 2000 years. Earliest records are of dynasty rule and domination by the Chinese (111 BC to AD 938). There were 900 years of independence until the French came in 1858. Throughout the French domination (until 1954), the Vietnamese continued to work toward independence.

The country was divided into the Communist north and the non-Communist south by the Geneva Accords in 1954, when it became clear that the "Nationalist" movement in the north had been monopolized by leaders leaning toward Communist ideology. The struggle between the Soviet-assisted North Vietnam and the United States–assisted South Vietnam ended in 1975 when Vietnam was reunited under the victorious Republic of North Vietnam. More than 30 years of war had physically, economically, and socially devastated the country. There was a great deal of turmoil and isolation during the next 15 years as the Communists attempted to rebuild the country under a new philosophy. Floods and drought added to the crises and poverty. Thousands of people left the country for hope in the outside world, especially France, the United States, Canada, and Australia. By the late 1980s however, the need and opportunity for economic exchange helped ease restrictions, and there was a pronounced influx of economic interests and business with countries around the world. Dollars carried in by friends and family provided welcome help for improving the quality of life for many Vietnamese.

By 1993 the country had a trade surplus and was the world's third largest exporter of rice. Political and economic advisors agree that there were many "Miles to Go" (Hiebert, 1993b), but the clear direction was encouraging Vietnamese to stay at home. A 1995 estimate of the gross national product was $97 billion with a per capita income of $1300 (Information Please Almanac, 1998). Citing Vietnamese coopera-

tion in returning remains of U.S. solders killed in the Vietnam War, the United States announced an end, on Feb. 3, 1994, to the 19-year-old U.S. embargo on trade with Vietnam. The United States extended full diplomatic recognition to Vietnam on July 11, 1995 (World Almanac, 1997). By 1998, "going back" to visit Vietnam was a common occurrence in most U.S. Vietnamese communities. Today tourism provides many jobs for the people of Vietnam.

IMMIGRATION TO THE UNITED STATES

There are 615,000 Vietnamese persons in the United States today representing 0.2% of the U.S. population (Information Please Almanac, 1998; U.S. Department of Commerce, Bureau of the Census, 1993a). Of this number, 60,509 reside in the Northeast, 51,932 in the Midwest, 168,501 in the South, and 333,605 in the West (U.S. Department of Commerce, Bureau of the Census, 1993b). The highest concentrations of Vietnamese Americans are in California, Virginia, Texas, and Florida. Approximately 79.9% of Vietnamese persons in the United States today were born in a foreign country (U.S. Department of Commerce, Bureau of the Census, 1993b). The number of Vietnamese who immigrate to the United States continues to increase dramatically. Between 1980 and 1990, 69.7% of all Vietnamese residing in the United States were immigrants, compared with 27.1% between 1975 and 1979. The median age for Vietnamese Americans is 25.2 years, compared with 33.1 years for the rest of the U.S. population (U.S. Department of Commerce, Bureau of the Census, 1993c). Approximately 48% of Vietnamese Americans are females, compared with 51% for the total nation (U.S. Department of Commerce, Bureau of the Census, 1993d).

First-wave immigrants

The first group of refugees, who began arriving in 1975, included many lowlanders, professionals, ranking South Vietnamese military personnel, and those with close U.S. connections. This group also included those who had the means to get out of the country and those who would stand to lose the most under the new regime. A high percentage of these immigrants were educated in Vietnam or abroad, and some spoke English. Many were young and single, or married with small children. The children moved into the school systems and could soon speak English more fluently than their parents, and in some cases more fluently than they could speak Vietnamese. (Today, some Vietnamese communities are sponsoring classes in Vietnamese for their children to study Vietnamese.)

Some of these immigrants had been exposed to European cultures or to the American culture for years and had economic or vocational assets. They generally did not go through a long stressful period of economic and psychological deprivation that affected their health and psyche. Of the 145,000 Vietnamese persons who came to the United States in 1975, 14% lived in single-family households, 42% were under 18 years of age, and 11.6% were over 44 years of age. Approximately 90% were employed 1 year after arrival (Coelho & Stein, 1980).

Second-wave immigrants

A higher percentage of the second-wave refugees (1979 to 1980) were Chinese-Vietnamese extended family groups who left Vietnam under duress and pressure from the government. Again, these people often were educated and part of the business community in or near Saigon, with as much social status as was permitted under the new regime. For many persons in the second wave of refugees, however, Vietnamese was a second language, and fewer spoke English than in the 1975 group. These immigrants also included elderly persons and other extended family members who had varying health needs and problems.

Third-wave immigrants

Most of the Vietnamese refugees during the 1980s were "boat people," who in many cases had lived through not only economic struggles, but also political and social change while at home. In addition, the boat people had survived life-threatening situations for days at sea. Persons in the third wave often spent months or even years in refugee camps along the way, and these earlier experiences caused turmoil that needed to be dealt with once they ar-

rived and got settled in the United States. Third-wave immigrants were even more diversified than those in the two former groups. Many were in poorer physical condition than those arriving earlier, and generally the adjustment was more difficult and more complex. Although many refugee education programs and school systems had organized effective programs to absorb the newly arrived children and adults in the first and second waves (and these persons tended to be motivated, highly literate, and able to do well quickly in the school system), the programs were not so effective with persons in the third wave. Life in camps did not encourage rigorous study habits or academic excellence, and many children in the third wave were not able to read or write well in either Vietnamese or English. For the boat people education needed to be much more comprehensive to assist adjustment to the new environment.

Approximately 850,000 Vietnamese, Cambodian, and Laotian refugees have come to the United States since the end of the war in Vietnam (Poss, 1989). In 1986 nations surrounding these countries tightened laws for illegal travelers on their shores, and the traffic of boat people slowed down. At the same time the government of Vietnam gave new economic life to the country by allowing the people some private marketing and land use. In 1989 the government agreed to voluntary repatriation of Vietnamese who had left the country, and during the next 3 years with United Nations' help more than 32,000 boat people returned from camps, especially in Hong Kong (Balfour, 1993).

COMMUNICATION
Language

In the United States, Vietnamese is the language of most of the 3 million people who call or have called Vietnam their home. In 1993, 65.0% of all Vietnamese 5 years of age or older could not speak English well (U.S. Department of Commerce, Bureau of the Census, 1993a, 1993c). Vietnamese is not mutually intelligible with any other Asian language. It is monosyllabic and disyllabic and polytonal (five to six tones), and so a syllable when spoken with different tones has an entirely different meaning each time. The language is flowing and musical, and for the most part, pronunciation is consistent and the grammar is simple.

Until the 1960s French was the language of educated Vietnamese people, along with Vietnamese; therefore, much of the scientific and technical vocabulary was borrowed from French or, more recently, English. After 1975 in Vietnam, English was more common as the choice for a second language in high schools and colleges. Three distinct dialects of Vietnamese separate the northern, central, and southern regions of Vietnam. Dialects identify the speaker's origins and are understood by others regardless of region.

For many years before the Vietnam War, Vietnam had a large Chinese minority with their own schools where classes were conducted in Chinese. In the Chinese suburb of Saigon called Cholon, many older Chinese persons spoke only Chinese, and the children learned Vietnamese as a second language. This explains why many persons in the large Chinese-Vietnamese refugee group can speak both Chinese and Vietnamese or only Chinese. In contrast to this, the ethnic mountain people, or Montagnards, have their own tribal languages (usually of Austronesian type and, in the north, Miao-Yao type) and often do not understand Vietnamese.

Style

As a cornerstone of Vietnamese society, respect is very evident in communication (Huynh, 1987). The Vietnamese language demonstrates the cultural focus on respect by a proliferation of titles. For example, when describing family relationships, English users have titles reserved for family members that include "mother," "father," "sister," "brother," "uncle," "aunt," "cousin," "grandmother," and "grandfather." However, the language and style of the Vietnamese not only encompass family descriptors such as "uncle," but also designate which side of the family a family member represents (mother's or father's) and further indicate whether that relative is the eldest brother or sister. Grandparent titles also reflect paternal or maternal side. When a sister or brother is being described, the term used indicates if the sister or brother is younger *(em)* or older *(chị or anh)*.

Context

The word "yes" is used in English to express agreement and does not reflect an attitude of respect or disrespect. For Vietnamese people *ya* indicates respect and not necessarily agreement. Therefore a troubling verbal communication between health workers and Vietnamese-American clients is the polite *Ya, ya, Tha Bà, ya, ya,* response, which Americans interpret as "Yes, yes, I understand, and I'll do it." For the Vietnamese the "yes" of *ya* is simply being respectful, indicating "I'm listening, and I respect what you're saying" (even though the request may not be within the realm of possibility). Nurses often reflect later, "But he said, 'Yes, yes,' and agreed to. . . ." Noncompliance by Vietnamese Americans can often be traced to this misinterpretation of *ya*.

Vietnamese people will often use personal pronouns to describe various roles held. For example, the speaker may refer to self as *"con"* (referring to a child) when addressing parents, and as *"em"* to the nurse, or any superior. However, this same individual may refer to himself or herself as *thầy* ('teacher') when addressing students. Except with family and close friends, it is very common for Vietnamese persons to use only the title of a person: "Uncle," "Teacher," etc. Especially when there is considerable distance between the speaker and the listener, the title alone is most correct. This custom is even practiced in the United States. For example, people often say "Madam Chair" or "Mr. President," indicating that the title is more important than the name.

A distinct feature of the Vietnamese culture and consequently the language is moderation and caution (Huynh, 1987). Vietnamese people are taught from childhood to think before speaking. High value is placed on modesty of action and speech. A Vietnamese proverb suggests that "bragging reflects an empty soul." There is also concern that a slip of the tongue may bring discord and be disruptive to harmony and respect. Ethnic Vietnamese lowlanders as well as those from the mountain tribes place high value in showing respect: communication should always be in a formal, polite manner (Rairdan & Higgs, 1992). Box 18-1 highlights some differences between Oriental and American communication styles.

Box 18-1

COMMUNICATION STYLE AND EXPRESSION OF EMOTION

ORIENTAL	AMERICAN
Nonverbal	Verbal
Subtle, indirect	Open, direct
Serene, stoic, suppress negative emotions	Expressive, spontaneous
Indirect expression of affection by fulfilling obligations, needs	Direct verbal and physical expression of affection

From Nilchaikovit, K., Hill, J., & Holland, J. (1993). *General Hospital Psychiatry, 15*, 41-50.

Touch

Traditionally the high value of emotional self-control and the general esteem for correct behavior has limited the use of touch in communicating. Physical behavior, including backslapping, is not considered proper for the well bred. The young people have been less formal, and in the 1970s in Vietnam it was not uncommon to see groups of Vietnamese boys jostling each other in the street or girls walking arm in arm on the sidewalk. Today in the United States, many Vietnamese youths are taking some cues from their American counterparts.

Kinesics

In the Vietnamese culture, respect is also conveyed by nonverbal communication. By the time they can stand alone, children are taught to cross the arms over the chest, lower the head, and bend the upper torso slightly forward when greeting an elder or a guest coming into the house. Forms of this behavior continue throughout life in situations requiring respect. Deference to others shows a Confucian and Buddhist influence in that how something is done is often more important than what is done. Nonetheless, posture can give clues about an individual's self-esteem, and an individual's walk may give indications about self-concept (Sideleau, 1992). For example, if the client has a robotlike cog-wheeled gait, it is possible that the client has a phenothiazine side effect. A client who has rigid boundary movements could be a schizophrenic with a fragmented and fragile self-concept (Sideleau, 1992). Although it is essential to understand the psychodynamic implications related to posture, the gait of an individual may be related to a cultural phenomenon.

Respect is also shown by avoiding eye contact when talking with someone to whom one is not equal in education, social standing, age, or gender. A student avoids eye contact with a teacher, an employee with the boss, a younger member of the family with the elders, and so on. Direct eye contact in these settings generally means a challenge or an expression of deep passion. Bowing the head slightly when entering the presence of an elderly person conveys respect. Using both hands to give something to an adult, especially an elder, does the same. The head may be considered sacred, and care should be taken in touching and patting. Feet are the lowliest body members and should be kept on the floor.

In contrast to the usual palm-up position used by persons in the dominant culture in the United States, Vietnamese persons beckon for someone to come by turning the palm downward and waving the fingers. The upturned palm is used to call a dog or other animal, or as an insult. It is never proper to snap one's fingers or wave violently to gain the attention of another.

Open expression of emotions is considered in bad taste, except in very private circumstances. Emotions interfere with self-control and can be considered weaknesses. Romantic overtures are reserved for home or private settings, and wildly joyous scenes in public are not considered appropriate. One exception to the usual restraint is the expected behavior of a widow at the grave on the burial of her husband, when she may wail or attempt to throw herself into the grave.

Implications for nursing care

Because respect and harmony are highly valued in relationships, there is a great desire in the Vietnamese culture not to disappoint, upset, embarrass, or cause another person to lose face. The desire to maintain harmony takes precedence over what the actual truth of a situation may be. When a

Vietnamese-American client is confronted with a difficult or delicate question, particularly if the answer is negative, such as "Did you take your medication?" the client may choose not to give a direct answer in favor of the higher good of keeping peace with the nurse. In the Western culture this avoidance might be considered an attempt to avoid the truth; however, in the Vietnamese culture the answer would be considered the correct way to handle a delicate situation.

The nurse should recognize that negative emotions or expressions of disagreement are usually conveyed by silence or a reluctant smile. For the Vietnamese a smile may express joy, but more often it is used to convey many other messages, such as stoicism in the face of difficulty or an apology for a minor social offense. A smile may be a proper response to a scolding to show sincere acknowledgment for the wrongdoing and to convey that there are no ill feelings. A smile is also a way to respond when it is improper to say "thank you" or "I'm sorry" because of age or status. The smile is often present in Vietnamese-American clients, regardless of their situation. Even if angry, neglected, or in need, the Vietnamese-American client will rarely express this to the nurse or physician but will speak quietly and smile. Instead of asking questions that allow an answer, "Are you having pain?" or "Do you want something for pain?" the nurse should acknowledge the likelihood of pain and state, "Please let me get you something for pain."

The nurse may experience difficulty with information gathering as well as in relating to Vietnamese-American clients. Vietnamese-American clients tend to be discreet and passive, quietly understanding problems and rarely expressing feelings. Usually there is even more difficulty obtaining information in areas such as emotional problems or sexual difficulties. These topics are considered private and to be avoided in public conversation (Nilchaikovit, Hill, & Holland, 1993). In short-term relationships, it is crucial to have a good same-sex Vietnamese interpreter with whom the patient can identify; for the long term, the health professional should work toward a trusting relationship. For the Vietnamese client a caring, accepting attitude bridges the gaps where true understanding is not possible.

Because most Vietnamese-American clients entering the health care system in the United States do not speak medical English, an interpreter or bicultural medical translator may be essential to assist in accurate communication. It is important that the translator be culturally aware and conscientious to bridge the gap between the culture of the client and members of the health care team. Accurate translation can be assisted if the interpreter is Vietnamese because of the built-in cultural awareness. However, the Vietnamese interpreter may be hesitant to translate certain complaints that are unacceptable to Western practitioners, such as symptoms the client states are "caused by the wind," a common problem. Other important factors to consider are the effect of differences in social class between interpreter and client, the possible effect of a male interpreter with a female client, and the need for a female interpreter or companion when a physical examination is done on a female client. When an interpreter is unavailable, it is important for the nurse to choose vocabulary carefully and keep instructions simple and brief. Medical jargon should be avoided (Tran, 1980).

The nurse should be aware that English phonetic practices applied to Vietnamese names often result in pronunciations that are unintelligible to the Vietnamese. Nguyên Thị Hồng, who has been responding to approximately /Wee-un Tee-hung/ for 23 years can hardly be expected to appear at the clinic desk when she hears /Hung Thigh Nugooen/ summoned. (In Vietnamese, the family name, i.e., Nguyên, is spoken first and always appears first on listings. In the United States the family name is always *spoken* last, though it appears first on listings.) In a clinic where clients must be called, it may be useful to have the clients take numbers because numbers are more readily understood. It is important for the nurse to appreciate that pronunciation may also cause difficulties with questions regarding addresses and phone numbers. It may be easier for the client to write answers to such questions. Such a client should be encouraged to carry this information in written form.

A question about age may also be difficult for the Vietnamese-American client. A Vietnamese mother may be able to indicate the year a child was born but may not be able to state the child's exact age. In Vietnam individual birthdays are not usually celebrated; rather, everyone becomes a year older at the beginning of each new year *(Tết)*. Thus a newborn who arrives during the week before New Year would be considered 1 year old following the first *Tết* celebration. Another reason for confusion about age, especially for persons who immigrated as teenagers, is that new birth certificates may show an age adjustment of 2 or 3 years earlier. This adjustment may have been done in Vietnam to avoid the draft or in the United States to facilitate entrance into high school. After 18 years of age the student was not usually accepted into high school regardless of educational level attained in Vietnam. The slight build of many Vietnamese persons facilitates this age adjustment. Elderly Vietnamese persons without birth certificates usually know the year of their birth and are officially assigned, on arrival in the United States, a birthday of January 1. Finally, the nurse should be cognizant of the fact that for many Vietnamese Americans the numerous questions asked by health professionals in the United States raise doubt about the competency of the health professionals. The nurse should attempt to communicate both acceptance of varying cultural practices and genuine concern in order to bridge the gap between the cultures and to increase the trust of the client in the caregivers.

SPACE
Intimate zone

Beliefs about space are rooted deep in the Vietnamese culture. For traditional Vietnamese persons, intimate-zone activities are carefully confined to private settings. Holding hands in public, especially with members of the opposite sex, is considered in poor taste, and hugging or emotionally touching in public, even by close friends or family members, is embarrassing to the traditional Vietnamese onlooker. For some Vietnamese people the head is considered the "seat," and touching it, even in the process of giving care, may cause some vital force to escape (Hoang & Erickson, 1982).

Beliefs about space also influence how Vietnamese people feel about care given to females. Until the early 1900s, traditional practitioners were not to touch the bodies of their female clients except to take their pulse. Figurines were used for the female client to indicate where she was having problems. Today, many Vietnamese persons still place an emphasis on virginity at the time of marriage, especially for the woman, and continue to have strong feelings about unmarried young women having pelvic examinations.

Personal, social, and public zones

Vietnamese individuals are likely to feel more comfortable with more distance during personal and social relationships than that required by persons in the dominant culture. Social exchanges generally do not involve physical contact other than handshaking, which may be practiced between men.

Living space

In Vietnam extended families live comfortably in relatively small areas. The moderate or warm climate allows many of the family activities to be carried on outside. Often the kitchen is separate from the rest of the house, and the two or three main rooms double as living rooms and bedrooms, with the mosquito nets neatly tied back during the day. Even in spacious homes family members often prefer to spend much of their time in proximity to each other. In Vietnam, homes are typically arranged in communities and villages with several homes near each other.

Although many Vietnamese persons were used to living in proximity, refugee camps brought a new kind of cramped and confined closeness. As refugees, many Vietnamese persons lived for several months to years with 8 to 10 persons occupying a one-room space, sometimes enclosed only by a blanket curtain. Special adjustment was required by most refugees when they received housing in the United States because many well-intentioned sponsors made special efforts to provide single-home dwellings for the refugees because "they've been so crowded so long." Unfortunately this space lacked the familiar sounds, smells, and people and soon brought feelings of loneliness. Today, many Vietnamese Americans have homes with room for parents and additional family members and usually feel comfortable having relatives and friends in proximity.

Implications for nursing care

When caring for Vietnamese-American clients, the nurse should be cognizant of the effect that issues related to space may have on client care. For example, the nurse should be aware that if a pelvic examination is to be conducted, it is important for a female translator to explain carefully why it is necessary and what will be done and to remain with the client during the examination. If the head of a Vietnamese-American client is accidentally touched or must be touched in the process of care and the client believes that the head is sacred, the nurse should also touch the opposite side of the head or the shoulder (and thus preventing any vital forces from escaping) (Hoang & Erickson, 1982).

The nurse should also be aware that a back rub could be an "uneasy" experience when given by a stranger. The nurse should use discretion in including a back rub as a routine part of nursing care if it is not a critical component of the care.

SOCIAL ORGANIZATION
Family

In the past in Vietnam, the family was the basic institution of society and provided lifelong protection and guidance for the individual. The roles and structure of the family were well defined, with extensive terminology designating kinship relationships. The father was the head of the household but usually shared the rights and authority with his spouse.

The immediate family included the parents, unmarried children, sometimes the husband's parents, and sons with their wives and children. In addition, the extended family included other close relatives (with the same family name and ancestors) who lived in the same community (Box 18-2). The oldest son had the heavy responsibility of carrying on the family name, of taking over for the parents when they became elderly, and of following through with religious and ancestral observances.

The Vietnamese concept of family and extended family that has existed across generations as a "superorganic unit" is profoundly different from the individualism of the nuclear family in the United States (Indochinese Refugee Action Center, 1980). For Vietnamese people the family has been the

chief source of cohesion and continuity for hundreds of years. In the United States the family continues to be the basic unit of the Vietnamese society. Interestingly, today in their new locations, when Vietnamese individuals are asked for choices about associates, the highest percentage first choose family members or persons from their own village in Vietnam; second, they choose other Americans; and third, they choose other Vietnamese persons (Huynh, 1987).

Married-couple families account for approximately 73% of all family structures within the Vietnamese-American population, compared with 83% for the rest of the general U.S. population. There are approximately 4.4 persons per family in Vietnamese-American families, compared with 3.3 for the rest of the U.S. population. Today 21.3% of all Vietnamese-American families have three or more members in the work force. The median family income for Vietnamese-American families is $12,800, compared with $19,900 for the rest of the general U.S. population. Therefore, it is not surprising that 35% of all Vietnamese Americans live in poverty, compared with 12% for the rest of the U.S. population. Nevertheless, 27% of all Vietnamese Americans own their own homes, which is not an impressive statistic when compared with the rest of the U.S. population, 64% of which own their own homes. Despite this fact, the median value of homes for Vietnamese Americans is $56,800, compared with $47,200 for the rest of the U.S. population (U.S. Department of Commerce, Bureau of the Census, 1993b).

Family rules and structure

The crux of family loyalty is filial piety, which commands children to obey and honor their parents. According to Huynh (1987), the worst insult a Vietnamese person can receive is to be accused of failure in fulfilling the obligation of filial piety. Filial piety is also encouraged and reinforced by Christian teaching, that is, "Honor your father and mother."

Obedience and honor are shown in several ways: by obedient behavior and attitudes, by contributing to a good family name through outstanding achievement in some aspect of life, and by using

Many Vietnamese family names originated during the various dynasties that ruled in Indochina during the past 3000 years. There were about 100 family names for over 56 million people, and of those 100 names, "only a score" are in common usage today (Huynh, 1987). "*Nguyên*" (near pronunciation is /Nwee-un/) is the family name for more than 25% of the Vietnamese family units in the United States and Canada. With so many persons having the same family name, it has limited usefulness in identification; therefore, given names are used.

Names in Vietnam are always written family name first, middle name (or names) second, and given name last, for example, "Nguyên Thi Hông" or "Trân Văn Hai." The same names may be used for males and females, and the middle name can be a clue as to gender. "Văn" used as a middle name usually indicates male gender (Trân Văn Hai) compared with "Thị" (pronounced /Tee/), which is used for females (Nguyên Thị Hông). Sometimes several middle names are used, and therefore there is no gender indicator.

After marriage a woman keeps her maiden name and does not combine it with her husband's name. Informally she may be called by her given name or her husband's given name ("Mrs. Hai"), but formally she uses her full maiden name preceded by "*Bà*," which can be used as a respectful 'Mrs.' Children take their father's family name. Customs are changing in the United States, but to avoid confusion, many Vietnamese-American wives are adopting their husband's family name. Either name may be used depending on the setting, and children have interesting choices when asked for "mother's name."

Given names usually have special meanings, often describing the baby or expressing the hopes of the parents for the baby. Names can be chosen from virtues or from nature or music; for example, "Hông" means 'rose' and "Xuân" means 'spring'. At home or in the village, people may be called by their number in the sibling ranking, rather than by their given names, which explains the "nicknames" of "Nam" ('fifth') or "Bây" ('seventh').

Today, many babies born in the United States are given both an American name and a Vietnamese name. This is not a new practice for the Vietnamese. During the past half century, for example, the Chinese Vietnamese were commanded by law to change their Chinese given names to Vietnamese names. These persons may also have taken a Christian name when they converted to Christianity. In this resettlement period almost every Vietnamese child who has an English first name can also give a Vietnamese name if asked.

Except for close friends and coworkers, Vietnamese custom dictates that a person's name is used with a title, never alone. An example of this in English would be "Mr. Bill," "Mrs. Mary," "Director James," or "Uncle John." Titles are important and therefore should be selected carefully by the speaker to convey appropriate respect as well as sometimes to place emotional distance between the conversationlist and the listener.

the detailed kinship terminology that carefully designates the place of each person in relationship to the others. Parents consider it very important to train their children, and this responsibility is usually shared by members of the extended family living in the household, especially the grandparents. Personal interests and destiny are seldom considered outside the framework of the immediate and extended family. Behavior or misbehavior (juvenile delinquency, academic failure, mental disorders, and so on) reflects on the entire family and has great significance beyond the person involved. If personal feelings or ambitions might disrupt family harmony, the individual could be expected to restrain from taking action and to sacrifice personal wishes.

Socialized role of children

Children are similarly socialized at a very early age as to roles in the family. If a very young child is made to feel guilty or ashamed of his or her role, the child will likely develop a poor self-concept.

Role reversals are common in United States society because of the pluralistic nature of the country. When families, out of dictated needs, are forced to reverse roles, a great deal of stress and anxiety will likely accompany the reversals. For example, many Vietnamese Americans after arriving in the United States were forced to reverse traditional roles. Those who were traditionally the providers became the "recipients." For example, Vietnamese-American women, initially on arriving in this country, are more likely to find employment (Gold, 1992). Jobs that are traditionally identified as "women jobs" such as maids, sewing machine operators, and food service workers are more plentiful than male-oriented unskilled jobs. Thus the Vietnamese-American male was forced to reverse roles with the wife, becoming the recipient instead of the provider. Likewise, Vietnamese American children often assume the role of translator for non–English speaking parents. Because Vietnamese-American children are assimilated very rapidly into the U.S. society, they are more likely than their parents to find gainful employment (Gold, 1992). Such role reversals have caused intergenerational conflicts for Vietnamese-American families (Gold, 1992).

Education

In Vietnam, the Vietnamese experienced tremendous competition for the limited places in the high schools and universities. Before 1954 Hanoi was the educational center for Vietnam, and most of the institutions of higher learning, including the medical and dental schools, were there. Some 10 years after the Geneva Accords, South Vietnam had its own educational centers in Saigon, Hué, and Can Tho, but the demand far exceeded the supply, and many students had to either delay their education, go abroad, or, for the men, be drafted.

Today in the United States, education continues to be highly valued in the Vietnamese community. The number of Vietnamese Americans with at least a high school education decreased slightly from the 1980 census. Nevertheless, approximately 68.5% of all Vietnamese Americans 25 years of age or older have a high school education: 53.3% of Vietnamese women 25 years of age or older and 71% of Vietnamese men have at least a high school education. This compares with 78.3% of women in the same category and 78.5% of men in the same category for the rest of the general U.S. population. Vietnamese Americans continue to gain ground regarding a college education. Today, at least 12.2% of all Vietnamese women (up from 8% in 1980) 25 years of age or older and at least 22.3% of all Vietnamese men (up from 18% in 1980) 25 years of age or older have a college education (U.S. Department of Commerce, Bureau of the Census, 1993b), compared with 23.0%

of women in the same category and 23.5% of men in the same category for the rest of the general U.S. population (U.S. Department of Commerce, Bureau of the Census, 1993d). This statistic is remarkable, considering that either these students or their families have come to this country within the past 15 years.

Religion

Vietnam has a history of religious tolerance except for the period immediately before the French takeover, when Christians were suspected of being spies. Religious beliefs in Vietnam have been strongly influenced by several different religions, including Buddhism, Confucianism, and Taoism. Buddhism was introduced from China and India by the second century of our era. Buddhism is considered less an organized orthodoxy than a state of mind using the Four Noble Truths taught by Buddha: (1) life is suffering, (2) suffering is caused by desire, (3) suffering can be eliminated by eliminating desire, and (4) to eliminate desire, one must follow the eightfold path of right understanding, purpose, speech, conduct, vocation, effort, thinking, and meditation.

The Buddhist truths have played a large part in molding the Vietnamese characteristics of stoicism, strong self-control, and apparent passivity. Some clients, by implication, may attribute physical pain and suffering to failure to be righteous. There is much variation in specific application of Buddhist thought in Vietnam because of the many forms of Buddhism and a wide range of commitment.

Confucianism also came to Vietnam from China and is a code of ethics rather than a true religion. Confucianism emphasizes hierarchy of society, worship of ancestors, and respect for age, customs, teacher, and family.

Taoism originated from a Chinese philosopher in the sixth century BC and has been very influential in the Vietnamese culture. *Tao* (or *dào*), or 'The Way', is a creative principle that orders the physical universe. Taoism emphasizes that when things are allowed to take their natural course, they move toward harmony and perfection. Therefore individuals should attempt to blend into the natural world rather than trying to conquer it.

Two minor religious sects, Cao Đài ('high-tower') and Hòa Hảo ('harmony'), began in Vietnam in 1919 and 1939. The former is a combination of the three chief religions (Buddhism, Confucianism, and Taoism) along with teachings of Jesus, Victor Hugo, and others. Hòa Hảo is a reformed Buddhist sect. In Vietnam these religions have a combined total of about 3 million followers. Another belief system, animism, continues to have a strong influence in Vietnam, especially among the tribal people. Animism includes many practices to deal with demons, evil spirits, angry gods, and elements of the natural world that are not understood.

The first Catholic missionary arrived in Vietnam in 1513, and the Jesuits came in the early 1600s. Protestantism came to Vietnam in the early 1900s. Today in Vietnam, Catholics and Protestants number over 2 million, with Protestant membership doubling to near 500,000 since 1975. Buddhists claim approximately two thirds of the country's 71 million people (Hiebert, 1993a).

Death beliefs and practices

The religious beliefs of many Vietnamese-American people are often a rather vague synthesis of the three traditional "religions," along with one or more forms of ancestral worship or veneration of the dead. Through such rites as cleaning the ancestral graves and celebrations on the anniversary of a death, the family ties are reinforced and strengthened. In fact, part of family loyalty for the Vietnamese is an obligation that extends even beyond death in the form of properly remembering their parents and caring for their tombs. Many of these practices are so woven into the fabric of Vietnamese life that it is difficult to separate them into either religious or cultural practices. In any case, because most of the ancestors are buried in Vietnam, the custom of gathering the family in the family home around the family altar or at the tombs in celebration is impossible to duplicate in another country, and this leaves a painful void for many refugee-generation Vietnamese persons who are serious about filial piety and properly honoring their ancestors.

When the health care team anticipates that a Vietnamese client may die, the head of the family, usually the parents or eldest child, should be informed first. A priest or monk may be called to provide assistance. The decision to not resuscitate is a sensitive issue and a decision that should be made by the entire family. If a Vietnamese patient is terminally ill, the client will prefer to die at home with dignity and with his or her family. If the client dies in the hospital, some families may cry loudly and uncontrollably while others may pray. Some families will want to wash the body (Ferrales, 1996; Shanahan & Brayshaw, 1995). Box 18-3 compares Oriental and American views on the meaning of life, illness, and death.

Values

Respect and harmony are the two most important values in the Vietnamese culture and are based on the three major religious belief systems that have dominated the country. When the beliefs common to the Oriental, or Eastern, system found in Vietnam and those of the Occidental, or Western, system found in the United States are compared (Box 18-4), the nature and extent of the conflict and frustration experienced by Vietnamese undergoing acculturation in the United States become readily apparent (Cao, 1986; Nguyen, 1988a).

Implications for nursing care

Because of the high priority on respect, harmony, filial piety, and material sharing built into the Vietnamese family and extended family system, both the immediate and the extended family serve a significant role in providing emotional, physical, and economic support for the Vietnamese people. The nurse must include family members in planning care and use the family to assist the client in regaining physical and mental health. For the Vietnamese-American client, family members provide a network that provides a feeling of interdependence, belonging, and support (Cook & Timberlake, 1984).

TIME

The Vietnamese culture dates back thousands of years, and this antiquity is reflected in an orientation to time with an emphasis on the past. Emphasis is placed on ancestors and their wishes, memories, and

---

Box 18-3

MEANING OF LIFE, ILLNESS, AND DEATH

ORIENTAL	AMERICAN
Life	
Life = suffering	Life = happiness, health, opportunity
One's life is determined by various factors out of one's control.	One has control over one's own life
Your life is not yours	Your life is your own
Death and illness	
Part of normal life cycle	Disruption of normal life cycle
Bad luck, result of former deeds and so forth	Personal failure
Something to be accepted and dealt with calmly	Something to be beaten
Response to illness	
Ideal response: serenity, stoicism	Seeking control, fighting (beating) illness, heroic self-healing
Possible problems	
Helplessness	The burden of having to be positive
Denial	Sense of personal failure
Depression	Anger, depression, difficulty letting go
Sick role	
Permission for regression and dependency	Little permission for regression and dependency
Cooperation	Participation
Conflicts over unmet expectations and dependency needs	Conflicts over losing independence and control

From Nilchaikovit, K., Hill, J., & Holland, J. (1993). *General Hospital Psychiatry, 15,* 41-50.

Box 18-4

COMPARISON OF EASTERN AND WESTERN VALUE SYSTEMS

ORIENTAL, OR EASTERN, SYSTEM	OCCIDENTAL, OR WESTERN, SYSTEM
Harmony with nature	Mastery of nature (skyscraper)
Tradition	Change, innovation
Hierarchy	Mobility, upward or downward movement
Age	Youth
Extended family (few family names)	Nuclear family, small, individualistic
Convergent thinking	Divergent thinking
Cyclical concept of time	Specific point, schedules, clocks
Group orientation and reward	Self-concept and self-actualization
Rote learning	Discovery learning
Conformity	Competition

---

graves. Most Vietnamese people have been oriented to think of time in terms of cycles, events, or occurrences (Hoang & Erickson, 1982). Many Vietnamese individuals, even those who are not Buddhist, have some belief in reincarnation. This cultural heritage makes time less of a fixed point (here and gone) and more of a recurring reality. In other words, there was yesterday, there is today, and there will be tomorrow . . . which will in fact be today, followed by tomorrow . . . and so on. This belief results in a less stressful and less time-conscious pace than that commonly experienced in the West. Being late or early is not considered a problem.

As refugees, Vietnamese people practiced a present and future orientation as they struggled to survive and focused on food, housing, employment, transportation, child care, and education. Today, Vietnamese Americans have goals for the future and save for the future, and for many the motivation to live wisely may not only be to please the ancestors (past), but may also be connected with "the good life" (present) or the anticipation of heaven or reincarnation (future).

Implications for nursing care

The nurse should be aware that the concept of illness prevention requires both a future and a present time orientation. Illness prevention is a difficult concept if a person lacks a scientific understanding of disease processes. The nurse should also be aware that Vietnamese-American clients may believe that luck and fate play a significant role in suffering and that illness may be considered a result of spiritual failure or punishment. For Vietnamese Americans the act of seeking medical care is influenced by many factors, including time orientation.

Time orientation also affects a client's tendency to return for clinic or medical appointments. Because Vietnamese Americans think of time more in terms of cycles than as a specific point of reference, arriving at an exact time for an appointment may be considered less important than some other things. However, through assimilation and acculturation, many Vietnamese Americans have developed an understanding that punctuality is very important to persons in the United States and often arrive for appointments ahead of the designated time.

Noncompliance with keeping appointments is often a result of other factors in addition to time orientation. Some noncompliance can be traced to not understanding oral or appointment card communications or not being able to read the instructions. It is important for the nurse to review carefully the appointment card and any instructions given to the client to clarify what is written and to ensure that the client can read the information given. When a client is given a phone number to call for an appointment or for assistance, it is also important that the nurse ascertain whether the client knows how to use the available telephone and has the clinic telephone number. Understanding and arriving at a clinic appointment on time can be a complex transcultural assignment for a Vietnamese-American client.

Time orientation also contributes to the frustration of the nurse attempting to obtain a chronological sequence of the history of an illness. Especially rural Vietnamese may think of occurences in relation to important life events such as births, marriages or deaths, rather than a specific date on the calendar. Sometimes the nurse can move through an impasse by referring to one of these, "Did you start having these stomach pains before your husband died or since then?"

ENVIRONMENTAL CONTROL
Concepts of Illness

The medical system in Vietnam is a complex one, providing various options for health care from which the Vietnamese person may choose. Many traditional Vietnamese individuals tend to combine Chinese medicine with scientific techniques brought in from the West (Tran, 1972, 1980, 1989). For most the choice is usually deliberate and purposeful but rarely rigid or restricted in any single direction. "The baseline is often a set of time-honored beliefs, customs, and usages that are faithfully followed by some, fiercely contested by others, but more or less consciously incorporated by the majority. . . ." (Tran, 1989).

Tran (1980, 1989) divided the explanations of cause of illness into three types: naturalistic (folk medicine), supernaturalistic (animistic beliefs), and metaphysical (the theory of hot and cold). None of these theories excludes the others, and a client may explain illness by aspects of all three. A fourth explanation of illness (germs) is offered by some.

Natural causes The naturalistic explanation for illness encourages a search for a natural or obvious cause of the symptoms, such as rotten food, "poisonous water," or an obvious cause-and-effect relationship. To counteract the effects of these natural elements, an informal body of knowledge has been collected about indigenous medicinal herbs, therapeutic diets, and simple medical and hygienic measures. The information is usually transmitted orally and often treated with secrecy, remaining inside the clan or extended family. Vietnamese folk medicine may fall into the category of either *thuốc nam* ('southern medicine') or *thuốc bắc* ('northern medicine'), which more closely resembles Chinese medicine (Box 18-5).

Supernatural causes The supernaturalistic explanation for disease lays the blame on supernatural powers, such as gods, demons, or spirits. The illness is considered a punishment for a fault, for a violation of religious or ethical codes, or for an act of omission causing displeasure to a deity. In the supernaturalistic theory, disease may be caused by black magic or an evil incantation of an enemy who has bought the services of a sorcerer (Westermeyer & Winthrop, 1979).

The supernatural explanation for illness is the more likely choice of the mountain tribes people or peasants from the rural areas. The Hmong (meaning 'free'), for example, believe the individual's spirit is

---

Box 18-5

COMMON FOLK PRACTICES

1. *Cạo gió* ('rub-wind': skin rubbing with a coin) is a folk practice used for diseases caused by wind entering the body, a common cold, flulike symptoms, and so on. A layer of balm or ointment is spread on the skin over the affected area—often the chest, upper back, or shoulders. A coin (preferably the size of a nickel or quarter) is pressed on the skin and drawn in one direction, and the coin is moved a short distance on the skin without breaking the skin. This is repeated several times, and if dark blood appears under the skin, the treatment is considered to be working. Often these ecchymotic stripes are continued in symmetrical rows down the back or chest. The purpose is to create areas where the offending wind or air may escape from the body. It is usually not a painful procedure for children or adults, and most report feeling improved by the procedure (Lan, 1988; Rosenblat & Hong, 1989).

2. *Bắtgió* ('catch-wind': skin pinching) is a folk practice used for a headache. Fingers and thumbs are pressed on both temples in an attempt to move the blood across the forehead toward a spot between the eyes. After this has been repeated several times, the area on the forehead between the eyes is pinched between the thumb and forefinger and twisted slightly. If petechiae or ecchymoses appear, the treatment is considered successful. Skin pinching is also used on the neck for sore throat.

3. *Xông* is a folk practice in which Vicks VapoRub or a similar agent or herb is stirred into scalding water. Depending on the reason for the treatment, the patient may simply inhale the vapor or may be treated under a blanket as in a steam tent.

4. Inhalation of aromatic oils or liniments, such as menthol, eucalyptus, or mint-based aromatic oils, is used as a folk practice for symptoms such as motion sickness, indigestion, or cold or wind illness. The oils and liniments may be carried in vials in a pocket or purse for ready access and may be smelled when necessary; rubbed on the temple, under the nose, or on the abdomen; or taken internally in small amounts.

5. Balm and medicated plasters are a folk practice involving direct application to the skin. Many common balms, such as Red Tiger Balm, *Củ-Là-Mắc-Su*, or *Nhị Thiên Đường* oil, are available in Oriental shops, with certain balms obtainable only from an Oriental pharmacy. *Salonpas* is a Japanese preparation (Hisamitsu Pharmaceutical Co., Tosu Sagu, Japan) with widespread availability and use. Many of the ointments have a mild "deep heat" quality on application and are used for bone and muscle problems as well as a variety of other ills.

6. Herbal decoctions, soups, and condiments are used as a folk practice for a variety of symptoms and to maintain health (Spector, 1996). The more complex, involving a variety of ingredients and combinations, are prepared by a pharmacist, whereas the simpler ones are prepared at home. The recipes may be generations old and have a mystical or secret quality about them. Many medicines are prepared to be given as soups. A treatment that may have a familiar ring is the use of garlic for hypertension. There is increasing interest and experimental evaluation of Eastern herbs in Western pharmaceutical firms.

7. *Giác hơi* ('cup-vapor': cup suction) is a folk practice in which small, heated, cuplike forms applied to the skin cause a suction on the skin as the cups cool. The suction is used to remove unwanted wind or other elements from the body and is a favorite remedy for joint and muscle pains.

8. String tying is a folk practice to control spirits. This practice is more common among the mountain people. Although the string, which stays on the arm, leg, or around the neck for long periods, may become dirty, it is relatively harmless and is a source of security for the wearer and significant others. Usually it can be left on without difficulty for anyone except health care workers, who may not understand the possible significance of this practice.

---

the guardian of the person's well-being. If the spirit is happy, the person is happy and well. A severe shock or scare may cause the individual's spirit to leave, and the individual will become ill. The shaman then must come and call the spirit to return. Copper or silver bracelets, necklaces, or anklets lock the soul to oneself so that it cannot leave.

Metaphysical causes A metaphysical explanation for illness may be found in areas of Vietnam heavily influenced by the Chinese (Box 18-6). The meta-physical explanation is built on the theory that nature and the body operate within a delicate balance between two opposite elements: the *yīn* and the *yáng*, such as female and male, dark and light, or hard and soft. In medicine the opposites are expressed as "hot" and "cold," and health is the result of a balance between hot and cold elements, which results in harmonious functioning of the viscera, and harmony with the environment. An excess or shortage in either direction causes discomfort and illness.

Box 18-6

CHINESE MEDICINE

Any attempt at probing into the nature of Asian health practices must begin with a search into the age-old philosophy from which they, and indeed all Eastern concepts of health and illness, cure, and death, evolved (Branch & Paxton, 1976).

"Chinese medicine is a 5000-year-old system of medicine in which an 81-volume classic on the philosophy of life became the primary medical textbook. Body, mind, and soul are integrated and never separated. Man is seen in relationship to the environment. The system encompasses all of the following (in order of their importance as preventive concepts): philosophy, meditation, nutrition, martial arts, herbology, acumassage, acupressure, moxibustion, acupuncture, and spiritual healing (Branch & Paxton, 1976; Huard & Wong, 1968).

Part of the theoretical and philosophical basis for Chinese medicine comes from the Taoist concept that nature maintains a balance in all things and that as part of the universe, man interacts with this balance. The balance is measured in terms of energy and is articulated by the principle of *yin* and *yang* (negative/positive, dark/light, cold/hot, feminine/masculine, and so on).

An important difference between Chinese and Western medicine is the emphasis on prevention rather than disease and crisis intervention. This difference can be illustrated by the Chinese story of the "old days" when people would go to their physician to have their energy balanced. The physician, knowing the client well, would prescribe the specific approach to life, type of meditation, exercise, diet, and occasional herbs to keep the client healthy. For this service the doctor would be paid regularly. If the client became ill, however, the client stopped paying, and the treatment was free of charge. This may not be as true for Chinese medicine today, but it does underline a major difference in approach from Western medicine.

Disease theory and "germs" is another area where the basic approach separates the two systems. Western medicine has spent the past 200 years identifying disease-causing organisms under the microscope and finding ways of destroying them, in many cases with dramatic success. The goal of the treatment is to destroy the microorganisms causing the illness.

In Chinese medicine when illness results in an imbalance caused by faulty diet or strong emotional feelings, body harmony can be restored through self-restraint and the use of a corrective diet, often aided by herbs. Action is taken not to kill organisms but to restore a balanced state, countering the effects of unwise life-styles or food. When the *yin-yang* balance is disturbed, the body is more likely to become ill. Use of message, steambaths, or the application of Tiger Oil are methods to protect health and prevent illness (Spector, 1996).

All illnesses, foods, medications, and herbs are classified along a continuum according to their "hot" and "cold" qualities. Hot medications and food are used to balance the need in cold diseases and vice versa. Fever, ulcers, and infections are usually hot, though some febrile illnesses are cold. Severity, cause, and duration can influence where diseases are placed. Hot usually includes strong, rough, spicy, and oily foods. Beef, eggs, cheese, and chocolates are usually hot; chicken, fish, honey, and fresh vegetables are cold. Some fruits are hot; tropical fruits are cold. The source and how food is prepared can be significant. Almost all Western medicines are considered hot and Oriental herbs, cold. Water is usually cold but is not always advised for treatment.

Different countries and locales develop their own version of the Chinese system, and there is considerable variation in application. Knowledgeable practitioners seem reluctant to construct "lists" of hot and cold specifics, possibly because of the complexities involved in correct use. Lay people, on the other hand, often seem quite certain of what should be used and when, probably because of what their family has practiced for generations. These ideas are strongly integrated into the thought systems of many Vietnamese and can cause major stress and conflict for the client and family in the Western setting.

Germs

Some Vietnamese believe in another possible cause for illness—germs. Western medicine, with a germ-disease causation philosophy, was introduced in Vietnam by the French in the nineteenth century. Western medicine was practiced and thus available in most cities and in the military but was expensive. By 1975 there were about 2000 Western-trained physicians in Vietnam, and 70% of these were in the military. The Indochinese modern medical model that evolved, which was often described as "shotgun therapy," was based more on clinical findings than on laboratory tests and was more pragmatic than strictly scientific. Often many medicines were prescribed in the hope of conquering the offending organism. Generally, treatment plans included at least one or two injections. After the initial office visit, the client would go to a pharmacy to purchase the medications. After purchasing the medications, the next step was to visit an "injection nurse," who gave the subcutaneous intramuscular or intravenous medication the client had purchased. Tiredness or recuperation from surgery was reason enough to purchase a bolus of dextrose solution and have it injected intravenously.

Until 1975 many Vietnamese pharmacies sold any Western medicines they had, including antibiotics, over the counter without a prescription. Because Vietnamese either treated themselves or were treated by physicians with over-the-counter antibiotics, a high incidence of bacterial resistance to common antibiotics, as well as cases of agranulocytosis, developed. In the late 1960s chloramphenicol (Chloromycetin) was commonly bought as an over-the-counter drug to treat common colds and upper respiratory tract infections.

Implications for nursing care

It is important for the nurse to understand that Vietnamese-American clients sometimes do not understand illness or diagnostic and treatment procedures encountered in the Western medical system (Box 18-7). In addition, Vietnamese-American clients who adhere to Eastern practices may explain illness by disease entities that may be totally unfamiliar to Western practitioners, such as problems caused by the wind *(phong)*, an encounter with an "evil eye," or toxic substance problems, bad *karma*, problems caused by spirits, or an imbalance of hot and cold. A client who has such beliefs may use approaches that are contradictory to the recommendations of Western practitioners. For example, a client who has a febrile disease or diarrhea will be encouraged by the Western practitioner to increase fluids, whereas the theory of hot and cold may mandate that because these illnesses are cold diseases, fluids should be restricted. External use of either hot or cold water may also be restricted

according to this theory, and therefore a treatment such as a cold sponge bath may invoke dire consequences.

Another example of conflict between the theory of hot and cold and Western medicine is the requirement during illness of carefully restricting food to correct an imbalance. Fresh fruits and vegetables, which are considered cold, are often banned. Meats such as pork or chicken, but not beef, are added to the diet slowly. Milk is usually not used. Maternity clients are told to eat a very salty diet with almost no fruits or vegetables. Nutritional deficiency or starvation can inadvertently result, especially during long illnesses.

Because the theory of hot and cold has been used by Vietnamese people for generations with some success, it is important for the nurse to understand that belief in this theory is not likely to be discarded simply because Western health care practitioners do not approve of it. Rather, the nurse should assist the client and the family in combining approaches from tradition with those from Western medicine to facilitate a high level of wellness. The nurse must remember, however, that in an effort to be culturally aware there is the potential danger of responding to assumed but no longer existing cultural differences (Webster, 1991).

The nurse who conducts physical assessments of Vietnamese-American clients should be able to recognize ecchymotic areas that may result from *cạo gió* ('rub-wind': coin rubbing) and should understand that this folk practice is not harmful. Yeatman and Dang (1980) reported a study that was done with 50 Vietnamese persons 4 years after their arrival in the United States to determine the prevalence of *cạo gió* and problems created by it. The sample included students, professionals, housewives, and others. The data from the study indicated that 94% of the respondents had practiced *cạo gió* before arriving in the United States and that all the respondents claimed to have felt better after the treatment. None of the respondents reported any harm as a result of *cạo gió*. All but one of the respondents reported having practiced *cạo gió* in this country, and 26% of the respondents reported being criticized by physicians, teachers, spouse, or foster parents. One respondent

Box 18-7

COMMON MISUNDERSTANDINGS ABOUT ILLNESS AND DIAGNOSTIC OR TREATMENT PROCEDURES

1. Drawing blood for diagnostic purposes may cause a crisis for a Vietnamese-American patient. The patient may complain, though often not to the health care worker, of feeling weak and tired for varying periods after the procedure. Such symptoms may last for months. A Vietnamese-American client may feel that any body tissue or fluid removed cannot be replaced and that once it is removed, the body will continue to suffer the loss, not only in this life but also in the next life.

2. Donating blood may be a major decision for Vietnamese. In one rural hospital in Vietnam, Western staff members made an effort not only to teach the Vietnamese staff the "facts" about donating blood, but also to have the Vietnamese staff assist as the Western staff donated blood and, after a short recovery time, rejoined the medical team. Vietnamese staff members were invited to have their blood typed and to place their names on a possible donor list for emergency situations. Some did donate blood when the need arose (though, because Vietnamese often weigh less than 100 pounds, only one half or three fourths of a unit was drawn).

3. Donation of body parts, such as the donation of an eye after death, is an act that is often viewed with much skepticism by many Vietnamese individuals who have been heavily influenced by Buddhist beliefs that a body part cannot be replaced once it is removed and that the body may suffer in the next life. Even those who have been Christians for several generations may be very serious about care given to the body after death and are unlikely to feel comfortable with such practices.

4. Hospitalization and surgery were often considered a last resort in Vietnam. Unless insurance considerations are important, outpatient care for the refugee is likely to cause much less anxiety and should be offered as an option when possible.

5. Clergy visitation is usually associated with "last rites" by the Vietnamese, especially those who have been influenced by the Catholic religion. A visit by the clergy may be considered an indication that the situation is grave, and the common practice of chaplains visiting clients in hospitals in the United States can be quite upsetting for Vietnamese-American clients. It is important to provide the client with a careful explanation of a visit by the hospital clergy.

6. Giving flowers to the sick is a practice that may surprise and upset a Vietnamese-American client who has not been given an explanation of this practice. In Vietnam flowers are usually reserved for the rites of the dead.

7. American medicines are considered by Vietnamese to be much more concentrated than Eastern medicines. American medicine is likely to be given in tablet form, rather than in tea or soups. Also, Americans are often much larger than the average Vietnamese; therefore, medication needs to be carefully titrated so that it will not harm the Vietnamese-American client. It is important for the professional to let the client know that small stature has been considered when the dosage was calculated, which can be done by either weighing the client or by orally discussing this when the prescription is written. It is not an uncommon practice for some Vietnamese-American clients to take only half of their prescribed dosage.

8. The germ theory is very confusing to Vietnamese individuals who have no knowledge of this concept. Many clients with animistic beliefs have a supernatural or spirit-world disease-cause orientation. In an effort to move the client's understanding into the scientific, or natural, world, germs are presented as the cause of disease because they are a component of the real Western world. For all practical purposes, however, germs cannot be seen and are far less real to the refugee with animistic beliefs than the spirits and demons that the client knows can cause trouble.

---

had been reported by a teacher for child abuse. Today, the nurse should be aware that many Vietnamese Americans no longer practice *cạo gió* because of fear of societal condemnation, though many continue to believe in its validity. Yeatman and Dang (1980) advocate that Western practitioners should accept *cạo gió* as a "nurturant folk practice."

Although the benefits of folk medicine are likely to outweigh the risks, the nurse who provides care to

Vietnamese-American clients must be aware of possible risks for clients including the following:

1. Toxicity may result from the use of remedies containing heavy metals (lead, mercury, arsenic). In 1983, 24 Hmong children were found in the St. Paul, Minneapolis, area with excessively high lead blood levels.

2. Inadequate labeling of Chinese medicines may result in excessive use of potentially harmful

chemicals. In 1984 four cases of agranulocytosis were diagnosed in one facility in clients who had been taking one or more Chinese medicines containing phenylbutazone or aminopyrine, neither of which was listed as an ingredient.

3. Toxicity may result from human error. For example, many herbs and plants such as mushrooms and seeds found in the United States are new to Southeast Asians, and some have been mistaken for familiar ones "back home," resulting in poisonings.

4. Problems may result from misidentification of folk medicine treatments when seen by Western health professionals. For example, a child with ecchymotic areas on the back or abdomen caused by *cạo gió* may be examined and diagnosed as having been abused (Lan, 1988; Yeatman & Dang, 1980).

The nurse must be cognizant that the client's use of folk medicine practices may cause delay in seeking Western medical treatment, with dire results. For example, if a Vietnamese-American parent uses folk medicine practices for an extended period of time in the treatment of a dehydrated baby, the baby may be brought for treatment too late for Western medical practices to be effective. If a Vietnamese-American client waits until gangrene has spread too far to save the limb or if oxygen deprivation has been severe for a long time, Western medicine will probably not be beneficial. As Vietnamese-American clients experience success with Western medicine and develop positive relationships with health care providers, these clients will be less likely to retain the "old ways" and more likely to seek help before symptoms become severe.

BIOLOGICAL VARIATIONS
Body size and structure

Vietnamese people generally have small frames and build, with average body weights between 80 and 130 pounds. An overweight Vietnamese person is uncommon, except among the Vietnamese-Chinese population (Williams & Westermeyer, 1986).

Skin color

The skin coloring is usually light to medium with yellow tones. Newborns are usually fair skinned. In the United States there appears to be a higher-than-average incidence of newborn icterus among Vietnamese Americans, as compared with the rest of the general population.

Other visible physical characteristics

Noses may be small and "classically Oriental" or larger with a less-defined bridge. The eyelids usually have an epicanthic fold and a slight droop over the cartilage plate. Both variations are common to Orientals.

Teeth are usually proportionately large, with a high incidence of mandibular torus (lump on the inner side of the mandible near the second molar). Some dentists who have treated Vietnamese clients estimate that at least 40% of Vietnamese Americans have these tori, compared with 7% of the White U.S. population (Nguyen, 1988b).

Enzymatic and genetic variations

The incidence of dizygotic twin births among the Vietnamese is only one half of 1%, compared with 2% for Whites and 4% for Blacks in this country (Overfield, 1985).

Although some Vietnamese people enjoy milk, cheese, and ice cream, an unknown percentage, possibly as high as 50%, have a congenital lactase deficiency. For most Vietnamese people, the intolerance is not a total one, and many Vietnamese persons can digest milk in small amounts without incidence. For some Vietnamese individuals with some degree of lactose intolerance, a glass of milk can be an inexpensive solution for constipation (Tran, 1989). Vietnamese babies show a lesser degree of the deficiency by their ability to accept the usual formula preparations without difficulty (Bayless, 1975).

Medical problems among Vietnamese refugees

Medical problems identified in 594 persons in two groups of refugees (400 in one; 194 in the other) studied by Hoang and Erickson (1982) included the following:

1. *Skin:* superficial fungal infections and scabies, 10% to 15%.
2. *Teeth:* moderate to severe dental problems, 90%.

3. *Endocrine system:* thyroid diseases, especially goiters, 10% in the group of 400 and 6% in the group of 194.
4. *Cardiovascular system:* mitral valve prolapse, 1.7%; hypertension, 7% of adults over 30 years of age; rheumatic heart disease, 1%.
5. *Renal system:* microscopic hematuria may be present with no specific cause.
6. *Blood:* anemia, 16%.
7. *Parasites:* ascariasis, hookworm infestation, giardiasis, trichuriasis (most common), and amebiasis.
8. *Hepatitis Bs antigen (HBsAg):* 13%.
9. *Malaria:* 2.5% of the sample of 194 persons had a history of malaria, and 1% of this number developed an acute episode.
10. *Psyche:* 5% in the sample of 194 persons had "significant" psychiatric problems.

Tuberculosis risk

Although bacillus Calmette-Guérin (BCG) was widely used in Vietnam during the 1960s and was given to babies shortly after birth in hospitals across the country, the living conditions and general upheaval during the past 25 years have reduced the long-term effectiveness of any type of preventive effort. In the early 1970s there were an alarming number of active cases of tuberculosis in the South Vietnamese army, where "early TB" (stage 1) was rarely sufficient reason for discharge, and almost all cases seen at private hospitals or tuberculosis clinics were either moderate or advanced.

Between 1968 and 1974, the movement of people from the less secure countryside to the cities, with their accompanying overcrowding and poor nutritional status, simply exacerbated an already precarious situation. The case load of children with active tuberculosis being diagnosed and treated in a private tuberculosis clinic in an area of Saigon (1969 to 1970) doubled in less than 1 year, partly from newly detected cases and partly from new cases developing in crowded rooms shared with adults with active disease. Hoang and Erickson (1982) recommended the use of isoniazid prophylactically for 1 year for all refugees under 35 years of age with positive skin tests and that children with negative skin readings

on arrival in the United States be checked in 3 to 6 months to single out false-negative readings.

Cancer

The problem of utilization of screening and diagnostic services by American Vietnamese is well documented. Analysis of breast and cervical cancer among Vietnamese women provides information concerning reasons for lack of preventive care (Fry & Nguyen, 1996; Pham & McPhee, 1992; Rossiter, 1994). Records from the Cancer Hospital of Ho Chi Minh City (formerly Saigon) from 1976 to 1981 showed that cervical cancer accounted for 53.3% of all cancers diagnosed; breast cancer for 10.4%. A preliminary study of the same period in San Francisco suggested that fewer Vietnamese women were diagnosed with in situ cancer and more with advanced stages than White cancer patients were. Additionally, it was noted that there was less screening done and fewer mammograms and Pap smears among Vietnamese patients. The Vietnamese population in California increased 212% from the early 1980s to the early 1990s. With multiple life changes and crises in adjustment to breast self-examination and an annual Pap smear, if the women had the information on these screening tests, they were likely a low priority. Further, the incidence of these types of cancer in this population was not available to the doctors treating these clients. Yet another factor compounding the fatal outcome was the reticence of Vietnamese females to discuss these kinds of problems with their new doctors. A later study of Vietnamese women in the San Francisco area found these five reasons given for not having breast and cervical screening tests: (1) lack of physician recommendation, (2) patient lack of knowledge, (3) embarrassment, (4) cost, and (5) language difficulty. More than half said that they did not know the risk factors and a third did not know the common signs. Even when the women were given a screening invitation in writing, often they were unable to read it because it was in English.

Nutritional preferences

A common staple in Vietnam is rice, which is eaten from large bowls with chopsticks several times a day, often with dark green leafy vegetables. Fish sauce is added for saltiness and flavor. One way a client may describe a medical problem to a doctor is to hold a hand up in the form of a bowl and say, "Now I eat only one bowl of rice at a meal instead of three the way I used to do."

Rice, as well as many other cooked dishes, is seasoned with the unique Vietnamese condiment *nước mắm* ('fish sauce'), which is made by marinating small fish in salt in kegs for a month or more. When this condiment is used on rice, water, sugar, fresh lime juice, garlic, and chili peppers are added. In Vietnam dark green leafy vines or plants are gathered from the countryside or from gardens and brought in to the local village or small-town markets in truckloads each morning. Although not served in large quantities, the regular presence of these greens with rice contributes to a diet with adequate nutrients despite the lack of meat or meat substitutes. Meat, when served, is cut into slivers and eaten with rice and vegetables. Chicken and duck eggs are used as available. Bean curd is used, but (dry) bean dishes are uncommon. For the most part, milk and milk products are imported, expensive, and generally discouraged because a large percentage of the population has lactose intolerance.

During the long French occupation, bread was introduced into Vietnam and was widely consumed in the form of small tasty French rolls, available fresh daily on the street corners in cities and towns. French pastries were also available. Today, many Vietnamese people replace some of their rice with fresh white bread.

According to the U.S. Department of Agriculture, Food and Nutrition Service, the traditional Vietnamese diet is low in fat and sugar, high in complex carbohydrates, and moderate in fiber. These levels compare very favorably with the dietary guidelines of the U.S. Department of Agriculture and the U.S. Department of Health and Human Services (Burtis, Davis, & Martin, 1988).

Depending on where the Vietnamese refugees live in the United States and Canada, the traditional diet has changed considerably. With more meat and fat available, many Vietnamese persons are increasing their fat intake. In cities with large concentrations of

Vietnamese Americans, the ingredients to prepare almost all the ethnic foods, including *nước mắm*, are likely to be available. Many Vietnamese Americans enjoy preparing native Vietnamese dishes as well as dining in Vietnamese restaurants. In Vietnam, brown, unpolished grains were considered the food of the mountain people and were almost never eaten by the more sophisticated lowlanders; in the United States, except for those Vietnamese Americans who take nutrition facts seriously, polished rice and white bread continue to be a favorite among the Vietnamese people (Tien-Hyatt, 1989).

A favorite Vietnamese dish is a variation of Chinese noodle soup called *phở* (pronounced /phuh/). The dish is made by placing cooked rice noodles in a delicately flavored, clear, boiling broth, adding thinly sliced beef or chicken that is rare or fully cooked (or both kinds), and finally topping the mixture with scallions and black pepper. At the table a lime slice, bean sprouts, and *quế* ('cinnamon') leaves may be added to taste. Although *phở* was a morning meal in Vietnam, in the United States it may be served in *phở* shops at any hour of the day.

Although in Vietnam tea was associated with social etiquette (all guests were served tea) and potable cold water was a luxury many did not enjoy, because of immigration many Vietnamese Americans have begun to drink water, other soft drinks, coffee, and some milk and have begun to drink less tea. Among Vietnamese in Vietnam and Vietnamese Americans, poor liquid intake has been related to bladder stones in small boys and in men (Hoang & Erickson, 1982).

Psychological characteristics

Mental health The term "psychiatrist," or "mental doctor," has no direct Vietnamese translation. There is a slightly better understanding with the term that translates as "nerve doctor," but by far the best comprehension comes with an explanation of "a specialist who treats crazy people" (Tran, 1989).

In the Vietnamese culture there is recognition of two possible sources of mental disease: the organic model, which considers damaged nerves or the brain, and the inorganic model, in which the less comprehensible phenomena of bizarre behavior may be attributed to various causes such as disobedience, sin, or demon possession.

Vietnamese often believe the nervous system to be the source of all mental and physical activities. Therefore, when there is a disturbance in mental or physical activity, the nervous system is considered central to the malfunction. Neuroses are called "weaknesses of the nerves," a term used to describe many kinds of anxiety, depression, weariness, mental deterioration, and retardation. Psychoses, on the other hand, are known as "turmoil of the nerves," more accurately reflecting the client's behavior or feelings (Tran, 1989).

For some Vietnamese people, most illnesses associated with the nerves precipitate optimistic feelings about the possibility of treatment with folk remedies: a nerve tonic to restore strength to weak nerves or a calming medicine to quiet inner turmoil. For some Vietnamese people, medication is the logical answer, although there is concern about dependency, oversedation, or mind-altering medicines. Most Vietnamese seek help from a Western psychiatrist or health professional only after their problems have become too obvious to be ignored (Westermeyer & Winthrop, 1979).

Evaluation of severity and decisions on treatment of refugee psychiatric problems by Western psychiatric professionals is extremely difficult. Language is only one major hurdle; understanding "normal behavior" expected and making acceptable social responses to stress, family decisions, or interactions contribute significantly toward workable solutions. In response to problems created by the language barrier in assessing Vietnamese-American clients, Kinzie, Manson, Do, et al. (1982) developed a Vietnamese Language Depression Rating Scale that can assist the practitioner in the evaluation of the severity of the depression. Because many Vietnamese refugees are not used to verbal expression of emotion and thought, "amobarbital interviews" are used by some psychiatric practitioners to both assess and treat symptoms of depression (Lee, 1985; Owen, 1985). The variables affecting the mental health of Vietnamese refugees arriving in this country are profound and complex, and establishing a healthy equilibrium takes time and effort.

Emotional and behavioral manifestations of distress in refugees Immigration is a complex circumstance that exacts a serious toll in terms of mental turmoil and distress, which may be referred to as "culture shock" (Pickwell, 1989; Williams & Westermeyer, 1986). Hoang and Erickson (1982) reported that psychiatric problems may become more obvious 6 to 12 months after immigration. Psychologically the distress is often experienced as a combination of depression and anxiety (Lin, Masuda, & Tazuma, 1982; Rumbaut, 1977; Tyhurst, 1977). As is often noted, individuals going through a life crisis, such as immigrating to a new land as a refugee, tend to exhibit behavioral disturbances (Lin, Masuda, & Tazuma, 1982; Nguyen, 1981). Somatic preoccupations, marital conflicts, intergenerational conflicts, substance abuse, and sociopathic behavior may all be manifestations of the stress of adjustment to a new culture.

The emotional and behavioral problems of refugees are often related to (1) loss of immediate and extended family, (2) overemployment or underemployment, and (3) stresses of adaptation. Because of the great differences between the Eastern and Western cultures and the traumatic conditions under which the immigration occurred, the culture shock experienced by many Vietnamese refugees is profound. Because Vietnamese people place a high value on self-control in speech and behavior and are used to dealing with family problems within the family structure, the refugee situation, in which family structure is incomplete or missing, has contributed to feelings of isolation, helplessness, and disorganization. Additional problems are found when families go through the acculturation process together, yet members react individually. Nguyen (1988b) stated that "prolonged closeness often creates friction; compulsory intimacy may generate irritation; exposure of the younger generation to the American culture often is the origin of conflict; and constant expectations of mutual dependency may turn into hateful obligations and be a source of mental illness."

Often compounding this problem is the language barrier between Vietnamese refugees and those who try to help them. With so much change and often with the very foundations of the Vietnamese society under attack (that is, deterioration of the ties with the family unit: the ancestors, grandparents, or parents), the conflicts may become overt crises that move "toward outcomes which are more likely to be radical and disruptive" (Nguyen, 1988b).

General patterns of coping and adaptation A general pattern of coping and adaptation is experienced by many persons in their cultural adjustment to immigration (Cook & Timberlake, 1984).

Stage I For the first few months there is a positive attitude and high expectations; energy is focused toward language, employment, and meeting basic needs. The excitement of a new physical environment and "things" helps suppress the pain of the multiple losses.

Stage II The period of "psychological arrival" occurs 6 to 18 months after immigration, when the person becomes more aware of losses and "the past" becomes idealized. Survivor's guilt must be faced. (Why did I survive and my child did not?) Posttraumatic stress disorder (PTSD) is common, and all the normal tensions of close family life are magnified. Interpersonal conflict is common. Other symptoms may be feelings of hopelessness, acute distress and grief, fatigue, and mood instability. The period may be transitory or long lasting, mild or severe, and seems to occur regardless of how much help or support has been given. It is usually a very frustrating time for sponsors and "helping persons," who feel inadequate to help. During this period somatization is common.

Stage III After 18 to 24 months the person is able to reformulate the grief and get involved with the tasks at hand. There is less idealizing of the past, and helping those left behind becomes important. Adaptation moves ahead at a more rapid rate as former ways of coping are given up for more effective ones. A new self-identity emerges.

Cook and Timberlake (1984) list denial as the defense mechanism most often used by Vietnamese refugees. The authors believe that denial is congruent with the values of the culture: submission to the common good (and to fate), harmony, and self-sacrifice. Denial is needed to lessen the profound effect of losses and to allow the refugees to go on with the task of survival. When denial fails, facing

the hard realities without the needed support systems sometimes causes "uprooting psychosis," withdrawal, and inappropriate behavior (Cook & Timberlake, 1984).

Posttraumatic stress disorder The stress of immigration has been found to be particularly difficult for Southeast Asian women. Fox, Cowell, & Johnson (1995) identify that the chief role of Southeast Asian women is meeting the needs of husband, children, and the extended family. Many Southeast Asian women, especially those who came to America as "boat people," suffered the atrocities of Pol Pot, lost family through sickness, separation, starvation, drowning, or even killing, and experienced great trauma. For many, premigration experiences have continued to produce great emotional stress years into the resettlement period (Fox, Cowell, & Johnson, 1995).

The exact relationship between premigration and postmigration experiences and adaptation continues to be unclear (Fox, Cowell, & Johnson, 1995). There is a continuing debate regarding the relationship to high rates of mental health disorders among the South East Asian refugees. Empirical testing is difficult because of factors such as communication barriers and varying perception of mental health concepts (Fry & Nguyen, 1996). Nicholson (1997) noted that current stressors allowed more strongly the prediction of mental health outcomes. However, experienced events did allow prediction of posttraumatic stress disorder (PTSD) more strongly than either anxiety or depression did (Nicholson, 1997). Symptoms of PTSD include sleep disturbances, inability to form close relationships, anxiety, compulsive thoughts, and startle reactions (Fox, Cowell, & Johnson, 1995). By 1984, Southeast Asian refugees were being diagnosed with PTSD, and by 1987 half the Southeast Asian refugee outpatients at a psychiatric clinic were found to have diagnosable PSTD (Fox, Cowell, & Johnson, 1995). The percentage of Cambodians who have been diagnosed with PSTD is unusually high (Fox, Cowell, & Johnson, 1995).

Somatic preoccupation Somatization is viewed as being common among Southeast Asian refugees. In a Chinese-influenced culture where overt expression of anxiety, disappointment, or anger is considered failure, a high value is placed on suppressing negative feelings; therefore, expressing mental distress through various physical ailments may be an acceptable option. One study reported that among Chinese clients with mental disorders, as many as 88% of the respondents complained of somatic ailments without admitting to feelings of anxiety or mental discomfort, compared with 4% in a group of clients without the influence of the Chinese culture (Eyton & Neuwirth, 1984). These data are suggestive that Vietnamese immigrants may be more agreeable to seeing a physician for physical problems (Eyton & Neuwirth, 1984).

Drug interactions and metabolism

Alcohol is metabolized differently in different groups and in different races. For example, in Whites, alcohol is metabolized by the liver enzyme alcohol dehydrogenase. In Asians, it is metabolized by acetaldehyde dehydrogenase, which works faster, often causing circulatory and unpleasant effects such as facial flushing and palpitations (Kudzma, 1992). With alcohol use, facial flushing occurs in 45% to 85% of Asians, compared with 3% to 29% of Whites (Chan, 1986). In addition, caffeine, a component of many drugs as well as coffee, tea, and colas, appears to be metabolized and excreted faster by Whites than by Asians (Grant, 1983).

Implications for nursing care

The small body size of many Vietnamese-American clients has an important implication in terms of nursing treatment. Some nurses have delayed giving pain medication to a Vietnamese-American client in pain "since the client is so tiny" (Tien-Hyatt, 1989). Because Vietnamese-American clients may be stoic, it is important for the nurse to evaluate carefully the need for pain medication and to provide sufficient medication without delay (Lin & Finder, 1983; Tien, 1984; Tien-Hyatt, 1989). Some studies have suggested that the Vietnamese individuals have a pharmacodynamic difference in therapeutic response to psychotropics. In a study by Lin, Poland, Nuccio, et al. (1989), the Asian client's mean required dose was significantly lower than the average for optimal clinical therapeutic response as well as the emer-

gence of extrapyramidal symptoms, when haloperidol was administered. This study and others have suggested that Asian clients generally respond to substantially lower doses of neuroleptics (Murphy, 1969; Rosenblat & Tang, 1987).

Smither and Rodríguez-Giegling (1979) have noted that within the first 5 years after leaving Vietnam, personality and coping are the more important determinants of which acculturation patterns develop. Other significant factors are level of income and social class (Smither & Rodríguez-Giegling, 1979). Crystal (1989) has suggested that an additional complicating factor is the myth of the model minority. According to the model-minority myth, Asian Americans' cultural traits, which include diligence, frugality, and willingness to sacrifice, propel their upward mobility and win them public accolades. In reality, the model-minority myth has obscured many serious problems in the Asian community and has been used to justify omitting Asian Americans from federal funding and some special minority programs. The Asian-American success story for some has been an obstacle rather than the norm.

In the difficult everyday situations needing translations in psychiatric evaluation and counseling, the use of bilingual paraprofessionals is gaining increasing attention (Leung, 1988). Professionals and clients readily recognize that the person communicating between them is indeed a key person in determining the outcome of this effort. When the inherent potential of the "translator" is recognized, persons can be selected and trained in techniques of information gathering, importance of not screening the reporting, confidentiality, and so on. When this interpreter is welcomed as a colleague on the team, the client also comes to see this person not only as a member of "my team," the only possibility of communicating my problem, but also as a respected member of "their team" who is trying to help. Trained or untrained, the paraprofessional often becomes the first source of help Vietnamese-American clients turn to because they are hesitant to contact the professional with personal or family matters.

The nurse should also recognize that for many

Vietnamese-American clients, food is medicine. Many Vietnamese Americans are able to practice their food beliefs without difficulty. However, if a client develops a health problem and encounters Western medical practitioners, the need to adopt Western food practices may be considered necessary for survival, such as the need for fluids, the restriction of salt, the need for specific medications (such as cardiac medications), and the need for specific nutrients in the diet. Helping the client to understand why dietary restrictions have been recommended is essential. A client may be willing to limit the amount of *nước mắm* in the diet when health care professionals carefully explain the reason for this request. For many Vietnamese Americans, eating habits are changing. Children are learning to eat hamburgers, french fries, pizza, spaghetti, and tacos in school lunch programs. Vietnamese Americans are pragmatists, and teaching about dietary practices in relation to Western medicine can result in changed behavior.

Another important health care issue for the nurse who provides care for Vietnamese-American clients is utilization of health care resources. Tran (1980) suggested that utilization of health care services is related to the identification of a problem and the availability of an appropriate service. A study by Strand and Jones (1983) found that health services utilization is not directly correlated with education and English-language skills but is related to a variety of factors. For example, working two jobs makes it difficult to take time for a clinic appointment. The person who speaks English best and those persons who should accompany the client to the health facility are usually at work or at school. A car or a baby sitter may be unavailable. Choosing health care may be difficult. The options for health care are fewer than they were in Vietnam, and even wealthy Vietnamese persons may have problems finding health care providers who understand the Vietnamese language. *A Model for Providing Health Maintenance and Promotion to Children from Low-Income, Ethnically Diverse Backgrounds* (Phan, 1996) reports how taking the clinic to the community and working with individual families in their own environment helped eliminate many of the utilization problems.

Another deterrent for some Vietnamese Americans in the utilization of health services is integration into ethnic subcommunities. For a minority group that has found learning English and the process of acculturation difficult, surrounding themselves with familiar life-styles, language, friends, or family has made loneliness less of a problem. For such individuals, traditional beliefs and superstitions survive far more readily in these subcommunities than in the "outside world." In such situations decisions are more likely to be made by the client's extended family and community.

The majority of health care problems do not occur or at least are not reported by Vietnamese refugees during the initial settlement period. This may result from the fact that immediately before or after arrival the refugees are routinely screened and treated for existing problems. After the excitement of arriving and getting settled, however, previously untreated health problems often become evident. Silverman (1977) reported that in Denver 80% of Vietnamese-American clients waited 5 days after the initial onset of illness before seeing a physician and at least 75% failed to return for follow-up care.

SUMMARY

It is important for the nurse to recognize that although many similarities exist among Vietnamese Americans, many variations also exist among subgroups and generations. Geographic origin, sex, age, and individual idiosyncrasies may all contribute to variations in response to the American health care system. The customs, values, and health beliefs and practices of Vietnamese-American clients are an important consideration for the Western health care professional (Tripp-Reimer & Thieman, 1981). Most Vietnamese Americans have retained some folk medicine beliefs that affect not only explanations for causes of symptoms, but also the type of treatment that will be selected. The nurse who develops a knowledge and understanding of these beliefs, as well as sensitivity to the refugee's lack of familiarity with the American health care system, will promote more effective health care delivery and will ease the Vietnamese-American client's adjustment to the new country.

The importance of the nurse in teaching, modeling, and encouraging health promotion and illness prevention practices among children of the Vietnamese immigrants cannot be overemphasized. As Nguyen et al. (1988, p. 176) state, "Children can learn to make positive health behaviors an integral part of their lives." Understandably for their parents, ideas of illness and treatment are deeply ingrained. However, Vietnamese-American children who are immersed in new ideas and change, who understand the new language, and who can be taught germ theory and the benefits of immunization can learn to make important health decisions that will influence their lives and the lives of their children.

Case Study

Mr. Yen Van Nguyen is a 26-year-old man who has recently arrived in the United States from Vietnam with his wife and 2-year-old son, Tran. Yen arrives at a local emergency room one evening carrying his son, Tran, and gesturing that his son needs medical attention because he has been running a low-grade fever, sneezing, and coughing for the past 2 days. Yen speaks very poor English and appears to be somewhat excited.

The emergency room nurse takes Tran back to an examination room where she can get him undressed and into a gown for examination by the physician. While undressing Tran, the nurse notices bruising over the sternum and along the spine and immediately summons the physician. On examination the physician notices that the bruised areas do not appear tender but nevertheless suspects child abuse. The child's father, Yen, is escorted back to the child's room by a hospital security officer, where he is questioned by the physician. Yen speaks very poor English, and communication is difficult. The harder the physician tries to communicate with Yen, the more frustrated both the physician and Yen become.

A young Vietnamese woman who works in housekeeping is requested to report to the emergency department to help with the communication problem between the emergency room staff and Yen. After a short discussion with Yen, the young Vietnamese woman explains the custom of *cạo gió* ('rub-wind'), or "coin rubbing," to the emergency room staff. On further examination the physician can find no other evidence of child abuse. The emergency staff realize that the bruising is from the coin rubbing and not from child abuse as initially suspected. The child is given an injection of an antibiotic and discharged.

CARE PLAN

 Nursing Diagnosis   Communication, impaired verbal, related to foreign-language barrier

Client Outcomes

1. Parent will be able to communicate more effectively customs and beliefs used in treating illnesses, and nurse will better understand these customs.

Nursing Interventions

1. Determine parent's understanding and ability to communicate in English.
2. Talk slowly, enunciating words.
3. Face parent and speak in a slow, clear voice.
4. Use gestures to convey meanings, but do not use excessive "touching."
5. Attempt to locate a translator for assistance.
6. Provide parent adequate space to communicate without "crowding."
7. Keep language simple.

Nursing Diagnosis Fear related to Americans' misunderstanding of Vietnamese culture with a potential for prosecution for child abuse

Client Outcome

1. Parent will experience reduced fear with awareness of nurse's understanding of Vietnamese cultural folk medicine.

Nursing Interventions

1. Allow parent to explain Vietnamese traditional folk medicine.
2. Provide parent with a quiet area to help reduce fears.
3. Attempt to communicate in a nonthreatening manner.
4. Recruit others familiar with Vietnamese culture to help parent explain.
5. Remove persons perceived as threatening to parent.

 Nursing Diagnosis Knowledge deficit related to modern medical practices secondary to cultural differences

Client Outcome

1. Parent will demonstrate an understanding of importance of modern medical treatment in conjunction with traditional folk medicine.

Nursing Interventions

1. Explain to parent importance of modern medical care in conjunction with cultural folk medicine.
2. Determine parent's perception of medical model of treatment.
3. Keep language simple; avoid long medical terms.
4. Explain importance of compliance with medical treatment ordered.
5. Keep instructions simple and brief.
6. Arrange for an interpreter to help explain importance of seeking medical attention for illness or injury.

 Nursing Diagnosis Parental role conflict related to child's present illness and need to seek "foreign" medical attention

Client Outcome

1. Parent will demonstrate an understanding of importance of seeking qualified medical attention for betterment of child's well-being.

Nursing Interventions

1. Educate parent on importance of seeking medical attention to treat illnesses.
2. Provide parent the opportunity to describe how similar situations were handled.
3. Assess past medical practices and folklore that the parent normally uses in similar situations.
4. Allow parent time to ask questions related to child's health care.
5. Provide information in a clear, concise, easy-to-understand manner.

Nursing Diagnosis Noncompliance (risk for) related to misunderstanding of the prescribed treatment secondary to the belief that medications in the Western world are much stronger than those found in the Far East

Client Outcomes

1. Parent will demonstrate an understanding of prescribed treatment and importance of following prescribed medical regimen.

Nursing Interventions

1. Assess parent's fear of prescribed treatment.
2. Promote health teaching to educate parent on the effects, desired outcome, and side effects of prescribed medicine.
3. Warn parent that some medications may make the client sleepy and that this is an expected occurrence.
4. Teach parent about importance of adhering to prescribed medical treatment.
5. Reassure parent that prescribed medication is appropriate and safe for client.
6. Review medication, dosage, and proper administration technique to help parent feel more comfortable with the treatment.

 Nursing Diagnosis Coping, ineffective family: compromised, related to illness of a family member and the necessity to seek culturally unfamiliar medical treatment

Client Outcomes

1. Family members will be better able to cope with illness-related problems after obtaining information on prescribed medical treatment.

Nursing Interventions

1. Reassure parent of appropriateness of prescribed medical treatment.
2. Provide parent the opportunity to express fears and concerns.
3. Encourage parent to verbalize familiar treatments that family sought in Vietnam, including customs and folk medicine.
4. Direct parent to areas of potential help (such as churches, Vietnamese communities, social workers).
5. Instruct parent on how to perform prescribed treatment to increase feelings of being needed.

 Nursing Diagnosis Role performance, altered (risk for), related to undue stress of an ill family member in an unfamiliar culture

Client Outcomes

1. Parent will discuss feelings of altered role performance and identify areas of undue stress.

Nursing Interventions

1. Encourage parent to talk openly about actual or potential areas of stress.
2. Provide quiet area for parent to gather thoughts.
3. Help parent to understand what resources are available in the community (such as self-help groups).
4. Reassure client.
5. Avoid negative criticism.
6. Encourage parent to discuss openly concerns about the health of child and about the care that child will receive.

STUDY QUESTIONS

1. List several ways that the nurse and the emergency room staff might better communicate with the Vietnamese-American client.

2. Should the client be told that his folk medicine treatment is foolish and that he should abandon it? Why or why not?

3. How could the nurse effectively teach the client about the benefits of seeking conventional medical treatment in the United States?

4. When asked questions, Yen answers, "Yes." Does this always indicate that he necessarily means 'yes'?

5. List some strategies and techniques to help the nurse communicate more effectively with the Vietnamese-American family.

6. Describe the misconceptions that Vietnamese Americans have concerning Western medical practices and medications.

7. In American society hospitalization and visitation by clergy is a common, almost expected, act by some. How do the Vietnamese view hospitalization and clergy visitation?

8. Describe the importance of folk medicine and folk healers to Vietnamese Americans.

References

Balfour, F. (1993). Return of the boat people. *World Press Review, 40*(7), 10-12.

Bayless, T. (1975). Lactose-milk intolerance: clinical implications. *New England Journal of Medicine, 292*(5), 1156-1159.

Branch, M., & Paxton, P. (1976). *Providing safe nursing care for ethnic people of color.* East Norwalk, Conn.: Appleton-Century-Crofts.

Burtis, G., Davis, J., & Martin, S. (1988). *Applied nutrition and diet therapy.* Philadelphia: W.B. Saunders.

Cao, A.Q. (1986). Linguistic and cultural issues in refugees. In The next decade: The 1986 conference on refugee health care issues and management. *1986 Refugee Health Care Conference Proceedings,* pp. 70-75. Miami: University of Miami.

Chan, A.W. (1986). Racial differences in alcohol sensitivity. *Alcohol, 21*(1), 93-104.

Coelho, G., & Stein, J. (1980). Change, vulnerability, and coping: stresses of uprooting and overcrowding. In Coelho, G., & Ahmed, P. (Eds.), *Uprooting and development.* New York: Plenum Press.

Cook, K., & Timberlake, E. (1984). Working with Vietnamese refugees. *Social Work, 29*(2), 108-113.

Crystal, D. (1989). Asian Americans and the myth of the model minority. *Social Casework, 70*(7), 405- 413.

Eyton, J., & Neuwirth, G. (1984). Cross-cultural validity: ethnocentrism in health studies with special reference to the Vietnamese. *Social Science and Medicine, 18*(5), 447-453.

Ferrales, S. (1996). Vietnamese. In Lipson, J., Dibble, S., & Minarik, P. (Eds.), *Culture and nursing care.* School of Nursing, University of California at San Francisco: UCSF Nursing Press.

Fox, P.G., Cowell, J.M., & Johnson, M.M. (1995). Effects of family disruption on Southeast Asian refugee women. *International Nursing Review, 42*(1), 27-30.

Fry, A., & Nguyen, T. (1996). Culture and the self: implications for the perception of depression by Australian and Vietnamese nursing students. *Journal of Advanced Nursing, 23,* 1147-1154.

Gold, S. (1992). Mental health and illness in Vietnamese refugees. *The Western Journal of Medicine, 157*(3), 290-294.

Grant, D.M. (1983). Variability in caffeine metabolism. *Clinical Pharamacology Therapy, 33,* 591-602.

Hiebert, M. (1993a). Answered prayers. *Far Eastern Economic Review, 156*(30), 24-26.

Hiebert, M. (1993b). Miles to go. *Far Eastern Economic Review, 156*(30), 24-26.

Hoang, G., & Erickson, R. (1982). Guidelines for providing medical care for Southeast Asian refugees. *Journal of the American Medical Association, 248*(6), 710-714.

Huard, P., & Wong, M. (1968). *Chinese medicine.* New York: McGraw-Hill.

Huynh, T. D. (1987). *Introduction to Vietnamese culture.* San Diego, Calif.: Multifunctional Resource Center, San Diego State University.

Indochina Refugee Action Center (per D. McGlauflin) (1980, March 20). Special report: physical and emotional health care of Indochinese refugees. Washington, D.C.

Information please almanac (1998). Boston: Houghton Mifflin.

Kinzie, J.D., Manson, S.M., Do, T.V., et al. (1982). Development and validation of the Vietnamese language depression rating scale. *American Journal of Psychiatry, 139,* 1276-1281.

Kudzma, E. (1992, Dec.). Drug responses: all bodies are not created equal. *American Journal of Nursing, 92,* 48-50.

Lan, L. V. (1988, Sept.). Folk medicine among the Southeast Asian refugees in the U.S.A.: risks, benefits, and uncertainties. *Journal of the Association of Vietnamese Medical Professionals in Canada, 98,* 31-36.

Lee, E. (1985). Inpatient psychiatric services for Asian refugees. In Owen, T. (Ed.), *Southeast Asian mental health.* Washington, D.C.: U.S. Department of Health and Human Services.

Leung, L. (1988). Training bilingual paraprofessionals for counseling services. *Hawaii Journal of Counseling and Development, 4*(1), 16-22.

Lin, K.M., & Finder, E. (1983). Neuroleptic dosage for Asians. *American Journal of Psychiatry, 140,* 490-491.

Lin, K.M., Masuda, M., & Tazuma, L. (1982). Adaptational problems of Vietnamese refugees: Part 3. Case studies in clinic and field: adaptive and maladaptive. *The Psychiatric Journal of the University of Ottawa, 7,* 173-183.

Lin, K.M., Poland, R., Nuccio, I., et al. (1989). Longitudinal assessment of haloperidol doses and serous concentrations in Asian and Caucasian schizophrenic patients. *American Journal of Psychiatry, 146*(10), 1307-1311.

Murphy, H.B. (1969). Ethnic variations in drug responses. *Transcultural Psychiatric Research Review, 6,* 6-23.

Nguyen, D. (1981, Sept.). *Psychiatric and psychosomatic problems among Southeast Asian refugees.* Paper presented at the Sixth World Congress of the International College of Psychosomatic Medicine, Montreal, Canada.

Nguyen, D. (1988a, Sept.). Culture shock: a study of Vietnamese culture and the concept of health and disease. *Journal of the Associates of Vietnamese Medical Professionals in Canada, 98,* 26-30.

Nguyen, D. (1988b). Personal communication.

Nicholson, B. (1997). The influence of pre-emigration and postemigration stressors on mental health: a study of SEA refugees. *Social Work Research, 21*(1), 12-15.

Nilchaikovit, K., Hill, J., & Holland, J. (1993). The effects of culture on illness behavior and medical care. *General Hospital Psychiatry, 15,* 41-50.

Overfield, T. (1985). *Biological variations in health and illness.* Reading, Mass.: Addison-Wesley.

Owen, T. (Ed.) (1985). *Southeast Asian mental health.* Washington, D.C.: U.S. Department of Health and Human Services.

Pham, C., & McPhee, S. (1992). Knowledge, attitudes, and practices of breast and cervical cancer screening among Vietnamese women. *Journal of Cancer Education, 7*(4), 305-310.

Phan, T. (1996). Ethnic and cultural specificities of domestic violence: a research and clinical discourse with references to the Vietnamese emigrant community. *The International Journal of Psychiatric Nursing Research, 2*(2), 187-197.

Pickwell, S. (1989). The incorporation of family primary care for Southeast Asian refugees in a community-based mental health facility. *Archives of Psychiatric Nursing, 3*(3), 173-177.

Poss, J. (1989). Providing health care for Southeast Asian refugees. *Journal of the New York State Nurses Association, 20*(2), 4-6.

Rairdan, B., & Higgs, Z.R. (1992). When your patient is a Hmong refugee. *American Journal of Nursing, 92*(3), 52-55.

Rosenblat, H., & Hong, P. (1989). Coin rubbing misdiagnosed as child abuse. *Canadian Medical Association Journal, 140*(4), 417.

Rosenblat, H., & Tang, S.W. (1987). Do Asian patients receive different dosages of psychotropic medication when compared to Occidentals? *Canadian Journal of Psychiatry, 32,* 270-274.

Rossiter, J. (1994). The effect of a culture-specific education program to promote breastfeeding among Vietnamese women in Sidney. *International Journal of Nursing Studies, 31*(4), 369-379.

Rumbaut, R.D. (1977). Life events, change, migration and depression. In Fann, W.F., Faracan, I.J., Pokorny, A.D., & Williams, R.L. (Eds.), *Phenomenology and treatment of depression.* New York: Spectrum.

Shanahan, M., & Brayshaw, D.L. (1995). Are nurses aware of the differing health care needs of Vietnamese patients? *Journal of Advanced Nursing, 22*(3), 456-464.

Sideleau, B. (1992). Space and time. In Haber, J., Leach McMahon, A., Price-Hoskins, P., & Sidleau, B. (Eds.), *Comprehensive psychiatric nursing* (ed. 4) (pp. 193-209). St. Louis: Mosby.

Silverman, M.L. (1977). United States health care in cross-cultural perspective: the Vietnamese in Denver. Master's thesis, University of Denver, Colorado.

Smither, R., & Rodríguez-Giegling. (1979, Dec.). Marginality, modernity, and anxiety in Indochinese refugees. *Journal of Cross-cultural Psychiatry, 10,* 469-478.

Spector, R. (1996). *Guide to heritage assessment and health traditions.* Stamford, Conn.: Appleton & Lange.

Strand, P., & Jones, W. (1983). Health service utilization by Indochinese refugees. *Medical Care, 21*(11), 1089-1098.

Tien, J.L. (1984, Dec.). Do Asians need less medication? Issues in clinical assessment and psychopharmacology. *Journal of Psychosocial Nursing and Mental Health Services, 22,* 19-22.

Tien-Hyatt, J. (1989, May). Keying in on the unique care needs of Asian clients. *Nursing and Health Care, 11,* 269-271.

Tran, T.M. (1972). The family and the management of mental health problems in Vietnam. In Lebra, W.P. (Ed.), *Transcultural research in mental health.* Honolulu: University of Hawaii Press.

Tran, T.M. (1980). *Indochinese patients.* Falls Church, Va.: Action for Southeast Asians.

Tran, T.M. (1989, Oct.). Personal communication.

Tripp-Reimer, T., & Thieman, K. (1981). Traditional health beliefs/practices of Vietnamese refugees. *Journal of Iowa Medical Society, 71*(12), 533-535.

Tyhurst, L.J. (1977). Psychosocial first aid for refugees. *Mental Health and Society, 4,* 319-334.

U.S. Department of Commerce, Bureau of the Census (1993a, June 12). *News Release,* Commerce News.

U.S. Department of Commerce, Bureau of the Census (1993b). *Population profile of the United States, 1993* (Publication No. 23-185). Washington, D.C.: Government Printing Office.

U.S. Department of Commerce, Bureau of the Census (1993c). *We the Americans . . . Asians.* Washington D.C.: Government Printing Office.

U.S. Department of Commerce, Bureau of the Census (1993d). *Current population reports, U.S. population estimates by age, sex, race, and Hispanic origins, 1980-1991* (Publication No. P25-7025). Washington, D.C.: Government Printing Office.

Webster, R. (1991, March). Asian patients in the CCU. *Nursing (London),* 4(31), 16-19.

Westermeyer, J., & Winthrop, R. (1979). Folk criteria for the diagnosis of mental illness in rural Laos. *American Journal of Psychiatry, 136,* 136-161.

Williams, C., & Westermeyer, J. (1986). Refugee mental health in resettlement countries. New York: Hemisphere.

World almanac (1997). Mahwah, N.J.: World Almanac Books.

Yeatman, G.W., & Dang, V.V. (1980). *Cạo gió* (coin rubbing). Vietnamese attitudes toward health care. *Journal of the American Medical Association, 244*(24), 2748-2749.

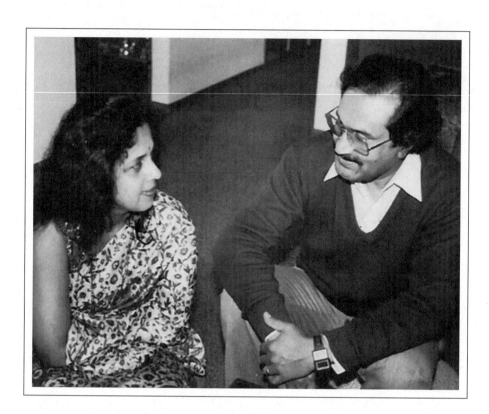

CHAPTER 19

East Indian Hindu Americans

Scott Wilson Miller and Jill Nerala Goodin

BEHAVIORAL OBJECTIVES

After reading this chapter, the nurse will be able to:

1. Identify two important East Indian Hindu cultural values that influence the behavior of East Indian Hindus living in the United States or Canada.
2. Describe concepts of health and illness influencing East Indian Hindus in relation to illness and health-seeking behaviors.
3. Outline the characteristics of the three waves of immigrants who have come to the United States and Canada from India.
4. Describe the effect culture has had on symptoms of mental illness experienced by the East Indian Hindu in India and after immigration.
5. Understand the unique beliefs about touch held by East Indian Hindus and explain how these beliefs may influence attitudes and reactions of East Indian Hindu Americans to caregivers.
6. Describe the beliefs and values held by East Indian Hindus concerning the family.
7. Explain the past, present, and future time orientation held by East Indian Hindus.
8. Describe the Ayurvedic system and the way this system explains illness.

OVERVIEW OF INDIA AND HINDUISM

India is a subcontinent that is a vast, wedge-shaped triangular peninsula jutting south from the mainland of Asia into the Indian Ocean. India includes an area of about 1,262,000 square miles and stretches about 2000 miles from north to south. It has three major land regions: the Himalayas and associated mountain ranges to the north, the Indus-Ganges-Brahmaputra Plain in the north central, and the Deccan Plateau in the south. The country contains a large part of the great Indo-Gangetic plain, extending from the Bay of Bengal on the east to the Afghan frontier and the Arabian Sea on the west. This plain is the richest and most densely populated part of the subcontinent.

The climate of India varies according to region. The Himalayas shield the Indian subcontinent from the main body of the Eurasian land mass, resulting in a unique climate. High-pressure winds moving down the Gangetic Plain into the Bay of Bengal result in winters that are generally dry on most of the continent. The Ganges River valley is noted for summer monsoons and rain, though rainfall may vary considerably. In the Ganges-Brahmaputra delta and surrounding areas, rainfall may exceed 80 inches per year, whereas in the northeastern portions of the

459

Deccan region and along the southeastern coast, the total rainfall ranges from 40 to 80 inches per year. In the areas around the western half of the Deccan region, the annual rainfall is 20 to 40 inches per year. In the southern half of the country, temperatures are tropical and vary little from month to month. In northern India, however, the annual range is considerable, and in January the average temperature in the north may be 30° F lower than in the south (Simons, 1976).

About 70% of India's working population is engaged in agriculture. Living in small villages, working farms that average 2 acres per family, and using age-old cultivation techniques based on human or animal power, the average Indian farmer lacks efficiency and is seldom able to provide more than bare subsistence for the family. Cultivation potential is further handicapped by lack of water, allowing only 50% of the land to be cultivated (McKay, Hill, & Buckler, 1988; Simons, 1976). The Indian constitution prohibits the slaughter of cattle. India has one of the largest livestock populations in the world, yet most of the animals are undernourished and diseased.

India is a democratic republic with a parliamentary system of government. The head of state is a president who is elected for a 5-year term by the members of the national and state legislatures. Effective executive power is exercised by a prime minister who is normally the leader of the majority political party. Prime ministers have included Jawaharlal Nehru (1889-1964); Nehru's daughter, Indira Gandhi (1966-1984); and Gandhi's son, Rajiv Gandhi (1984-1989); Prime Minister Shekhar (1989-1991); and P.V. Narasimha Rao (1991-   ). In 1991, Prime Minister Shekhar resigned. Two months after Shekhar's resignation (May 22, 1991), former Prime Minister Rajiv Gandhi was assassinated (World Almanac, 1997). In November 1991, an election was held and P.V. Narasimha Rao was chosen to form a new government. In May 1996, the ruling Congress Party lost the parliamentary elections. At the time, Atal Bihari Vajpayee of the Hindu nationalist Bharatiya Janata Party became prime minister for 13 days. After this short regime, Deve Gowda of the United Front coalition became prime minister. However, Prime Minister Gowda lost a confidence

vote in April 1997. At that time Foreign Minister Gujral was sworn in as prime minister (Information Please Almanac, 1998).

Despite a large land mass, India is overpopulated. Most of the population, crowded into the Ganges River valley and the eastern and western coastal regions, is of diverse racial genotypes. The people of India speak approximately 200 different languages, the principal languages including Hindi (official), English (official), Bengali, Gujarati, Kashmiri, Malayalam, Marathi, Oriya, Punjabi, Tamil, Telugu, Urdu, Kannada, Assamese, Sanskrit, and Sindhi (all recognized by the Constitution), including 1652 dialects.

In 1989, the Indian subcontinent numbered more than 685 million people (United Nations, 1989). By 1997 the (estimated) population of India numbered 967,612,804 with a natural increase of 1.59% (Information Please Almanac, 1998). Similiarly, in 1997, the birth rate of India was 25.33 births per 1000 persons; infant mortality was 69.2 per 1000; and the density per square mile was 787.7 The Hindu population is increasing at the rate of 1.8%, or almost 13 million people, each year (Information Please Almanac, 1998).

In the slums of Calcutta, Mumbai (formerly Bombay), and other large cities, thousands die yearly from malnutrition and disease. Under the pressure of population increases, the economic, political, and social aspects of life are strained (Warshaw, 1988).

Today the situation in the region is further complicated by the forces of religion and nationalism. The people of the subcontinent are deeply divided by the Hindu and Muslim faiths. Their loyalties are divided between the nation-states of India, Pakistan, and Bangladesh, which share the subcontinent. Indian society is composed of many separate fragments coexisting through mutual tolerance and general agreement on the status and functions of various groups. The regions vary considerably in their historic traditions, cultural patterns, and complement of castes. Within each region contrasts in customs and traditions parallel class and caste differences. Cutting across linguistic and class divisions are the "communities," which are large aggregates of people defined by some common denominator, such as religion, ethnic affiliation, or area of origin (Melendy, 1977). Some Indians believe that there is no need for people in these diverse groups to conform to a single set of practices and beliefs. The underlying unity of the country is derived from the larger arena of cultural traditions shared by most groups and from the dominance of certain national elites.

Hinduism is the title given for convenience to the religion of most of the population of the Indian subcontinent (Warshaw, 1988). Consequently, approximately 85% of the population is classified as Hindu. Hinduism is a culture as much as it is a religion, and the balance of culture and religion forms the social structure of the Hindu society. Social and religious mores are so predominant that if the Orthodox Hindu were to abandon Hindu belief for another religion, this individual, like the Orthodox Jew, would become an outcast from the people.

Hindus agree on a philosophy rather than a doctrine. Although Hindus built magnificent temples, they developed no church. The priesthood is hereditary and can be achieved only through reincarnation. Of the few beliefs shared by all Hindus, respect for a priest is among the foremost. Hinduism evolved over the last 4000 years and has no single founder or creed; rather, it consists of a vast variety of beliefs and spiritually based health practices and customs. Formal organization is minimal and a religious hierarchy is nonexistent.

A common belief shared by most Hindus is veneration of life, especially regarding the cow, which is believed to embody fertility. Although rivers, trees, and other forms of life are also regarded as sacred, the cow is considered the holiest life form.

Early Hindus were united in other philosophical respects. The transmigration of the soul represented one essential element of faith. In the backward or forward movement of the soul, there existed an underlying moral responsibility (*dharma,* which may also be translated as 'law, religion, virtue, morality, or custom'). It was dharma that obliged each member of society to maintain the role that was assigned at birth. On the individual level, *dharma* required the pursuit of *nirvāṇa* in ways that were defined by the priests (Warshaw, 1988).

The doctrine of reincarnation, of which transmigration is an integral part, provided a vital link between the religion of Brahmanism and the social order in which it was practiced. The religion claimed a divine mandate to separate people by castes, otherwise known as the *varṇa* (color) system. At the same time, it suggested to members of the toiling lower castes that they might become reincarnated at a higher level in another life. To attain advancement in the other life, the individual must fulfill moral obligations in the present one. Thus the doctrine of reincarnation was an incentive for members of the lower caste to be dutiful. The ultimate bliss of final union with Brahma, though dim and distant, was a realizable goal. Although this union might be achieved through correct actions, the nature of action was limited by each caste (Warshaw, 1988).

The relationship between the people's belief concerning the causes of illness and attempts to seek relief from its effects is learned from local folk practitioners. Illness and its treatment are perceived as a biological as well as a social phenomenon (Kakar, 1977).

Many health care professionals do not recognize that the health beliefs and practices of Hindus evolved over the centuries and that every cultural trait has direct relevance to the environment. Although beliefs concerning the causes of prevalent diseases may appear illogical, they are difficult to dismiss or substitute with Western medical practices. Adequate knowledge about these beliefs can assist nurses in the formulation of nursing diagnoses and nursing interventions and guard against undue conflicts with the practice of folk medicine.

IMMIGRATION TO THE UNITED STATES AND CANADA
First-wave immigrants

The arrival of East Indians from the Indian subcontinent during the first two decades of the twentieth century caused considerable uproar along the Pacific Coast of Canada and the United States (Melendy, 1977). Although East Indians immigrated to these countries in very small numbers, their immigration coincided with increasing American hostility toward the Japanese. Before the nineteenth century, very few Hindu Indians migrated overseas from the Indian subcontinent because most Hindu Indians believed that crossing the "black waters" was dangerous to a Hindu soul. By 1900 the U.S. Bureau of the Census reported that 2050 East Indian residents had immigrated to the United States. Many of the immigrants in this group were non-Indians who were born in India, some were Indian students, and some were Indian businessmen (Melendy, 1977).

In 1901, East Indian students began arriving in the United States to enroll in various colleges and universities throughout the East Coast area. Many of these students enrolled in such prestigious institutions as Cornell University. It was not until about 1904 or 1905 that East Indian students began to immigrate to the western portion of the United States to enroll in such universities as the University of California and California Polytechnical Institute. Students were not the only immigrants who were included in this first major wave of Hindu Indians. During this period, U.S. ports of entry began to register major increases in East Indian immigrants; from 1904 to 1906, 674 East Indians immigrated, compared with only 9 in 1900. The majority of East Indian immigrants were unskilled agriculturalists and small entrepreneurs from the arid lands of the Punjab, the United Provinces, Bengal, and Gujarat (Melendy, 1977).

From the onset of the first wave of East Indian immigrants, these people were classified as Hindus (or Hindoos) regardless of their home, culture, or religion. The U.S. Immigration Commission in 1911 mandated that any native of India was to be considered a Hindu for immigration purposes (Divine, 1957; U.S. Immigration Commission, 1911). In 1917 Congress passed, over President Wilson's veto, an immigration restriction act for East Indians. This new law required a literacy test and also encompassed a barred zone for immigration. All Asians who resided in India, Southeast Asia, the Indonesian islands, New Guinea, or regions of Arabia, Afghanistan, or Siberia were excluded by the new immigration law (Melendy, 1977).

Second-wave immigrants

In 1909 Canada closed its doors to East Indian immigrants; however, immigration of East Indians to the United States continued for another 5 years. The Immigration Exclusion Act of 1917, which excluded most persons of East Indian descent, including Hindu Indians, severely curtailed the number of Hindus in the United States. The number of East Indian immigrants residing in the United States began to decline sharply in 1910. In 1910 the U.S. Commission reported that there were some 5000 East Indians residing in the United States, but in 1930 this number was disputed by the U.S. Bureau of the Census, which reported that there were only 2544 East Indians residing in the United States, with the vast majority of these people residing in California. In 1946 President Harry Truman signed into law a bill that allowed East Indian immigration on a quota basis and allowed naturalization of East Indians. This law is credited with beginning the second wave of migration of East Indian Hindus to the United States.

These new immigrants, who arrived after World War II and before 1965, were mostly professional Hindu people and their families. These immigrants came mostly from the large cities of Mumbai (formerly called Bombay) and Calcutta (Ramakrishna & Weiss, 1992).

Third-wave immigrants

In 1965 an immigration law marking the beginning of a third wave of immigrants to the United States was enacted. Although the first-wave immigrants were primarily agriculturalists with some students and the second-wave immigrants were primarily businessmen with their families, the third-wave immigrants were entirely different. This new generation of immigrants were very young, with three out of five under 30 years of age and one out of seven less than 10 years of age. In 1974 approximately 12,777 East Indians resided in the United States (U.S. Immigration and Naturalization Service, 1974).

In 1998, there were 570,000 people of East Indian descent residing in the United States (Information Please Almanac, 1998) with 107,954 living in the South, 85,245 in the Midwest, 159,641 in the Northeast, and 97,566 in the West (U.S. Department of Commerce, Bureau of the Census, 1993a, 1993b). The median age of East Indian Hindus in 1990 was 30.1 years, and the number of married-couple East

Indian Hindu American families represented 91% of that population, compared with 83% for the rest of the general U.S. population. In 1990, the per capita income of East Indian Hindu Americans was $17,777, compared with $14,143 for the rest of the general U.S. population (U.S. Department of Commerce, Bureau of the Census, 1993a).

COMMUNICATION
Origins of Hindustani dialect

Language is a means of communication, and it disseminates new ideas. It is the storehouse of tradition and literature that provides a people with a sense of pride, self-confidence, and emotional unity. The national elite groups of a culture emphasize the value of a common language as a unifying force and the necessity for the development of language and literature. The study of linguistic heritage not only is an end in itself, but also serves to establish the conditions for nationhood (Pye, 1962).

Hindustani (the name given by Europeans to an Indo-Aryan dialect), as a result of political causes, has become the great *lingua franca* of modern India. The name is not used by natives of India, except as an imitation of the English nomenclature. Hindustani is by origin a Hindi dialect of western India. Hindustani has been called a mongrel pidgin form of speech comprising contributions from the various languages spoken in a Delhi bazaar. This theory has not been disproved because of the discovery that the language is the actual living dialect of western India, which has existed for centuries in its present form (Singh, 1966).

Hindustani is the natural language of the people of Delhi. Because the origin of Hindustani began with the people in the Delhi bazaar, it became known as the "bazaar language." From the inception of Hindustani, this language became the *lingua franca* of the mongrel camp and was transported everywhere in India by the lieutenants of the empire. Several recognized forms of the dialect exist, such as Dakhini, Urdu, Rekhta, and Hindi. *Dakhini*, or 'southern', is the form in current use in southern India and the first to be employed in literature. It contains many archaic expressions now extinct in the standard dialect. Urdu, '(the language of the) camp',

is the name usually employed for Hindustani by natives and is now the standard form of speech used by Muslims. All the early Hindustani literature was written as poetry, and this literary form of speech was named *Rekhta*, or 'scattered', from the way in which words borrowed from Persia were scattered through it. Hindustani is the dialect used in poetry, with Urdu being the dialect of prose and conversation (Singh, 1966).

Style

The term "Hindi" is ambiguous and therefore the source of much controversy because it is not easily defined. It is considered a regional dialect with a variety of common structural and interchangeable content elements. Its usage depends on both the regional affiliation and the social background of the speaker. Hindi is a highly open language closely related to other Indo-Aryan languages; therefore the degree of stylization is determined by the degree of language-orientation consciousness in the speaker's mind (Corlett & Moore, 1980). Hindi encompasses three areas of stylization: high, medium, and low. An individual may shift between high and low stylization according to situational requirements, as in formal discourse, during conversation with equals, and in giving instructions to subordinates.

Volume and kinesics

East Indians are generally noted for their soft-spoken manner, almost considered mumbling by some. Frequently, head movements and hand gestures accentuate conversations, adding vitality to the speaker's content. Men maintain direct eye contact with each other when conversing, but women usually draw their eyes downward when addressing their husband, father, or grandfather. This gesture demonstrates a sign of respect.

Touch

Any display of public affection is prohibited and viewed as disrespectful in the eyes of the gods. Married East Indian couples may show signs of affection in the privacy of their own home but not in view of children or elders. Affectionate touching among friends, relatives, and acquaintances is not a socially acceptable Hindu practice.

Implications for nursing care

The use of Hindi among East Indian Hindus is the one culturally unifying trait these people possessed after immigration to the United States or Canada. Reluctantly, East Indian Hindus have recognized the need for adoption of English as a communicative norm in the Western culture. Still, most elderly family members are unwilling to abandon the native language, which is regarded as meaningful to their cultural identity, and find it difficult to learn and communicate in English. On the other hand, younger family members, especially children, easily adapt to the Western culture and are more inclined to incorporate English into their language skills. Whenever possible, translators, as well as younger family members who have a better conceptualization of English, should be utilized by the nurse and other health care personnel when administering care to persons in the East Indian Hindu American population.

When obtaining a health history from an East Indian Hindu American client or family, both Hindi- and English-speaking family members should be involved. Because of uncertainty with the English language, the client may feel frustrated and not communicate conditions thoroughly. When a Hindi-speaking client becomes frustrated, the client may first attempt to translate needs by using Hindi; therefore, it may be necessary to translate Hindi responses into English. This process preserves the client's cultural identity while promoting client confidence.

It is important for the nurse to remember that it is considered taboo for a man other than the woman's husband to extend his hand toward a woman in greeting. In introducing oneself to a female Hindu client, the greeting is first addressed to the husband or eldest female companion.

It is also considered taboo for a man other than the woman's husband to initiate or maintain direct eye contact with a woman. This may be perceived by the husband as a seductive gesture. The wife, as a show of respect and out of fear of reprisal, will divert her eyes downward during conversation.

SPACE

In countries that are vastly overpopulated, such as India, the time lag between a decline in the death rate and the acceptance and practice of rational control of fertility presents a serious strain on the economy of the country. India is making positive efforts to reduce the birth rate and thus reduce the phenomenon of overcrowding that currently exists (Moore, 1963). The automobile has been poorly adapted in India because the cities are so physically crowded, and the Indian society has elaborately architecturally designed buildings (Hall, 1966). Most Hindu Americans are surprised to find that internal ornaments such as ceiling fixtures do not fit in American houses because the ceilings are too low, the rooms are too small, and privacy from the outside is viewed as inadequate (Hall, 1966).

Most East Indian Hindus have become accustomed to extremely crowded spaces; therefore the assimilation of these people into the Western culture, where crowding is not the norm, may be difficult. Some East Indian Hindu Americans may perceive that their personal space is greatly overextended and may sense a need to have their personal space collapse inward to feel more in control of their environment.

Implications for nursing care

East Indian Hindus are a family-oriented people who do not view family as intrusive in personal space parameters. When an East Indian Hindu American becomes ill and is hospitalized, the entire family may gather at the bedside. It is important for the nurse to remember that the client may feel that the space in the hospital is overextended and that the family's presence is essential to collapse the space inward. In this case it is important for the nurse to involve family members in the plan of care and to ascertain which family member will provide personal care. This may eliminate feelings of overcrowding on the part of the nurse and other health care professionals.

SOCIAL ORGANIZATION
Family

In a traditional East Indian Hindu household, married sons live with the family under the parental roof and are subject to parental authority. Frequently the joint family includes approximately 25 individuals and may include up to 200 people. The average joint family is composed of six or seven family members, and the family may comprise several generations. The patriarch controls the finances of the group, giving the sons allowances from their earnings. The matriarch is the autocrat of the home, and her daughters-in-law are subject to her rule. Although this system provides the members of the family with security and sustenance, it has been suggested that it encourages dependence and lack of initiative among many family members (Reddy, 1986). In the past, East Indian Hindu girls have wept at the prospect of marriage, not because of objections to little-known bridegrooms, but in fear of their future mothers-in-law (Reddy, 1986). The joint family is a powerful social unit, whose pressures on the individual are greater than most Westerners can imagine. It has also been suggested that the East Indian Hindu family demands much sacrifice and devotion and consequently fosters timidity and lassitude in its members (Reddy, 1986).

The hierarchy of the joint family places the father or eldest brother at the highest level. However, the family relies heavily on a democratic system of governance, and decisions of prime importance are determined by a vote in which the heads of the family may be overruled. Although the head of the family (the patriarch) is the undisputed overseer of other male members of the household, the matriarch is responsible for the family's female members and is instrumental in determining other domestic concerns. Recent efforts to promote family planning to reduce the burden of the mushrooming population for the most part has resulted in action by women. Indian men appear to reject sterilization for both psychological and religious reasons, fearing it will destroy their male power or will interfere with God's will (McKay, Hill, & Buckler, 1988; Nossiter, 1970).

The East Indian Hindu father is perceived as being distant from his children, who prefer to bond closely with the mother (Kurian & Ghosh, 1983). The eldest son is destined to continue the family name and perform the holy death rites that will ensure peace for his father's soul. It is this expectation that places the eldest son in the position of being one of the closest family members to the patriarch.

Throughout his life the eldest son, even when fully mature, rises when his father enters a room or is near him and greets his father with the *pranām*, the sign of deference in which one touches the feet of a highly respected figure. East Indian Hindus tend to be respectful of authority figures but are more distant with male superiors than with their female counterparts. These people cherish courtesy, which is reflected in the traditional greeting, wherein the head is bowed, the hands are clasped, as if in prayer, and the Hindi word *namaste* ('I bow to thee') is uttered softly.

It is the family, above all other institutions, that is responsible for the implantation of social mores and values in the Hindu culture. Ancient traditions that are suggestive of the existence of external rituals are still strictly practiced, and it is the adherence to these ancient traditions that determines whether young East Indians become conservative or rebellious (Warshaw, 1988).

Marriage

In India, marriages of Hindu Indians have always been arranged by the parents or other intermediaries. Because marriage was regarded as a union of families rather than of individuals, the marriage traditionally took place when the husband and wife were only children. In 1955 in India, it became illegal to arrange for the marriage of girls under 15 and of boys under 18 years of age. However, this law is not easily enforced, and almost 20% of girls are married before they reach 18 years of age.

The long-standing practice of courtship rituals, which is primarily a Western phenomenon, is beginning to gain wide acceptance as traditional arranged marriages are being displaced. Now, only the educated elite are able to personally arrange marriages, and these marriages account for less than 10% of the total marriages in India (Warshaw, 1988).

East Indians have long considered marriage a financial and social arrangement designed to strengthen the position of the whole family, and traditionally one of the most important factors determining the choice of a bride has been the size of the dowry, that is, the property a woman brings to her husband at marriage (Warshaw, 1988). In India marriage proposals traditionally have been elicited through a third party who may or may not be a member of the immediate or extended family. In contrast to this, today in the United States, East Indian Hindus frequently place a classified advertisement in their search for a suitable candidate for a prospective bride or groom (Warshaw, 1988).

Position of women in the family and in society

In the past, East Indian Hindu women ranked far below men in social status. Marriage became obligatory because the unmarried woman was believed to have no place in heaven. Traditionally the belief has been held by East Indian Hindus that the role of a woman is faithfulness and servility to her husband. Because women were deprived of inheritance, a male descendant was essential (Reddy, 1986).

Traditionally the wife had few legal rights and could not publicly contradict or challenge her husband. Mentioning her husband's name in public also was not permitted. This taboo proved particularly confusing when she was required to identify herself for legal purposes (Warshaw, 1988). Among the upper class in the Hindu communities of the northern regions of India and in some areas of southern India, many wives practice purdah, the anglicized form of Hindi *parda*, meaning 'veil'. This tradition decrees that in public a wife hides her face behind a veil to ensure that she will be seen only by her husband. This custom is intended to protect her husband's rights over her (Warshaw, 1988).

Mahātma Gandhi was one of the first champions for women's political and social rights in India. In addition, the Women's Indian Association (1917) and the All-India Women's Conference (1927) were organized to unite women in their quest for status attainment through education, social reform, and politics. The association and conference included political picketing and voluntary social work. Although the Indian women's organizations provided tremendous support for the independence movement, it has been reported that they were unable to promote the essential issues related to women's emancipation. It has even been alleged that these organizations were a means of maintaining and gaining status to move into higher echelons of power

and that only upper- and middle-class women benefited from them (Reddy, 1986). Cumulatively, change in the status of women in postindependence Indian society has been moderate and not far reaching in its influence; for example, the issues of marriage (particularly regarding the remarriage of widows), divorce, and property inheritance serve to illustrate the inequities still occurring in India where women are concerned (Mukherjee, 1983; Sinha, 1977).

Caste system in India

For centuries East Indians had divided themselves by caste, by language, and by religion (Spear, 1972). The Hindu population was divided into four *várṇa*s (colors), which became castes (Box 19-1). These segregated castes were the *Brahmin*, or priestly caste; the *Kshatriya*, or warrior caste; the *Vaiśya*, or trading and farming caste; and the *Śūdra*, or artisan caste (*ś* is a palatal /sh/). Approximately 60% of the population held membership in one of these four castes. Outside the caste system, another group of people were referred to as "untouchables." Gandhi renamed the untouchables the "Harijans," or 'children of God'. These people were the handlers of slaughtered animals, garbage, and the dead. Although the members of the highest caste, the *Brahmin*s, were regarded as pure, Harijans were thought of as polluted and defiled (Spear, 1972). See Box 19-1 for a description of each caste's or noncaste's role in Hindu society.

An individual became a member of a caste at birth, and it was believed that only death could release an individual. Individuals were expected not to marry outside of the caste. The exception to this rule was when a man took a bride from a lower caste. Work, acquisition of property, and education could not enable an individual from a lower caste to move to a higher caste.

Historically in India, an intricate system of subcastes, known as *jāti*s, interlaced with the four main *varṇa*s. The members of a *jāti* ('caste, lineage') were closely united by family, village, and region. A *jāti* had more prestige and gained greater rewards for services than other people had. Often the members of a *jāti* would claim to have descended from a com-

Box 19-1

CASTE SYSTEM IN INDIA

1. *Brahmins*. The *Brahmins* ('possessing sacred knowledge') were the priests and occupied a position of prestige and influence. These priests performed scholarly pursuits. The distinguishing color of the *Brahmins* was white.

2. *Kshatriyas*. The *Kshatriyas* were the warriors, who in ancient times had been the head of society and later were ranked second to the priests. The color of their dress was red to symbolize their work of providing military and political leadership. Warfare was considered a duty of the *Kshatriyas*, and any hesitancy to fight, even against one's own kin, was considered a violation of the *dharma*, or 'law', of the caste.

3. *Vaiśyas*. The *Vaiśyas* ('community men settled on soil'), who made up the largest caste, were involved in commerce. The ritual color of this caste was yellow. The members of this caste had the more mundane tasks of raising cattle, tilling the soil, shopkeeping, and lending money. Although the *Vaiśyas* lacked the social, ritualistic, and political privileges associated with the *Brahmins* and the *Kshatriyas*, they ultimately gained great power and wealth as a mercantile order.

4. *Śūdras*. The function of the *Śūdras* was to perform menial tasks for the higher groups. Most members of this caste were poor tenant farmers and artisans. The most the *Śūdras* could hope for was that they would be reborn in a higher caste. The ritual color of this lower caste was black.

5. *Untouchables*. Untouchables were not allowed to live within the boundaries of a community or to have access to the village well. They had to perform those duties that were considered unclean, such as tanning leather, cremating the dead, and executing criminals.

From Spear, P. (1972). *India: a modern history.* Ann Arbor, Mich.: University of Michigan Press.

mon ancestor, whether they had or not, to proclaim kinship with one another. These people shared customs, traditions, and usually a dialect. Based on an occupation or a set of related occupations, the *jāti* did not encourage members to seek social relationships outside of the group. Tailors, sweepers, or moneylenders (some of the occupations included in *jāti*s) did business with one another but maintained a social distance from one another (Spear, 1972).

The caste system was officially abolished by the Indian constitution in 1950 (Warshaw, 1988). Today in most large cities, educated workers and professionals of many castes intermingle. Caste taboos on eating and drinking with others tend to be ignored. Schools, public transportation facilities, restaurants, and apartment houses have been almost entirely desegregated. Caste lines in major cities are so blurred that a person of the merchant caste may be an officer in the army, whereas a person of the military caste may be a prosperous business executive. However, although commercial practices are forcing East Indians to abandon the old castes, family life continues to use them.

Religion

The Hindu religion may be the oldest religion in the world (Eshelman, 1992). Over 80% of the persons in India practice the Hindu religion. There are at least 910,000 practicing Hindus in the United States including those of East Indian descent (Information Please Almanac, 1998; World Almanac, 1997). Hinduism, especially as learned and practiced in the United States, is a religion of disciplined acts, *karma yoga*, the path of deeds (Miller, 1995). Key teaching of Hinduism emphasize the importance of *satya* ('truthfulness, reality'), self-control and respect for others. Many practicing Hindus engage in meditation, *prāṇāyama* ('breathing exercises'), singing *bhajan*s ('sacred hymns'), yoga, and daily prayer.

The Hindu religion is polytheistic in the sense that there are numerous gods and goddesses, but there is an overriding sense of a supreme spirit. The origin of Hinduism is based on the *Vedas*, the sacred written scriptures. In Hinduism the belief is that *Brahma* is the principle and source of the universe and the center from which all things proceed and to which all things return. Reincarnation is a central belief in Hinduism. Life is determined by the law of *karma*, which states that rebirth is dependent on moral behavior in a previous stage of existence. In Hinduism life on earth is transient and a burden. The goal of existence is liberation from the cycle of rebirth and redeath and entrance into *nirvāṇa* (literally 'out-blowing'), a state of extinction of passion.

Hinduism is a common part of life for most Hindu Indians. Religious shrines are prevalent within many Hindu households and are located in various parts of the home, based on family preference. Each family has a set of specific gods and goddesses to whom they pray, and by popular account the Hindu pantheon numbers some 33 million gods. The shrines contain statues and pictures of the chosen gods, candles, incense, and offerings of milk, flowers, and fruits. Times for prayer and meditation are reserved for the early morning (after bathing) and early evening, as time permits.

The common Hindu custom of fasting is observed on specific days of the week, depending on which god the individual worships. This practice is predominant among the women of the family, and children are not allowed to participate. Based on the family's degree of compliance to Orthodox Hindu law, fasting rituals may vary from absolute abstinence to consuming only one meal a day. This practice may span over a 1-month period of time or merely be an observance of a holy day. Pittsburgh is a major center of Hindu cultural and religious strength. The first major Hindu temple in the United States, the Śrī Venkateswara Temple in Penn Hills (a suburb of Pittsburgh), is an internationally known pilgrimage site for Hindus. Other major temples have been established in Washington, D.C., Chicago, Austin, Berkeley, Los Angeles, and Boston. Temples serve as the center of the community promoting the retention of Hindu values and instruction in the scriptures and key teachings, such as *ahiṁsā* ('nonviolence'), vegetarianism, and self-control. The temples often sponsor cultural events, language classes, and secular activities (Miller, 1995).

Effect of immigration to the United States on social organization

The restricted immigration policies that were in place before 1965 in the United States created fear for many East Indian Hindu Americans because it appeared that the culture was losing its significance. Before 1965 there were so few East Indian Hindus residing in the United States that the few who did chose to remain culturally isolated. Those Hindu Indians who did choose to assimilate believed that there was no free access to the White community and therefore chose to assimilate the Mexican-American culture, particularly because there were so few East Indian Hindu women residing in the United States before 1965. Some sociologists concluded that the assimilation between East Indians and Mexicans occurred as a result of their similarities in physical characteristics. In addition, some sociologists believe that the East Indian Hindus may have lost their ethnicity entirely in the Mexican subculture, but others regard the fact of intermarriage between East Indian Hindu Americans and Mexican Americans as evidence of mutual acceptance (Melendy, 1977). In a classic study of 50 East Indian Hindu American men, 26 had wives in the United States, 22 of which were Mexicans. Consequently the children from these Mexican–East Indian marriages were raised predominantly in the Mexican culture (Dadabhay, 1954).

As a new wave of East Indian Hindu immigrants began to assert themselves in the 1960s, the sagging Hindu culture and traditions were revived and prospered. This was attributable in part to the fact that after 1965 more East Indian Hindu wives and families began to arrive in the United States, which facilitated a revival of the traditional culture. On arrival these wives continued to wear saris, the traditional dress, whereas only about 10% of the men continued to wear traditional garb because many of the men felt the need to conform to the business community in the United States (Wenzel, 1965). Most of the newer immigrants were more adaptable and moved more easily into the American way of life, whereas the older generation remained apart from the mainstream of American society. Although the older group of East Indian Hindus, who continued to live in rural areas, managed to adjust to economic demands, the social acculturation of this group remained significantly behind that of the newer generation of immigrants (Melendy, 1977). Some East Indian Hindu wives in the United States continue to practice *bindī* ('forehead dots', also *tilak*) as a sign of the husband's well-being and prosperity (Reddy, 1986).

Urbanization, industrialization, and education are major interacting forces disrupting the framework of the joint family system traditionally found in the East Indian Hindu culture and consequently are affecting the East Indian Hindus' family value system in the United States.

Education is so highly valued among East Indian Hindus that approximately 80.1% of East Indian Hindu Americans 25 years of age or older have a high school education, compared with 66% for the rest of the general U.S. population. Of the U.S. population 25 years of age or older, East Indian Hindus have the highest percentage of college graduates, with approximately 68% of Hindu men and 36% of Hindu women obtaining a college education as compared with approximately 20% of men and 13% of women for the rest of the general U.S. population (U.S. Department of Commerce, Bureau of the Census, 1993a).

Since the third-wave immigration period, East Indian Hindus have integrated into the U.S. labor force, with approximately 65.4% of all East Indian Hindus working. The per capita income for East Indian Hindu Americans is $17,777, compared with $14,143 for the rest of the general U.S. population. Consequently the poverty rate of East Indian Hindu Americans is considerably lower than that of the rest of the general U.S. population, with only about 9.9% of East Indian Hindu Americans residing in poverty. In addition, 51% of East Indian Hindu Americans own their own homes, which have an average value of $74,300, compared with 64% of the general U.S. population owning their own homes, which have an average value of $47,200 (U.S. Department of Commerce, Bureau of the Census, 1993b).

Politically the adult East Indian Hindu community in the United States tends to favor a low profile, with fewer members serving in public office. Relationships between East Indian immigrant and U.S. society vary, based on the community where they reside. According to Miller (1995), "discrimination against East Indian groups can be severe, ranging from the 'dot-buster' violence in New Jersey (perpetrated by white racist "skinheads") to subtle forms of job discrimination that are difficult to document statistically."

An increasing number of young East Indian Hindu Americans are relocating to large urban centers in New York, New Jersey, Pittsburgh, Texas, and California (Helweg & Helweg, 1990) and are living in apartments, and, as a result, the joint family system has been rendered impractical. In school and at work, more East Indian Hindu Americans have learned to depend on ability rather than the caste system formerly found in India. The development of individualism among family members has resulted in uncertainty about the need for the elaborate rituals of the past. Some of the values learned from the family are therefore becoming extinct, especially as more young people detach themselves from the traditions that previously controlled them.

Implications for nursing care

It is important for the nurse to appreciate that the traditional East Indian Hindu family is the basic unit wherein values, manners, and morals are learned as part of its social structure. The pursuit of individualism, which is so predominant in Western culture, is not the accepted norm. The nurse should appreciate that the father is highly regarded as the head of the family and is the primary spokesman concerning important family matters, including the health care of the individual members. It is unusual for East Indian Hindu Americans to seek medical care outside the confines of the family because of fear that the family will be subjected to public scrutiny by strangers.

The nurse who cares for East Indian Hindu American clients should expect that the wife will usually sit passively by her husband, expecting all questions and inquiries to be directed toward him. He in turn may consult with his wife regarding the health status of other family members. The nurse who ignores the husband and seeks information directly from the wife may precipitate, on the part of the husband, feelings of personal humiliation and disrespect in the eyes of his family. The major objective in developing an effective nurse-client relationship is to develop trust by gaining the husband's confidence so that the husband no longer views the nurse as an intruder but, instead, as a health care advocate.

TIME

The sense of time is an important concept for East Indian Hindus, who are past, present, and future oriented. East Indian Hindus are perceived as past oriented because of the traditions and rituals that are inherent to the culture. On the other hand, they are perceived as present oriented because of the view that they are "beings-in-becoming" (Kluckhohn & Strodtbeck, 1961). Finally, they are perceived as future oriented because life in the present is lived with an emphasis on the hereafter.

At the highest intellectual level, Hindus seek the one reality, whether this is conceived impersonally or theistically. Once they succeed in reaching this reality, they may continue to live in the world but without emotional attachment to it. They will have passed beyond sorrow and joy, pain and pleasure, and good and evil (Warshaw, 1988). In other words, the present is transcended by concern for the future and future reward.

Hindus, through the cremation of their dead, hope to release the individual's spirit for union with an all-pervading one. The act is suggestive of the existence of a timeless presence in which all Hindus may share. The doctrine of rebirth—that every living being, animal or heavenly, will again be reborn and for all eternity—is a popular Hindu belief. The precise form of each rebirth is determined by the balancing of the being's deeds, good and evil, in previous existences. Escape from the cycle of rebirth constitutes salvation, a state of perfect, blissful consciousness that may be gained by acquiring perfect knowledge and performing one's duty flawlessly. Most Hindus aim only to improve their condition in the next existence.

Implications for nursing care

Because East Indian Hindu Americans are perceived as being past, present, and future oriented, it is important for the nurse to remember that the client may place little or no value on some present things, such as being on time for appointments, but may place considerable importance on other present-oriented concepts, such as the spiritual atonement of the self. At the same time, the same client may place equal importance on past-oriented things, such as traditions and rituals, and on future-oriented concepts, such as the preparation of the soul for the life hereafter.

ENVIRONMENTAL CONTROL

According to Kluckhohn and Strodtbeck (1961), it is essential for a people to answer the question of whether humans are innately good or bad. In regard to this question, there exists a range of variabilities, including evil, good and evil, and good. Hindus believe that the goodness in the soul of man is recaptured by virtue of the process of reincarnation. In addition, they believe in the man-to-nature orientation, as proposed by Kluckhohn and Strodtbeck, that man is not only subjected to nature but also has a need to live in harmony with nature. Being a past-, present-, and future-oriented cultural group that subscribes to a multiple man-to-nature orientation, some Hindus believe that because man is a mixture of good and evil, there is a need for constant control and discipline of the self, if any real goodness is to be achieved.

Hindus are viewed as having both an internal and an external locus of control, meaning that some Hindu people believe that, although external forces control destiny, internal forces, such as feeling states or misuse of the body, can also control destiny. For example, Hindu Americans who subscribe to both an internal and external locus of control believe that internal conditions are influenced by psychological factors, such as anger, jealousy, envy, fright, and shame. This belief is supported by the premise that when an individual is unable to control internal conditions that are self-perpetuated, a possibility exists for a susceptibility to disease (Henderson & Primeaux, 1981). The external locus of control is evident in that illness is an external event or misfortune, the cause of which may be related to the fault of a family member or the wrath of a disease goddess against the entire family. It is not uncommon for Hindus to believe that malevolent spirits of dead ancestors, sins committed in a previous life, or jealous living relatives are responsible for one's ill health. Such phenomena as "soul loss," "breach of taboo," and "wrath of a goddess" are viewed as symbolic expressions of internal conflict. Hindus believe that people make themselves vulnerable to such calamities through conscious or unconscious transgressions against the ghosts and spirits. Agents empowered by evildoers to precipitate illness are numerous and varied; thus, to avert the evil intentions of these demons, Hindus wear charms, make offerings to the saints and their ancestors, and avoid visiting areas in the village where spirits are believed to reside.

Perception of illness

According to classical East Indian theory, the human body consists of five natural elements: earth (bones and muscles), water (phlegm, or *kapha*), fire (gall, or *pittá*), wind (*vāyú;* also breath, or *prāṇá*), and space (in hollow organs) (Andrews & Boyle, 1995). Water, fire, and wind are the three elements that interact in harmony to produce wellness. Illness results from an excess or deficiency of one of these elements, which are also referred to as the *tridosha,* or the 'three troubles'. *Prāṇá* deals not only with respiration, but also with a pneumatic element circulating in channels, distributing the "humors" and body fluids (bile, blood, and phlegm) throughout the body. In contrast to this view is that held by some other cultural groups, such as Puerto Ricans, that there are four bodily humors (blood, phlegm, black bile, and yellow bile) that must be in a state of balance for the individual to stay at an optimal level of wellness (Harwood, 1971). In addition to giving attention to the five natural elements, East Indian theory also identifies bone, flesh, marrow, fat, chyle, blood, and sperm as seven essential constituents of the body. Although the nomenclature of bones is extensive, the viscera are given less attention in East Indian theory.

A great deal of attention traditionally was devoted to the source of diseases and to hygienic prescription. The intention of medical treatment addressed not only the disease symptomology, but also the diagnosis of causes. For example, the treatment of fever consisted in giving antithermic drugs in addition to prescribing medication against *pittá* or the causative element involved (Dash, 1974).

Hindus believe that praying for health is the lowest form of prayer. Among East Indian Hindus, it is preferable to be stoic rather than pray for recovery (Peck, 1981).

Folk medicine

Significance of folk beliefs in the Hindu culture

Today there is a growing sense among psychologists, sociologists, and biologists that illness and its treatment are both biological and sociological phenomena (Kakar, 1977). It is believed that there are at least three different types of medical systems practiced at three different cultural levels. On the first level are primitive or preliterate people, who practice a form of primitive medicine based predominantly on a supernatural theory of disease causation. These people are believed to seek treatment through magicoreligious means. On the second level are people who belong to the folk culture level and practice folk medicine, which encompasses a theory of illness that involves both supernatural and physical treatments as well as causations. On the third level are people who subscribe to a modern theory of treatment and disease causation. At this level people recognize natural rather than supernatural causes of disease. When East Indian medicine is traced back historically, there is a magicoreligious mixture of theology. In early East Indian history, disease causation was attributed to gods and goddesses and was explained on the basis of a cause-and-effect relationship with these gods and goddesses or with ghosts and evil spirits. However, Indian folk beliefs have undergone centuries of transition and now include herbal medicines and the Ayurvedic system (Kakar, 1977).

The belief that certain diseases have natural or physical origins does not preclude the simultaneous role of a supernatural antecedent. For example, diarrhea in a child is generally attributed to consumption of a combination of incompatible foods. However, the possibility of someone casting an "evil eye" or "evil mouth" on the child is also recognized (Kakar, 1977).

Another system of beliefs is the Ayurvedic doctrine, which dictates that disease not only has a germ causation, but also occurs because of an imbalance of the essential body elements. *Āyurveda* is a term that is composed of two words: *āyus* and *veda*. The literal translation for the word *āyurveda* is 'science of life'. A primary concern for East Indian Hindus is knowledge of favorable or unfavorable conditions that assist in the introduction or resistance of the growth of harmful or nonharmful germs. East Indian Hindus believe that there are three fundamental elements in the body—*dosha, dhātu,* and *mála*—which must be in balance if a state of optimal equilibrium is to exist. *Dosha* ('disease') governs the physiochemical and physiological activities of the body; *dhātu* ('layer') forms the basic structure of the body cell; and *mála* ('dirt') consists of substances partly utilized in the body and partly excreted in modified form after their physiological function has been completed (Kakar, 1977; Ramakrishna & Weiss, 1992).

There are many medications that may be prescribed in the Ayurvedic system of medicine. For example, drugs for rejuvenation may be prescribed by an Ayurvedic physician (Dash, 1974). Another example of Ayurvedic medicine is found with the treatment of amebic dysentery, which is caused by the organism *Entamoeba histolytica.* In Ayurvedic medicine the belief is that the organism is not the major etiological factor of the condition; rather, the major cause is attributed to irregularity of diet; intake of heavy, indigestible foods; and emotional factors such as worry, anxiety, and anger (Dash, 1974). As a folk remedy for amebic dysentery, the drug *cyávana prâśa* ('disease causer–eating') is used, but this drug is considered more a food than a medicine. Two tablespoons of this medication are taken in a glass of milk, and the client is instructed to avoid salt in excess as well as sour things. Another part of the treatment includes avoidance of anxiety, worry, and sexual indulgence (Dash, 1974; Ramakrishna & Weiss, 1992).

Emphasis on the diet of a client is a unique feature of Ayurvedic medicine. The popular belief is that the client does not require any medication if he or she has a wholesome diet. According to this belief system, even if errors in diagnosis are made, most of the Ayurvedic herbal medicines will not produce any harmful effect; however, if a diagnosis of a disease is correct, these herbal medications will act instantaneously.

Diseases in Ayurvedic medicine are considered to be psychosomatic, involving both the body and the mind. This point is always kept in mind when medicines and regimens are prescribed for the client (Dash, 1974; Ramakrishna & Weiss, 1992).

Types of folk practitioners A majority of East Indians obtain their beliefs in relation to the cause, prevention, and elimination of illnesses from their families, their parents-in-law (particularly the mother-in-law), elderly women of the neighborhood, indigenous midwives, other folk practitioners, and government health care workers. Usually the decision to seek medical treatment is influenced by factors such as the client's sex, the economic condition of the family, the family's perception about the cause of the illness, and the family's relationship with the local practitioner (Kakar, 1977).

Therapeutic advice is generally obtained at five different levels: family level, *mohalla* (properly *mahalla*) level, caste level, village level, and beyond the village level (Kakar, 1977).

1. At the family level, the mother-in-law, regarded as the family practitioner and well versed in the use of home remedies, is the source of treatment for any illness. Her authority is highly regarded and usually unchallenged in the scope of maternal and child care. Acting as diagnostician and therapist, her healing techniques include such practices as the use of purgatives, massages, and various body-stretching devices.

2. At the *mohalla* (*mahalla* 'eunuch in palace or harem') level, there exist two or three highly respected *syānas* or *syānis* ('wise or holy men'), who are readily available and consulted only for certain illnesses. Intervention by the *syānas* is decided by the mother-in-law, and it is assumed that the importance of not relinquishing the family's secrets and affairs to the community is understood.

3. At the caste level, the intervention by one or two *syānas* is often sought. These practitioners cater to people's needs, especially members of their own caste. They are highly respected members of the caste and recipients of special treatment on socially important occasions.

4. At the village level, the faith healer, the most religious member, is a popular practitioner of

choice and is employed for his free services regardless of caste or creed.

5. Beyond the village level, consultation is sought with a variety of folk and indigenous practitioners, ranging from exorcists to spirit mediums. There have been instances where a simple reassurance of the client by the spirit medium, without any actual medication, has resulted in instant relief (Kakar, 1977).

Principles of hygiene

Personal hygiene is extremely important to East Indian Hindus. As part of the religious duty, a bath is required at least once every day. Some Hindus believe that bathing after a meal is injurious and that a cold bath may prevent a blood disease, whereas a hot bath may cause an alterative effect on blood diseases. East Indian Hindus also believe that if the bath is too hot, injuries to the eyes may occur. Hot water may be added to cold water, but cold water is not to be added to hot water when one is preparing a bath. When the bath is completed, the body is to be carefully rubbed dry with a towel and properly dressed (Jee, 1981).

Perception of death

Death, according to the Hindu belief, is perceived as a passage from one existence to another. From the scriptures and the inspiration of "seers," the Hindu learns that all creatures are in a process of spiritual evolution extending through limitless cycles of time. A person's lifetime is like a bead on a necklace whose other beads represent past and future lifetimes. Each *atmán* ('basic self') strives through successive rebirths to ascend the scale of merit until—after a life of rectitude, self-control, nonviolence, charity, reverence for all living creatures, and devotion to ritual—it wins liberation from worldly existence to achieve union with *Brahma* (Chakravarty, 1978).

In India the preparation of the body for cremation involves bathing the remains with a milk and yogurt solution, which symbolically cleanses the soul of the deceased. When a married woman dies, she is attired in a traditional white wedding sari, devoid of makeup or jewelry, the wearing of which is considered a bad omen. A man is attired in a plain off-white East Indian suit. Religious prayers and chanting are continually offered by friends, family members, and priests before and after death to promote safe passage of the soul. Outward displays of grief are accepted practices within the Hindu faith. Open grieving by family, friends, and acquaintances encompasses wailing, crying, and even fainting. Men are as expressive in their grief as women and do not project a stoic demeanor (Chakravarty, 1978). The eldest son of the deceased carries the body to the funeral pyre, and all other children are prohibited from approaching the funeral site. During the cremation ceremony a priest chants prayers while the body is cremated. The ashes are then placed in a container and transported by the eldest son to a designated holy ground and scattered.

Implications for nursing care

It is important for the nurse to remember when working with Hindu Americans that there may be a belief that self-control of strong feelings is one of the keys to balancing health or a wellness state. In addition, some Hindu Americans believe in a value orientation that encompasses the belief that man is subjected to nature and at the same time is expected to live in harmony with nature. Because of this belief, it is important for the astute nurse to keep in mind that the client may believe that illness has a twofold causation, which may include ill favor or overindulgence of self.

Because Hindu Americans have very strict beliefs regarding things such as bathing, it is important for the nurse to remember that a Hindu American may refuse to take a bath after breakfast, which may be a common policy in some health care facilities. In addition, because some Hindu Americans believe that it is not permissible to add cold water to hot water, if the water is too hot, the nurse should pour the water out and begin the process again rather than risk offending the Hindu client.

Because some Hindu Americans subscribe to a theory that encompasses the belief that there are three elements in the body that must be in harmony to produce wellness, it is important for the nurse to identify with the client those beliefs that are beneficial, neutral, or harmful. If the client has beliefs that are beneficial, it is important for the nurse to identify these beliefs and practices and incorporate them into the plan of care. It is equally important for the nurse to identify those beliefs and practices that are considered neutral, having no effect one way or the other on the outcome of treatment, and therefore do not need to be eliminated from the daily rituals of the client. Finally, it is extremely important for the nurse to identify those practices that could be considered harmful and therefore need to be eliminated from the practices and daily rituals of the client.

In a study reported by Kakar (1977), 98% of East Indian Hindus in a small village attributed specific diseases to the wrath of God. In this case many of these respondents believed that herbal preparations such as neem tree leaves and twigs were useful in the treatment of these diseases. It was difficult to convince these people that these practices did not alleviate or prevent the conditions. Although a successful vaccination program was launched, it was only successful because of education of the local leaders and folk practitioners. Therefore it is important for the nurse to remember that education of the client and the family is extremely important to develop shared goals about health and wellness.

When a Hindu-American client dies, the nurse should not be surprised by the religious rites after death. For example, the priest may tie a thread around the neck or wrist to signify a blessing, and this thread should not be removed. The nurse should expect that after death a priest will pour water into the mouth of the body and that the family will request to wash the body. Because Hindus are particular about who touches the body after death, it is essential that the nurse communicate respect and provide privacy for the family so that these rites can be carried out (Murray & Huelskoetter, 1991; Potter & Perry, 1996).

BIOLOGICAL VARIATIONS
Variations according to racial strain

The modern population of India can be classified into six major racial strains. Two of the six racial groups can be related to a geographical region, and the other four groups may be found throughout India. Persons in the upper classes are different in

physical type from those in the lower social strata. East Indians can be regarded as a separate racial group occupying an intermediate position between the peoples of Asia on the one hand and those of Europe on the other.

1. *Mediterranean strain.* These people are characterized by a long head, moderate stature, slight build, and dark skin. The face is narrow, the nose is small and moderately broad, and the hair is wavy or curly. These are the dominant features among the Dravidian-speaking people of southern India.

2. *Broad-headed strain.* This section of the population varies in stature from short to medium and in skin color from light to dark brown. The head is broad and sometimes high. The nose is prominent, and the hair is straight and usually abundant on the face and body.

3. *Nordic strain.* A distinguishing characteristic of these people is their long head. They are tall, long faced with a straight and narrow nose, and light skinned. This type of strain predominates in the upper castes in northern India.

4. *Mongoloid strain.* The head on these people varies from long to medium, and the skin color varies from light to dark brown. Their stature is medium, and the hair is sparse on the face and body. The face is short with predominant cheekbones, and the eye sockets are slanted, giving a slitlike appearance to the eye.

5. *Negritos.* These people represent earlier inhabitants of India. Their stature is less than 5 feet, and frizzy hair is among the chief distinguishing feature.

6. *Proto-Australoids.* This strain is predominant with tribal people of central, western, and southern India. A long head; short stature; broad, short face with strongly marked brow edges and a small, flat nose; and wavy to curly hair are features of the lowest social strata of the population. The skin is dark to black. The strain is so named because of certain resemblances between people of this type and the Australian aborigines (Guha, 1945), but genetic evidence of such a relationship is exceedingly weak (Cavalli-Sforza, Menozzi, & Piazza, 1994).

Enzymatic and genetic variations

Thalassemia, a genetic condition that can result in various degrees of anemia, is believed to have a high incidence in people from the Mediterranean region, the Middle East, and Southeast Asia. It is believed that thalassemia has a range of variability in occurrence in people of Indian descent (Overfield, 1985). In addition, G-6-PD deficiency, which also causes anemia, is believed to have a high occurrence among people in high-risk malarial areas. What is believed to occur in high-risk malarial areas is that the malarial parasite attacks red blood cells that contain the G-6-PD enzyme. Therefore, cells with the deficiency are less likely to be parasitized, which lowers the parasite load and consequently lessens the severity of G-6-PD deficiency.

Lactose intolerance is another condition that affects persons of East Indian descent. Lactose intolerance is believed to occur among African and Asian populations because of genetic selection that may lead some groups of people to have adequate levels of intestinal lactase and others to have inadequate levels (Bayless, Rothfield, Massa, et al., 1975; Overfield, 1995). It is believed that, although lactose intolerance varies by race, at least 80% to 90% of the world's population become lactose intolerant in adult life, except for some Whites (Overfield, 1995).

Susceptibility to disease

Current United States data on life expectancies and susceptibility to disease by race do not allow an adequate perspective of all racial groups residing in the United States. The data available on life expectancy are suggestive that White women in the United States have a life expectancy of 74 years and White men have a life expectancy of 70.5 years, compared with non-Whites such as Asian Americans and East Indian Americans, who have a lower life expectancy than White Americans but a higher life expectancy than Black Americans, Native Americans, and American Eskimos (National Center for Health Statistics, 1993; Overfield, 1985). However, statistical data giving empirical support to this contention are limited.

It is believed that susceptibility to heat stress is influenced by factors such as age, race, body build, body fat, climatic experience, and possibly gender (Wagner, 1972). According to Frisancho (1981), there is a possibility that certain races have the ability to withstand heat stress better than other races do; however, the racial effect is compounded by climatic exposure. Frisancho (1981) concluded that persons brought up in hot climates, such as that in India, are better able to tolerate heat than those persons raised in cooler regions, such as certain regions of the United States. In general, it is believed that Blacks, southwestern American Indians, Asian Indians, East Indians, and Australian aborigines have the ability to withstand heat better than their White counterparts (Frisancho, 1981; Riggs & Sargent, 1964). The belief is that these people have lower sweat rates than Whites with similar body temperatures and therefore may possibly have more efficient sweat production (Dill, Yousef, & Nelson, 1983). It is believed that part of the climatic influence on heat tolerance is directly related to the effect of heat on the development of the body during childhood. Eveleth (1966) concluded that children who grow up in hot climates, such as the conditions found in India, have a tendency to be more slender than their counterparts raised in more temperate areas. In addition, these children also have thinner arms and legs.

Nutritional preferences and deficiencies

Most caste Hindus are vegetarians. However, strictness in adherence to the vegetarian diet varies. In most cases the vegetarian diet consists primarily of grains (wheat, rice, millet, and barley) and legumes (grains, beans, and pulses, the edible seeds of plants having pods). In northern and western India baked or fried cakes made with wheat are common. *Chapātī*, a popular form of bread, is a round, flat cake made of whole wheat flour and water and baked on a convex iron plate. *Pūrī* is similar to *chapātī*, except for the addition of shortening and being fried in deep fat. *Parāṭhā*, a third form of bread, is cooked on a convex metal pan.

In eastern and southern India, rice is the staple food. It is usually boiled, but it can be combined with ghee (*ghi*, clarified butter) and spices to become *pilau (or pilaf)*. Corn, barley, and millet are served alone or as supplements to wheat and rice dishes. The primary sources of protein are the grains and pulses, which include *chanā* (chick-pea) and *arhar* (pigeon pea), which when split and dried is referred to as *dāl*. Vegetables include most of the green leafy vegetables, especially spinach, mustard, and radish greens, as well as gourds, eggplant, okra, cucumbers, cabbage, turnips, and potatoes.

Most East Indians eat a very light breakfast on rising in the morning, a heavy meal at midday, and a lighter meal between 7 and 9 PM (Ashraf, 1970). Before partaking of the meal, traditional Hindus chant the name of their god of preference, as if offering food to him or her before they eat. East Indian Hindu dietary law dictates that the right hand is used for eating, whereas the left hand is used for personal hygiene and toileting.

Psychological characteristics

Community tolerance for mental illness is high in India, and in many cases any idiosyncrasies are channeled into occupations or life-styles in which the behavior can be carried out. For example, a marginally schizophrenic Indian person may wander around the country doing odd jobs and living off handouts. Approximately 500 years ago ambalams were built throughout India to house travelers. Today, these ancient buildings are used by many persons who wander through India, including the mentally ill, as places to obtain food, beg, get water, and bathe.

For the East Indian Hindu, environment has a significant effect on mental illnesses that may develop (Ali, 1989). For example, because of the strong belief in supernatural forces, when a client becomes psychotic, delusions and hallucinations are often related to possession by a god, demons, or a witch, rather than to the mind being influenced by equipment being placed or fears that the place is "bugged," which is more often the case in Western societies. An East Indian immigrant who has difficulty with English and with understanding what is occurring in the environment and who becomes psychotic will often manifest a paranoid reaction rather than one of the other psychotic illnesses. The delusions of the new immigrant frequently relate to the supernatural and reflect the culture of India. However, as East Indian

Hindus have become assimilated into the Western culture, the nature of these delusions has changed to more "Western" symptoms.

Because mental illness is consistent with the sociological beliefs of the people, the treatment is also sociologically based and must be appropriate for the belief about the cause of the illness, such as exorcism of a spirit, demon, or god. The most effective exorcism is dramatically performed in a room with others in the family or in front of neighbors and friends (Ali, 1989).

Many drugs that are restricted in the United States are legal in India, such as cocaine, opium, and marijuana. Although these drugs are cheap and available, abuse is much less common than in the United States. Drugs that are commonly abused in the United States may be used in India for therapeutic purposes; for example, marijuana leaves in water may be used for a baby's cramps, and opium may be used for diarrhea. Although Judeo-Christian beliefs regarding drug use as wrong have been present in India since the British arrived and to some extent have been adopted by upper-class people, most East Indian Hindus still retain the value that although drug use may not be "good" it is not "wrong."

Implications for nursing care

The most crucial aspect for practicing proper nutrition is to make Hindus aware of the advantage of diet in relation to the survival of children. As East Indian Hindu Americans become assimilated into the Western culture, it is important for them to understand the significance of using available foods in a nutritious manner. The nurse must keep in mind that a Hindu person may be reluctant to use Western foods because of sociocultural restrictions. Therefore because dietary considerations are of utmost importance to some Hindu Americans, the astute nurse will involve the nutritionist or dietitian in the development and implementation of a culturally appropriate plan of care. The nurse should also be aware that fasting is an important part of religious practice and that this practice can have consequences for persons on special diets or with diabetes or other diseases related to food (Murray & Huelskoetter, 1991).

Nurses and other health care workers must be aware that the joint family is an important characteristic of the East Indian Hindu community and that the paternal grandmother has great authority because of her important role in decision-making matters related to health and nutrition. In planning culturally relevant nutritional programs for East Indian Hindu Americans, the nurse must understand the nutritional patterns in relation to other aspects of the culture and to identify those elements that can be changed without disorganization of the whole cultural scheme. The nurse also needs to explore the beliefs and attitudes of not only the people, but also the authorities from whom these beliefs are derived. It is also important for the nurse to remember that because some East Indian Hindu Americans have a genetic predisposition for G-6-PD deficiency, thalassemia, and lactose intolerance, alternative methods of supplying calcium in the adult diet may be necessary. Therefore the nurse may need to teach the client to supplement calcium by incorporating foods such as buttermilk, yogurt, and sharp cheeses in place of whole milk. Another consideration for the nurse is the theory that people from warmer climates have a more efficient heat-production system and thus can better tolerate heat. In this case, it is important to teach the client that overexposure to heat does have profound effects on the body. East Indian Hindu Americans must be taught to recognize the signs and symptoms of heat exhaustion regardless of this biological or climatic adaptation.

Because of the concept that health results from the body's ability to help itself, the traditional East Indian Hindu American may discount Western medical practices while responding positively to traditional folk healing practices. It is important for the nurse to appreciate that these clients may believe that the treatment they receive for an illness is more likely to be effective if both a pill and a solution are prescribed. A physician who is aware of this belief may prescribe both types of medication because this is what the client expects will effect a cure (Ali, 1989).

SUMMARY

Nurses who work in a transcultural setting providing health care services to clients of East Indian descent and Hindu affiliation are challenged by the multiplicity of norms, mores, and values, all of which influence and shape the delivery of nursing care. It is essential that the professional nurse and other health care providers use a holistic approach toward the assessment, planning, intervention, and evaluation of nursing care activities.

Case Study

Vaidya Chuttani is admitted to the hospital with a diagnosis of Cooley's anemia (thalassemia major). Although Vaidya is only 14 years old, she is a student at the local university. Vaidya speaks English, but she is experiencing difficulty communicating her needs to the health care team. Her family, which consists of her mother and father and five brothers and sisters, all reside in Bombay, India. Vaidya has not seen her family or talked with them for the 3 months that she has been enrolled in the American school. She tells the nurse that it is not unusual for some Indian families to allow their children to come to the United States to study at such a young age. In addition, she relates to the nurse that after she receives her degree, she will return to her country to assist her family by working and contributing to the family's monetary resources.

On admission, Vaidya's presenting complaints include (1) cholelithiasis as revealed on radiographic examination, (2) a right leg ulcer about 1 inch in diameter, (3) jaundice, and (4) an enlarged spleen as revealed on radiographic examination. The nurse notes the following on examination: blood pressure, 140/70; pulse, 88; respirations, 20; and temperature, 99.2° F.

CARE PLAN

 Nursing Diagnosis   Communication, impaired verbal, related to recent arrival from India and use of English as a second language

Client Outcomes

1. Client will be able to communicate basic needs to health care personnel.
2. Client will relate feelings of acceptance, reduced frustration, and decreased feelings of isolation.

Nursing Interventions

1. Use gestures or actions instead of words to communicate information.
2. Use visual aids that will communicate to client necessary procedures to be done.
3. Write down messages in the hope that client can understand written English better than spoken English.
4. Obtain a translator, if necessary, to communicate important information.

 Nursing Diagnosis   Tissue perfusion, altered peripheral circulation, secondary to Cooley's anemia

Client Outcomes

1. Client will define peripheral vascular problems in own words.
2. Client will identify factors necessary to improve peripheral circulation.
3. Client will verbalize an understanding of medical regimen, diet, and medications.
4. Client will verbalize an understanding of activities that promote vasodilatation.
5. Client will verbalize an understanding of factors that inhibit circulation.
6. Client will communicate existence of pain from right leg ulceration to health care professionals.

Nursing Interventions

1. Assess causative and contributing factors of right leg ulceration as related to Cooley's anemia.
2. Promote factors that will improve arterial blood flow.
3. Encourage client to keep right leg in a dependent position.
4. Encourage client to change position every hour when in bed.

Nursing Diagnosis   Health maintenance, altered, related to lack of information about Cooley's anemia (thalassemia major)

Client Outcomes

1. Client will verbalize desire to learn more about condition and preventive techniques to reduce symptoms.
2. Client will verbalize a willingness to comply with treatment regimen.

Nursing Interventions

1. Identify sociocultural factors that affect health-seeking behaviors.
2. Determine present knowledge of illness severity and prognosis.
3. Determine client's level and stage of adaptation to present condition (such as disbelief, denial, depression).
4. Using appropriate visual aids, describe necessity for blood transfusions to correct Cooley's anemia.

 Nursing Diagnosis   Family processes, altered, related to separation from family because of schooling in another country

Client Outcomes

1. Client will verbalize fears and anxiety related to separation from family.
2. Client will identify support systems available within school and community and from external resources that will facilitate return to optimal health.
3. Client will verbalize desire to be involved in health care and scheduling of client-centered activities.

Nursing Interventions

1. Determine client's understanding of present condition.
2. Determine support systems available in school and community and from external outside resources that will facilitate return to optimal functioning.
3. Involve client in care and scheduling of client-centered activities (such as wound care for right leg ulceration).

STUDY QUESTIONS

1. List other nursing interventions that can be implemented to facilitate communication between Vaidya and the health care team.
2. Describe the family structure of some East Indian Hindu families and the effect the family organization may have on health-seeking behavior as well as how this may affect nursing interventions for Vaidya.
3. Describe why Cooley's anemia is perceived as a biological variation for East Indian descent.
4. Identify at least two other biological variations that are common to East Indian descent.
5. Identify how Vaidya's health-seeking behavior may be affected by time and space variables.

References

Ali, S. (1989, Nov. 1). Personal communication. (Dr. S. Ali was former district medical officer in Silon, Madhya Pradesh, India.)

Andrews, M., & Boyle, J. (1995). *Transcultural concepts in nursing care.* Hagerstown, Md.: Lippincott Co.

Ashraf, K.M. (1970). *Life and conditions of the people of Hindustan.* Delhi, India: Munshiram Manoharial.

Bayless, T.M., Rothfield, B., Massa, C., et al. (1975). Lactose and milk tolerance: clinical implications. *New England Journal of Medicine, 292,* 1156-1159.

Cavalli-Sforza, L.L., Menozzi, P., & Piazza, A. (1994). *The history and geography of human genes.* Princeton, N.J.: Princeton University Press.

Chakravarty, A. (1978). Quest for the universal one. In *Great religions of the world.* Washington, D.C.: National Geographic Book Society.

Corlett, W., & Moore, J. (1980). *The Hindu sound.* New York: Bradbury Press.

Dadabhay, Y. (1954). Circuitous assimilation among rural Hindustani in California. *Social Forces, 33,* 141.

Dash, V.B. (1974). *Ayurvedic treatment for common diseases.* Delhi, India: Delhi Diary.

Dill, E., Yousef, M., & Nelson, J. (1983). Volume and composition of hand sweat of White and Black men and women in desert walks. *American Journal of Physical Anthropology, 61*(1), 67-73.

Divine, R. (1957). *American immigration policy, 1924-1952.* New Haven, Conn.: Yale University Press.

Eshleman, J. (1992, Nov.). Death with dignity: significance of religious beliefs and practices in Hinduism, Buddhism, and Islam. *Today's OR Nurse,* 19-20.

Eveleth, P. (1966). The effects of climate on growth. *Annals of the New York Academy of Sciences, 134*(2), 750-759.

Frisancho, A. (1981). *Human adaptation.* Ann Arbor, Mich.: University of Michigan Press.

Guha, B.S. (1945). *Racial elements in the population of India.* New York: Oxford University Press.

Hall, E. (1966). *The hidden dimension.* New York: Doubleday.

Harwood, A. (1971). The hot-cold theory of disease. *Journal of the American Medical Association, 216*(7), 1153-1158.

Helweg, A.W., & Helweg, U.M. (1990). *An immigrant success story: East Indians in America.* Philadelphia: University of Pennsylvania Press.

Henderson, G., & Primeaux, M. (1981). *Transcultural health care.* Reading, Mass.: Addison-Wesley.

Information please almanac (1998). Boston: Houghton Mifflin.

Jee, H.H. (1981). *Aryan medical science: a short history.* Delhi, India: Maharaja of Gundal.

Kakar, D. (1977). *Folk and modern medicine.* New Delhi, India: New Asian Publishers.

Kluckhohn, F., & Strodtbeck, F.L. (1961). *Variations in value orientations.* Evanston, Ill.: Row, Peterson.

Kurian, G., & Ghosh, R. (1983). Child-rearing in transition in Indian immigration families in Canada. *Journal of Comparative Family Studies, 83,* 132-133.

McKay, J., Hill, B., & Buckler, J. (1988). *A history of world societies.* Boston: Houghton Mifflin.

Melendy, H. (1977). *Asians in America.* Boston: G.K. Hall.

Miller, B.D. (1995, Spring). Precepts and practices: Researching identity formation among indian hindu adolescents in the United States. *New Directions for Child Development,* no. 67. San Francisco, Calif.: Jossey-Bass, Inc., Publishers.

Moore, W. (1963). *Man, time and society.* New York: John Wiley & Sons.

Mukherjee, P. (1983). The image of women in Hinduism. *Woman's Studies International Forum, 6,* 375-381.

Murray, R., & Huelskoetter, R. (1991). *Psychiatric nursing.* East Norwalk, Conn.: Appleton & Lange.

National Center for Health Statistics. (1993). *Health, United States 1992.* Hyattsville, Md.: Public Health Service.

Nossiter, B. (1970). *Soft state: a newspaperman's chronicle of India.* New York: Harper & Row.

Overfield, T. *(1995). Biological variation in health and illness: race, age, and sex differences* (ed. 2). New York: CRC Press.

Peck, M.F. (1981). The therapeutic effect of faith. *Nursing Forum, 22*(2), 153.

Potter, P.A., & Perry, A.G. (1996). *Fundamentals of nursing: concepts, process, and practice* (ed. 3). St. Louis: Mosby.

Pye, L. (1962). *Politics, personality, and nation building: Burma's search for identity.* New Haven, Conn.: Yale University Press.

Ramakrishna, J., & Weiss, M. (1992, Sept.). Health, illness, and immigration: East Indians in the United States. *Western Journal of Medicine, 157,* 265-270.

Reddy, G. (1986). Women's movement: the Indian scene. *The Indian Journal of Social Work, 46*(4), 507-514.

Riggs, S., & Sargent, F. (1964). Physiological regulation in moist heat by young American Negro and White males. *Human Biology, 36*(4), 339-353.

Simons, B. (1976). *The volume library.* Nashville, Tenn.: Southwestern Company.

Singh, B. (1966). *The dialect of Delhi.* New Delhi: Lakherwal Press.

Sinha, D. (1977). Ambiguity of role-models and values among youth. *Indian Journal of Social Work, 38,* 241-247.

Spear, P. (1972). *India: a modern history.* Ann Arbor, Mich.: University of Michigan Press.

United Nations (1989). *Population and vital statistics report.* New York: United Nations.

U.S. Department of Commerce, Bureau of the Census (1993a). We the Americans . . . Indians. Washington, D.C.: Government Printing Office.

U.S. Department of Commerce, Bureau of the Census (1993b). *Population profile of the United States, 1993* (Publication No. 23-185). Washington, D.C.: Government Printing Office.

U.S. Immigration Commission (1911). *Dictionary of races of people.* 63rd Congress, 3rd Session, pp. 52-54, 75-76.

U.S. Immigration and Naturalization Service (1974). *Annual report,* pp. 3, 59.

Wagner, J. (1972). Heat intolerance and acclimatization to work in the heat in relation to age. *Journal of Applied Physiology, 33*(5), 616-622.

Warshaw, S. (1988). *India emerges.* Berkeley, Calif.: Diablo Press.

Wenzel, L. (1965). East Indians of Sutter County. *California Living, 17,* 3-15.

World almanac (1997). Mahwah, N.J.: World Almanac Books.

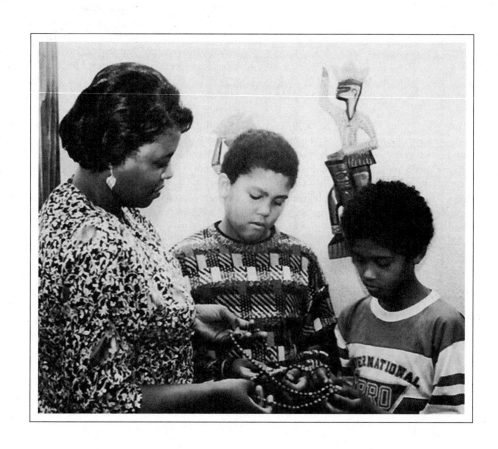

CHAPTER 20

Haitian Americans

Robert E. Cosgray

BEHAVIORAL OBJECTIVES

After reading this chapter, the nurse will be able to:

1. Understand the dynamics of using culturally appropriate nursing care for Haitian Americans.
2. Understand the Haitian family structure and the relevance to assimilation of Haitian Americans into the Western culture.
3. Identify diseases that are prominent in Haitian-American people.
4. Identify the religious beliefs of the Haitian culture and how they pertain to healing.
5. Understand beliefs of Haitian Americans related to the postpartum period.
6. Formulate a workable nursing care plan for a Haitian-American client with tuberculosis.

The small republic of Haiti in the West Indies has a colorful but tormented history. To provide appropriate care to Haitian-American clients, the nurse needs to have knowledge about the social and political turmoil that Haiti has experienced. In addition, the nurse should be aware of the difficulties that have surrounded migration as Haitians have sought sanctuary from their troubled homeland. It is only through an understanding of Haitian culture and health beliefs that the nurse can adequately meet the needs of Haitian-American clients. In addition to discussing the land of Haiti and the immigration process and the influence of the six cultural phenomena on nursing care of Haitian-American clients, this chapter explores the struggles that Haitians have experienced in their attempts to assimilate cultural traits of the dominant culture in North America.

OVERVIEW OF HAITI
Social history

Haiti (République d'Haïti) is situated in the western third of the island of Hispaniola. The other two thirds of the island is occupied by the Dominican Republic. Haiti is in the Caribbean Sea with Cuba to the northwest, Jamaica to the southwest, and Puerto Rico to the east. Haiti, about the size of Maryland, is two thirds mountainous, and the rest of the country is characterized by great valleys, extensive plateaus, and small plains (Information Please Almanac, 1998). Columbus discovered the island of Hispaniola on Christmas Eve in 1492 when his flagship, the Santa María, ran aground and was wrecked at Cap Haitien, a historic town on Haiti's northern coast. As the French took over the island, the native Indians were either exterminated or removed to Mexican gold mines. Black slaves were imported from Africa as the French became owners of flourishing sugar cane plantations. By 1681 there were 2000 slaves in St. Domingue, the French name for

Haiti. A little more than 100 years later, there were at least 500,000 African slaves and some estimate as many as 700,000, compared with 40,000 Whites and 28,000 freemen of color—offspring of masters and slaves (Wilentz, 1989). Many slaves were newly imported because many died of overwork, beatings, disease, and undernourishment. The masters were obviously outnumbered, necessitating harsh measures to keep the slaves in line.

Interestingly the African religions were seen as a source of resisting the French. Although night ceremonies and dances were often forbidden, they continued and fomented the desire for power and freedom. Legend has it that one night the slaves on half a dozen plantations rose up and burned down their masters' homes, killing their masters. This revolt spread throughout the country, continuing for some 13 years. In 1802 Napoleon's troops landed at Cap Haitien, planning to recapture the island from the slaves and use it as a jumping-off place for an invasion of the United States. However, because of yellow fever epidemics, which assisted the Haitians in killing the French soldiers, the Haitians altered the course of world history, and the French admitted defeat. In 1804 Haiti was freed from France and became the second independent nation in the Western Hemisphere and the first independent Black republic in the world. According to Hobsbawn (1962), the failure of Napoleonic France to recapture Haiti was one of the main reasons why France liquidated its entire remaining American empire, which was sold by the Louisiana Purchase to the United States. Thus a consequence of the revolution in Haiti was to make the United States a continental world power.

Unfortunately, independence from France did not end the misery for the poor in Haiti. Although they were no longer slaves, the poor soon found that the oppressive French rulers had been almost immediately replaced by equally oppressive new Black rulers, the mulattos. With the advantage of money inherited from their French fathers, the mulattos became educated and wealthy and continued to monopolize Haiti's resources with little regard for the social conditions of the poor (Seligman, 1977).

The American occupation, from 1915 to 1934, resulted in reorganization and improvements of the country regarding its road system, telecommunications, health care system, universities, banking system, and so on but did not effect permanent change. This assistance failed to solve the economic and social problems, and when the majority of Americans left in the 1930s, the country once again regressed.

In addition to the attempt at revitalization by the Americans, François Duvalier, who came to power in 1957 and was the self-proclaimed "president for life," can be credited with initiating comprehensive programs to alleviate economic and technological problems. Unfortunately, Duvalier, preoccupied with wealth and power and the programs that were initiated, failed to have long-lasting effects, and the country's money was squandered. In 1963 Duvalier murdered countless enemies and managed to incur the wrath of Haiti's neighbor, the Dominican Republic, by harboring enemies of its new president. When François Duvalier died in 1971, his son, Jean-Claude, came to power (Wilentz, 1989). In 1980 a sizable portion of the country's financial resources were spent on the wedding of Jean-Claude Duvalier and Michèle Bennett, a mulatto whose large family suddenly started to do better socially and economically. Michèle Duvalier's lavish spending contributed to her total alienation by the people, and resentment toward the new dictator increased. Eventually, Jean-Claude Duvalier and his wife were forced to flee the country because of massive rioting and murders occurring throughout the country (Bordeleau & Kline, 1986). Democracy was attempted, but the country was soon taken over by a military coup (Masland, 1992). In 1991, the United States joined members of the Organization of American States in a regional embargo aimed at reinstating Haiti's first democratically elected president, Jean-Bertrand Aristide. The economic blockade led to a sharp downturn in an already poor economy. In July 1991, Aristide and the army signed an accord to return the exiled president to power. When the military leaders failed to resign, the UN reimposed an embargo. The embargo had a severe effect on the health of the population because it created difficulties in distributing aid and health care in Haiti (Chelala, 1994). Although food and medicine are exempt from United Nations sanctions, an increase in AIDS, tuberculosis, and malnourishment among children occurred (Chelala, 1994). After Aristide's return to Haiti in October 1993, he quickly replaced the police force, downsized the military, and purged the officer corps (Information Please Almanac, 1998). In 1996, René Préval, the winner of the second free election in the country's history, was sworn in as President of Haiti with the UN Security Council remaining in the country to assist in maintaining peace (Information Please Almanac, 1998).

Not only has there been social and political unrest in Haiti, but this has also contributed to despoiling of the land. Today only 2% of the country is forested and more than half of the land has been destroyed by erosion (United Nations Program Development, 1996). The remaining agricultural land is capable of producing food for only half of the population. Still, Haitian farmers continue to despoil remaining land by removal of roots and stumps for charcoal manufacture to heat their cooking stoves in order to survive. The lack of farming land in the country has resulted in dependence on food from foreign aid (Hiebert, 1997). There are presently efforts in the country by charitable groups to assist the country economically. One example of this is the Mennonite Economic Development Association which has 20 paid staff who assist Haitians in developing their own small business by giving them small loans for start-up money. This organization has been very effective in helping hard-working Haitians have a chance to be self-supporting (Claude, 1997).

Life in Haiti

Today, Haiti is an independent republic of 6,611,607 (1997 estimate) inhabitants (Information Please Almanac, 1998). Between 90% and 95% of the population are descendants of West African slaves. Sixty-eight percent live in rural settings. Haiti is considered to be the poorest nation in the Western hemisphere with a gross domestic product in 1995 of $6.5 billion and a per capita income of $1000 (Information Please Almanac, 1998). However, for most of the rural Haitians the per capita income is more realistically estimated at $100 (Claude, 1997). Less than 1% of the people take in 40% of the income. Unemployment is 60% with most people living in destitute

poverty (United Nations Program Development, 1996). Some 92% of the population live in small, rural hamlets in small straw shacks without light, water, or windows. In sharp contrast to the destitute living situations is the pride of the Haitians, their value of self-respect, and their hard-work ethic. Much time is spent daily in washing clothes, and at the beginning of each day the typical Haitian has clean and often ironed clothing (Hiebert, 1997). Although the issues and problems confronting the people of Haiti are similar to those of many other countries, they seem to be more numerous and more intensified. The country is drastically overpopulated with a density of 617.1 persons per square mile (Information Please Almanac, 1998). The annual population growth rate is 2.08% with a natural growth rate of 23% and a gross birth rate of 34%. The reproduction rate is 2.24. The mortality for children of less than 5 years of age is 130 per 1000, and the maternal mortality is 457 per 10,000. The gross death rate is 11% with an infant mortality of 102.4 per 1000. Only 67.8% of the population have access to prenatal care. The rate of immunization availability for children of less than 1 year of age is 30%. The life expectancy is 59 years of age (Information Please Almanac, 1998; United Nations Program Development, 1996).

Haiti has numerous unresolved obstacles to public hygiene, including an inadequate water supply for 77% of the rural population and 62% of the urban population. There is inadequate access to sanitation for 64% of the rural population and 59% of the urban population. Some 80% of the population suffer from malnutrition. Health care services are lacking throughout Haiti. A national health service is responsible for the medical care of the population, but only 50% of the population have access to health care with only 47% of the rural population having access to health care. There is one physician for 8800 people and one nurse for 8600 people. This is even more problematic than it appears because most of the physicians are on the government payroll and are disproportionately concentrated in the capital city, Port-au-Prince (United Nations Program Development, 1996).

Health care is also provided by private foundations such as the Mellon Foundation, which sponsors the Hôpital Albert Schweitzer in central Haiti. To make health care more available to the people, small medical teams go out from this hospital into the rural areas to provide village-based health services. In this program, rural farmers, both men and women, are trained in primary health skills and provide direct services to clients. Health service delivered to the natives has resulted in a significant decrease in tetanus, which formerly ranked with tuberculosis and malnutrition as the three major health problems (Grant, 1989; Reichman, 1989; Stauffer, 1989; Westphal, 1989). However, although this hospital operates as a charity to the local people, it is not without exposure to the unrest in Haiti. For example, administrators are sometimes threatened that their family members will be harmed if they do not hire certain Haitians who come seeking employment (Venton, 1997).

IMMIGRATION TO THE UNITED STATES

Most of the immigrating Haitians in the early years were upper-class individuals who came to the United States as resident aliens. These upper-class Haitians were able to obtain permanent residence and citizenship with little difficulty and became assimilated into the dominant culture.

In 1980 an explosion of Haitian immigration took place as a result of a short-lived (April to October 1980) change in the U.S. immigration policy. More than 14,000 Haitian refugees landed on the shores of southern Florida during 1980 (Dempsey & Gesse, 1983), which includes the Mariel boatlift from Cuba. The influx of Cuban refugees required that a special status be created by the U.S. State Department, called "Cuban-Haitian entrant, status pending." Haitian refugees were included in this status to prevent the policy from being discriminatory (Metropolitan Dade County, 1981; Walsh, 1980). The "entrant" status described a temporary status and was used rather than granting the new arrivals political asylum. However, this "entrant" status placed the Haitian immigrants in a bureaucratic limbo that cannot lead to citizenship (Wilk, 1986).

The immigration policies changed in October 1980. A maritime interdiction program was initiated to turn back Haitian refugees at sea. Haitians who arrived in the United States were not classified as entrants but as parolees and were subject to deportation. Haitians were kept in detention along with Cubans while their cases were processed in the courts. Unlike other refugees arriving at the time (such as Indochinese refugees), resettlement was not guided by the federal government. The federal government's refusal to grant asylum deprived the refugees of benefits under the new 1980 Refugee Act. Emergency aid was limited, and most of it had lapsed by 1983 (Holcomb, Parsons, Giger, & Davidhizar, 1996). Lacking either jobs or government assistance, many refugees were compelled to rely on private charity and to invent jobs in a burgeoning "informal" economy in Miami. In 1991 mass migration of Haitians led to 34,000 Haitians being held at the U.S. Naval Base in Guantánamo Bay, Cuba, while their immigration status was determined (Lillibridge, Conrad, Stinson, & Noji, 1994). Numerous health problems were addressed by the uniformed-service medical support personnel including active tuberculosis and AIDS (Granich, Sfeir, & Jacobs, 1994; Bonnlander, 1996). In 1993 the Supreme Court of the United States ruled that repatriation was legal and illegal aliens could be returned to Haiti (Holcomb, Parsons, Giger, & Davidhizar, 1996). Despite this ruling, thousands of Haitians still attempt to enter the United States each year by trying to travel from Haiti to the United States by boat. Some have given all their money to private entrepreneurs and boarded barely seaworthy crafts for a chance to escape to a better life in the United States (Portes & Stepick, 1985). Many Haitians do not survive because the conditions at sea are too harsh or the boat is too full to permit safe travel. When weather conditions are too harsh, older Haitians have been thrown into the sea to lighten the load (Veeken, 1993). Still, perilous as the journey may be, many Haitians would rather try for the hope of the opportunities of living in the United States. Of those that do arrive, only a fraction (5%) are allowed to stay under the status of political refugees. The United States has steadfastly clung to a policy that makes it difficult for Haitians to meet the requirements for political-refugee status. For example, since the immigration act of 1990, mandatory HIV testing with indefinite detention without treatment in HIV-positive detention camps has discriminatively singled out Haitians from other immigrants (that is, Cubans, Vietnamese, Chinese) and required that persons with HIV be held rather than "paroled" (Annas, 1993).

These waves of immigrants have resulted in four classifications or categories of Haitians in the United States: (1) citizens, (2) residents or legal aliens, (3) entrants, and (4) illegal aliens. Illegal aliens have all the pressures and fears of discovery, which could result in sudden deportation. Entrants, on the other hand, suffer from the uncertainty of whether they will be able to remain and from being unable to make permanent plans or feel entirely settled (Wilk, 1986). Because possibly half of the Haitians in the United States are here illegally, few programs exist to provide assistance. Some Haitians are understandably reluctant to discuss their difficulty and attempt to maintain a low profile with government agencies that might return them to Haiti. Another effect of an uncertain status in North America is infrequent use of health care services after immigration. The nurse should be aware that the Haitian immigrant probably will not seek medical treatment until the condition is severe or has become chronic (Bryan, 1988).

Despite these difficulties and the possibility of deportation, many, primarily poor, Haitians continue to try to enter the United States. Those who do make it to North America are in one of the most at-risk populations now living in the United States. This high risk becomes actualized in several ways; for example, a study by Moskowitz, Kory, Chan, et al. (1983) reports unusual cases of death among Haitians residing in Miami and a high prevalence of opportunistic infections. The nurse should expect, when caring for a Haitian, that the client may never have had immunizations. If a client needs a tetanus immunization, it is unlikely that a tetanus booster is appropriate because the client more than likely has not received the series.

Adaptation of post-1980 Haitians to the dominant culture in the United States and Canada has been especially problematic because the proportion of refugees having a high school or college education and skills in English has declined. With limited education and money, many Haitians arriving in North America have been restricted to occupations such as migrant agricultural work and service industry jobs in restaurants and hotels (Eshleman & Davidhizar, 1997). Only a few of the more educated Haitians have been able to find work as mechanics and construction workers. Gaining the requirements needed to adjust to the urban, industrialized culture encountered in the United States and Canada is for most Haitians a stressful, overwhelming, and slow process because the people continue to cling to their cultural values and beliefs. Potocky (1996) noted that, although many other refugees are faring moderately well in the United States, Nicaraguans and Haitians tend to be faring poorly. Assimilation to the United States culture for Haitians has been particularly difficult. When they are compared to other groups, Potocky (1996) noted that Haitians on the average in regard to yearly earnings, percentage employed, and percentage never employed and living in poverty had a significantly lower economic status. A substantial proportion of Haitians arriving in the United States are children who often arrive without their parents and are placed with extended family or in foster care (Office of Refugee Resettlement, 1993). Children who are with families face intergenerational problems. Children often experience a role reversal as they tend to more quickly adopt the language and culture of the United States and then must translate English for their parents. Because most of the asylum cases of Haitians are denied (U.S. Committee for Refugees, 1995) many Haitians in the United States are considered illegal aliens. Children who are denied asylum but remain in the country illegally have suffered even into their adult years and in general suffered from nonhumanitarian treatment. Whereas other immigrants have been welcomed, the lack of welcome experienced by many Haitians has had a negative effect (Fernández-Kelly & Schauffler, 1994). Haitians have not consistently received the same treatment as other asylum-seeking refugees. It was not until May 1995 that the Clinton administration reversed the de facto policy that granted virtual blanket asylum to all Cubans (Epstein, Lantigua, & Cavanaugh, 1995).

In 1975 Haitians could be found in 45 of the 50 states (Seligman, 1977). Large settlements of Haitian people are located in the southern and eastern parts of the United States, with from 75% to 95% residing in Florida (Boswell, 1982; Wilk, 1986). New York City (especially Brooklyn) and Montreal have large, established Haitian communities that have mushroomed during times of revolution and political unrest in Haiti. For example, in 1960 there were reported to be 2584 Haitians living in New York City (Rosenwarke, 1972; Laguerre, 1984). In 1968 it was estimated that 34,000 Haitians had arrived in the United States during that year, and in 1970 it was estimated that 50,000 Haitians were living in New York City alone (McMorrow, 1970). According to the U.S. Census Bureau, there were 289,521 people of Haitian descent residing in the United States in 1993 (U. S. Department of Commerce, Bureau of the Census, 1993). This census figure may be underrepresented because of the number of illegal aliens from Haiti.

COMMUNICATION

Issues related to communication present a variety of problems for Haitians living in the United States or Canada. In Haiti there are two official languages: Haitian Creole (*Kreyòl*) and French. French is the official national language and is understood and spoken only by the upper or wealthy class. Although Haitian Creole is the language of the rural or poor population, it is also the primary language and is understood and spoken throughout the country (Weil, 1973). Speaking only Haitian Creole, a hybrid of old French vocabulary and African grammar, is perceived as a sign of poverty and a lack of education. Both Haitian Creole and French are often spoken so fast that one word is slurred into another. Because many Haitian immigrants in the United States continue to combine Haitian Creole and French, a dialect undergoing further creolization has been created, and it creates language barriers for some Haitian immigrants because most people in the dominant U.S. society are unfamiliar with it.

Haitians frequently use hand gesturing to complement their speech. Hand gesturing and tone of voice become more pronounced during communication. Primarily, hand gesturing is used as an addition to verbalizations. Touch and direct eye contact are also used in both casual and formal conversation. The Haitians' use of touch in conversation is perceived as friendship and does not violate personal space. Direct eye contact is used to gain the attention and respect of the other person during conversation. The Haitian cultural uses of touch and direct eye contact and the perception of friendship through conversation are much like those used throughout the United States.

Implications for nursing care

Language is often an area where problems arise between refugees and health care providers. One reason Haitians have received limited health care in the United States is the failure of many Haitians to speak either of the dominant languages: English or Spanish. Many schools in the United States have extensive bilingual programs for native Spanish speakers but have paid little attention to other non-English speakers. The problem of providing bilingual education for Haitians is complex and begins with a lack of materials for teaching English to Haitian Creole speakers. There are also varying opinions on the best way to teach literacy skills. Some persons believe that Haitians who have immigrated to the United States must be taught literacy in their native language. The view is that if Haitian Creole is used as a teaching tool, it can facilitate acquisition of reading and writing skills in English (Dejean, 1983).

The nurse should promote the Haitian-American client's interest in gaining English-language skills to facilitate the client's adjustment to the dominant culture. Although most Haitians are eager to learn English, learning to read and write as an adult is often difficult and time consuming, and support from health care professionals can encourage the Haitian individual to stick with this difficult task. Many Haitians who use French as their primary language have retained it, even though they have made a permanent move to the United States or Canada. Although many in the United States and Canada share the French-speaking Haitian's view that French is the language of the culturally elite, it should be noted that French-speaking Haitians have as much difficulty learning English as any other non-English speakers do.

If the client does not speak English, the nurse should first determine what language the client does speak. If the nurse does not know Haitian Creole or French, an interpreter may be necessary. When possible, a bilingual family member can help convey to the client and nurse information essential to health care. The nurse may find that Haitian Americans with children are more likely to speak correct English because speaking correct English is a status symbol and parents who know English will usually speak correct English in the home. The nurse caring for a Haitian-American client should be aware that Haitians value a touch or a smile by the nurse as a sign of friendship. Nonverbal communication can assist in bridging gaps between the differences in language because it can facilitate an understanding of client needs.

SPACE

Personal space to the Haitian can be defined as a public zone. Haitians as a cultural group are a sharing population. If they possess something that another person could or might benefit from, it will be shared. Another factor that tends to make the culture a public zone is the closeness of the living arrangements or dwellings. As a result, the Haitians are a public-oriented society. Haitians in the United States, for the most part, usually socialize with other immigrants arriving from their own town in Haiti and maintain primary loyalty to family members, many of whom remain in Haiti. Legal immigrants look forward to spending holidays in Haiti and regard the allowed time each year as a focal point. Illegal aliens are more isolated because they cannot maintain family contact. This represents a great change from the lifestyle led in Haiti, where extended family and the closeness of the community are emphasized.

Implications for nursing care

It is important for the nurse caring for a Haitian-American client to know that data from studies have indicated that Haitians find touch by caregivers to be supportive, comforting, and reassuring (Dempsey & Gesse, 1983). In a study of 10 women, Dempsey and Gesse noted that there were diverse views on whether these women preferred to be touched during delivery and if the preference was for a man or woman to touch them. In the study two

women specified a preference for being touched by a woman, three preferred to be touched by a man, and three did not have a preference. Nine stated that the father should be present. What is implied by this is that Haitian women may be less likely than women from some cultural groups to insist on having female nurses in the delivery room.

Although Haitians and African Americans share a heritage that extends back to Africa, the two groups do very little social mixing and tend to mistrust each other (Dempsey & Gesse, 1983). It is important for the nurse to understand that just because two clients may be Black does not mean they will share common interests or find each other suitable companions for sharing a hospital room. Some Haitians, like some other people from other social groups, are not free of social prejudice. Appreciation of these cultural socioeconomic issues by the nurse will facilitate assignment of staff to care for Haitian clients as well as room assignments of clients.

Because of the large gap in social classes, it is important for the nurse to consider the economic background of Haitian-American clients before placing them in the same area. For example, a poor client and a wealthy client with a Haitian background, though being from the same country, may find a room assignment together in a hospital very distasteful.

SOCIAL ORGANIZATION
Social class

The Haitian masses are essentially divided into two class structures: the wealthy and the poor. Statistically, 85% of the Haitian population is classified as poor, 10% as middle class, and 5% as wealthy (Bell, 1981). Class is demonstrated in many interesting ways. Wearing shoes is a requirement by law in the capital city, but many Haitians, especially in the small towns and villages, go barefooted. This is by no means a matter of choice but a mark of social standing. As an illustration of this, a Haitian physician who was enjoying a little recreation in one of the small towns was told that a client was waiting for him nearby. The physician asked if the client had shoes on. What was implied in this question was that, if the client had shoes on, the physician would be obliged to go immediately. On the other hand, if the client did not, the client would be in for a wait (Jeanty, 1989). Regardless of class, Haitians are a proud and independent people.

Education

Education in Haitian schools differs greatly from that in American schools. Until 1979 the only officially recognized language and the language that was required to be used in school was French. The educational system and schools are strict and authoritarian. Children who are financially able to attend must wear starched uniforms. The Haitian teacher has the right to use corporal punishment on a misbehaving child. Thus the lack of structure and discipline of many American schools meets with disapproval from Haitians. Much of the information given to students in the Haitian schools is memorized; memorization through repetition is the primary source of learning. Haitian children can be heard reciting multiplication tables through rhyme and song throughout the community. Sheer repetition of the same formula, problem after problem written on the blackboard, manages to register the information in the student's mind. Haitian teachers enunciate clearly when communicating with their students (Verdet, 1985).

Rather than attend the public high schools, Haitian Americans prefer to remain out of the mainstream of education and often strive to accelerate the educational process and obtain the credentials they value by seeking a high school–equivalency diploma. Haitian Americans view a college education as a form of prestige and status.

Family

The commonality among Haitians in Haiti and Haitians in the United States, whether wealthy or poor, is family. The family structure or system is very different from that of the American system. The practice of common-law marriage is predominant, particularly among the poor. Most legal marriages occur among the wealthy as a result of their economic status. Common-law marriage gives the father of the family much freedom and imposes much of the responsibility of caring for and meeting the needs of the family unit on the mother. The father,

perhaps dividing his time between several family units, becomes a powerful but unreliable figure. The concept of a single-parent family, primarily the single mother, is similar to that in the United States but is more prevalent in Haiti. The Haitian mother is commonly left to raise the children without the support system of the father.

The term *plaçage* may be defined as the union of a man and woman who desire to live together and who fulfill certain obligations and perform certain ceremonies at the home of the woman's parents, after which a new household is established. These unions are said to endure as long as recognized church marriages and constitute two thirds of all unions in Haiti (Herskovits, 1971; Schaedel, 1962). Haitian women involved in *plaçage* can be classified into four groups according to their relationship with Haitian men:

1. *Femme caille* (common-law): a woman who shares her home with a man in a common-law marriage situation.
2. *Mama petite* ("mother of my children"): a woman who is the mother of some of the man's children but does not share his house. This is similar to some *plaçage* unions with children, but in this situation the husband continues to live with his first wife while maintaining the second relationship.
3. *Femme plaçage* (woman whom a man "goes with" or a friend): a woman who neither lives with nor has had children by a man but who shares his bed intermittently and often maintains a garden, usually furnished by him.
4. *Femme avec* (woman who is lived with): a woman with whom the man cohabits for pleasure and without firm economic ties (Williams, Murthy, & Berggren, 1975).

Affection from both parents is readily given to children, and physical punishment is given as a form of discipline. Haitian mothers rely less on parent-child dialogue and more on physical punishment to effect changes in the child's behavior and to instill proper attitudes and values (Charles, 1979). Although Haitian mothers are extremely affectionate with their children, the children are taught from infancy that there is an unquestioned obedience to adult wishes. Haitian children do not presume to question parents or seek information concerning matters such as sex education because this would be seen as disrespectful of adult authority (Bestman, 1979). Child-rearing is shared by siblings as well as by the parents.

The Haitian family is traditionally extended, with each dwelling or residence paralleling a small community. Outside of the extended family, godparents play a very important role in the family organization and are generally considered part of the natural family. Rural or poor families tend to be matriarchal and child centered, with parents exercising a strong influence and authority over their offspring, even when the children are grown. Haitians view their children as direct reflections of themselves and the family. If children fail to fulfill obligations or meet expectations, they are seen as having failed the family and as having brought disgrace on the parents (Desantis & Thomas, 1987). Because of the parent-child ties, many Haitian couples separate only temporarily when immigrating. The wife usually immigrates with the younger children, and the husband remains in Haiti with the older children until the entire family can obtain authorization to relocate. One-parent families are quite common among this immigrant group in the United States.

DeSantis and Ugarriza (1995) investigated Haitian mothers and their child-rearing practices. They identified the need for psychiatric mental health nurses to assist immigrant Haitian families in handling intergenerational conflict because there are significant differences between the culture of origin and the culture encountered in the United States. Conflicts arise for children between what their parents say and what they see in the culture around them. Adolescent Haitians tend to fit the profile of high school leavers in that they are often poor and Black and live in households with high levels of stress. Social support for education is necessary if the adolescents are to remain in school (Rosenthal, 1995).

Traditionally, Haitian parents have a strong voice in their children's selection of a mate and in their choice of a career. Haitians tend to be an extremely status-conscious group and desire marriages or careers that enhance the status of the family. For most Haitian immigrants in the United States, home ties to Haiti remain strong. Even though there may be little opportunity for travel back and forth because of cost and the illegal status of many, ties to the mother and home remain. Letters, packages, and money are sent regularly. Because many Haitians are illiterate, sending cassettes to relatives in the United States or home to Haiti is a common form of communication (Jeanty, 1989).

Some older Haitian immigrants have been found to depend more on the members of their social support network than other Haitian age groups (Degazon, 1994; Seabrooks, 1992). The older immigrants experienced more changes in life events and loss of network members because of age in addition to problems associated with migration. The older Haitian immigrants also reported that they encountered hostility and stress because of their African heritage and skin color (Seabrooks, 1992). On the other hand, Robinson (1994) reported that aides in nursing homes caring for Black clients from three cultural groups were generally positive toward the elderly but negative toward the families of the elderly residents who did not take care of the elderly at home. Findings indicated the need for education for aides related to differences among people in different cultural groups.

Implications for nursing care

Cultural factors related to social organization have an important influence on health and health care behavior. Fundamental norms, such as the desirability of having many children and the traditional roles of men and women, affect reproductive behavior. Because the legal status of many is either questionable, as for entrants, or undesirable, as for illegal aliens, Haitians frequently use different names, giving one name at one clinic and another name at another clinic. In addition to causing confusion to health care providers, this practice leads to people "falling through the cracks" because of records not being available. Consequently there is a loss in continuity of care for some Haitian clients. In addition, because of the repeated intake procedures on the same client, health care services may be delayed (Wilk, 1986).

An astute nurse should keep in mind that because the Haitian family is traditionally extended the opinions and ideas of the family must be incorporated into a culturally sensitive plan of care. It is also important to remember that because Haitian children are taught from infancy to be unquestionably obedient to adult wishes it is especially important to provide parents with adequate health education if children are to benefit from improved and knowledgeable health care.

The nurse should also be aware that bisexuality may be an occurrence among Haitian men. Even when this information is important, the client may not readily offer this information. The nurse may need to elicit this information by asking if the client has ever had sex with another man rather than using the labels of homosexuality or bisexuality (Randall-David, 1989; Laguerre, 1981).

Immigrant Haitian mothers have been found to believe that little can be done to avoid childhood illnesses considered medically preventable in the United States (DeSantis & Thomas, 1992). Many Haitian mothers adhere to the beliefs and practices of Haitian folk medicine because they have not been taught or do not believe in preventive health care. This has important implications for health education of parents and for health teaching of children (DeSantis & Thomas, 1992). DeSantis and Thomas (1992) found that nurses were considered the best persons to do health teaching. Teaching was valuable when it is understandable, is practical, reinforces parenting abilities, and allows time for questions.

TIME

Traditionally, Haitians have not been committed to time or a schedule. It is not considered impolite to arrive late for an appointment. Everyone and anything can wait. Haitians compensate for lack of time orientation by manipulating timing of activities. For example, a wedding invitation will show a starting time of 6 PM when the actual starting time is actually 7 or 7:30 (Colin & Paperwalla, 1996).

The time orientation of Haitian Americans is related to social class. Poor or lower-class Haitian Americans tend to be relatively past and present oriented because they find it necessary to live from day

to day looking for food and trying to sustain a meager living. Because of their economic and educational status, the future for some of these people remains bleak. If a poor Haitian American has little to no chance of getting ahead, it is unlikely that a future orientation will be developed.

On the other hand, wealthy Haitian Americans may perceive time from a totally different perspective. For these people time orientation may be a combination of both present and future orientations. It would appear that as a result of adequate financial resources, upper-class Haitians and Haitian immigrants do make plans for the future. Because wealth may ensure educational attainment, which may translate into status and prestige, it is likely that a well-educated upper-class Haitian may have a future-time orientation.

Implications for nursing care

Because Haitians may have different orientations to time, depending on their social status and class, it is important for the nurse to adequately assess each individual client. It is also important for the nurse to remember that personal ethnocentric attitudes toward time may negatively affect the planning of care for clients. Persons with a present-time orientation may view future-oriented tasks as irrelevant or unimportant to present situations. Thus a present-time orientation may restrain a Haitian from gaining upward mobility because future orientation is required in gaining an education and planning to achieve future goals. It is also important to remember that when a Haitian immigrant does not keep an appointment or does not arrive for a clinic appointment on time it may be a result of a present-time orientation but may also be the result of economic constraints. It is important for the nurse to assess not only the time variable, but also other socioeconomic variables, including the availability of transportation to and from clinic appointments. If a Haitian American is to meet clinic appointments on time, it is very important for the nurse to emphasize the importance of adhering to the clinic's schedule. The nurse should be aware that Haitian Americans frequently stop a treatment regimen as soon as the symptoms appear to be relieved. It is also very likely that the Haitian American will fail to follow through with a treatment regimen or preventive health care because cultural beliefs do not relate personal actions to health status.

ENVIRONMENTAL CONTROL

Although Haitians and African Americans share a lineage that extends back to Africans who were seized from their countries and enslaved, some individuals have surmised that these two cultural groups fraternize very little socially and tend to mistrust and be suspicious of each other (Wilentz, 1989). It is believed that Haitians place a high value on personal liberty and are therefore resentful and at times indignant of American prejudice and critical of African Americans, whom they discern as being too submissive and accepting of discrimination (Wilentz, 1989). At the same time, African-American militancy and violent protest seem to be contrary to the Haitian personality and are generally regarded by Haitians with disapproval (Wilentz, 1989).

Traditionally the upper classes in Haiti have been the lighter-skinned Blacks, whose skin color results from crossbreeding with other, lighter-skinned people. Light skin traditionally has been regarded as more prestigious than dark skin in Haiti (Leyburn, 1980), with the upper-class, lighter-skinned Haitians dealing with the lower-class, darker-skinned persons in an authoritarian manner. Therefore, because of indoctrination regarding the color of the skin and its perceived relationship to social status or class, some Haitians have developed social prejudice that causes difficulty in the assimilation process in the United States. As a result of social prejudice formed by such variables as color grading and social status, some Haitians living in the United States or Canada continue to have trouble adjusting to other groups and thereby choose to remain in isolated areas, socializing only with other Haitians and family members.

Some Haitians view illness and disease as natural or unnatural events. Natural events keep balance between nature and humankind and as such are believed to be designed by God. Natural laws are believed to give life predictability (Snow, 1981). Unnatural events are believed to upset the balance of nature and at their worst represent forces of evil and the devil. Unnatural events lack predictability because they exist beyond the parameters of nature and are beyond the control of "mere mortals." This view is in sharp contrast to traditional Western medical beliefs. It is essential that the nurse remember that some Haitians believe illness is a result of witchcraft. People who supposedly possess supernatural power are believed to be able to alter the health status of others (Snow, 1981).

Voodoo practices

The practice of voodoo, the primary religion in Haiti, is prevalent throughout the country. Voodoo is a religious cult practice that dates back to the preslavery days of Africa. Christianity, particularly Catholicism, is becoming more prevalent but is slow to emerge because of the deep-seated roots of the voodoo culture and conviction. From their West African homelands, Haitians brought the belief that man is surrounded or enveloped by a variety of powerful, dominant spirits. Some Haitians believe that it is essential to invoke spirits. In the Haitian culture the invoked spirits are called *loas, mystères,* or *saints.* Some Haitians believe that voodoo spirits manifest and reveal themselves by possessing or "riding" the devoted believer. It is believed that the personality of the *loa* "mount" may change; he or she may be calm and subdued one minute and then suddenly become violent. Such transformations may be caused primarily by nervous instability under the influence of compelling drum rhythms and mass emotion (Logan, 1975). Haitians trust and depend on their voodoo beliefs and also rely on "readers" or "diviners," who predict the future by reading cards or hands and cure by means of being possessed by the voodoo spirit. The readers, or diviners, also considered voodoo priests, are organized into independent cults.

Voodoo priests may be either male *(hungan)* or female *(mambo)* and are categorized in five classes: shaman (voodoo practitioner), herbalist *(docte fey,* literally 'leaf doctor'), midwife *(matronn,* or *fam saj),* bonesetter *(docte zo),* and injectionist *(pikirist).* Healers are often not well defined, and a Haitian may go to a neighbor who has "extra" medicine or a healing practice in hopes of relief. In terms of the number of practitioners and frequency of use, the herbalists constitute the most significant class of healers. Herbalists are the most generalized caregivers, and thus their role characteristics overlap to a certain extent with all other healer types (Coreil, 1983). Haitians often use home remedies and herbs for treating illnesses that are suggested by healers or priests. Many Haitians believe that tea made from leaves of the Bible will cure rheumatism. In this case, the Bible serves as protection against black magic, which is believed to cause rheumatism (Nida, 1954).

Magic powers may be used for purposes other than destroying enemies or healing the sick. The voodoo sorcerers of Haiti claim to be able to change themselves into animals, to pass through locked doors, and to raise the dead and make them slaves (*zombies*). Almost everyone who is a native Haitian claims to know someone who has been a genuine *zombie*. One man requested his family to cut his corpse into two pieces to be buried in separate graves for fear that the local sorcerer, who was his enemy, would bring him to life as a wretched slave. Although the Haitian government has no valid evidence of the existence of *zombies,* it sanctioned the belief by passing a law against the supposed practice (Nida, 1954).

In Haiti voodoo is sometimes actualized as fetishes, which are shared by groups of native Haitians. For example, a Haitian might have a small bottle containing some reddish liquid and a small mirror backed by cardboard facing the bottle, and all this wrapped in coarse red cloth with yards of black thread. This object is safeguarded in the most remote part of the house, with its location kept secret from visitors. If the Haitian could be induced to talk about this, he might explain that his father, who was a kind of voodoo priest, captured his soul when he was very young and put it in the bottle. As long as the bottle is preserved, the person will live, but once the bottle is broken, the soul will depart and the man must die. Not only would this fetish be held by this individual, but identical or similar fetishes might be shared by others in the community (Nida, 1954).

Many Haitian influences regarding voodoo practices are evident in the mainstream of American society. For example, in some cities and towns in Louisiana, the Haitian influence is extremely prevalent

and is perceived or felt by persons from other cultural groups as well. Louisiana is renowned for its voodoo society, which is a carryover from Haitian slaves who were brought to areas such as New Orleans for various domestic duties. Even today, because of early Haitian influence, voodoo and mystical thought remain evident regardless of ethnic or cultural background in cities such as New Orleans (Snow, 1981).

Childbearing beliefs

Although health care is a significant problem in urban Haiti, it is even more of a problem in rural Haiti, with pregnant and postpartum women being particularly vulnerable (Wiese, 1976). Many Haitians know nothing about prenatal care and do not routinely seek such care. Some may never have seen or been to a physician in their life. Healers are related to protection, and physicians are related to sickness. Use of a midwife is culturally permissible and is much more likely among Haitian people than other cultural groups in the United States. When a nurse is interacting with a pregnant Haitian woman or is providing care for a baby, using the phrase "We will help you have a strong baby" will often elicit cooperation. Staff who are willing to help the mother have a "strong baby" (rather than a "healthy baby") are more likely to be accepted (Jeanty, 1989).

Some pregnant Haitian women who experience an increase in salivation do not believe they should swallow the saliva. Sometimes they carry a "spit" cup with them and are not embarrassed to use it in public (Colin & Paperwalla, 1996). Many dietary precautions are followed by the Haitian pregnant women.

Pregnant women are viewed as special and are likely to be treated with more kindness and respect than nonpregnant women. Chants or sounds of a woman in labor include praying, singing, crying, and moaning in various combinations, which is done to call on their voodoo protectors (Dempsey & Gesse, 1983).

A study conducted by Scott in 1978 identified the postpartum period as the most crucial and decisive period of childbearing for the Haitian woman. During the postpartum period of 6 to 11 weeks, the Haitian woman follows a cultural regimen of baths, teas, vapor baths, and dressing warmly. This practice is supposed to make the client healthy and clean again after the birth. For the first 3 days the mother bathes in hot water in which herb leaves have been boiled. She also drinks a decoction made from boiled herb leaves. (Also during the first few days after childbirth, the mother takes "vapor baths." She sits above a pot of steaming water with leaves in it, especially orange tree leaves, and drapes a cloth over her head and shoulders.) For the next 3 consecutive days the mother takes her second series of baths, which are prepared with leaves in water warmed by the sun. At this point the mother drinks only water warmed by the sun or an infusion made with leaves steeped in water warmed by the sun. The mother takes constant special care to keep her body warm. She stays inside her dwelling for at least 3 days after the birth and keeps the doors and windows closed to keep out the cool air. She wears long sleeves, keeps her head covered, and wears heavy socks and shoes.

After 2 weeks to 1 month, the mother takes another bath. She may take a cold bath or perhaps jump into a cold stream. After this ritual, she may self-induce vomiting to cleanse her inner body. After all of this is completed, she can again resume normal activities and is considered clean (Harris, 1987).

The Miami Health Ecology Project (Scott, 1978) reported beliefs about menstruation among Haitians, a majority of whom believed the function of menstruation was to rid the body of "unclean," "waste," or "unnecessary" blood. Many Haitians also described menstruation in this manner: "It means you are a woman," with "woman" meaning that the individual has sexual feelings or needs and is not sterile. The Haitian girl reportedly learns about menstruation at a median age of 10 years. For 85% of the sample, this information was obtained from their mothers or in classes at school.

Implications for nursing care

It is important for the nurse to understand that for many Haitians, leaves have a special significance. When the client comes into the hospital or the clinic for an examination, leaves may be found in the clothes and on various parts of the body. Leaves are believed to have mystical power, and therefore keeping them close to the body is related to regaining or keeping health (Jeanty, 1989). The nurse should be accepting of this practice and avoid being shocked if leaves are found in the luggage or on the body of a client being treated. The nurse should also appreciate that religious medallions, rosary beads, or figures of a saint to whom the Haitian client is devoted may have special significance and be felt to offer protection and should be left with the client (Colin & Paperwalla, 1996).

If Haitian Americans do use conventional means of health care, they tend to use emergency rooms or clinics and to seek health care only when they are quite ill (Orque, Bloch, & Monrroy, 1983; Samet, Retondo, Freedberg, et al., 1994). Haitian Americans may also seek relief from their symptoms through a physician and at the same time consult a cultural healer. The client's having both a faith healer and a physician should not be perceived as incongruent (Jeanty, 1989). A client's fear and anxiety that he or she has been "hexed" may be alleviated or reduced if the therapist combines conventional treatment with the assistance of a cultural healer who is believed to be able to remove the hex or spell. Nurses, as primary health care providers, must formulate and use a treatment plan that displays respect and understanding of the client's cultural healing system or systems and must accept that a Haitian-American client may use a variety of sources to obtain relief when sick.

Haitians have grown accustomed to receiving some direction from authority figures in their lives—parents as well as religious and social leaders. The nurse, as an authority figure, will usually find that Haitian Americans respond well to counseling approaches that foster self-help and independence and should consider the need for heightened self-esteem, which is manifested by the pride and willingness to work that is present in most Haitians.

Haitian Americans need to have occupational options expanded for them and need to understand the steps involved in achieving an occupational goal. Because Haitians have not traditionally had the freedom to set goals, the nurse may be of assistance in this process, as well as in problem solving, to achieve the established goals.

A variety of tools has been used to measure beliefs of Haitians about illness and wellness (Neilson,

McMillan, & Díaz, 1992). Neilsen (1989) used a semi-structured interview for three Black cultures including Haitian. This work is ongoing (Neilsen, 1989).

BIOLOGICAL VARIATIONS
Body size and structure, skin color, and other visible physical characteristics

Haitians and African Americans are similar biologically. As with some other racial groups, the body size and structure of Haitians vary greatly. Haitians have no specific or distinctive size that can be linked genetically. This phenomenon may be a result of crossbreeding with other races throughout history. For this reason, Haitians can be short or tall, light skinned or dark skinned. Haitians are characterized as having shades of brown to black skin as well as brown to black eyes. The hair on the head is often tightly curled, and the body hair is sparsely distributed. The "true" Haitian is tall and exhibits an erect stature. The skull is dolichocephalic in form, being long and relatively narrow. The eyebrow ridges are scant or absent, and the forehead is moderately wide. The form of the orbits is almost square, and their margins are strongly built. The cheeks are wide and, with their supports or zygomatic arches, are bowed laterally in keeping with the powerful jaw musculature. The eyes are set widely apart by the broad and flattened nasal bones. The nose is flat, and the nostrils are widely expanded. The face is large and prominent. The jaws are prognathic and are covered by full, fleshy lips, the prominent mucosae of which are reddish black or purple in color (Godsby, 1971).

Some years ago, anthropologists and scientists discovered that two different types of earwax are present among the human race and that the composition of the earwax determines racial origin. Haitian earwax is described as moist and adhesive (Godsby, 1971).

Susceptibility to disease and other health concerns

Several major areas of health concerns have been identified in the Haitian culture, including intestinal problems, malnutrition, venereal disease, high birth rate, tuberculosis, sickle cell anemia, hypertension, and cancer. AIDS has also become a serious and increasing health issue since the 1970s for Haitians both in Haiti and in the United States.

Intestinal problems and malnutrition Intestinal problems stemming from malnutrition and ranging from stomach ailments to peptic ulcers are common. The peasant Haitian suffers more from these types of ailments than the wealthy or elite Haitian does. Typically, the Haitian diet tends to be very spicy and greasy. Haitians cook almost everything in oil or grease. Even after immigration to the United States, some Haitians continue to prepare foods that are spicy and greasy.

In Haiti the poor Haitian will consume virtually any type of food to sustain human life. Because many Haitians who have immigrated to the United States have remained at or below the poverty level, they will most likely continue to consume any type of food available. Chronic abdominal discomfort is primarily caused from parasites that are common to the Haitian population (Wilk, 1986).

Venereal disease Another problem is venereal disease. Haitian men tend to be more susceptible to different kinds of venereal diseases as a result of promiscuity (Jeanty, 1989). Because most marriages are common-law, the man of the family generally lacks commitment to one woman and usually has more than one sexual partner. In addition, the venereal disease is difficult to treat because the medication is usually taken only as long as the symptoms persist. Premature discontinuation of medication results in an incomplete cure. The problem of venereal disease is also extremely difficult to treat because Haitians do not equate venereal disease with sexual intercourse.

Because there are numerous illegal Haitian immigrants, the prevalence of venereal disease among Haitians in the United States is likely, but the extent is unknown. Testing for syphilis has been required since the Immigration Act of 1990 (Herip, 1993). When Haitians had been interdicted at sea and subsequently tested, 5% of Haitians had serological evidence of past or present syphilis (Herip, 1993).

High birth rate The high birth rate has many health and cultural implications for Haitians. One factor contributing to the population explosion is the lack of contraception, which is virtually nonexistent in the conventional manner. This is attributed to a lack of education and technology. An unusually large number of very young Haitian women become pregnant (Jeanty, 1989), and Haitian women also tend to become pregnant at older ages. Pregnancy in women 35 years of age and older in Haiti is fairly common (Wilk, 1986). Williams, Murthy, and Berggren (1975) reported that Haitian women between 35 and 49 years of age have an average of eight pregnancies. Because of this pattern, the nurse must be aware of the high risk among Haitian women in relation to their childbearing habits. Furthermore, family spacing is not an option, and a series of pregnancies within a short time leaves the women's body unable to fully recover or to replenish iron levels.

Tuberculosis Tuberculosis is another concern to the Haitian population. As a result of the poor economic levels, which lead to poor living conditions and malnutrition, Haiti has one of the world's highest rates of tuberculosis (Wilk, 1986). Another factor is overcrowding, which results in poor sanitation. The majority of the population has no waste facilities. Garbage and human excrement are thrown into the streets or placed in community pits and the water for drinking is contaminated, resulting in a vast majority of diseases, including tuberculosis. Malnutrition complicates the situation. The poor cannot afford the cost of examination or the medication to treat the illness if it is diagnosed. Of the number of Haitians who have attempted to immigrate to the United States from November 1991 to April 1992, 55% tested positive for tuberculosis on a purified protein derivative. Chest radiographs confirmed pulmonary tuberculosis in approximately 5% of this group (Herip, 1993). Approximately one third of those testing positive had findings suggestive of active infection. In 21% of the cases, culture and sensitivities for tuberculosis isolates were found to be resistant to medication. Because there is a high incidence of tuberculosis among Haitian immigrants assessment for symptoms of tuberculosis is an important part of health screening when the nurse is caring for Haitian clients.

Sickle cell anemia Sickle cell anemia, or Hb SS disease, is a chronic hereditary hemolytic disorder mainly affecting the Black populations of the world and is characterized by the presence of erythrocytes that primarily contain Hb S instead of Hb A. The red blood cell assumes a sickle shape when exposed to lower oxygen levels. Persons who are homozygous for Hb S are estimated to have erythrocytes that contain 80% to 100% abnormal Hb S and only up to 20% normal Hb A. The erythrocytes of persons with sickle cell trait contain approximately 25% to 40% Hb S and 60% to 75% Hb A.

Sickle cell anemia develops as a result of a genetic mutation that is transmitted from parent to child. Laboratory testing is available to determine if the sickle cell trait is present (Sorensen, Luckmann, & Bolander, 1994). It is important for the nurse to have a working knowledge of sickle cell anemia when assessing Haitian-American clients and to be able to refer the client to a sickle cell association or support group. It is important to provide the client with information about this illness because most of these clients know little about it (Jeanty, 1989).

Hypertension Little is known about hypertension among Haitians. A pilot study was conducted with 88 Haitian clients by Preston, Materson, Yoham, and Anapol (1996). This study indicated that hypertension was highly prevalent and unusually severe in terms of blood pressure level, refractoriness to treatment, and target organ consequences.

Malaria *Plasmodium falciparum* malaria was a major problem among displaced Haitians in temporary camps at the U.S. Naval Base, Guantánamo Bay, Cuba. From December 1991 to March 1992, 235 cases of unmixed falciparum malaria were diagnosed, giving a cumulative attack rate of 160 per 10,000 camp residents. Health professionals in treating Haitian immigrants should plan for malaria, and preventive medicine measures are indicated (Bawden, Slaten, & Malone, 1995).

Cancer Cancers reported in Haiti include cervical, hepatic, stomach, and intestine and Kaposi's sarcoma (Mitacek, St. Vallières, & Polednak, 1986). Cervical cancer accounts for 39% of all cancers among Haitian women and may be related to poor feminine hygiene as well as early sexual activity with multiple partners (Sebastian, Leeb, & See, 1978). Failure to have Pap smears, which would allow early detection, may relate to the high incidence of cervical cancer.

Fruchter, Wright, Habenstreit, et al. (1985) reported that approximately 50% of Haitian women had never had a Pap smear compared to 25% of the English-speaking Caribbean immigrants and 10% of United States–born Black women studied. Liver, stomach, and intestinal cancers are high among Haitian males. From 1979 to 1984, cancer of the liver (23.4%) and stomach and intestines (20.5%) accounted for 43.9% of all cancers (Mitacek, St. Vallières, & Polednak, 1986). Gastrointestinal cancer is related to the poor nutrition and low vitamin intake. Kaposi's sarcoma is found in some Haitians who are HIV positive.

AIDS Cases of AIDS in Haiti are believed to date back to the late 1970s. Actual incidence is unclear, though Herip (1993) noted that 7% of Haitians interdicted at sea tested positive for HIV. Pape, Verdier, Boney, et al. (1994) conducted a study from 1990 to 1993 with 2400 persons in Haiti with HIV who have diarrhea for the prevalence and clinical manifestations of *Cyclospora* bacteria. It was determined that *Cyclospora* was common in Haitian clients with HIV infection, that it responded to trimethoprim-sulfamethoxazole therapy, and that the high recurrence rate could be largely prevented with long-term trimethoprim-sulfamethoxazole prophylaxis. Samet, Retondo, Freedberg, et al. (1994) noted that most Haitian-American clients presented for primary care with advanced immune dysfunction. Many had waited a year to initiate medical care after testing positive for HIV. Women presented with significantly higher CD4+ cell counts than men did.

Because of the publicity of AIDS originating in Haiti (which has never been proved), Haitians who have immigrated to the United States face constant discrimination, though the combination of fear and the stigma about AIDS in the Haitian population is reported to be gradually decreasing (Laverdière, Tremblay, Lavallée, et al., 1983). Testing of Haitian immigrants for AIDS has been required since the Immigration Act of 1990 (Herip, 1993). Martin, Rissmiller, and Beal (1995) conducted a qualitative study of health-illness beliefs and practices of Haitian Americans with HIV disease living in Boston. Five themes were identified: (1) incorporation of traditional health-illness beliefs into beliefs about HIV disease, (2) a perceived need to hide HIV disease to avoid rejection, humiliation, and isolation, (3) use of spirituality to help cope with HIV disease, (4) history of limited contact with doctors before diagnosis of HIV disease, and (5) use of traditional healing practices for HIV disease. These findings have implications for improving cross-cultural communication between Haitians with HIV disease and their health care providers.

Nutritional preferences and deficiencies

There is a critical problem with malnutrition in the agricultural areas of Haiti among the poor (Rodman, 1961). Some estimate that 80% of Haitians suffer from malnutrition (National Catholic Reporter, 1983). For the Haitian peasant, environmental, technological, and economic factors alone account for a substantial amount of poor nutrition.

Haiti's rugged topography combines with a generally limited system of mass transport to accentuate the regional and seasonal nature of many of the crops. The economic status of most Haitians confines their food expenditures to a survival level of foods chosen from among locally produced foodstuffs. In addition, the humeral medical beliefs that classify food into "hot" and "cold" categories further restrict dietary selection (Wiese, 1976).

The nurse should be aware of food preferences customary to the Haitian culture (Box 20-1). As a result of the lack of ready availability of food items, Haitians have learned many poor nutritional habits, which have persisted even after immigration to the United States, particularly if similar economic conditions prevail.

Dietary habits for childbearing Haitian women Childbearing Haitian women are very particular about their dietary habits both before and after delivery. These dietary cultural habits include foods that a woman should and should not eat (Box 20-2). The nurse should assess these foods to ensure that the client maintains adequate nutrition (White, Linhart, & Medley, 1996).

Breast-feeding has traditionally been very common among Haitians because bottle-feeding was

Box 20-1

COMMON CULTURAL
FOOD REFERENCES

FRUITS AND NUTS	MEAT, VEGETABLES, AND OTHER FOODS
Rice	Beef
Avocados	Beets
Cashews	Okra
Coconuts	Biscuits (from imported white flour)
Granadilla flesh	
Mangos	Cabbage
Pineapples	Carrots
Soursop (guanabana) fruit	Imported cheese
Star apples (Chrysophyllum)	Chicken
Cassava (manioc, tapioca) bread	Milled corn
	Eggplant
Bananas	Fish
Limes	Goat meat
Grapefruits	Kidney beans
Oranges	Lima beans
Tomatoes	Peas
Watermelons	Pork
	Sweet potatoes
	Pumpkin
	Sugar cane

Box 20-2

CHILDBEARING WOMEN
AND FOOD PREFERENCES

FOODS EATEN BY CHILDBEARING WOMEN	
Cornmeal porridge with bean sauce	Black mushrooms
	White beans
Rice and beans	Okra
Plantains	Lobster
Vegetables	Fish
Red Fruits	Eggplant
FOODS AVOIDED BY CHILDBEARING WOMEN	Black peppers
	Milk
Lima beans	Bananas
Tomatoes	

considered unnatural (Jeanty, 1989). However, as traditional beliefs are changing among Haitian Americans, breast-feeding is decreasing (Thomas & DeSantis, 1995).

Psychological characteristics

Psychiatric care is also limited in Haiti. In 1956 Kline (Bordeleau & Kline, 1986) reported the presence of one psychiatrist and one psychiatric hospital in Haiti. In 1989 Gustafson reported less than a dozen psychiatrists in Haiti and all were located in the capital.

The first modern psychiatric hospital was opened in 1959, amid prejudice and resistance, by two psychiatrists from Canada and the United States. Because perphenazine (Trilafon) was donated by the three founding pharmaceutical companies and was used abundantly, the psychiatrists were called "Tri-

lafon doctors." Although psychiatric treatment has improved, the frequency of mental illness in Haiti is unknown, and the psychiatric services remain undeveloped. Bordeleau and Kline (1986) have reported that psychiatric symptoms do not appear to be much different from those found in other countries. Projection has been identified as a frequent defense mechanism because paranoid delusions often appear in clients who are psychotic. Delusions are profoundly colored by voodoo religious beliefs. Aggressivity is seldom directed toward others, with psychomotor hyperactivity being more often noisy than destructive. Affective disorders are more often of the hypomanic or manic type than depressive, and suicide among Haitians is rare. More recently, psychiatric care has advanced with the development of outpatient clients (Bordeleau & Kline, 1986). However, in 1986 the Pan-American Health Organization reported no listing of psychiatric diagnoses in Haiti in a study involving the years 1981 to 1984. Rather than psychiatric care, most emotionally disturbed clients sought native healers who treat with amulets, packets of herbs and spices, liquids, baths, powders, rubbing, and massage (Gustafson, 1989).

Laguerre (1981) has studied patterns of bereavement among Haitian-American families. Death arrangements are usually taken care of by a male kinsman of the deceased who has had experience with American bureaucracies. Death appears to mobilize the entire extended family, including matrilateral and patrilateral members. Because Haitians frequently believe that illness and death can be of a supernatural as well as natural origin (Metraux, 1953), death is often accompanied by feelings of guilt and anger. The surviving relatives may believe that the death was a result of failure to relate appropriately to the voodoo spirit. Recurrent dreams of the deceased person, so much a part of grief work, take on a particular meaning to the Haitian. Haitians commonly evaluate illness in terms of symptoms previously experienced by close kin (Laguerre, 1981), and grief work frequently includes taking on symptoms of the deceased person's last illness (Eisenbruch, 1984).

Possession crisis, which has been diagnosed in some Haitian clients, is not unique to Haitian voodoo but has also been observed in many African countries and on rare occasions among American Indians. This belief has much similarity with the early Greek Dionysian mysteries, the evil possession of the European Middle Ages, the witch possession in the New England colonies, and the contemporary African-American religious services of certain extreme groups in the South. See Box 20-3 for the conditions that must be present to have a possession crisis (Bordeleau & Kline, 1986).

Implications for nursing care

Because stomach ailments are a major problem for Haitians, the astute nurse will carefully assess the Haitian-American client for various stomach ailments, including worms, which may be the result of spoiled food. In fact, a nurse may assume that if a Haitian-American family has poor nutritional habits and at the same time cannot afford nutritious food, the likelihood that the family members will have worms is increased. Garlic is considered a folk remedy for worms and is boiled and eaten to prevent and treat worms. When a Haitian-American client brings in a specimen and hands it to the clinic nurse, it is important for the nurse to understand that this

---

Box 20-3
POSSESSION CRISIS

1. The general population of the local community must believe that a human being can communicate with the deities.
2. The person being "mounted" by the spirit (*loa*) is one of a group involved in a religious ceremony where the drums control the rhythm of the dance and the *hungan* behaves at first as a ritualistic priest.
3. Some spirits "participate" only at a certain time of the year and with a similar type of personality; that is, a gentle *loa* mounts a calm person and a fighting *loa* chooses an aggressive person.
4. The group considers being possessed to be a privilege, not a shameful event.
5. The possession crisis is stereotyped in the sense that someone mounted by a specific loa will talk like the loa, ask for the needed symbolic ornaments, and generally behave and dance in the way traditions in the region have dictated.

From Bordeleau, J.M., & Kline, N.S. (1986). *World Mental Health*, pp. 170-183.

---

may be a communication about a problem with worms and that the specimen should be analyzed with this in mind. The nurse will be better able to assist the Haitian-American client by not trying to convince the client that garlic is inappropriate. The folk remedies should be accepted and combined with Western medicine.

The nurse should appreciate that in addition to diet being important in relation to the health of pregnant women, dietary practices are generally related to health. Eating well and eating fresh foods is related to maintaining health. Drinking tea every day made with *sorosi* ('mulberry juice') is believed by many Haitian Americans to increase appetite and protect health and prevent illness. One can treat fever by mixing castor oil, alcohol, and shallot (*Allium ascalonicum*), heating the mixture, rubbing it together, and rubbing it all over the fevered body (Spector, 1996).

It is important for the nurse to know that many Haitian Americans have very little information about disease or medical problems. Therefore an illness is more commonly considered a "hex" or the result of an evil curse. The nurse should collect information from the client about the possible cause for the medical problem and should remain nonjudgmental even when voodoo is provided as a possible explanation. Health teaching (such as regarding diarrhea or pneumonia) is essential to help the Haitian client understand that the illness is not an evil curse imposed by a neighbor but an illness with natural physical causes.

The nurse cannot assume that all Haitian Americans will have the same beliefs. It is useful to ask Haitian-American clients how long they have been in the United States, which will provide an indication of how Americanized the client may be. The age of the client is also a consideration when health beliefs are being assessed. Younger people are more likely to have made an effective adjustment to the Western culture, whereas older people often continue to find such things as American food strange and unacceptable.

Haitian-American clients are more likely to believe that they are receiving effective treatment when a nurse is seen. In Haiti a nurse is given more authority and status than a physician, and the client will often be more cooperative with directions given by a nurse (Jeanty, 1989). When nursing procedures are being implemented (such as taking the client's blood pressure), the nurse should tell the client orally what is being done and that this is for the client's benefit. Actions by the nurse are related to being helped.

Some Haitian Americans associate wheelchairs with being sick. Therefore on discharge the client who is allowed to walk out of the hospital will be more likely to feel that care has been effective (Jeanty, 1989).

Great stress has been placed on Haitians as they have attempted to adjust to life in the United States and Canada. Coming from a disadvantaged background and often arriving in the United States with a history of poor health care, Haitians have been hesitant to reach out for health care. For some of these people, a hospital is perceived as a place to go to die, which may contribute to large numbers of visitors when a Haitian is ill (Jeanty, 1989). Health professionals at all levels must communicate a nonjudgmental attitude while trying to encourage the Haitian-American client to take advantage of available health services. Not only do Haitian Americans need to be educated regarding health care agencies, but they may also need information on health insurance, on how to use health benefits, and on finding a job that has medical benefits. Conway and Buchanan (1985) suggest that what is most helpful to Haitians' adjusting to life in the United States is to focus on the strengths from their cultural heritage, such as attitude, perseverance in the most arduous circumstances, deep religious faith, high self-respect, reliance on the extended family, and the tradition of sharing.

SUMMARY

Haiti is an independent, underdeveloped republic that continues to face many critical issues such as a poor economy, lack of technology, high mortality, inadequacy in food and water supplies, and lack of adequate or quality health care. With the ever-growing Haitian population immigrating to the United States, the nurse must constantly keep these issues in mind when formulating a treatment plan for a Haitian-American client. The holistic approach must be a priority approach when the nurse is assessing, treating, and evaluating the Haitian-American client. The Haitian cultural method of health care delivery must be included with conventional methods of treatment, and transcultural issues in nursing must be recognized before quality care can be rendered. Cultural behavior is meaningful and should not be ridiculed, judged negatively, or ignored. The nurse must be aware of cultural and behavioral considerations that affect the care of the Haitian immigrant and use this understanding in implementation of the nursing process. Quality health care that is culturally sensitive to the needs of Haitian refugees is possible when knowledge of their culture and beliefs is used as a basis for intervention.

Case Study

A 33-year-old Haitian man is admitted via the emergency room with symptoms of persistent coughing and spitting up small amounts of blood. Through the nursing assessment and by talking with the client and his family members, the nurse determines that the client has been experiencing a progressive lack of appetite and is visibly underweight. Radiographic examination reveals that the client has an active and communicable case of tuberculosis. When the client and the family are informed that the diagnosis is tuberculosis, there is little reaction. The nurse is informed by the client's family members that the client was initially diagnosed as having a positive Mantoux test in Haiti approximately 2 years previously. At that time the client was given a prescription for isoniazid (INH) by a clinic physician but was noncompliant with his medication regimen.

CARE PLAN

 Nursing Diagnosis Gas exchange, impaired, related to tuberculosis as evidenced by viscous secretions and coughing

Client Outcomes

1. Client will have no further coughing or viscous secretions.

Nursing Interventions

1. Maintain adequate hydration (increase fluid intake to 2 to 3 quarts per day).
2. Maintain adequate humidity of inspired air.
3. Minimize irritants in inspired air (such as dust, allergens).
4. Provide periods of uninterrupted rest.
5. Administer prescribed medication such as cough suppressant or expectorant as ordered by physician.

 Nursing Diagnosis Nutrition, altered, less than body requirements, related to tuberculosis as evidenced by anorexia and weight that is below normal for age, sex, and body stature

Client Outcomes

1. Client will gain weight to be within normal range for body size.

Nursing Interventions

1. Maintain good oral hygiene (make sure client brushes teeth, rinses mouth) before and after ingestion of food.
2. Arrange to have foods with the most protein and calories served at times the client feels most like eating.
3. Use dietitian for meal planning.

 Nursing Diagnosis Medication noncompliance related to communication barriers as evidenced by previous noncompliance, cultural beliefs, and religious beliefs

Client Outcomes

1. Client will take prescribed medication as ordered.

Nursing Interventions

1. Allow client an opportunity to make decisions about his own health care; assume an advisory approach when counseling, rather than one that is dictatorial.
2. Consult with an interpreter who speaks both English and Haitian Creole to provide instructions on how to take medication.
3. Consult with an interpreter who speaks both English and Haitian Creole to help client vent his feelings of anxiety and frustration.

Nursing Diagnosis   Medication noncompliance related to referral process

Client Outcomes

1. Client will keep scheduled follow-up appointments.

Nursing Interventions

1. Whenever possible, allow client to make own appointments.
2. Shorten referral waiting time.
3. Personnel handling referral appointment should inquire about transportation, suggesting help if needed.

 Nursing Diagnosis   Family processes, altered, related to an ill family member as evidenced by ambivalent feelings of family members to the disease process and lack of support from family members

Client Outcomes

1. Family will achieve functional support for client.

Nursing Interventions

1. Include family members in group education sessions about tuberculosis.
2. Refer family members to support and self-help groups.
3. Obtain Haitian Creole–speaking interpreter to facilitate communication.
4. Facilitate family involvement with social supports.

STUDY QUESTIONS

1. If a Mantoux test is given incorrectly and no wheal appears (because the injection was made too deep), should the nurse repeat the test at another site that is at least 2 inches away from the first injection?
2. What does erythema without induration mean?
3. In tuberculosis, treatment is continued until when?
4. The physician says the client has induration. What does this mean?
5. List the possible side effects of isoniazid (INH).
6. What preventive steps can be taken to avoid the spread of a diagnosed case of tuberculosis?
7. Why is proper nutrition important with a client diagnosed as having tuberculosis?
8. Why is the Haitian population at high risk for being infected by tuberculosis?
9. What is the nurse's role when caring for a client with tuberculosis?
10. Compare the similarities and differences in family structure between the American and Haitian cultures.
11. What are the contributing factors that lead to the high birth rate in Haiti and among Haitian immigrants?
12. Why are Haitian women at risk during pregnancy?
13. Describe the practice of healers and their importance to the Haitian population.
14. Describe the role of the Haitian man as it pertains to family.

References

Annas, G. (1993). Detention of HIV-positive Haitians at Guantánamo. *New England Journal of Medicine, 329,* 589-592.

Bawden, M.P., Slaten, D.D., & Malone, J.D. (1995, Nov.-Dec.) Falciparum malaria in a displaced Haitian population. *Transactions of the Royal Society of Tropical Medicine and Hygiene, 89*(6), 600-603.

Bell, I. (1981). *The Dominican Republic.* Boulder, Colo.: Westview Press.

Bestman, E. (1979). *Cultural, linguistic and racial barriers in providing health services to Haitian refugees.* Paper presented at a workshop on improving health services to Haitian refugees, sponsored by the U.S. Health Service Administration, Metro-Dade County, Florida.

Bonnlander, H. (1996, Sept.). Migrant TB treatment in Haiti resulting in U.S. policy change at Guantánamo Bay, Cuba. *Bulletin of the Pan-American Health Organization, 30*(3), 206-211.

Bordeleau, J.M., & Kline, N.S. (1986). Experience in developing psychiatric services in Haiti. *World Mental Health,* pp. 170-183.

Boswell, T. (1982). The new Haitian diaspora. *Caribbean Review,* 11(1), 18-21.

Bryan, S. (1988). *Ethnic diseases.* Paper presented at a workshop sponsored by the U.S. Health Service Administration, Metro-Dade County, Florida.

Charles, C. (1979). *Anthropological consideration of barriers affecting delivery of health services to Haitian refugees in Florida.* Paper presented at a workshop on improving health services to Haitian refugees, sponsored by the U.S. Health Service Administration, Metro-Dade County, Florida.

Chelala, C. (1994, Aug. 20-27). Fighting for survival. *British Medical Journal,* 309(6953), 525-526.

Claude, Jean (1997, Nov. 7). Presentation on Haiti at the Mennonite Economic Development Conference in Kansas City, Missouri.

Colin, J., & Paperwalla, G., (1996). Haitians. In Lipson, J., Dibble, S., & Minarik, P. (Eds.), *Culture and nursing care: a pocket guide.* School of Nursing, University of California, San Francisco: UCSF Nursing Press.

Conway, F., & Buchanan, S. (1985). Haitians. In Haines, D. (Ed.), *Refugees in the United States* (pp. 95-109). Westport, Conn.: Greenwood Press.

Coreil, J. (1983, July). Parallel structures in professional and folk health care: a model applied to rural Haiti. *Culture, Medicine and Psychiatry, 70,* 131-151.

Degazon, C. (1994). Ethnic identification, social support and coping strategies among three groups of ethnic African elders. *Journal of Cultural Diversity, 1*(4), 79-85.

Dejean, Y. (1983). *Revisiting the issues of the native language as a natural medium of instruction.* Master's thesis. New York: Bank Street College of Education.

Dempsey, P.A., & Gesse, T. (1983). The childbearing Haitian refugee: cultural applications to clinical nursing. *Public Health Reports, 98*(3), 261-267.

Desantis, L., & Thomas, J. (1987, Aug.). Parental attitudes toward adolescent sexuality: Transcultural perspectives. *Nurse Practitioner, 12,* 43-48.

Desantis, L., & Thomas, J. (1992). Health education and the immigrant Haitian mother: cultural insights for community health nurses. *Public Health Nursing, 9*(2), 87-96.

Desantis, L., & Ugarriza, D. (1995, Dec.). Potential for intergenerational conflict in Cuban and Haitian immigrant families. *Archives of Psychiatric Nursing, 9*(6), 354-364.

Eisenbruch, M. (1984). Cross-cultural aspects of bereavement: Part 2. Ethnic and cultural variations in the development of bereavement practices. *Culture, Medicine and Psychiatry, 8,* 315-347.

Epstein, G., Lantigua, J., & Cavanaugh, J. (1995, May 7). U.S. ship taking rafters to Cuba. *Miami Herald,* p. 1A.

Eshleman, J., & Davidhizar, R. (1997, Spring). Life in migrant camps for children—a hazard to health. *Journal of Cultural Diversity, 4*(1), 13-15.

Fernández-Kelly, M., & Schauffler, R. (1994). Divided fates: immigrant children in a restructured U.S. economy. *International Migration Review, 28,* 662-689.

Fruchter, R.G., Wright, C., Habenstreit, B., et al. (1985). Screening for cervical and breast cancer among Caribbean immigrants. *Journal of Community Health, 10,* 121-135.

Godsby, R. (1971). *A race and races.* New York: Macmillan.

Granich, R., Sfeir, M., & Jacobs, B. (1994, Feb. 3). Detention of HIV-positive Haitians and Cubans. *New England Journal of Medicine, 330*(5), 372.

Grant, W. (1989, Aug. 6). *The prevalence of antibodies to HTLV-I virus in the Aribonite Valley.* Paper presented at the annual reunion of the Hospital Albert Schweitzer Alumni Association, Burlington, Vermont.

Gustafson, M. (1989). Western voodoo: providing mental health care to Haitian refugees. *Journal of Psychosocial Nursing, 27,* 22-25.

Harris, K. (1987). Beliefs and practices among Haitian American women in relation to childbearing. *Journal of Nurse-Midwifery, 32*(3), 149-155.

Herip, D. (1993). Health status of Haitian migrants - U.S. naval base, Guantánamo Bay, Cuba, November, 1991–April, 1992. *Journal of the American Medical Association, 269,* 1395.

Herskovits, M.J. (1971). *Life in a Haitian valley.* New York: Doubleday.

Hiebert, C. (1997, Nov. 8). Presentation on Haiti at the Mennonite Economic Development Conference in Kansas City, Missouri.

Hobsbawn, E.J. (1962). *The age of revolution: 1789-1848.* London: Weidenfeld & Nicolson.

Holcomb, L.O., Parsons, L.C., Giger, J.N., & Davidhizar, R.E. (1996). Haitian Americans: implications for nursing care. *Journal of Community Health Nursing, 13*(4), 249-260.

Information please almanac (1998). Boston: Houghton Mifflin.

Jeanty, M. (1989). Personal communication at Logansport State Hospital, Logansport, Indiana.

Laguerre, M. (1981). Haitian Americans. In Harwood, A. (Ed.), *Ethnicity and medical care.* Cambridge, Mass.: Harvard University Press.

Laguerre, M. (1984). *American Odyssey: Haitians in New York City.* Ithaca, N.Y.: Cornell University Press.

Laverdière, M., Tremblay, J., Lavallée, R., et al. (1983). AIDS in Haitian immigrants and in a Caucasian woman closely associated with Haitians. *Canadian Medical Association Journal, 129*(11), 1209-1212.

Leyburn, J.G. (1980). *The Haitian people.* New Haven, Conn.: Yale University Press.

Lillibridge, S., Conrad, K., Stinson, N., & Noji, E. (1994, Feb.). Haitian mass migration: uniformed service medical support, May 1992. *Military Medicine, 159*(2), 149-153.

Logan, M. (1975). Selected references on the hot-cold theory of disease. *Medical Anthropology Newsletter, 6*(2), 8-11.

Martin, M., Rissmiller, P., & Beal, J. (1995, Nov.-Dec.). Health-illness beliefs and practices of Haitians with HIV disease living in Boston. *Journal of the Association of Nurses in AIDS care, 6*(6), 45-53.

Masland, T. (1992, Feb. 24). Haiti: "We could turn our back." *Newsweek,* pp. 30-32.

McMorrow, T. (1970, Nov. 15). Haitians try to adopt U.S. with three strikes on them. *Daily News,* p. B1.

Métraux, A. (1953). Médecine et voudou en Haïti. *Acta Tropica, 10,* 28-68.

Metropolitan Dade County. (1981). *Social and economic problems among Cuban and Haitian entrant groups in Dade County, Florida: trends and implications.* Miami, Fla.: Metropolitan Dade County.

Mitacek, E.J., St. Vallières, D., & Polednak, A.P. (1986). Cancer in Haiti 1979-1984: distribution of various forms of cancer according to geographical area and sex. *International Journal of Cancer, 38,* 9-16.

Moskowitz, L., Kory, P., Chan, J., et al. (1983). Unusual causes of deaths in Haitians residing in Miami. *Journal of the American Medical Association, 250*(9), 1187-1191.

National Catholic Reporter (1983, March 2). p. 1.

Neilsen, B. (1989). Beliefs towards a diagnosis of cancer—a transcultural approach. In Prichard, A. P. (Ed.), *Proceedings of the Fifth International Conference on Cancer Nursing* (pp. 129-132). London: McMillan Press.

Neilson, B., McMillan, S., & Díaz, E. (1992). Instruments that measure beliefs about cancer from a cultural perspective. *Cancer Nursing, 15*(2), 109-115.

Nida, E. (1954). *Customs and cultures.* New York: Harper & Brothers.

Office of Refugee Resettlement (1993). *Refugee resettlement program: Annual report to Congress, FY 1992.* Washington, D.C.: Government Printing Office.

Orque, M.S., Bloch, B., & Monrroy, L.S.A. (1983). *Ethnic nursing care: a multicultural approach.* St. Louis: Mosby.

Pape, J.W., Verdier, R.I., Boncy, M., et al. (1994, Nov.). *Cyclospora* infection in adults infected with HIV. Clinical manifestations, treatment, and prophylaxis. *Annals of Internal Medicine, 121*(9), 654-657.

Portes, A., & Stepick, A. (1985, Aug.). Unwelcome immigrants: the labor market experiences of 1980 (Mariel) Cuban and Haitian refugees in South Florida. *American Sociological Review,* 493-515.

Potocky, M. (1996). Refugee children: how are they faring economically as adults? *Social Work Journal of the National Association of Social Workers, 41*(4), 354-373.

Preston, R.A., Materson, B.J., Yoham, M.A., & Anapol, H. (1996). Hypertension in Haitians. *Journal of Human Hypertension, 10*(11), 743-745.

Randell-David, E. (1989). *Strategies for working with culturally diverse communities and clients.* Washington, D.C.: U.S. Department of Health and Human Services.

Reichman, L. (1989, Aug. 5). Treating tuberculosis in developing countries. Paper presented at the annual reunion of the Hospital Albert Schweitzer Alumni Association, Burlington, Vermont.

Robinson, A. (1994, Winter). Attitudes toward nursing home residents among aides of three cultural groups. *Journal of Cultural Diversity, 1*(1), 16-18.

Rodman, S. (1961). *Haiti: the Black republic.* New York: Devin-Adair.

Rosenthal, B. (1995, Jan.). The influence of social support on school completion among Haitians. *Social Work in Education, 17*(1), 30-39.

Rosenwarke, I. (1972). *Population history of New York.* Syracuse, N.Y.: Syracuse University Press.

Samet, J., Retondo, M., Freedberg, JG., et al. (1994, Oct.). Factors associated with initiation of primary medical care for HIV-infected persons. *American Journal of Medicine, 4,* 347-353.

Schaedel, R. (1962). *The human resources of Haiti.* Unpublished manuscript.

Scott, C. (1978, Nov.). Health and healing practices among five ethnic groups in Miami, Florida. *Public Health Report, 55,* 524-532.

Seabrooks, P. (1992). *Social supports of older Haitians in Port-au-Prince and Miami: effects on health practices and perceived health status.* Doctor of Nursing Services dissertation, University of California, San Francisco.

Sebastian, J.A., Leeb, B.O., & See, R. (1978). Cancer of the cervix: a sexually transmitted disease. *American Journal of Obstetrics and Gynecology, 131,* 620-623.

Seligman, L. (1977, March). Haitians: a neglected minority. *Personnel and Guidance Journal, 2,* 409-411.

Snow, L.F. (1981). Folk medical beliefs and their implications for the care of patients: a review based on studies among Black Americans. In Henderson, G., & Primeaux, M. (Eds.), *Transcultural health care.* Reading, Mass.: Addison-Wesley.

Sorensen, K., Luckman, J., & Bolander, V. (1994) *Sorenson and Luckmann's basic nursing: a psychophysiologic approach.* Philadelphia: W.B. Saunders.

Spector, R. (1996). *Guide to heritage assessment and health traditions.* Stamford, Conn.: Appleton & Lange.

Stauffer, R. (1989, Oct.). Personal communication with the former Assistant Director of Nursing at Hôpital Albert Schweitzer, Deschapelles, Haiti.

Thomas, J., & DeSantis, L. (1995, Winter). Feeding and weaning practices in Cuban and Haitian immigrant mothers. *Journal of Transcultural Nursing, 6*(2), 34-42.

United Nations Program Development (1996). *Rapport de Coopération au Développement—Haïti.* United Nations Program Development: Haiti.

U.S. Committee for Refugees (1995). Asylum cases filed with INS, April 1991—Sept. 1995. *Refugee Reports, 16*(12), 12.

U.S. Department of Commerce, Bureau of the Census (1993). *Population profile of the United States, 1993* (Publication No. 23-185). Washington, D.C.: Government Printing Office.

Veeken, H. (1993). Hope for Haiti: *British Medical Journal, 307,* 312-313.

Venton, D. (1997, Nov. 7). Report on volunteer experiences in Haiti at the Mennonite Economic Development Association Conference in Kansas City, Missouri.

Verdet, P. (1985, Winter). Trying times: Haitian youth in an inner city high school. *Social Work in Health Care,* 228-233.

Walsh, B. (1980, May 17). The boat people of South Florida. *America,* pp. 420-421.

Weil, T.E. (1973). *Area handbook for Haiti.* Washington, D.C.: Government Printing Office.

Westphal, R. (1989, Aug. 5). *Transfusion transmitted infectious diseases.* Paper presented at the annual reunion of the Hospital Albert Schweitzer Alumni Association, Burlington, Vermont.

White, J., Linhart, J., & Medley, L. (1996, Sept.). Culture, diet and the maternity. *Advance for Nurse Practitioners,* 26-29.

Wiese, J. (1976). Maternal nutrition and traditional food behavior in Haiti. *Human Organization, 35*(2), 193-200.

Wilentz, A. (1989). *The rainy season.* New York: Simon & Schuster.

Wilk, R. (1986, Winter). The Haitian refugee: concern for health care providers. *Social Work in Health Care, 11,* 61-74.

Williams, S., Murthy, N., & Berggren, G. (1975, Nov.). Conjugal unions among rural Haitian women. *Journal of Marriage and the Family, 37,* 1022-1031.

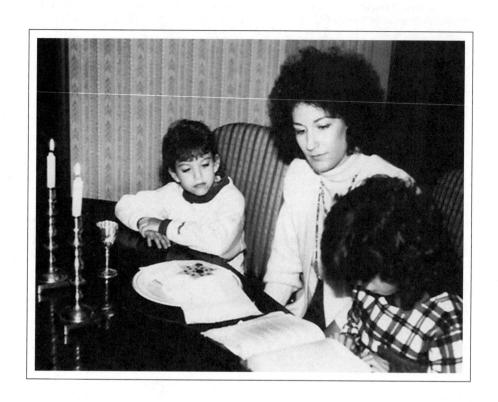

CHAPTER 21 Jewish Americans

Enid A. Schwartz

BEHAVIORAL OBJECTIVES

After reading this chapter, the nurse will be able to:

1. Identify how the religion of Judaism affects the cultural behaviors of Jewish Americans.
2. Identify some of the differences between health-oriented behaviors demonstrated by various religious groups within Judaism.
3. Identify how the various ethnic backgrounds of Jewish Americans affect their cultural behaviors.
4. Describe attitudes and beliefs affecting health care within and across individuals in various Jewish groups.
5. Identify how the verbal and nonverbal communications of Jewish individuals may affect health care.
6. Identify implications or precautions for providing effective nursing care to Jewish Americans.
7. Recognize those health care practices that are mandated by Jewish law for people who are Jewish.

Explaining what it means to be Jewish is not easy. It is more than just belonging to a religious organization; it is also being a part of a specific people (Glazer, 1957; Popenoe, 1977; Trepp 1980). It is a shared feeling of "Jewishness." Jewish people are linked together by a common history, common ethical teachings, a common language of prayer (Hebrew), a vast quantity of literature, common folkways, and, above all, a sense of common destiny (Kertzer, 1978). Jewish people share centuries of history as a minority subjected to hostility wherever they go.

The Jewish-American culture has many subcultures because of the different areas of the world in which Jews live as well as a diversity of religious observances. Jews came to the United States predominantly from Spain, Portugal, Germany, and Eastern Europe. There are three main reli-

gious groups: orthodox, conservative, and reform. Within the orthodox group are the Chassidic (or Hasidic) and Lubovitch subgroups, which are the largest subgroups in the United States today.

Despite differences, there are some cultural similarities that are indigenous to this group of people. To understand the culture, one must have knowledge of some of the religious dictates. Through a discussion of the six common variables found within and across cultural groups as they apply to Jewish Americans, this chapter attempts to clarify some behaviors that are commonly found among Jews in order to assist nurses in developing an effective plan of care for the Jewish-American client. Attention is also placed on Jewish rituals and the effects of assimilation on their cultural traits.

509

OVERVIEW OF THE JEWISH PEOPLE IN THE UNITED STATES

The history of American Judaism encompasses three distinct waves of immigration. The first wave of people, who began arriving in the middle 1600s, was relatively small. They were Sephardic Jews from Spain and Portugal, and they had little effect on the development of modern American Judaism (Sachar, 1964). The beginning of the nineteenth century saw a steady German immigration, which swelled after 1836, when Jews sought to escape persecution in Bavaria and other German states (Glazer, 1957). The last tide of immigration began slowly in 1845, when Polish Jews began arriving in the United States, but swelled to tens of thousands in 1881 as a result of a wave of pogroms and a series of new anti-Jewish decrees in Russia. This last wave, consisting of Eastern European Jews and German Jews, has had a profound effect on modern Jewish-American culture and religious practices.

To understand Jewish-American culture today, it is necessary to consider Europe during the Middle Ages. At that time, most of the internal law in European Jewish communities was strongly controlled by the Talmud (the Rabbinic code). Talmudic law not only governed the religious behavior of Jews, but also governed almost every other aspect of life, such as birth, marriage, and death, as well as the proper foods to eat and the proper clothes to wear. The Jews were kept separate from the general population not only by persecution from others, but also by the rigidity of these laws.

In the nineteenth century not all German Jews were isolated in their communities; some were involved in non-Jewish communities. Many of these Jews were embarrassed by the ancient laws and found them distasteful, especially if they desired the status of full members of the German nation (Glazer, 1957). To maintain their beliefs and yet not appear different from the general culture, German Jews of high social status attempted to start the Reform movement. The freedom experienced in the United States allowed the Reform movement to flourish. The German Jews who immigrated into the United States and wished to become part of the American community were willing to rid themselves of the old traditions and become increasingly "Americanized." They were insistent, however, that the Jews be maintained as a people.

The Eastern European immigrants came predominantly from Russia, Romania, Poland, and Austria. In contrast to many of the German Jewish immigrants who had lived predominantly in nonsegregated areas, most of the Eastern European Jews came from all-Jewish villages, known as *shtetls*, where a Jewish culture was created that was almost totally unaffected by the cultures of the people around them. Life was dictated by the religious traditions Eastern European Jews followed and was much the same as it had been during the Middle Ages.

Along with these pious Jews came the radical political and socialist Jews, who believed that the only way to survive was through complete abandonment of religion. A third group who immigrated during this time represented the "middle-of-the-road" Jews, who were both religious and radical (Glazer, 1957).

It is important to understand the differences in religious behavior when caring for Jewish clients. All Jewish beliefs derive from the Torah (the five books of Moses) and the Talmud (the Rabbinic code). From the Torah come 613 commandments. The combination of the Torah and Talmud results in codes of law. Rather than referring to a body of doctrine, Judaism refers to a body of practices (Glazer, 1957).

Four main religious Jewish groups exist today: orthodox, conservative, reform, and reconstructionist. The Orthodox Jew maintains a strict code of interpretation of the law; the Conservative Jew maintains a less strict code of interpretation; and the Reform Jew follows a more liberal interpretation of the law. Reconstructionist Judaism is a little difficult to explain. Reconstructionists do not necessarily believe in God as a personified deity, or that God chose the Jewish people. If they follow the laws of Judaism, they do so because of their cultural value. An example of the differences deals with the head coverings worn by men: the Orthodox Jew is obligated to keep his head covered at all times in reverence to God, the Conservative Jew keeps his head covered during times of worship, the Reform and Reconstructionist Jews are not obligated to keep their heads covered.

The division between Jewish practices started in Germany in the nineteenth century, but it was not until Jews experienced the religious freedom of the United States that the conservative and reform movements thrived. The freedom experienced in the United States allowed the Jewish immigrant to question the narrow confines of orthodoxy and led to a desire to express religious beliefs and traditional practices in a less confining environment. The German Jews had begun to practice Reform Judaism. However, to the Eastern European Jew, Reform Judaism seemed empty (Howe, 1976). A movement known as "Conservatism," which had begun in nineteenth-century Germany, had a small beginning but appealed to the children of many Eastern European immigrants. According to Glazer (1957), Conservatism offered a compromise between the blind religious teachings of the Orthodox Jews and the scholarly endeavors of the Reform movement to break from tradition completely. Today, the Reform temples are moving toward more traditional practices but maintain the belief that a person should be able to make choices based on knowledge of customs and their meanings.

In regard to religion, Jewish identity has changed through the generations. In the United States today, the sense of Jewish identity does not lie in the Old World religious observances. Most Jewish Americans do not observe the traditional Jewish Sabbath, nor are they active in their temple or synagogue. According to Sowell (1981), their identity lies not with the historical religious aspects of Judaism, but with their ethnic or racial identity.

Changes in immigration laws have decreased the number of Jews entering the United States. However, since the time of the large immigration of Eastern European Jews, Jews from other countries have come to the United States under different circumstances. There are Jews who escaped or lived through the Holocaust, Jews who have emigrated from communist Russia, and Jews who have arrived from many other countries of the world, including Ethiopia and Israel. Each group has added to the cultural diversity of the Jewish people. All have brought with them the culture of the land from which they emigrated. Because of the close ties that have developed between Jews of all nationalities, cultural traits have begun to blend. For example, descendants of Eastern European Jews talk about their *falafel,* a food made from ground chick-peas, which originated in the Middle East.

A fear of many Jewish Americans is the effect of assimilation on their children. Jewish-American people do not want to appear different from other Americans because being different has led to thousands of years of persecution. However, many Jewish Americans do not want to lose the common thread that binds them to one another.

Although Jewish Americans make up only about 3% of the United States population, they are visible in many areas of the United States culture. It is estimated that today the total number of Jews residing in the United States is approximately 6 million people (U.S. Department of Commerce, Bureau of the Census, 1993; Yearbook of American and Canadian Churches, 1993). They are distinguished members of the arts, academia, the sciences, medicine, law, and the political arena. Education is a large part of the Jewish culture, which has helped Jews in the United States succeed as they never could in other countries.

The desire to succeed, plus intermarriage, has caused some loss of Jewish identity. Some Jews today in the United States do not wish to be identified as Jewish for fear of discrimination in the workplace. Discrimination against Jews does exist in the United States, and many Jews are sensitive to anti-Semitism.

COMMUNICATION

Today the primary language of Jewish Americans is English. In the late 1800s the primary language of the Jews was Yiddish, which is a combination of German, Slavic, Old French, Old Italian, and Hebrew languages (Rosten, 1968). The freedom experienced in the United States led to the desire for assimilation. Many Jewish Americans of German descent were embarrassed by the use of Yiddish. To them, Yiddish was vulgar, represented the lower socioeconomic class, and above all was un-American. The children of first-generation Jews, born to Eastern European parents, wanted to be accepted by the other children. Although Yiddish may have been spoken in the home, these children spoke English outside the home. Very few second-generation Jewish Americans understand Yiddish. However, almost all Jewish Americans know some Yiddish, and many Jewish conversations are sprinkled with Yiddish words. Some of these words have become a part of American English, such as *shtick* (or *shtück*) and *tush*.

Hebrew, which is the language of Israel, is not spoken by most Jews who do not live there. However, Hebrew is the language of the Torah, and many Jews can read it. An important part of Jewish religious education is the reading, speaking, and writing of Hebrew. *Shalom* is a Hebrew word that is commonly used by Jewish people to mean 'peace', 'hello', or 'good-bye'.

The Sephardic Jews have a language of their own, Ladino, which is similar to Old Spanish. It is not commonly spoken in the United States today.

Style

Jews tend to be expressive when communicating, and they tend to be very verbal about how and what they are feeling. Most Jewish people use their hands to express their thoughts; as they talk, their hands emphasize what is being said. They not only punctuate their conversations using hand and arm movements, but also use voice inflections. By changing the emphasis on certain words, the Jewish person changes the meaning of the message being conveyed (Rosten, 1968). This change in emphasis is done easily in Yiddish and has been carried over into English. As an example, changing the emphasis on the words, "Him you trust?" changes the meaning: "Him you *trust*?" versus "*Him* you trust?" The first questions a person's judgment; the second implies that anyone who would trust the character of such a scoundrel must be an idiot.

Humor is used frequently by Jews, and often the humor is directed at themselves. This self-directed humor has led to comments that Jewish humor comes out of self-hatred. Although Jewish humor may appear to be self-critical and sometimes self-deprecating, it does not stem from a form of Jewish masochism. One of the most popular beliefs is that Jewish humor arose as a way for Jews to cope with the hostility they found around them, sometimes using that hostility against themselves. It appears as if

a Jewish person is telling enemies, "You don't have to attack us. We can do that ourselves—and even better" (Novak & Waldoks, 1981).

Jews today are sensitive to humor from "outside" sources. Jokes that are not appreciated when told by non-Jews include "JAP" (Jewish American Princess) jokes and those about "Jewing people down" (referring to Jews being cheap or unmerciful at bartering).

As Jews become more acculturated with each generation, the communication styles change. Jewish people who are third- or fourth-generation Americans will more likely demonstrate the same communication style as their neighbors rather than that of their parents, grandparents, or great-grandparents. This type of acculturation is part of the history of Jews all over the world (Patai & Wing, 1975).

Touch

The use of touch varies among Jewish people; however, the use or nonuse of touch can be a critical issue with Orthodox Jews and must be carefully considered by the nurse. Because of the Jewish laws regarding personal space and touching others of the opposite sex, it is important to ascertain to which religious group the client belongs. If the client is orthodox, he or she will be very modest. Overexposure of or touching the parts of the body associated with sexual activities can cause a great deal of distress. When caring for strictly Orthodox Jewish clients of the opposite sex, the nurse should use touch only for hands-on care. To touch the client at any other time could be offensive because of the sexual connotations attached to casual touch. It is also important to note that, according to Jewish law, religious observances are not to be followed if doing so will endanger the person's health.

Implications for nursing care

Because older Jewish clients may be very verbal about what and how they are feeling, they may appear to be chronic complainers. Although it is difficult to remain nonjudgmental with a client who is considered a chronic complainer, it is important to remember that letting others know feelings is part of the Jewish culture. It may be difficult to assess pain levels of Jewish clients because they are very emotional when expressing their discomfort, and it may take persistence and patience to pinpoint the problem and its extent. Younger Jewish clients may be more articulate and may also complain less than their parents or grandparents as a result of acculturation.

SPACE

The Orthodox Jew is keenly aware of religious dictates regarding personal space that may or may not be invaded by members of the opposite sex. Many Orthodox Jewish men and women will not shake hands with a member of the opposite sex. This practice stems from the ruling in the Code of Jewish Law that forbids a man to smell the scent of a strange woman, to look upon her hair, or even to gaze upon her little finger (Kolatch, 1985). A very Orthodox Jewish man will not usually touch his wife in public.

Traditionally, Jewish people have also had practices about personal and social space. In times of sickness and during their elderly years, Jewish individuals have an acute desire to have members of their family and other Jews around them. This desire has been illustrated in studies of the elderly that indicate that elderly Jewish people in nursing homes adjust better if they have other Jews around them (Kaplan, 1970).

Implications for nursing care

Judaic laws can lead to some misinterpretation by nurses and other health care providers. For example, during childbirth, if a very Orthodox Jewish husband decides to participate in the delivery, his participation will only be verbal. He will not touch his wife during labor. This practice is associated with the laws of separation that dictate that avoidance is necessary during the time a woman has any vaginal bleeding. He will not view the birth because he is not permitted to view his wife's genital area. After the birth, he may lean over his wife (being careful not to touch her), smile, and say, *"Mazel tov"* ('good luck, congratulations') (Bash, 1980; Lutwak, Ney, & White, 1988). Some very Orthodox husbands elect to participate only spiritually. If this is the case, they will sit with their prayerbook and recite from the Book of Psalms. It is important to remember that this practice does not mean the man loves his wife any less than the man who actively participates.

Among the Orthodox Jews there are different groups. The "modern" Orthodox Jew cannot be distinguished by his or her dress though some traditional Orthodox Jews are often recognizable by their appearance. The men usually have long earlocks and beards and wear a *yarmulke* (skull caps) or large black hats and long black frock coats. The women are modestly dressed in long-sleeved dresses and have wigs or scarves covering their heads.

With the increase of male nurses, the question arises regarding the assignment of a male nurse to a female Orthodox Jewish client. The Code of Jewish Law (Ganzfried, 1927) states that "a male is not permitted to attend to a woman who is suffering with a belly ache . . . but a woman may attend to a male who is so suffering. . . ." This passage may be interpreted to mean that a male nurse should not be assigned to care for a female client. If, however, there are only male nurses available, this law would probably be waived because all laws are suspended in the case of severe illness. A law that addresses attendance of a male physician with a female client states that a physician is permitted to let blood and to feel the pulse or any other place of a woman, even if she is married, even the pudenda (external genital organs), as is customary with physicians, because he is merely following his profession (Ganzfried, 1927).

The nurse should be aware that since elderly Jewish clients in non-Jewish hospitals or nursing homes may adjust better with other Jews around them, it may be advantageous to have Jewish clients room together or at least be in proximity. This closeness will allow for increased comfort and offer the Jewish client the chance to interact with someone who "understands" him or her.

SOCIAL ORGANIZATION

The foundation of the Jewish culture is the nuclear family and the greater Jewish community. Controversy exists as to whether the Jewish community or the Jewish family has had the bigger influence on maintaining the Jewish faith and the Jews as a people (Schneider, 1985).

Jewish families tend to be closely knit and child oriented (Schlesinger, 1971). Jewish parents tend to "want better" for their children than they had themselves. It is not unusual to hear parents say that they have given up something they really wanted for the "sake of the children."

Family life of the Jewish Americans has changed through the years. The earlier Jewish family was male dominated, and the father made the major decisions. The mother's job was to care for the home, the children, and her husband. Today the delineation of duties is more obscure. Usually both parents work, often at jobs of equal financial and professional status.

The Jewish family structure is seen as protective. The Eastern European mother of the past got the reputation of being overbearing and overprotective. In the *shtetls* of Europe, the mother was the cohesive force in the home. This is still the case today, though younger women are not considered as overbearing or overprotective as their mothers and ancestors were.

In the Jewish family the child is seen as the means of maintaining Jewish existence. Therefore education of the child in the Jewish faith and traditions is often seen as the most important thing a community, as well as the family, can do. The fear of assimilation and annihilation increases the importance to the community of "sticking together" and educating the children.

Among the commandments that Jews are expected to follow are those that dictate the social relationships of family and community. These commandments dictate expected behavior toward parents and people within the community, such as the poor, teachers, rabbis, neighbors, ill people, the dying, and the dead.

Social orientation has helped maintain the Jewish people. When the Eastern European immigrants arrived in the United States, they were an embarrassment for the German Jews. However, commandments that control social behaviors dictated that the German Jews reach out to help the newcomers. This sense of kinship was so strong that Jews felt obliged to help one another, both in the United States and abroad.

Eastern European Jews brought with them a strong sense of community, which arose from their restricted lives within the *shtetls*. Furthermore, they were often held responsible for political events that occurred outside the Jewish quarters. Even though each Jew developed his or her own individuality, there was an intense feeling of groupness, an identification with a common cultural heritage (Kolatch, 1985).

When the immigration laws of the 1920s resulted in decreased numbers of Eastern European Jews entering the United States, increased assimilation began to occur. Several significant events have helped slow the rate of Jewish-American assimilation. The event that seems to have had the largest effect was the rise of Nazi anti-Semitism and its American counterparts. The Holocaust caused all Jews to realize that they were indeed brothers (Janowsky, 1964), and the memory of the Holocaust continues to have this effect on Jewish people. Other events that have had an effect on Jewish identification were related to the development of the state of Israel and the struggle of Israel to continue to exist despite a hostile environment. When Israel won the "Six-Day War" in 1967, the feeling of pride in the Jewish State was almost tangible. There seemed to be a stronger sense of "Jewishness" and an increased willingness to admit to being Jewish.

Today, the Jewish-American community is much more mobile than it was in the past. It is not unusual for the children to move away when they leave for college or marry. When a Jewish individual moves, often one of the first things looked for is Jewish affiliation. A Jew may not join a synagogue until the children are ready for Sunday school, but often he or she desires the company of other Jews despite the inability to join a synagogue until that time.

Implications for nursing care

When a Jewish person becomes ill, family and community resources are mobilized to assist the client. The Jewish faith contains a commandment to visit the sick. Therefore, friends, relatives, and neighbors will visit an ill Jewish client. If the client is very ill, the visitors will act as client advocates. It is important for the nurse to recognize the cultural implications of these visitors and to expect them to ask about the client.

Because of the protective attitudes of Jewish parents, they will make arrangements to have someone with their child at all times if the child is hospitalized. Jewish parents may appear demanding and aggressive if they believe their child is not getting the care he or she "deserves." Handling the concerns of the parents may take patience on the part of the nurse. The nurse needs to remember that this cultural group highly prizes their children and see the survival of the Jewish people as a responsibility of the next generation. This view places a large responsibility on the child to get well and on the parents to see that the child does get well.

TIME

The best way to classify Jewish people in relation to time orientation is to say that they are past, present, and future oriented. Jews are aware of their past—all 5000 years of it. They are also concerned about the present and are very involved with current social concerns, both Jewish and non-Jewish. They also look toward the future by insisting that their children be educated, religiously and secularly, and by participating in philanthropic activities to help the future of Israel.

The Jewish concern with the past is very obvious in American society, especially in relation to the Holocaust. Every Jewish person believes that this kind of atrocity should never happen again. By continuing to remind the world of the horrors that happened, not only to Jews, but to people of all faiths and ethnic origins, the Jewish people hope the world will never again let that type of event occur.

During happy occasions, such as a wedding, there is always something to remind Jews of their past. As an example, at the end of the wedding ceremony the groom breaks a glass. One reason for this custom is to symbolize the destruction of the Jewish temple during the Roman invasion.

Past orientation is also seen following the death of a loved one (such as a parent, sibling, or spouse). On the anniversary of the death each year, a candle is lit and a prayer, *kaddish* (meaning 'holy'), is recited in honor of that person. In addition, the *kaddish* is recited at special times during the year for a loved one. In some congregations the *kaddish* is recited by the whole congregation in memory of those who have recently died or those who have no one to say the

prayer for them. In relation to present-time orientation, Jews tend to be very social minded and are often involved in social movements. In many communities, Jewish congregations help run soup kitchens. In a southwestern city a rabbi was involved with the sanctuary movement.

From the Talmud comes the requirement that Jews care for all who are in need whether they are Jewish or non-Jewish. Because the concepts of charity and righteousness are so intertwined, the Hebrew word for righteousness (justice), *tzedaka,* has become the Hebrew word for 'charity' (Kolatch, 1985). This concept has had an influence on the social system in New York City (Howe, 1976).

Another way that Jewish present-time orientation is apparent is in relation to an afterlife. Although Jews may believe that the spirit continues to live or reside with God after death, they are not concerned about an afterlife. What is considered important is doing good deeds on earth. During an interview regarding the belief in a soul, one woman summed up what has been written by other authors when she stated that it is the memory of one's good deeds that causes one to be immortalized (Schwartz, 1984).

Future-time orientation is apparent in issues concerning the education of children. Establishing schools, supporting schools, and furthering education are top priorities. Throughout the ages education of the children in the Torah has been regarded as a duty. Originally it was the duty of the parents. Eventually it became the duty of the community (Janowsky, 1964). Today, not only religious but also secular education is seen as important. In most Jewish households the children hear, from the time they are very young, that someday they will go to college. Education is highly prized as a way of securing the future for the child as well as for the Jewish community as a whole.

Another way that future-time orientation is apparent relates to concerns during illness. Jewish people not only want immediate relief, they also worry about what the future implications of their illness will be. They worry about the effect of their illness on the future of their family members, their jobs, and their lives. According to Zborowski (1969), the intensity of their concern is greater than that of other Americans.

Many Jews tend to be punctual when it comes to appointments and become very upset when they arrive on time and have to wait for their appointment to begin. However, some Jewish people also talk about "Jewish standard time," which is at least 10 to 15 minutes later than regular time. Although there are many Jews who are very punctual (especially when it comes to appointments), general Jewish functions, such as weddings or bar mitzvahs, often begin late.

Implications for nursing care

Because Jewish people are past, present, and future oriented as well as emotionally expressive, they appear to feel joy, sorrow, illness, and so on with great intensity. They become very anxious when they do not feel well and may appear to be impatient about finding a cure. Jewish people have a tendency to worry about what the illness means in the present as well as the implications it has for the future.

Patience and honesty are necessary qualities for a nurse to display when dealing with Jewish clients. Demonstrating interest and concern will convey the message that the nurse cares about the ill person and may help decrease the amount of anxiety the client is feeling. Until a diagnosis is made, trying to help the anxious Jewish client put events into proper perspective may not work because the client reasons that the nurse cannot know what the future will hold if the physician does not know what is wrong.

It is important to understand that the high degree of outward anxiety the Jewish person may feel is probably more apparent in the older generation of Jews than in the younger generation because assimilation has caused more "acceptable" behavior patterns to be exhibited in the younger generation.

ENVIRONMENTAL CONTROL

Many Jewish people tend to be fatalistic about life. They may believe that they do have some control over their health, but God has the final say. This belief is apparent during Rosh Hashanah and Yom Kippur (the New Year and the Day of Atonement),

when Jews pray to be written in the Book of Life for another year.

Health care beliefs

Jewish people have a religious requirement to maintain the health of the body as well as the soul. The origin of Jewish health care beliefs dates back to the Torah. Many of the 613 biblical commandments appear to be hygienic in intent. Several chapters in the Book of Leviticus (12 to 14) as well as other books in the Bible are devoted to the control of disease (Kolatch, 1985). The Talmud continues to stress this concern for health. There are passages that deal with proper exercise, getting enough sleep, eating breakfast, and eating the proper diet.

Physicians are held in high esteem by people in the Jewish culture (Feldman, 1986). In biblical times the priests were physicians. When a Jewish person is ill, it is a duty to go to a physician, and it is the duty of the family to make sure the individual goes. The importance of health care is so great in this culture that Talmudic scholars stated that a person should not settle in a city without a physician (Feldman, 1986).

Jewish people realize that physicians cannot heal without the participation of the client. It is permissible for the Jewish client to question the physician if the client believes the physician is wrong about a diagnosis or treatment (Feldman, 1986; Zborowski, 1969), and the Jewish client may decide not to follow the physician's orders. However, if the client chooses not to listen to the physician or does not agree with the physician, this individual is expected to seek the knowledge of another physician (Feldman, 1986). Seeking the best medical care, even obtaining a second opinion, is a religious dictate.

Health is one of the most frequent topics of conversation among Jewish people. With some Jewish people, especially older ones, health is seen as an exception rather than the rule. The older individual may become preoccupied with the issue of good health because life may be viewed as a temporary lapse between one illness and another (Zborowski, 1969).

The Jewish person believes that prevention of illness is important. Each family member tries to protect and warn the other members of dangers that may cause illnesses, which can make client teaching easier for the nurse. It is important to remember that client teaching in the Jewish family requires the cooperation of all the immediate family members.

There is an increased interest among Jewish adults in alternative or collaborative health care. It is not unusual to hear a group of Jews discussing the issues of fat content in food or the use of herbs to maintain health. In recent years, two healing centers that address prayer and healing have been developed in San Francisco and New York City. Healing services are held periodically in temples throughout the United States.

Illness behaviors

When a member of a Jewish family is ill, the whole family suffers with the person. Each individual is expected to become a part of the process of helping the ill person feel better.

Complaining about discomforts is expected and accepted, especially in the older generation. Complaining fulfills several important functions: it gives relief through its cathartic function, it is a means of communication, it mobilizes the assistance of the environment, and it reaffirms family solidarity (Zborowski, 1969).

When Jewish clients are admitted to the hospital, they may continue to behave as though they were at home. The Jewish client may attempt to mobilize the attention and sympathy of those in the new environment by using the same methods that worked in the home, so that what the nurse encounters may be a client who complains, cries, moans, and groans. When this behavior does not result in the reactions that would be received from the family, the client may attempt to temper reactions so that feelings of acceptance and being cared for are experienced.

If the client does not verbalize pain, another member of the family will usually do so. The reasoning is that the client may be too ill to tell the physician or nurse and that it is the family member's responsibility to communicate to obtain the attention the family member believes the loved one should have.

Zborowski's (1969) study of first-generation Jewish Americans in pain noted that these clients responded to questions in details that sometimes seemed to relate only marginally to the topic. In the study a simple question released a flow of responses that led to information about pain, illness, anxieties, intrafamily relationships, and so on. Probing was necessary to pinpoint specific information rather than to elicit a fuller answer to a question.

Second-, third-, and fourth-generation Jewish Americans seem to be a little less expressive about their pain. However, they do consider it wrong not to express their feelings. The expressive behavior of Jews seems to indicate that Jewish people believe that one cannot get help unless a complaint is made.

If oral complaining does not result in the type of behavior the client wishes to elicit from those around him or her, crying may be used. Crying, with many first-generation Jewish Americans, is acceptable behavior and is seen as an expression of frustration or pain and often results in the attention desired (Zborowski, 1969).

With increased American acculturation, each succeeding Jewish-American generation appears to be less expressive when in pain. The women may cry easily, but the men have adopted the American view that crying is not proper behavior for men. Second-generation Jewish-American male clients tend to be less verbal about their pain than their fathers (Zborowski, 1969). For some Jewish people, however, the meaning of pain does not change, just the outward signs. For a Jewish person, pain, discomfort, and change in the state of good health are seen as a warning that something is wrong and that professional health care system needs to be utilized.

Utilization of the health care system may involve getting the opinions of several physicians. The Jewish client recognizes that the physician is only another human, with the possibility of being incorrect. By getting at least one other opinion, the client can decide if the physician was correct or not. Not only is a Jewish client likely to get a second or third opinion, but also may check the medical literature. Zborowski (1969) has noted that these activities seem to be based on a feeling that the client is the final judge and authority in matters pertaining to his or her health. In this case the physician is seen in the role of consultant and advisor.

Once the Jewish client accepts the physician's opinion the client will also accept the prescribed treatment. The cultural belief is that, to get well, one must cooperate with all therapeutic measures. Although the Jewish client will follow the prescribed regimen, the client expects the medication regimen to be individualized because illness is viewed as being individualized.

In many cases, the client will want to know all about the prescribed treatment: what is expected of the client, what the side effects are, and, if a drug is being prescribed, the name of the drug. The client is unlikely to be content with "It's good for you."

The Jewish client tends to observe carefully the effects of the drug or treatment on the system. Since many Jews believe that they are the ultimate judge of their condition, they may change the time they take a drug, increase or decrease the number of drugs taken, or reject the drug completely if they decide it is not helping or is harmful. Many times these decisions are made without consulting the physician. Careful, thorough explanations about the drug, its purpose, side effects, and why it was ordered are essential.

The future-oriented Jewish client may become hesitant to take analgesics because most drugs are viewed as "dope" and Jewish persons often fear addiction. This fear increases the problem for the client in pain who wants to receive pain relief but is afraid of addiction (Zborowski, 1969).

Wellness behaviors

Jewish-American people tend to be more educated than most other American ethnic groups (Sowell, 1981), and the thirst for knowledge is apparent in their wellness behaviors. They tend to be well read on issues of health, and it is not unusual to hear Jews discussing the latest information on maintaining healthy diets, preventing disease, or following health-oriented regimens.

In years past, it was rare to see Jewish children involved in physical activities. Eastern European Jews tended to deemphasize physical activity in favor of more intellectual activities that kept the children closer to home. This practice may have stemmed from the fears of child abduction that they brought with them from the "old country" (Sowell, 1981).

However, this trend seems to be changing. Jewish children are now involved with soccer teams, baseball teams, and so on. Their parents are also more involved in physical exercise. Jogging, tennis, racquetball, and aerobics are some of the activities that are attracting more Jewish people as the importance of physical exercise is discussed in the media.

Maintaining certain laws is included in the wellness behaviors seen in Orthodox Jewish people. Many of these laws have been incorporated into the everyday habits of most Jewish Americans because they are good hygiene or they have been proved to be medically prudent. The following are examples of these laws taken from the Code of Jewish Law (Ganzfried, 1927):

1. The hands must be washed on awakening from sleep, after elimination of bodily wastes, after hair cutting, after touching a vermin, and after being in proximity of a dead human body.
2. The proper way of washing oneself is to take a bath regularly every week.
3. It is advisable for one to accustom himself to having breakfast in the morning.
4. One is forbidden to eat or drink out of unclean vessels, and the individual should not eat with hands that are not clean.

Kosher diet, religious holidays, and illness

Maintaining a kosher (*kasher* 'fit, proper') diet may pose a problem for some Jewish clients. As mentioned in Chapter 7, kosher meat is usually salted to help drain all the blood. This process presents a problem for a client on a low-salt diet unless the meat is soaked in water to remove as much of the salt as possible.

It is important for the nurse to consider what can be done for the Jewish client following a kosher diet if the hospital does not have a kosher supplier nearby. In this case it is possible to serve any fish that meets the dietary requirements of having fins and scales. It is also possible to serve dairy products as long as they are not contraindicated on the person's diet. These meals should be served on paper plates with plastic utensils because meat and milk products or dishes prepared with milk products should not be mixed.

If, because of medical dietary restrictions and unavailability of kosher food, maintaining a kosher diet is impossible, the client must decide to wave the dietary restrictions. All commandments are suspended whenever a life is in danger, no matter how remote the likelihood of death (Feldman, 1986). Food is essential to maintain life; therefore the client would be directed by the rabbi to eat whatever the hospital could provide that would help sustain life.

Yom Kippur (the Day of Atonement) and Passover (Easter, based on Hebrew *pesah*, 'passing over') are two holidays that require special consideration. On Yom Kippur Jewish people are required to fast for 24 hours. If this fast is considered physically or medically dangerous, however, the individual is required by law to put aside the law and eat. Passover requires that special foods be served. Passover, which falls in or near the spring of the year, is an 8-day holiday that celebrates the freedom of the Jews from Egypt. During these 8 days, certain foods must be "kosher for Passover" *(kasher le-pesah)*. In addition, there are other foods that are forbidden, including any foods with leavening (bread, cakes made with baking soda or powder) or foods made with even a small amount of a grain product or by-product that is not specifically prepared for Passover. This prohibition includes many drugs and medications, such as those containing starch or grain alcohol. These drugs may be refused by the client unless they cannot be replaced and are urgently needed by the client.

Procreation

The use or nonuse of contraceptives is dictated by Jewish law, which requires one to "be fruitful and multiply." This can cause special problems for the woman who is unable to conceive or the woman who may have physical problems making conception dangerous. There is a lengthy discussion of this issue in the Mishnah (a part of the Talmud containing the oral law). The final analysis is that the man is commanded to procreate, but the woman is not, because, it is believed, God would not impose on the "children of Israel" a burden "too difficult for a person to bear" (Gold, 1988). Since childbirth is painful and may be physically dangerous, it would be unfair for the Torah to impose the commandment for procreation on the woman.

When Jewish men were allowed two wives, this commandment was not a problem. Today, because monogamy is the rule in the Jewish community, procreation is seen as the couple's obligation. However, outside of the very orthodox community, Jewish couples today decide on how many children they want, and most practice some form of birth control. Within the very orthodox community, the use of birth control is discouraged unless pregnancy or delivery would be dangerous for the woman.

Couples who have a problem with fertility are encouraged to seek medical help. For the very Orthodox Jewish man, however, a problem arises in the collection of semen. Rabbis have declared that masturbation and the use of male contraceptives such as condoms are not permitted because the Talmud outlaws the spilling of seed. For this reason, the woman is usually tested first, and then, if no problem can be detected, the man may be tested. The very Orthodox Jewish husband will have to consult his rabbi before he consents to a sperm count. Since masturbation is considered taboo, it may be emotionally difficult for the man to collect his semen. This is not a problem for most nonorthodox couples.

It is interesting to note that the role of companionship is given an equal place with procreation in the purpose of a Jewish marriage (Gold, 1988). To add to this idea of companionship, rabbis have also addressed the idea of sexual satisfaction being the right of both men and women within the bonds of marriage (Lutwak, Ney, & White, 1988).

Organ transplants

According to Jewish law, all body parts should be buried with the body after death (Jakobovits, 1959). However, if an organ transplant would save the life of another human being, it is permissible to donate the organ (Feldman, 1986). Even removal of the heart for transplantation is allowed so long as the dying person has experienced total brainstem death (Feldman, 1986; Kolatch, 1985).

Life-support measures

According to Jewish law, nothing may be done to hasten death; a client must be given every chance for life. However, if the use of mechanical systems would delay death rather than prolong life, they should not be used. If mechanical systems have been connected and they are not helping to prolong life but are delaying death, they may be removed (Feldman, 1986).

The dying Jewish client

As there are commandments that control living for the Jew, there are also commandments that control dying. These commandments are usually followed strictly only by Orthodox Jews, but some of the behaviors that the nurse may see in non-Orthodox Jews are a result of the cultural knowledge that these commandments have created.

According to Jewish law, a person who is very ill and considered to be dying should not be left alone. One reason for this law is that the spirit is believed to depart from the body at the time of death, and if no one were present, the soul would feel alone and desolate (Sperling, 1968). To satisfy this commandment, family members will often take turns sitting with the critically or terminally ill client. Asking family members to leave may cause family distress.

Jewish law also dictates that a client should be informed that death is near. However, because of two controversial passages in the Torah, some rabbis believe it is important to inform a dying individual about serious illness but not that death is near. Informing a person about a serious illness allows the individual time to put worldly affairs in order, as Isaac and Jacob did when they were told they would die (Heller, 1975). However, to tell a person that death is imminent removes all hope, and some Jewish people fear that this information may hasten death.

Judaism teaches that it is important to lead a good, decent, and helping life on earth. Since good deeds must be done on earth, the law requires a Jew to ask God to forgive those deeds that may have been against God or not in keeping with His commandments. To fulfill this commandment, the dying person is encouraged to recite the confessional. If the individual is too sick to say the whole confessional, the individual is encouraged to recite the affirmation of faith, the *Shma*. If the dying person cannot repeat any of the confessional, the law says that it is up to the family or friends who are with the person to recite it.

Once death has been established the eyes and mouth are closed by the son or nearest relative. In some Orthodox Jewish families it is customary to remove the body from the bed and place it on a straw mat on the floor with the person's feet toward the door through which the body will be taken. A candle is placed at the person's head to symbolize the "light," or joy and love the departed brought to others while alive (Trepp, 1980). A sheet is placed over the person's face because it is disrespectful to the dead to permit others to see the ravages of death on the face (Sperling, 1968). The dead body is viewed as being contaminated by Orthodox Jews and is placed on the floor because the bed is viewed as being defiled by contact with the dead body; however, the ground is not considered defiled by contact (Sperling, 1968). It is important to understand that this behavior is rarely seen in most hospitals or nursing homes today.

Autopsy is not allowed by Orthodox Jews unless (1) it is required by governmental regulations, (2) the person had a hereditary disease and autopsy may help safeguard the health of survivors, or (3) another known person is suffering from a similar deadly disease and an autopsy may yield information vital to that person's health (Jakobovits, 1959). If an autopsy is performed, all parts that are removed must be buried with the body. Autopsy does not pose a religious problem for the non-Orthodox Jew.

AIDS

It has been stated that "AIDS will cause psychological and social reactions that may change the character of human social life" (Edelheit, 1989). In the Jewish community AIDS poses a psychological, social, and religious problem. The problem lies in the traditional belief system of the Jewish people: according to the Torah, homosexuality is an abomination, and premarital sexual activity is not permitted by the traditional rabbinate. This belief system is a potential cause of distress for the Jewish homosexual, or for any Jew who tests HIV-positive. They not only have to live with their disease, but also have to live with being an outcast of their culture.

Patient education in an Orthodox Jewish environment may be very difficult, and rabbis in all the religious groups are still trying to decide how to handle this situation. Some of them are addressing it and trying to teach about the disease and safe sex. It appears that Orthodox rabbis are handling the issue of "safe sex" by going to the law that states that methods to destroy or block the passage of the seed are not permitted. Rabbi Yonassan Gershom (1998) notes that the issue of safe sex should not be a problem for Orthodox Jews because sex outside of marriage is not permitted. When asked about issues of finger sticks or blood transfusions, Rabbi Gershom responded that each case would be considered on an individual basis. Homosexuality among Reform Jewish rabbis is recognized and accepted. There are Reform synagogues that have predominately homosexual congregations. In 1997 the Reform Jewish movement agreed to openly ordain homosexual Jewish rabbis.

AIDS and the Jewish client is an area requiring great sensitivity for the nurse. The most important thing that the nurse can do for the Jewish AIDS victim is to be there for support. These victims not only need to deal with a terminal illness and rejection by the general society, but also need to deal with possible cultural and religious ostracism.

Circumcision

According to Jewish teaching, God made a covenant with Abraham in which God promised to bless Abraham and make him prosper if Abraham would be loyal to God. This covenant was entered into and sealed by the act of circumcision. Jewish people honor this covenant by having a *brit* (which means 'sign of the Covenant', *běrith*) on the eighth day of the baby's life. If the child is ill or was born prematurely, the *brit* is postponed until the infant is in good health. The circumcision is usually done by a *mohel*, who is trained to do circumcisions. This is a time of celebration, and usually the entire family and friends gather at the home of the baby's parents for this important occasion. Since the circumcision is performed in the home, the nurse should review the principles of circumcision care with the mother before discharge. The postcircumcision care is usually managed by the *mohel*. L'Archevesque and Goldstein-Lohman (1996) note the importance of offering parents information about the different methods of circumcision, types of pain control measures, and symptoms of possible complications. Parents should be educated about the expected amount of bloody staining and what would be excessive bleeding as well as signs and symptoms of infection.

Implications for nursing care

Caring for Jewish clients may be viewed as difficult by the nurse. Jewish clients tend to be vocal about feelings, anxieties, and pain, but they may not be direct about what is bothering them. This type of verbalization can be difficult for health care providers who expect the client to be compliant, noncomplaining, and direct about needs. Nurses with judgmental attitudes may label the Jewish client as childish, which leads to treating the client as a child or ignoring the client as much as possible. It is important for the nurse to remember that for the Jewish client, this childlike behavior may be part of the culture. The nurse must be patient and let the client know that the nurse cares about needs because this will lead to feelings of trust and may decrease what is seen as demanding behavior.

Demanding behavior is less likely to occur in second-, third-, or fourth-generation Jewish Americans, who are more aware of what is considered acceptable behavior by the general American culture. This awareness does not mean that they feel pain or anxieties any less.

Illness is often viewed by Jews as a family affair. Because the whole family is involved with the ill person's suffering, the whole family wants to know what is happening with or to the client. The family members often do not appear to trust the word of another family member and instead want to get the information directly from the physician or the nurse. To assist the family and decrease the amount of time numerous explanations may take, it may help to have a family conference. However, not all the members may show up at the same time, and the nurse may need to repeat the information. The most important message to convey to the family of a Jewish client is that of caring, not only about the client, but also about each family member and the pain they are going through.

Assisting the client who is dying, as well as the family, requires knowledge of Jewish cultural practices and beliefs. The nurse needs to remain sensitive to the need for a confessional if death is imminent and the client is Orthodox. Studies have shown that following cultural practices helps decrease the amount of distress and disorganization felt by loved ones during the death and dying period (Dempsey, 1975; Ross, 1981). Therefore it is the duty of the nurse to assist families in following customs related to death and dying. When an Orthodox Jew dies, the body must not be touched by a person of the opposite sex. One nurse recounted the story of a young Chassidic boy who died and was washed by the nurses on the floor before the father arrived. The father became so upset that a female had touched his son's body that he told the nurses not to touch him, left the hospital, and returned a few minutes later with some dirt and a bag. He covered the boy's body with the dirt, put him in the bag, and carried him out of the hospital. He did this because the body was considered contaminated.

Jewish people are interested in health prevention and may ask in-depth questions to clarify what is being said. They may ask many questions to weigh information for personal effect, and these questions should not be misconstrued to indicate mistrust of the health care professional.

When caring for a Jewish client, it is helpful for the nurse to know what form of religious practice is adhered to because the Orthodox Jewish client will follow religious practices more strictly than any other group. Unless the nurse works in an area that has a large number of Orthodox Jews, most Jewish clients cared for will be nonorthodox and may not be affiliated with any group.

BIOLOGICAL VARIATIONS

Some people believe that a Jewish person can be recognized by physical appearance, and the "Semitic appearance" is occasionally related to cultural patterns (Goodman, 1979). However, Jews differ greatly in physical appearance depending on what part of the world they migrated to when forced out of Israel. Jews are not uniformly the same as far as

height, hair and eye color, body structure, or shape of the nose is concerned. European Jews are White, Falashas (Ethiopian Jews) are Black, and Chinese Jews have Oriental features. The differences among Jews from different parts of the world are the results of biological adaptation to the area of the world resided in, intermarriage with non-Jews, and converts to Judaism (Goodman, 1979; Mourant, Kopec, & Domaniewsks-Sobczak, 1978).

For determination of the extent of genetic similarity among Jews as opposed to non-Jews, studies of blood phenotypes have been done (Goodman, 1979; Mourant, Kopec, & Domaniewsks-Sobczak, 1978). As opposed to outward appearances, blood characteristics are unaffected by the environment.

Enzymatic and genetic variations

Although skin color, body size, and body structure vary depending on the part of the world resided in, fingerprint patterns indicate a relatedness among Jews from Germany, Turkey, Morocco, and Yemen. The patterns of fingerprint whorls, loops, and arches are similar to those of non-Jews living in the Mediterranean area. This seems to indicate that the Jewish people, though appearing to be diversified genetically, still maintain a remnant of the Mediterranean gene pool.

To classify genetic differences of peoples, polymorphic blood groups, serum and cell proteins, and enzyme variants that have altered catalytic activity, kinetic properties, stability, or electrophoretic mobility are used. Since anthropological structures and simple genetic traits of Jews are difficult to define, Jewish genetic studies have concentrated on the genetic polymorphisms (Rothschild, 1981). Data from these studies have concluded that (1) Jewish groups from different parts of the world are very different genetically, (2) Jews of a certain area tend to resemble the surrounding non-Jews more than they resemble Jews from other parts of the world, and (3) European Jews have a residue of non-European genes that resemble Mediterranean genes (Patai & Wing, 1975).

A study by Stevenson, Schanfield, and Sandler (1985) on immunoglobulin allotypes had interesting results. The multivariate analyses indicated that the Jewish populations may be derived from a common gene pool. When the results were plotted, all the Jews, except the Yemenite group, were genetically similar to each other. The European Jewish cluster is the most closely knit in similarity and the Asian and North African Jewish clusters are closer to Middle Eastern groups than to European non-Jews.

In relation to genetic disorders, the Jewish population is divided into Sephardic Jews, Oriental Jews, and Ashkenazi Jews. Since the largest number of Jews in the United States are Ashkenazi Jews (European), the rest of this discussion involves genetic disorders most prevalent in this group.

Of all the genetic disorders that occur most frequently in Eastern European Jews, the one receiving the most publicity is Tay-Sachs disease. This disease is recessively inherited and is characterized by the absence of an enzyme involved in fat metabolism, resulting in the accumulation of fatty substances in the brain and leading to gradual neural and mental degeneration, with death occurring around 3 or 4 years of age. Couples in which both partners are Jews of Eastern European descent should be counseled to have genetic screening done to prevent the possibility of having a child with this deadly disease.

Susceptibility to disease

Susceptibility to disease for Jewish people depends on geographical origin. Some beliefs about Jewish susceptibility have no real scientific basis, such as the belief that Jews are more likely than others to have diabetes mellitus. Some studies have shown that Jews are no more susceptible to this disease than non-Jews from the same area of the world, as had been originally believed (Goodman, 1979).

Cancer Certain cancers are more frequent in certain groups of Jews than in others. Stomach cancer is more prevalent among Jews from Europe and the United States. Colon and prostate cancer is prevalent in Jews of Eastern European descent. Breast cancer, the most frequent type of cancer for all Jewish female groups except those from Iran (Patai & Wing, 1975), has been found to be higher in Jewish women from Europe and the United States

than in those from Asia. Cancer of the ovary is generally higher in Jews from Europe than in those from Asia or Africa.

Studies indicate that Ashkenazi Jewish women have a high incidence of specific mutations of BRCA1 and BRCA2. These changes have been associated with an increase in breast and ovarian cancer, with a higher risk in breast cancer. A specific alteration (185delAG) appears to be found in Ashkenazi Jews and is considered to be ethnic specific (Key, 1997).

Historically, cancer of the cervix has been lower in Jewish women than in non-Jews (Patai & Wing, 1975). However, as Jews become more acculturated and the incidence of multiple sexual partners, as well as partners who are not circumcised, increases, so does the incidence of cervical cancer. Cervical cancer is an area of concern for some Jewish individuals and is an area where client teaching is helpful.

Heart disease Data from a classic 1952 study of serum cholesterol levels in New York indicate a higher frequency of elevated serum cholesterol levels among Jews than among non-Jews. It is believed that elevated serum cholesterol levels may be caused by a single gene (Patai & Wing, 1975). If this is true, Ashkenazi Jews may have a higher frequency of the gene than Oriental Jews, who seem to have a relatively low rate of elevated serum cholesterol levels.

It is commonly believed that Ashkenazi Jews are more prone to coronary disease than other Jewish ethnic groups or non-Jews are. In international comparisons of the rate of first-time myocardial infarctions among men, Israel ranks among the highest in the world if all types of infarcts (including clinically unrecognized infarcts) are included (Mourant, Kopec, & Domaniewsks-Sobczak, 1978). Although there is a relatively high incidence of infarcts in Israel, there is a low mortality. After numerous studies, the conclusion regarding heart disease in the Jewish population is that further studies need to be done to determine the frequency of the disease among Jews as well as the interplay between heredity and environment (Mourant, Kopec, & Domaniewsks-Sobczak, 1978).

Polycythemia vera Evidence indicates that polycythemia vera is more common in Ashkenazi Jews than in other ethnic groups. In addition, there seems to be a higher prevalence of polycythemia vera in Jewish men than in Jewish women (Mourant, Kopec, & Domaniewsks-Sobczak, 1978).

Diabetes mellitus Diabetes has been referred to as the "Jewish disease" in Germany. Through ethnic Jewish studies done in Israel, an interesting phenomenon has been noted. A slightly higher percentage of Ashkenazi Jews than Sephardic Jews have diabetes. Also, in Yemenite and Kurdish newcomers to Israel, there are almost no cases of diabetes. However, in Yemenite and Kurdish settlers who have lived in Israel for more than 25 years, the same frequency of diabetes as with Ashkenazi Jews has been identified (Mourant, Kopec, & Domaniewsks-Sobczak, 1978; Patai & Wing, 1975). The results of this study indicate that dietary habits have an influence on the development of diabetes. The main dietary change in the older settlers as compared with the new arrivals has been an increased intake of sugar.

Although the incidence of diabetes in Jewish people has been indicated as being higher than in the general population, there has been no study to confirm this belief. Most of the studies on diabetes among Jews have been done in Israel. For a truer assessment of the prevalence of diabetes in the Jewish community, further studies outside Israel need to be conducted (Mourant, Kopec, & Domaniewsks-Sobczak, 1978).

Crohn's disease Studies indicate that Crohn's disease occurs in Jewish males more often than in Jewish females, and in Jews more often than in any other White ethnic group (Mourant, Kopec, & Domaniewsks-Sobczak, 1978). Although the number of young people diagnosed as having this disease has been increasing (Thompson, McFarland, Hirsch, et al., 1989), it is unknown if the increase is a result of a better awareness of the disease and improved diagnostic techniques or if there is an actual increase in the number of cases.

Ulcerative colitis Ulcerative colitis is seen more frequently in Ashkenazi Jews than in non-Jews or any other Jewish ethnic groups. It has many similarities to Crohn's disease and may even be seen with Crohn's disease. The cause of ulcerative colitis

is unknown, but familial tendencies have been noted; it occurs 10% to 15% more often in families of clients with ulcerative colitis than in families of control clients without the disease (Mourant, Kopec, & Domaniewsks-Sobczak, 1978).

Myopia Jews seems to have a larger incidence of myopia than the general population, and it occurs more often in boys than in girls. It is important to understand that myopia is not caused by close book work, as was believed many years ago, but by a prevalence of low hypermetropia and factors that allow for a greater or longer development of the length of the eye. Vision screening is an important part of a physical examination for Jewish people, particularly Jewish children.

Nutritional references and deficiencies

Jewish people tend to eat a lot of dairy products, which becomes a concern in patients with a history of lactose intolerance. Lactose intolerance has been identified among some Jewish ethnic groups, and a study done in Israel identified approximately two thirds of the Jewish population in Israel as being lactase deficient. However, the researchers also noted that most of these clients were not aware of their milk intolerance, leading to the conclusion that the condition was relatively benign and asymptomatic in the Jews studied (Mourant, Kopec, & Domaniewsks-Sobczak, 1978). Any Jewish client with a history of diarrhea, nonspecific lower gastrointestinal symptoms, and abdominal pain should have a good dietary history taken to check for a history of milk intolerance. The nurse needs to determine any family tendency toward lactose intolerance as well as the relationship between foods and the onset of abdominal symptoms.

It is important for the nurse to remember that not all Jews maintain a kosher diet and that some Jews are more strict about their diet than others. If the nurse is caring for an Orthodox Jewish client who is not eating properly because of the conflict between maintaining a kosher diet and eating institutional food, the nurse should consult with the family about bringing food from home. If the family cannot help with this situation, the client's rabbi may be consulted.

Psychological characteristics

Jews have been labeled with certain personality traits for over 3000 years. According to the Bible, the Children of Israel, following their exodus from Egypt, were "stiff necked," quarrelsome, disobedient, and rebellious. In Talmudic literature the Jews are described as the "merciful sons of a merciful father." Greek and Roman authors, who were usually anti-Semitic, made derogatory comments on the Jewish character.

It was not until the 1930s that studies began to explore Jewish personality characteristics (Patai & Wing, 1975). All these studies involved Jewish Americans, and most involved college students. The conclusions derived from these studies are as follows (Patai & Wing, 1975):

1. Studies indicate that Jews are superior in intelligence to comparable groups of non-Jews, especially in verbal intelligence. It is questionable whether Jews are genetically more intelligent than non-Jews; the apparent superiority in intelligence may be attributable to the pressures from the Gentile world for Jews to rely on their brains in order to survive.

2. In scholarly, intellectual, literary, and artistic pursuits, Jews seem to be proportionately overrepresented. Whether this phenomenon is proof of special Jewish talent or the result of extraneous circumstances that attracted Jews to concentrate on certain areas is open for debate.

3. As far as character traits are concerned, it is difficult to pinpoint differences between Jews and non-Jews. Character traits seem to be formed more by personal experiences in the immediate environment than by historical conditioning. As an example, Jewish Americans have been characterized as being aggressive, and this aggressiveness may be attributable to the pressure placed on Jewish children by their parents to "have a better life" than they did.

Anti-Semitism is a concern for Jewish people. Within the Jewish community mention is often made of Jewish fear in regard to anti-Semitism. Although the relative freedom experienced in the United States has led to a decrease in the practice of many Jewish rituals and possibly to the increased numbers of nonpracticing Jews, there are constant reminders that Jews are different and not always accepted by the general public. Today, in addition to constant reminders of the Holocaust, some Jewish people are also concerned about events in Israel.

Mental health The older medical literature indicates that the rate of occurrence of a variety of mental illnesses in Jews is high. In discussing this issue with numerous psychiatrists and leaders in the mental health field, Mourant, Kopec, and Domaniewsks-Sobczak (1978) have concluded that necessary data are lacking to confirm that the old medical literature is correct.

One concern among psychiatrists and mental health workers in Orthodox Jewish sections is the apparent need for but lack of use of mental health facilities. To determine what discourages Orthodox Jews from seeking psychiatric professional help, a study was conducted with 20 Orthodox Jewish mental health outpatients; it revealed that Orthodox Jews attach a stigma to mental health treatment and to Jews who avail themselves of it. This stigma is partly the result of an association of mental health treatment with insanity and partly because of the fear that this knowledge will have a negative effect on matrimonial prospects (Wikler, 1986).

It is important for the nurse to remember that Orthodox Jews do not enter mental health treatment easily. In the case of an Orthodox Jew who may need psychiatric counseling, there may be resistance to overcome before treatment can be started. The prospective client may display a real concern about confidentiality that may be seen as paranoia. This paranoia needs to be understood within the context of the social risk involved.

Orthodox Jews who do seek mental health care usually choose the agency or therapist based on reputation. One agency that opened its office in the Williamsburg section of Brooklyn, New York, in the heart of the Chassidic and Orthodox Jewish sections, was picketed and threatened. Today, however, this center has earned the "grudging" respect of the community (Meer, 1987).

Alcoholism The literature reports that Jews have had a low incidence of alcoholism in the past (Mourant, Kopec, & Domaniewsks-Sobczak, 1978). This assumption is questionable, and the incidence of cross-addiction, to both alcohol and another substance, may be higher among Jews than among non-Jews (Steinhardt, 1988). Lieberman (1987) has noted that Jews do not acknowledge a problem with alcohol because of their perception of what an alcoholic is. Many Jews view the alcoholic as a skid-row bum, not a person who gets drunk and acts silly at a wedding or maybe drinks too much when celebrating a holiday or festival, even if this behavior occurs on a regular basis.

All the behaviors that characterize the alcoholic in general—denial, isolation, ignorance of the disease, and guilt—seem to be intensified in the Jewish alcoholic because of the myth of Jewish sobriety. Orthodox Jews seem to suffer the greatest from these symptoms (Steinhardt, 1988).

Studies done in the United States indicate that drinking disorders tend to increase in Jews as religious affiliation shifts from orthodox, to conservative, to reform, to secular (Mourant, Kopec, & Domaniewsks-Sobczak, 1978). Some sociologists have suggested that alcoholism among Jews may increase as acculturation increases.

Of greatest concern to the Jewish community and to health care workers is the increasing alcohol and drug abuse among the Jewish youth. It is important to educate the Jewish community on the facts that alcoholics are not just skid-row, homeless people and that the ceremonial and social drinking of the Jewish community can increase the potential for alcoholism if it is not tempered.

Holocaust survivors Although the Holocaust has had a profound effect on Jewish feelings regarding "Jewishness" and persecution, the Holocaust survivors have had very little effect on the Jewish culture in the United States as a whole. The reason for this is that a relatively small number of Jewish Americans are Holocaust survivors. Many studies have been done on the effects of the Holocaust on survivors (Kren & Rappoport, 1980; Rose & Garske, 1987). These studies have helped the medical profession, especially the psychiatric medical profession, to determine the effects of war atrocities on survivors.

Many Jews have a difficult time discussing the effects of the Holocaust and its devastation on Jewish families and communities. Jewish individuals sometimes leave the room when the Holocaust is mentioned or joke to relieve their distress or feelings of anger and bewilderment at how this type of event could occur in modern times in a country that was supposed to be "civilized."

The effects of the Holocaust on the survivors and their children are still being studied. From the literature comes evidence of anger, depression, withdrawal, and anxiety in the survivors (Krystal & Niederland, 1971; Steinitz & Szonyi, 1979). Bearing children was seen as a means for the survivors to replace their loved ones who were lost during "The War," and the children were seen as a source of new hope and meaning. Because of this transference, the children of the survivors were usually overprotected and placed in situations that placed unrealistic expectations on them (Nadler, Kav-Venaki, & Gleitman, 1985).

Numerous studies have been done on children of Holocaust survivors. The results of these studies indicate that, on the whole, this population is well adjusted, with few significant psychopathological problems (Nadler, Kav-Venaki, & Gleitman, 1985; Rose & Garske, 1987; Steinitz & Szonyi, 1979). The biggest problems for these children seem to be related to the pressures they feel to protect their parents from any further physical or psychological pain and to the desire to fulfill their parents' unrealistic need to have the child compensate for what has been lost. These feelings lead to feelings of guilt when the children attempt to become emancipated from their parents.

Personality characteristics that most studies have discovered in Holocaust survivors are repressed anger, feelings of guilt, depression, fears of abandonment, worries of personal injury, feelings of being different, strong feelings of Jewishness (even if they are nonpracticing Jews), concern for Jewish survival (often more intense than in non-Holocaust survivors), and desires to maintain Jewish traditions that may border on obsession (Nadler, Kav-Venaki, & Gleitman, 1985; Rose & Garske, 1987; Steinitz &

Szonyi, 1979; Sorscher, 1994). Daughters of survivors have been found to be more susceptible to Holocaust-related symptoms than sons, and daughters whose parents did not talk about their experience had more problems than those whose parents talked about the experience (Sorscher, 1994).

Some Jewish people believe that it is important that the memory of the Holocaust never die and that no event like this should ever happen again. These same people believe there should never be mass destruction of any people. Perhaps protecting the memory of the Holocaust is one plausible explanation for the vast amount of literature that has been published regarding the Holocaust and its effect on the survivors. Some Jewish people believe that the Holocaust was just one more act of persecution against a people who have endured thousands of years of being victims of ignorance and misunderstanding.

Implications for nursing care

The nurse caring for a Jewish-American client should get a careful history of the client's eating habits. Many ethnic Jewish foods are high in animal and saturated fats. Since these are known to influence the amount of cholesterol in the body and since high cholesterol is known to be a factor in heart disease, dietary education is important in this cultural group. In addition, many prepared kosher foods are made with eggs as well as palm or coconut oil. Jewish clients who maintain a kosher diet must be cautioned to read labels carefully on all prepared kosher foods.

Because of the use of dairy products by this cultural group as well as the high incidence of Crohn's disease and ulcerative colitis, a history regarding bowel habits and abdominal problems should be carefully obtained. The nurse needs to remain alert for any symptoms that may indicate lactose intolerance. In addition, the nurse needs to remain alert for signs of drug or alcohol abuse. Since alcohol consumption is considered permissible at religious and secular functions, excessive drinking on a routine basis may not be viewed as a problem by the individual or the family. Cultural beliefs and taboos may make educating the client about the potential for alcohol abuse difficult.

Assisting Orthodox Jewish clients in areas of psychological needs takes patience and understanding on the part of the nurse. Not only may clients have concerns about personal acceptance by peers, but they may also worry that knowledge of psychiatric problems in the family will lead to potential problems in finding a suitable mate for themselves or future children. Going to counseling is equated with being "crazy," and being "crazy" is seen as a hereditary problem. Further education on psychiatric and emotional problems is needed to change negative attitudes about treatment.

SUMMARY

It is crucial that the nurse remember that not all Jewish clients are alike. Although some Jewish patients are orthodox and follow the commandments strictly, other Jewish people, with each successive generation, have become more acculturated to the behavior of the people around them.

Caring for the Jewish-American client can be a challenge. Although nursing education traditionally has prepared nurses to view health from a singular professional perspective, health must also be understood from a cultural perspective when care is being provided to clients whose cultural background differs from that of the nurse (Leininger, 1985). Many educational programs are seeking to address this issue by providing transcultural experiences for student nurses. Other health care facilities are offering educational programs to new nurses and nurses already in practice. One such experience related to the Jewish client is at Baycrest Centre for Geriatric Care in Toronto, Canada (Gorrie, 1989; Gould-Stuart, 1986; Rose, 1981). This program provides a transcultural experience for nurses in orientation and for selected nurses on a continuing care unit of the hospital. During this experience, differences between the Jewish culture and the secular culture are examined. Such educational programs can assist nurses in developing increased understanding of the universality of various cultural attributes and the importance of culture to all individuals.

Case Study

Esther Rosenbloom was admitted to a nursing home after a fall that resulted in a fractured hip. Esther, age 87, immigrated from Russia with her family in 1910, at 8 years of age. She was brought to the nursing home by her son-in-law, Nat, and her daughter, Bernice. Esther was admitted for physical therapy and is expecting to be discharged to her home after learning to walk with a walker. Her home is a block away from her daughter and son-in-law's.

Esther was raised in an Orthodox Jewish home in Brooklyn, New York, but joined the Conservative movement when she married at 24 years of age. Bernice, age 61, informs the nurse that although Esther follows Conservative Jewish thought, she maintains a kosher diet. The nursing home she is admitted to has very few Jewish clients and is unfamiliar with kosher diets. Bernice also mentions that her mother has abdominal difficulties if she ingests too much cheese or milk.

Esther appears worried, is moaning, and is complaining of pain in her hip. Bernice's eyes appear red, as if she has been crying. Bernice is wringing her hands and mentions that her mother has been uncomfortable and that she hopes the nurses at the nursing home will be able to keep Esther comfortable.

When the nurse asks Esther how she is feeling, she states in a whining tone of voice, "My hip hurts, and I want to go home. How are you going to feed me here? What do you know about kosher foods?"

When moving Esther from wheelchair to bed, the nurse notes that Esther does not seem to want to assist, despite the fact that the transfer sheet notes that Esther can move from wheelchair to bed with minimal assistance. When asked why she did not help, Esther replies, "I'm just too tired." Esther is usually self-sufficient and very busy with her volunteer activities, despite decreased visual acuity, for which she wears glasses. Although Bernice mentions that her mother always worries about her bowels, Esther does not have a history of constipation. She is continent of urine and stool.

CARE PLAN

 Nursing Diagnosis   Pain related to fractured hip and anxiety
Supportive data: complains of pain, appears upset and tense, has difficulty transferring from chair to bed

Client Outcomes

1. Pain will decrease.

Nursing Interventions

1. Medicate as ordered.
2. Use comfort measures (such as relaxation techniques, diversional activities) to promote relaxation.
3. Assist client to a comfortable position.
4. Spend at least 10 minutes per shift, while client is awake, to allow for expression of feelings.

 Nursing Diagnosis   Nutrition, altered, less than body requirements, related to religious and cultural dietary restrictions, plus possible lactose intolerance

Client Outcomes

1. Client will maintain weight within normal limits.

Nursing Interventions

1. Determine client's likes and dislikes in foods that the institution can provide that meet with client's religious restrictions.
2. Request that family bring ethnic foods from home that client would enjoy.

3. Serve foods on paper plates with plastic utensils to avoid serving permissible foods and nonkosher foods on same set of dishes.
4. Offer cheese or milk products in small amounts until tolerance can be determined.
5. If milk products are ingested, assess for abdominal cramps and diarrhea.

 Nursing Diagnosis   Anxiety related to situational crisis

Client Outcomes

1. Client will adjust to new living arrangements with minimal difficulty.

Nursing Interventions

1. Spend time with client to allow verbalization of fears, discomforts.
2. Find activities client is interested in and attempt to have client participate in facility activities.
3. Encourage independence.
4. Include client in decisions related to her care whenever feasible.
5. Allow family to spend as much time as desired with client.
6. Give client clear, concise explanations of anything that is about to occur.
7. Introduce client to other Jewish clients and encourage them to visit with each other.
8. Remain nonjudgmental toward family and client.
9. Contact rabbi and ask him to visit if client wishes.

 Nursing Diagnosis   Anxiety related to maturational crisis

Client Outcomes

1. Client will identify potential and actual sources of anxiety.

Nursing Interventions

1. Encourage client to identify stressful life events experienced within the last year.
2. Spend specific amount of uninterrupted time with client to listen to her concerns.
3. Allow family to spend as much time with client as desired.
4. Involve family in client's care if desired.
5. Assist client in identifying sources of fear or tension.
6. Assist client in identifying activities that help decrease anxiety and encourage the use of these activities.

 Nursing Diagnosis   Mobility, impaired physical, related to discomfort, fractured hip, and possible fear

Client Outcomes

1. Client will be able to transfer easily by self from bed to chair and ambulate with walker with minimal assistance.

Nursing Interventions

1. Provide physical therapy daily.
2. Reinforce what client is learning in physical therapy.
3. Observe client's functional ability daily.
4. Encourage and compliment client liberally.
5. Encourage verbalization of fears and feelings regarding altered state of mobility.
6. Remain nonjudgmental when client is unwilling to perform to her ability.
7. Provide comfort measures, such as medication as ordered and padding of extremities where they may be prone to skin breakdown.

8. Do range-of-motion exercises to increase strength; instruct family in these exercises and encourage them to encourage client.
9. Promote progressive ambulation.
10. Discuss use of distraction and other nonpharmacological pain relief.
11. Explain necessity of moving, even when in pain, to prevent arthritic conditions or contractions and increased stiffness.

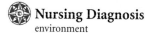 **Nursing Diagnosis**   Injury, risk for, related to impaired mobility, decreased visual acuity, and new environment

Client Outcomes

1. Client will sustain no injury.

Nursing Interventions

1. Encourage use of a walker, with assistance.
2. Assist client when getting short of breath, getting out of chair, or walking.
3. Be sure floor is dry and furniture and litter are out of the way when client is engaging in activities that may cause falls.
4. Instruct client and family regarding safety practices when client is using walker or transferring.
5. Keep side rails up when client is in bed.
6. Maintain bed in low position.

 Nursing Diagnosis   Constipation related to decreased mobility

Client Outcomes

1. Client will not develop constipation.

Nursing Interventions

1. Monitor frequency and characteristics of stools, and record.
2. Recognize that client may have concerns about bowels because of age and culture.
3. Ask client if she has a specific routine at home, such as a normal time for defecation or use of prune juice (a favorite "remedy" for Eastern European Jews).
4. Encourage fluid intake of 2000 mL per day.

 Nursing Diagnosis   Spiritual distress (risk for) related to separation from religious and cultural ties

Client Outcomes

1. Client will express feelings of spiritual distress.

Nursing Interventions

1. Listen for cues that client may be having spiritual distress (such as, "Why did God do this to me?").
2. Remain nonjudgmental.
3. Acknowledge spiritual concerns and encourage expression of thoughts and feelings.
4. Find ways to help client maintain kosher diet.
5. Encourage client to continue her religious practices during hospitalization and do whatever is necessary to help facilitate this.
6. Ask client if she desires rabbi to visit, and contact synagogue if necessary.
7. Introduce client to and help foster friendships with other Jewish clients.
8. If client can have pass, and family and client desire it, make arrangements for client to attend Friday night or Saturday services.

STUDY QUESTIONS

1. List ways that a kosher diet can be maintained while a client is in the hospital.
2. List religious needs a Jewish client may have while being hospitalized with which nursing staff can assist.
3. Identify three communication barriers that a nurse may encounter when giving care to a Jewish-American client.
4. List biological variations a Jewish client may have that will affect care given by a nurse.
5. Explain relationship characteristics that families of Jewish clients usually display toward a hospitalized relative.
6. Explain how Jewish people may react toward the impending death of a relative.

References

Bash, D.M. (1980, Sept.-Oct.). Jewish religious practices related to childbearing. *Journal of Nurse-Midwifery, 25,* 5.

Dempsey, D. (1975). *The way we die.* New York: Mac-Millan.

Edelheit, J. (1989, July-Aug.). The rabbi and the abyss of AIDS. *Tikkun, 4*(4), 67-69.

Feldman, D.M. (1986). *Health and medicine in the Jewish tradition.* New York: Crossroad Publishing Co.

Ganzfried, S. (1927). *Code of Jewish law: a compilation of Jewish laws and customs.* New York: Hebrew Publishing.

Gershom, Y. (1998). Personal communication, Douglas, Arizona.

Glazer, N. (1957). *American Judaism.* Chicago: University of Chicago Press.

Gold, M. (1988). *And Hannah wept: infertility, adoption and the Jewish couple.* Philadelphia: Jewish Publication Society.

Goodman, R. (1979). *Genetic disorders among the Jewish people.* Baltimore: Johns Hopkins University Press.

Gorrie, M. (1989). Reaching clients through cross cultural education. *Journal of Gerontological Nursing, 15*(10), 29-31.

Gould-Stuart, J. (1986). Bridging the cultural gap between residents and staff. *Geriatric Nursing, 7,* 319-321.

Heller, Z. (1975). The Jewish view of death: guidelines for dying. In Kubler-Ross, E. (Ed.), *Death: the final stage of growth.* Englewood Cliffs, N.J.: Prentice Hall.

Howe, I. (1976). *World of our fathers.* New York: Harcourt Brace Jovanovich.

Jakobovits, I. (1959). *Jewish medical ethics.* New York: Philosophical Library.

Janowsky, O. (1964). *The American Jew: a reappraisal.* Philadelphia: Jewish Publication Society.

Kaplan, R. (1970, May 26). *An experience with residual populations in Detroit.* Paper presented at the annual meeting of the National Conference of Jewish Communal Service, Boston, Massachusetts.

Kertzer, M. (1978). *What is a Jew* (ed. 4). New York: World Publishing.

Key, S.W. (1997, June 2) Three breast cancer gene alterations in Jewish community carry increased cancer. *Cancer Weekly Plus,* pp. 14-17.

Kolatch, A.J. (1985). *The second Jewish book of why.* New York: Jonathan David.

Kren, G.M., & Rappoport, L. (1980). *The Holocaust and the crisis of human behavior.* New York: Holmes & Meier.

Krystal, H., & Niederland, W.G. (1971). *Psychic traumatization: aftereffects in individuals and communities.* Boston: Little, Brown & Co.

L'Archevesque, C. I. & Goldstein-Lohman, H. (1996) Ritual circumcision: educating parents. *Pediatric Nursing, 22*(3), 228, 230-244.

Leininger, M. (1985). Transcultural nursing: an essential knowledge and practice field for today. *Canadian Nurse, 80*(11), 41-45.

Lieberman, L. (1987). Jewish alcoholics and the disease concept. *Journal of Psychology and Judaism, 13*(3), 165-179.

Lutwak, R., Ney, A.M., & White, J.E. (1988, Jan.). Maternity nursing and Jewish law. *Maternal and Child Health, 13,* 3.

Meer, J. (1987, April). An open door. *Psychology Today,* p. 17.

Mourant, A.E., Kopec, A.C., & Domaniewsks-Sobczak, K. (1978). *The genetics of the Jews.* New York: Oxford University Press.

Nadler, A., Kav-Venaki, S., & Gleitman, B. (1985). Transgenerational effects of the Holocaust: externalization of aggression in second generation of Holocaust survivors. *Journal of Consulting and Clinical Psychology, 53*(3), 365-369.

Novak, W., & Waldoks, M. (1981). *The big book of Jewish humor.* Philadelphia: Harper & Row.

Patai, R., & Wing, J.P. (1975). *The myth of the Jewish race.* New York: Charles Scribner's Sons.

Popenoe, D. (1977). *Sociology* (ed. 3). Englewood Cliffs, N.J.: Prentice Hall.

Rose, A. (1981). The Jewish elderly: behind the myths. In Weinfield, M., Whaffer, W., & Cotler, I. (Eds.), *The Canadian Jewish mosaic* (pp. 199-200). New York: John Wiley & Sons.

Rose, S.L., & Garske, J. (1987). Family environment, adjustment, and coping among children of Holocaust survivors: a comparative investigation. *American Journal of Orthopsychiatrics, 57*(3), 332-342.

Ross, H.M. (1981, Oct.). Societal/cultural views regarding death and dying. *Topics in Clinical Nursing, 3*(3), 1-16.

Rosten, L. (1968). *The joys of Yiddish.* New York: Pocket Books.

Rothschild, H. (& Chapman, C.F.) (Eds.) (1981). *Biocultural aspects of disease.* New York: Academic Press.

Sachar, A.L. (1964). *A history of the Jews.* New York: Alfred A. Knopf.

Schlesinger, B. (1971). *The Jewish family: a survey and annotated bibliography.* Toronto: University of Toronto Press.

Schneider, S. (1985). *The non-Orthodox Jewish perspective of dying and death.* Master's thesis submitted to the University of Arizona, Tucson, Arizona.

Schwartz, E. (1984). *The non-Orthodox Jewish perspective on dying and death.* Master's thesis, University of Arizona, Tucson, Arizona.

Sorscher, N. (1994, May) Children of Holocaust survivors may inherit their parents' trauma symptoms. *The Psychology Letter, 6*(5).

Sowell, T. (1981). *Ethnic America*. New York: Basic Books.

Sperling, A. (1968). *Reasons for Jewish customs and traditions*. New York: Bloch.

Steinhardt, D. (1988, Feb.). Alcoholism: the myth of Jewish immunity. *Psychology Today*, p. 10.

Steinitz, L.Y., & Szonyi, D.M. (Eds.) (1979). *Living after the Holocaust: reflections by children of survivors in America*. New York: Bloch.

Stevenson, J.C., Schanfield, M.S., & Sandler, S.G. (1985). Immunoglobulin allotypes in Jewish populations living in Israel and the United States. *American Journal of Physical Anthropology, 67*(3), 195-207.

Thompson, J.M., McFarland, G.K., Hirsch, J.E., et al. (1989). *Mosby's manual of clinical nursing* (ed. 2). St. Louis: Mosby.

Trepp, L. (1980). *The complete book of Jewish observances*. New York: Behrman House.

U.S. Department of Commerce, Bureau of the Census (1993). *Population profiles of the United States: 1993* (Publication No. 23-185). Washington, D.C.: Government Printing Office.

Wikler, M. (1986). Pathways to treatment: how Orthodox Jews enter therapy. Social casework: *The Journal of Contemporary Social Work*, 113-118.

Yearbook of American and Canadian churches (1993). New York: National Council of Churches.

Zborowski, M. (1969). *People in pain*. San Francisco: Jossey-Bass.

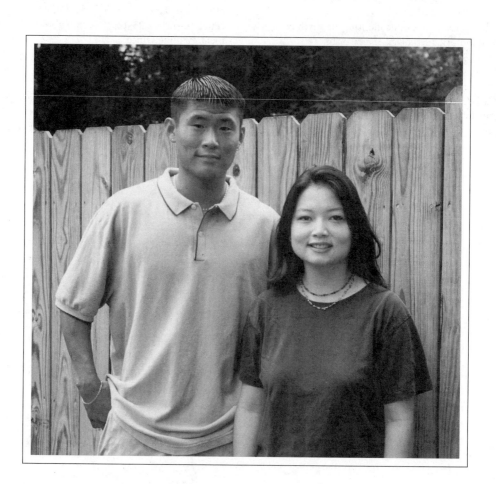

CHAPTER 22 Korean Americans

Jai Bun Earp

BEHAVIORAL OBJECTIVES

After reading this chapter, the nurse will be able to:

1. Describe the communication patterns of Korean Americans and the difficulties encountered when communicating in an English-speaking society.
2. Describe cultural values, beliefs, and practices of Korean Americans that affect health care.
3. Describe the communication patterns, the concept of time, and the dynamics of the family system in Korean Americans.
4. Describe the biological variations that affect health care in Korean Americans.
5. List a few Korean culturally bound illnesses found in the literature.
6. Describe the current status of health care practices among Korean Americans.

OVERVIEW OF KOREA

Korea, often referred to as the "Land of the Morning Calm" (Japanese *Chōsen*) is a nation with one of the richest and most original cultures in East Asia. Shaped like a sitting rabbit, Korea is a peninsula with about 4000 islands along the shoreline. The northern part of the country shares a border with the People's Republic of China and extends 625 miles to the southern tip of Cheju Island. The Yellow Sea separates the west coast of Korea from China. The Sea of Japan, which surrounds the east and south coasts separates Korea from Japan. The distance between Korea and China is only 129 miles. The peninsula is 125 miles wide at its narrowest point.

Unfortunately, the Korean War (1949-1953) left the country divided by the 38th parallel demilitarized zone (DMZ). Korea is one of the few nations in the world that is still affected by the Cold War. About 40,000 United States troops continue to guard Korea

against another communist invasion. The South Korean land mass is only 38,031 square miles and is slightly smaller than Indiana. In contrast, the North Korean land mass is 46,768 square miles and is slightly smaller than Pennsylvania (Information Please Almanac, 1998). The population of North Korea is 24,317,000 people. In contrast, the population of South Korea is 45,948,811 people (Information Please Almanac, 1998). If South Korea and North Korea were reunited, the country would be about the same size as Iceland or Portugal.

Today, North Korea remains under communist rule, isolated from the world. In contrast, South Korea has made great strides in developing its potential as one of the Far Eastern powers by blending nationalism, administrative efficiency, and semiauthoritarian rule (Czarra & Kaltsounis, 1988). The war left South Korea with no natural resources, and thus the Korean people were dependent on scarce farmland for basic subsistence (Kaltsounis & Shin, 1988). It can be safely said that the only natural resources South Korea has are human resources. In fact, South Korea's export successes have been the result of the sweat and skills of its people because it really has nothing else to sell (World Almanac, 1997). South Korea has made a remarkable economic transformation in the last three decades with its per capita gross national product (GNP) increasing from $87 in 1962 to $2300 in 1987 (Park, 1988) to $2900 in 1993 (Information Please Almanac, 1998). Today, South Korea is the sixth largest trading partner of the United States. Sponsorship of the Twenty-third World Olympics in 1988 and the International Council of Nurses (ICN) Nineteenth Congress in Seoul in 1989 represent a few examples of the economic confidence of the people of South Korea.

Mountains, valleys, and streams dominate the terrain of both North and South Korea. North Korea is almost completely covered by a series of north-south mountain ranges that are separated by narrow valleys. In North Korea, the Yalu River forms a part of the northern border with Manchuria (Information Please Almanac, 1998). South Korea is approximately 70% mountainous. In the north and east of South Korea, more than 10% of the land is 3000 feet above sea level. In South Korea, narrow plains and hills between the mountains provide the major land area for agriculture and other economic activities. In South Korea, approximately 22% of the land is cultivated for rice, barley, soybeans, and vegetables (Park, 1988).

South Korea has a clear delineation of four seasons and its climate is characterized by cold winters and hot summers. The average temperature in the coldest winter month is below 28° F and in the warmest month is over 86° F. A humid summer monsoon from the Pacific lasts about 6 weeks in June and July.

Of the 45,948,811 people in South Korea, 75% live in the cities. Predominant migration of population toward big cities, such as Seoul (the capital, which it also means) or Pusan ('cauldron-mountain'), is the most conspicuous phenomenon of population redistribution in South Korea (Park, 1988).

Because of its strategic location, Korea has been under foreign attack several times. Korea was under Japanese colonization for 36 years (1910-1945). Because of these attacks coupled with the Korean War and the division of the country, the Korean people are very conscientious about territoriality and communist invasion. Unification of the peninsula is a hope held very close to the hearts of most Korean people (Lee, 1988a).

OVERVIEW OF KOREAN AMERICANS

Although Korean immigration into the United States dates to before the Korean War, American military presence since the war has influenced Korean people to adopt Americanism. Those individuals who participated in the massive immigration into the United States after the war suffered extreme social wrath from those persons who stayed behind. However, because of the strict immigration laws, earlier Korean immigrants in the 1960s and 1970s were a chosen few in key professions. The massive immigration of highly talented and educated individuals left South Korea with what has become known as a "brain-drain" phenomenon. With the relaxation of the immigration laws, later immigrants have not been so well educated as the previous generations.

LIFE IN THE UNITED STATES TODAY

According to the U.S. Bureau of the Census, 837,000 Korean Americans reside in the United States, representing 0.3% of the total United States population (Information Please Almanac, 1998). Of the number of Asian Americans residing in this country, 54% live in the West, compared with 21% of the total U.S. population (U.S. Department of Commerce, Bureau of the Census, 1993a). A total of 66% of Asian Americans live in just five states: California, New York, Hawaii, Illinois, and Texas (U.S. Department of Commerce, Bureau of the Census, 1993b). The greatest concentrations of Asian Americans are in California, New York, and Hawaii.

Of the number of Korean Americans who resided in the United States before 1975, 16.4% were foreign born. Of the number of Korean Americans residing in the country between 1975 and 1979, 15.3% were foreign born, and between 1980 and 1990, 41.0%

were foreign born (U.S. Department of Commerce, Bureau of the Census, 1993c). Immigration has obviously contributed immensely to the growth of the Korean-American population over the past two decades. However, the percentage of Korean Americans who are foreign born differs considerably across time periods.

The median age of Korean Americans is 29.1 years, compared with the national median age of 33 years for the rest of the general U.S. population. In addition, only 6% of Asian Americans are 65 years of age or older, compared with 13% of the general U.S. population (U.S. Department of Commerce, Bureau of the Census, 1993c).

Korean Americans are noted for high educational standards. In 1990, 89.1% of Korean-American men 25 years of age or older and 74.1% of Korean-American women 25 years of age or older held a high school diploma. In 1990, 46.9% of Korean-American men and 25.9% of Korean-American women held a bachelor's degree. Children excel in school, particularly in science, which can be related to the struggle to achieve economic development after the Korean Conflict and the importance of education, which was ingrained in the minds of the people. Each year over 98% of elementary school students move into the middle schools and about 90% graduate from high school (Kaltsounis & Shin, 1988). The 30,000 Korean students constitute the third highest number of foreign students studying in United States educational institutions (U.S. Department of Commerce, Bureau of the Census, 1993c). Stress put on students to go to the top-rated schools has created some problems such as loneliness (Simmons, Klopf, & Park, 1991), depression (Crittenden, Fugita, Bae, et al., 1992; Park, 1988), and suicide.

Many Korean Americans view entering the work force after college graduation as a serious lifetime commitment. Because of limited job opportunities, some Korean Americans do not look favorably at moving from job to job. In addition, some Korean Americans believe that attendance at the right school plays a major role in landing a prestigious position because many elite companies scout capable people only from the top-rated schools. Korean Americans, as with other Asian Americans, are more likely to participate in the labor force. Of the number of Korean Americans in the United States, 63.3% participate in the work force. In general, Asian-American women are reported to have a higher participation rate than all other women in the work force. In fact, 69% of Asian-American women, compared with 57% of all other women in the United States, participate in the labor force (U.S. Department of Commerce, Bureau of the Census, 1993b). The proportion of families with three or more workers in the work force is 15.3%. Asian Americans—and Korean Americans are no exception—are more likely to work in jobs related to technical, sales, and administrative support (33.3%) and managerial and professional specialties (31.2%). The rest of Asian Americans work in jobs related to service (14.6%); farming, forestry, and fishing (1.1%); precision, production, craft, and repair (7.6%); and operators, fabricators, and laborers (14.9%). For Korean-American families, the per capita income is $9032, compared with $14,143 for the rest of the general U.S. population. In 1990, the poverty rate of Korean Americans was 13.7% (U.S. Department of Commerce, Bureau of the Census, 1993b).

One major issue that prompted Korean adults to immigrate to the United States was consideration for their children's future. However, many elderly Koreans came over without thorough awareness of what was to come (Messaris & Woo, 1991). Many Koreans found difficulty leaving behind old cultural and social norms and adjusting to new ones (Moon & Pearl, 1991). Many of these individuals faced problems, including financial struggles, poor health, poor care practices, difficulty with social interactions, mental problems such as *hwabyung* (which is a Korean culture–bound syndrome of suppressed anger), and depression (Lin, 1983; Pang, 1990).

Another major issue involved Korean-American men who suffer from loss of control and a sense of not belonging (Hurh & Kim, 1990). Many men followed their spouses who were nurses or physicians (it was easier for females to immigrate because of their professions) without adequate preparation for themselves.

COMMUNICATION
Language and culture

The Korean language, *Han-gul,* is spoken by more than 63 million people in many parts of the world. It is regarded as an isolated language without any near kin (Lee, 1988a). Many linguists, however, have shown that Korean has Ural-Altaic affinities, like Tungus, Mongolian, Japanese, and Turkic (Voegelin & Voegelin, 1977). Although the Korean language is entirely different and capable of standing on its own (14 consonants and 10 vowels), the language and literature have been greatly influenced by Chinese (Chang, 1991). More than half of the words now used in Korean are of Chinese origin. With continued emphasis on learning Chinese because of the ruling Neo-Confucian philosophy of the earlier Chosun Dynasty, Chinese characters and Chinese words in the Korean alphabet today occupy more than 50% of the text of Korean newspapers, magazines, and books.

The forced annexation of Korea by Japan from 1910 to 1945 prohibited the public use of the Korean language and forced Koreans to learn Japanese (Lee, 1988a). Thus, many words used in Korean also have a Japanese origin (many of which are also from Chinese).

Dialect and style

The usual commentary on dialect, style, emotional context, and kinesics does not apply to *Han-gul* as spoken by Koreans. Breadth of full language use and preciseness of pronunciation are most often the discriminators that identify and delineate higher class (educated) from lower class (less educated) Koreans.

Verbal communication

When abroad, a Korean being introduced to other Koreans, whether socially or professionally, will listen quite attentively before deciding to interact. This reserved behavior is related to the Korean equation of "reserved familiarity" until the individual has mastered the language and learned to know the individual. During conversation with an unfamiliar person, if there is a match between individuals, the individual is "in" and conversation will ensue. Of the number of Korean Americans residing in this country, 80.8% speak a (non-Korean) Asian or Pacific Islander language at home, 65% do not speak English well, and 43.9% are linguistically isolated (U.S. Department of Commerce, Bureau of the Census, 1993b).

Use of eye contact and kinesics

In public situations, Koreans are a "noncontact" group. In this sense, some Koreans have some difficulty making eye contact or engaging in physical contact on streets, at markets, on subways, and in the workplace. However, in one-on-one and "acquaintance" situations, Koreans are very similar to Americans in interactions. With a familiar acquaintance, some Korean Americans will engage in eye contact. When conversing with familiar individuals, they will speak in the first person. Some Korean Americans are comfortable in face-to-face situations. However, some Koreans are still offended if the sole of a shoe or foot is directed at them. Most Koreans who subscribe to this belief are willing to forgive "lack of knowledge" on the part of some Westerners in this regard. Basic courtesy, when sincerely exhibited by all parties, is a good faith gesture that overcomes traditional Korean mores.

Confucian philosophy forms the basis for behavior and position within the social hierarchy (Van Decar, 1988). Etiquette is very important to Koreans, and it is a mistake to appear too familiar or informal. First names are used only within a family or a circle of close friends. For some Korean Americans, addressing or referring to people by name is considered a lack of proper respect and is believed to invoke evil spirits and lead to ill fortune.

Social rank and language

The Korean language itself reinforces attention to rank or position. Different vocabulary and verb endings are used according to whether the person being addressed is of higher, equal, or lower rank or socioeconomic status than the speaker. Some Korean Americans are very sensitive regarding the feelings of others. In most instances, Korean Americans are generous, agreeable, and rarely say no to even an impossible request to prevent overt conflict and a breakdown of relationships (Fisher, 1996; Van Decar, 1988).

Implications for nursing care

Many elderly Korean Americans who immigrated late in life may be quite intelligent and trilingual, but they may not be able to communicate with health care professionals. Some elderly Korean Americans may have an attitude of "giving up on learning English." It is essential for the nurse to assess the linguistic abilities of the client. When translators are needed, and Korean interpreters are not available, a Japanese or Chinese translator may be used to communicate with the client. However, if the client speaks and understands only Korean, a Japanese or Chinese translator may not be helpful. In these instances, the nurse may seek the assistance of a family member who speaks English to serve as a translator. However, children should not be used as translators, because this may create a reversal in the parent-child relationship and cause conflict. When communicating with a Korean American client who has some knowledge of English, it is essential that the nurse speak slowly because this aids understanding. However, it is not necessary to speak loudly because the client is not deaf, but rather has an unfamiliarity with the language.

SPACE

Distal spacing, between elderly and young, seniors and juniors, bosses and subordinates is very subtle but quite distinct within the Korean community. If this spacing is ignored through ignorance or "cockiness," the person is considered a "black sheep" and will not be accepted socially.

Korean Americans, like some other Asian Americans (Chinese Americans, Japanese Americans), have a high tolerance for crowding in public spaces. For Korean Americans who immigrated from Korea, the ability to tolerate crowding probably developed in Korea as a result of the density of the population. In South Korea, it is so crowded that its 45 million people are packed 410 people per square mile. This rate is increasing by 1.5% each year (Information Please Almanac, 1998).

Although Korean Americans can tolerate crowding, some avoid physical contact if possible. These individuals are uncomfortable in situations where physical contact is likely to occur. In addition, although some Korean Americans can tolerate higher degrees of crowding, they do not necessarily desire to engage in eye contact with unfamiliar persons.

Implications for nursing care

Because Korean Americans are basically a "noncontact" cultural group until a relationship has been established, the nurse should attempt to establish an environment of trust and caring. Korean Americans are often perceived as extremely practical and thus, when confronted with sincerity, will respond in a manner of "Let's get the job done." When interacting with an elderly Korean who does not speak the language, a translator who can convey sincerity should be used. It is essential for the nurse to remember that, although some Korean Americans are reported to have a higher tolerance for crowding, physical contact may not be acceptable, despite the closeness to the individual.

SOCIAL ORGANIZATION
Family

The average family size for Korean Americans is 3.6 people. The percentage of Asian-American families maintained by a husband and wife is 82%, which is slightly higher than the national average of 79%. Of the number of Korean-American families, only 12% are female-headed households, compared with the national average of 17%. During the last 15 years, a watershed percentage that has both enhanced tradition and extended opportunity to family unit members, especially females, has been maintained (U.S. Department of Commerce, Bureau of the Census, 1993c).

Historically, the Korean-American family has been the cornerstone of the culture. In most cases, father and sons have enjoyed preeminence as the leaders and undisputed decision makers (Cho, 1996; Van Decar, 1988). The traditional Korean family has been fixated on the need for a male heir. A male heir is needed to guarantee the family line and lead the family in rituals that pay homage to ancestors, both in the home and at burial sites. The first-born son inherits the mantle of family leadership and a greater property inheritance. Other sons receive lesser portions. Daughters receive very little if any inheritance.

In Korea, marriages of daughters have been arranged, and elders have been respected and cared for. Gender biases may be held by some Korean Americans. However, since the Republic of Korea has leaped into the forefront of industrial export and partnership with the Western world, there has been a demand for qualified citizens with bachelor's, master's, and doctoral degrees, regardless of gender. This surge of national output and pride saw the competitive Korean educational system pushing those with potential to the top, regardless of gender. The movement toward equality in rights for women has threatened tradition both domestically and internationally. Although pure tradition is still found in the larger Korean rural society, the profound effect of this change is clearly visible in the matriculation picture at Korean universities. Essentially, modern mobility has strengthened relationships between couples and immediate family and has weakened traditional extended family obligations.

For some Korean-American families, problems have arisen when the wife has experienced professional upward mobility, and the educationally prepared husband has not been able to find employment. Some Korean-American males have not been able to accept this situation and as a result have experienced enormous stress and anxiety. Some Korean-American males have discouraged their partners from continuing competitive job tracks. This reaction should adjust with time because Koreans not only are rooted in tradition but also are very pragmatic.

Koreans as a whole are determined to increase their stock as an international economic partner. Korean Americans are an impressive example of how people can both assimilate and remain true to national heritage and family values. Korean-American communities have both become a part of the greater American society and begun to internalize to ensure homogeneity. Almost every major Korean community in the United States (that is, Los Angeles, San Francisco, New York, Baltimore, and Atlanta) and almost every city with a major university have Korean schools to ensure that the culture, history, language, and tradition are not lost.

Religion and social values

The social values of modern Korea reflect a blending of both old and new religious viewpoints. Shamanism, Taoism, Buddhism, and Confucianism were practiced in Korea long before Christianity (Eshleman, 1992; Lew, 1988). Christianity in Korea, though more recent, has been accentuated by the presence of 40,000 to 60,000 Westerners for more than 40 years. With the Westerners have come the missionaries. As a result, approximately 15% of Koreans are churchgoing Christians. In addition, even more are influenced by the "Christian way." Many Koreans honor and practice a blend of traditional and modern religion (Lew, 1988).

Although certain conflicts are recognized, that is, Confucianism versus Christianity, some Korean Americans are able to harmonize the best of "both" worlds. Korean Americans are generally more oriented to the future than the ancient past and will adapt consistent, provable change, whether religious or political.

Implications for nursing care

Although contemporary changes in traditional family customs have weakened the kinship and family structure, there is no question that Korean Americans are family oriented. Hospitalization of one client becomes an entire family concern. The increasing importance of conjugal family relationships rather than the son-parent relationship has put sons and daughters-in-law at risk of great guilt if the parents become ill. Some Korean Americans may blame the illness of the father or mother on inadequate attention and care on the part of the child. It is essential to remember that the family is the primary social unit. As the primary social unit, family members must be included in the plan of care if culturally appropriate care is to be rendered. In some instances, the client and the family may need counseling services to ensure proper intervention with the family.

TIME

According to Dodd (1987), time is an element of culture that belongs to a unique category in a nonverbal communication system. The organization of time is essential for some cultural groups. In other words, perceptions of time are culturally determined and are not culturally free (Dodd, 1987). Some Korean Americans believe that a person is in this world for only a brief time. For persons subscribing to this belief, life and living are viewed as a harmonious relationship between nature and the human being. Some Korean Americans, like some other Asian Americans, believe that every individual needs to learn to use time wisely. Thus they are likely to believe that time should be used for activities such as performance of service for another person (Dodd, 1987).

Many Korean Americans are future oriented, which is derived from a Confucian belief in reincarnation. In this sense, many individuals who subscribe to this belief are likely to believe that it is essential to finish a task before beginning another one.

By virtue of culture, individuals can be either polychronic or monochronic in the organization of time. Hall (1966) described the time orientation of Asians as polychronic in contrast to the monochronic orientation of Westerners. Monochronically oriented individuals believe that it is essential to do one thing at a time. Persons who are monochronically oriented believe that accomplishments should be achieved during each task (Dodd, 1987). These individuals have an increased need for closure (finishing a task, ending a relationship). Monochronically oriented individuals generally think in a linear fashion. People who think in a linear fashion tend to internally process information in a sequential, segmented, orderly fashion (Dodd, 1987). For example, these individuals would sequence a meeting in this order: arrival, meeting, conclusion, action. They are likely to cycle through this sequence all day (Dodd, 1987). In contrast, polychronic individuals tend to think about and attempt to do many things at one time (Dodd, 1987). Persons who are polychronic can experience a high degree of information overload because they are trying to process so many things at one time. These individuals may also procrastinate because of information overload (Dodd, 1987). They may also tend to struggle harder to articulate abstractions without visualizations. Dodd (1987) concludes that polychronic individuals are very visually oriented. This orientation appears to be in concert with some research that indicates that these individuals may have either a right-brain or left-brain orientation. Right brain–dominant people tend to think more creatively, visually, and artistically than left brain–dominated individuals do, whereas left brain–dominant people tend to think more mathematically and linearly (Dodd, 1987). Because Korean Americans tend to be polychronically oriented and appear to be visually oriented, they are very likely to be right brain dominant.

For some Korean Americans having children is an essential life task. Sacrifice to bring up children in the best possible environment is an indescribable quest. For example, parents may be maintaining a meager living by selling fish at the market, but they may send their children to the best private institution possible.

Many Koreans believe that people are reincarnated. They believe that those who perform good deeds and provide mercy for others in this world will be reborn as another human being and that if you are bad in this world, you will be punished and will be reborn as some sort of animal. Because of this belief, an intact body is necessary. Organ donation and transplantation are not seen as a virtue but as a threat to reincarnation.

Westerners tend to prioritize and schedule their lives. Compartmentalization of time occurs even in clinical settings such as the hospital. For example, in the hospital, rounds are made, temperatures taken, meals served, medicines dispensed—all on schedule.

Implications for nursing care

Time as viewed by Koreans is obviously a concept not held by Westerners in general. Nurses can expect cooperation in matters involving time, but when the client is suffering from anxiety and stress, the nurse must take time to communicate with the client to determine the client's needs.

ENVIRONMENTAL CONTROL
Illness and wellness behaviors

Several theories can explain the perceptions of illness by Korean people. One predominant health-illness theory governing Korean people is the equilibrium system which consists in harmony and balance. Health derives from the harmonious relationship among elements of the universe, the human environment, and the supernatural world. Health also derives from the balance of the two major forces: *eum* (cold/dark, Chinese *yin*) and *yang* (hot/bright, Chinese *yang*). Disruption in the harmony of nature and imbalance between the two forces causes illness.

Dominance of *eum* creates problems related to cold, which makes a person depressive, hypoactive, and hypothermic. Examples of diseases from this dominance of *eum* are abdominal cramps, indigestion, and vaginal discharge. In contrast, dominance of *yang* causes a person to be hyperactive, hyperthermic, and irritable. Febrile seizures, stroke, and pimples are some examples of conditions related to *yang* dominance. Treatment for a person with dominant *eum* includes its replacement with *yang* to achieve balance, which includes providing hot food such as onions, peppers, ginger, and scallion roots. Giving cold food such as ice water, myung bean curd, cold noodles, and crab are some of the treatment modalities for those who have dominant *yang* problems (Manderson, 1987).

Elderly Korean Americans consider drawing blood for laboratory work a very unfortunate event and may refuse. This idea stems from the fact that blood is considered life and removing blood from the body is considered as removing *ki* (Chinese *ch'i*), which is the very essence of life energy (Kim, 1992).

Many Korean Americans also believe that illness or death is fated and that they have no control over nature (Tien-Hyatt, 1987). Many Korean Americans equate admission to a hospital with a death sentence and may refuse to be admitted. This refusal may occur particularly in elderly Korean Americans, which in turn delays treatment.

Oriental herbal medicine

The use of herbal medicines (*Han-yak,* 'Chinese medicines') dates back to ancient Chinese practices. However, traditional Korean medicine has developed with its own characteristics (Pang, 1989). There are 396 distinct herbs and spices commercially available used either singly or in blended mixtures such as herbal decoctions (Lamba, 1993).

Today the power and influence of herbal medicine is evident in every city with a large Korean community, where many wholesale and retail herbal medicine shops may be found (Miller, 1990). Herbal medicine doctors practice their trade by four common treatment methods: herbal medicine shops, acupuncture, moxibustion, and cupping. They may use one method singly or several in combination to treat clients.

Oriental medicine is based on the visual observation of behavior, physical properties of the body such as build, illness history, verbal responses, and radial pulses. After assessment, symptoms of disease are interpreted and the treatment plan is devised on the basis of the metaphysical and cosmological philosophy of the concepts of *eum* and *yang* (Pang, 1989, 1990).

Oriental medicine doctors who have been assimilated into the American culture may incorporate biomedical technologies in making diagnoses. They may explain and make an analogy of their Oriental treatment in biomedical terms. It is likely that the number of Oriental medical doctors will increase as Korean communities become larger. In Atlanta alone, at least nine Oriental medicine doctors are in official practice (Pang, 1989).

Pregnancy and postpartum practices

Tae-kyo ('prenatal training') is commonly practiced among some Korean American women during pregnancy (Choi, 1986). Using *tae-kyo,* women are supposed to think only about good things in life and to maintain a calm attitude to ensure having a healthy baby. Pregnant Korean-American women are taught to eat only the right food in the right form, that is, an apple without nicks or spots.

During the postpartum period, women were instructed to have 21 days of bed rest with lots of seaweed soup for cleansing the body and providing fluid for adequate lactation (Giger, Davidhizar, & Wieczorek, 1993). However, this practice may be a dysfunctional health care practice because after delivery a woman is in a hypercoagulable state of pregnancy (Giger, Davidhizar, & Wieczorek, 1993).

General preventive health practices

During the hot summers in Korea, individuals tend to sweat more. Too much sweating is considered a loss of energy *(ki)* and negative to good health. Eating dog meat soup just before summer is believed to build stamina and strength by decreasing sweating. Restaurants specializing in dog meat soup are abundant and busy in Korea.

Sex is regarded as a high-energy consumer; therefore sex drains *ki* from the body. Traditionally, both Korean men and women have been highly considerate of their partner's state of health in that, if one's health were not at its best or if one were "weak," sex might be abstained from in consideration of the situation.

Chen, Wismer, Lew, et al. (1997) concluded that research collaboration between universities, community-based organizations, and ethnic communities may actually yield high-quality research and break through cultural barriers where Korean Americans are concerned. Further findings from this study are also suggestive that when Korean Americans are actively engaged in the research process community capacity may be enhanced, thereby laying the foundation for future projects that improve the health status of Korean Americans.

Implications for nursing care

Many Korean Americans embrace more than one belief about their health-illness systems. As a result of multiple beliefs in the health-illness system, a variety of health care practices may be encountered by nurses. Persons who believe that sickness is from the action of a supernatural being may delay seeking health care until it is too late. They also may project a guilty conscience about their past behavior and act as though they have given up recovering from the present illness. Nurses must be very authoritative in carrying out treatment plans for the Koreans who exhibit such attitudes. Healing practices utilized by Korean clients should not be rejected automatically. Careful assessment is essential to provide culturally appropriate care.

It is essential for the nurse to recognize that many Korean Americans who are admitted to acute care or other health care facilities may be using both modern and herbal remedies simultaneously. This creates a problem of allergic and synergistic effects. Several specific cases of herbal-use conflicts have been reported (Lamba, 1993). Some herbal decoctions contain mistletoe, shave grass, horsetail, or sassafras and are certainly unsafe. Mistletoe contains viscotoxin, a mixture of toxic proteins that can produce anemia, hepatic, and intestinal hemorrhage and fatty degeneration of the thymus in experimental animals (Lamba, 1993). Most of these ingredients are crude complex mixtures that are neither uniformly prepared nor assayed for purity. Many contain a variety of unidentified allergens that may cause many potentially adverse effects. Some of the known allergenic materials include pollen (particularly from flower herbs), insect parts, and mold spores. Nurses must monitor the clients closely for potential side effects as well as synergistic effects of medicines in case they are dual users.

If properly trained, Oriental medicine doctors have completed at least 6 years of education, with 2 years of premedical school and 4 years of Oriental medical school. To practice in Korea, they also must pass a national licensing examination. Because of the popularity of holistic and alternative forms of health care, it is not only Oriental people seeking herbal medicinal treatment in the United States, but also many Americans who are seeking to have their health monitored by the "herbal doctors" (Pang, 1989).

Health care practices that are based on the client's cultural beliefs must be honored when possible to ensure chances of success through client compliance. If a client desires and truly believes in herbal medicine, some sort of collaborative health supervision may be the best solution for the client. Open discussion to enhance rapport and trust is a key ingredient for successful client-oriented care. One of the herbal medicine ingredients that is gaining tremendous popularity in the United States is ginseng *(Panax quinquefolium* and *P. ginseng)*. Ginseng is used to raise stamina and power of thoughts, improve the tone of body organs, and increase longevity. The long-term properties of ginseng have been poorly researched. It is postulated, however, that long-term abuse of ginseng can cause hypertension. Other but less frequently seen side effects of ginseng include nervousness, sleeplessness, skin eruptions, morning diarrhea, and edema (Siegal, 1979). Nonetheless, despite the many hazards that have been alluded to, it should be understood that the majority of herbal products on the U.S. market are safe when properly used (Lamba, 1993).

BIOLOGICAL VARIATIONS
Body size and structure

Generally speaking, Korean Americans are shorter than other Americans. A direct correlation exists between age and height among Korean Americans in that the older they are, the shorter they are (Molnar, 1983). This correlation exists because in the old days in Korea, meager living and lack of food prevented people from consuming enough nutritious food for growth (Overfield, 1995). Children born since the industrialization of Korea are considerably taller, though they are not so tall as children in the United States. Korean Americans have longer trunks and shorter lower extremities in general (Overfield, 1995). This may be attributable in part to genetic factors but also from cultural habits. Koreans do not wear shoes in the house. They sit on *ondol* ('hypocaust') floors that are generally heated from beneath by coal, called *yun-tan* ('briquette'). Long years of sitting on the floor like Buddha prevents vertical blood circulation into the legs, which in turn prevents the legs from stretching and achieving adequate growth. Sitting also contributes to aches and weakening of the legs in many elderly Korean people because of the habitual stretching of thigh muscles above the knees (Overfield, 1995).

Adipose tissue deposition is smaller in Koreans than in Americans, which is largely a result of less fatty-food consumption. Shoulder-to-hip width is about the same in most Koreans (Giger & Davidhizar, 1990; Overfield, 1995). For Korean-American women breast-to-hip size is also about equal. Because of their small structure and body size, it is unusual for Korean-American women to wear large sizes of clothes.

Some Korean Americans tend to have less body hair than other Americans (Giger & Davidhizar, 1990; Overfield, 1995). In fact, some Korean-American women do not have to shave their legs. Usually, hair that does appear on Korean Americans is not shaved because of the Confucian belief that such hair means good luck and shaving it would be bad luck (Eshleman, 1992.)

Skin color

Koreans have a golden-brown skin tone as a result of a higher melanin composition in their skin (Molnar, 1983; Overfield, 1995). However, Korean Americans have a wide range of skin tones, mostly attributed to the degree of exposure to the sun. The majority of Korean and Korean-American infants have mongolian spots, which are dark pigmentations seen primarily in the posterior iliac crest and buttock areas (Giger & Davidhizar, 1990; Overfield, 1995).

Enzymatic and genetic variations

A majority of Korean Americans have lactose intolerance because of a lack of lactase in the body. The Korean-American diet may not necessarily include milk. After consuming dairy products such as milk, cheese, or ice cream, some Korean Americans experience a feeling of bloating, frequent burping, abdominal cramping, diarrhea, and vomiting. Lactose intolerance is a relatively common condition and is found in approximately 90% of Orientals (Giger & Davidhizar, 1990; Overfield, 1995).

Bone density among Korean Americans is lower than that in other Americans, creating a higher risk for osteoporosis (Ott, 1991). This low bone density is a result of both hereditary and dietary factors. Anemia is common among Koreans because of their predominant vegetarian diet (Ott, 1991).

Koreans and Korean Americans tend to have a higher prevalence of insulin autoimmune syndrome (Uchigata et al., 1992). Insulin autoimmune syndrome is characterized by spontaneous hypoglycemia without evidence of exogenous insulin administration. High serum concentrations of total immunoactive insulin and presence of insulin autoantibodies in high titer are found (Uchigata, Kuwata, Tokunaga, et al., 1992).

Hantavirus disease (HVD), which is characterized by fever, headache, hemorrhagic manifestations, shock, and renal failure, can trace its origin to Korea (Levins, Epstein, Wilson, et al., 1993) and is synonymous with Korean hemorrhagic fever (KHF) with its high mortality. Although found in other parts of the world, this disease in Korea is much more severe. Treatment consists mainly in the use of careful fluid balance and circulatory support to prevent shock (Levins, Epstein, Wilson, et al., 1993).

Diet

The Korean and Korean-American diets are known for high fiber content and spicy seasoning. Korean people consume large amounts of grains and vegetables high in fiber. The main food for Koreans is rice and *kimchee,* which is hot, fermented Chinese cabbage. Most of the food is prepared with garlic, ginger, red pepper, and soy sauce. Koreans generally eat only moderate amounts of protein, mostly from vegetables such as soybean curd, bean sprouts, and bean paste. Therefore sugar, fat, and calories are much lower in Korean diets than in the typical American diet. Obesity is not a common problem among the Korean and Korean-American people. Some Korean Americans tend to eat raw fish and vegetables, which encourages parasites to embed in the body and may cause liver cancer.

Drug interactions and metabolism

Korean Americans, like other Asian Americans, metabolize alcohol by aldehyde dehydrogenase (Kudzma, 1992). This is in stark contrast to White Americans who metabolize alcohol by the liver enzyme alcohol dehydrogenase. Since Korean Americans tend to metabolize alcohol by aldehyde dehydrogenase, alcohol tends to work faster, causing circulatory and unpleasant effects such as facial flushing and heart palpitations (Kudzma, 1992). Facial flushing occurs in 45% to 85% of Asian Americans after alcohol consumption (Kudzma, 1992).

Susceptibility to disease

Because Korean-American people have a tendency to consume high amounts of carbohydrates, including vegetables and high-roughage foods, health alterations such as diverticulosis or inflammatory bowel diseases are uncommon. Peptic ulcer diseases,

hypertension, and cerebrovascular accidents are prevalent among Korean and Korean-American people because of frequent consumption of spicy and salty food. Examples of spicy and salty foods include soybean mesh sauce *(dwen chang),* soy sauce *(gang chang),* or hot pepper sauce *(ko choo chang).* Consumption of salty food traces back to earlier days when refrigeration was unavailable and people were concerned about storing food for long times. Consequently, food was salted to preserve it.

Relatively few studies have been done regarding the cardiovascular risk factors among Asian Americans despite a considerable acceleration of the immigration rate since the 1960s (Lin-Fu, 1988). Asian Americans are often excluded from clinical trials on various cardiovascular conditions because of the assumption that they do not have cardiovascular risk factors because of their body weight and tendency to follow diets of consuming low animal fat. However, as a result of life-style changes after coming to the United States, available data are suggestive of more cardiovascular risk factors among Asian Americans, compared with those still in Asia (Yano, MacLean, Reed, et al., 1988).

Klatsky and Armstrong (1991) examined 13,031 Oriental people to determine if biological markers for cardiovascular risk factors existed. Findings from this study are suggestive that significant ethnic differences in risk factors exist and that health care professionals must target their public health efforts to reduce obesity, hypercholesterolemia, and hypertension among all Asian Americans. Findings from the study also are suggestive that smoking cessation among Asian-American women was imperative to reduce the potential for cardiovascular conditions (Klatsky & Armstrong, 1991).

It is speculated that, regardless of how low the blood cholesterol is, within 2 years of living in the United States the blood cholesterol level of Koreans will go up to 200 mg/dL unless they continue to follow the same diet as they did in Korea (Klatsky & Armstrong, 1991; Yano, MacLean, Reed, et al., 1988). Younger Korean Americans who have been living in the United States for at least 2 years and who are continuously exposed to high animal fat diets must be checked for cardiovascular risk factors. Elderly

Korean Americans who are set in their ways may be more prone to have salty vegetarian diets and must be monitored closely for cerebrovascular risk factors. When providing health teaching, health care professionals must remember that Korean Americans who were born in the United States may have the same risk factors as the rest of the U.S. population.

Psychological characteristics

Influenced by Confucian and Buddhism philosophy, Korean Americans are a very proud and independent people. Generally they do not ask for handouts in either the material or psychological realms. Korean Americans generally view psychological or psychiatric illness as shameful and do not usually reveal such afflictions to the public. *Hwa-byung* (an ailment caused by pent-up resentment) is common among Korean Americans, particularly among elderly Korean females (Pang, 1990). *Hwa-byung* is believed to be caused by *han*—a bitter feeling, an unsatisfied desire, a discontent caused by life's problems (Kudzma, 1992; Pang, 1990). Mental health interventions should be approached with insight, empathy, and patience.

Implications for nursing care

Korean-American clients may have food brought in by family members and friends while hospitalized. Some Korean Americans consider American food "too mushy," and many believe it has too many blended tastes. Knowledge of usual Korean diets will allow health care professionals to make informed choices about diet exchanges appropriate to the client's prescribed diet. For example, if the client is on a bland or full liquid diet, instead of orange juice and Jell-O, Korean clients will gladly take rice soup and corn decoction, which complements the prescribed diet. Instead of policing diets and creating conflicts, mutual understanding can promote client cooperation with satisfactory outcomes.

Health care professionals must also remember that Koreans talk very little during mealtime because of the Confucian belief that the quality of the food should be appreciated in silence by concentrating on eating. Providing a quiet mealtime without interruption is vital and will enhance the client's nutritional intake.

The nurse who attempts to develop a cultural appreciation of the Korean psyche can bring about more successful client outcomes and family and institutional economics and can improve public attitudes toward our health care system. The ability to be alerted by indicators, some obvious, some subtle, can transcend Asian-Western cultural differences and create opportunities for more desirable physical and psychological results.

If a health-restoration regimen requires Korean-American clients to consume milk or any other dairy products, lactose-free milk should be given. Comparable lactose-free food (such as *tōfu*) can be substituted for dairy products.

Korean women tend to avoid sunlight to prevent their faces from becoming darker. They use parasols *(yang-san)* to avoid the sun and often cosmetics to look lighter than their actual skin color. Most Korean women are sensitive about their skin color and allowing them in the medical setting to "fix" their faces to their satisfaction will ensure more positive client attitudes.

Because the development of insulin autoimmune syndrome is associated with a strong genetic predisposition, those Koreans who have insulin autoimmune syndrome should be instructed to carry sugar packs, chewing gum, or gum drops with them at all times.

Calcium intake during childhood has long been related to bone density. Korean-American female clients of childbearing age should be encouraged to take calcium supplements to increase bone density. Compliance with their drug regimen must be monitored because Korean Americans have a tendency not to take prescribed medicines if they do not have any obvious symptoms. Iron supplements also should be encouraged to prevent anemia.

For those with psychological or psychiatric problems, the best approach is to establish a relationship of trust with the client. Since Korean Americans are reluctant to reveal their feelings, time should be provided for them to sort through their problems. A consistent and caring approach will eventually cause the clients to open up and allow the health professionals to help them. If this approach is unsuccessful, they should be referred to appropriate psychiatric services. For the elderly, visits by a Korean of the same age group and background will often be the key to cooperation and problem-solving.

SUMMARY

Korean Americans, like other Asian Americans, vary in their degree of acculturation. The nurse should recognize this diversity and remember that as much diversity is present within any cultural group as across racial, ethnic, and cultural groups. Some Korean Americans have developed cultural behaviors that are integral to their past and complementary to their present. Therefore the nurse must develop a respect for the uniqueness of the individual. When the client is Korean American, illness or wellness behaviors should be considered from a cultural perspective so that culturally appropriate and competent care can be rendered.

Case Study

A 9-year-old Korean-American boy was admitted to the hospital after an automobile accident. Despite all efforts, he has been in a coma for 2 weeks. Basically, nursing care has been directed toward supportive and comfort measures. Throughout hospitalization, the mother maintained an obsessive-compulsive (rigid) behavior concerning nursing interventions. For example, if medications were not given on the dot, the mother was angry and hostile to the assigned nurse. She did not allow anyone to touch her son.

Because of the difficulty confronting the staff members, a Korean clinical specialist was called to provide inservice about Koreans in an effort to better understand the client and meet the client's needs. After speaking to the mother a few minutes, the nurse learned that this was the only son in her family. She was driving when the accident occurred, and the boy was not wearing his seat belt. She did not have health insurance. Thus she had tremendous guilt feelings, plus the normal anxiety and fear of having her son in the hospital and possibly losing him. In addition, the mother had the false idea that because her son was under indigent care, medications were not given on time and that this was the main reason so many different staff members were in and out of her son's room.

CARE PLAN

 Nursing Diagnosis   Communication, impaired verbal, related to inability to speak dominant language

Client Outcomes

1. Effective communication between provider and family will be established.

Nursing Interventions

1. Establish rapport with family members.
2. Assess family members' understanding of client's condition.
3. Encourage expression of feelings.
4. Support attempts to improve communication.
5. Assist in correction of faulty perceptions.
6. Speak slowly and in an unhurried manner.
7. Use translators to facilitate communication.

Nursing Diagnosis Coping, ineffective individual, related to situational crisis, guilt, and faulty perceptions

Client Outcomes

1. Client will display decreased levels of anxiety.
2. Client will verbalize need for more information or clearer understanding relating to the situation.
3. Client will demonstrate understanding of health status and verbalize any concerns.

Nursing Interventions

1. Involve other family members in care of client as much as possible.
2. Clarify misconceptions.
3. Expand social networks.
4. Seek to understand client's perspective of situation.
5. Encourage expression of fear of information given.

STUDY QUESTIONS

1. What are the two cultural values, beliefs, and practices unique to Korean Americans that affect health care?
2. Of which biological variations among Korean Americans should the nurse be aware?

3. How does culture affect illness and wellness behaviors exhibited by some Korean-American clients?
4. How can the nurse transcend a language barrier when a Korean-American client does not speak English?

References

Chang, K. (1999). Chinese Americans. In Giger, J., & Davidhizar, R. (Eds.), *Transcultural nursing: assessment and intervention.* St. Louis: Mosby.

Chen, A.M., Wismer, B.A., Lew, R., et al. (1997). "Health is strength": a research collaboration involving Korean Americans in Alameda County. *American Journal of Preventive Medicine, 13*(6), 93-100.

Choi, E. (1986). Unique aspects of Korean-American mothers. *Journal of Obstetrics, Gynecology, and Neonatal Nursing, 15*(5), 394-400.

Crittenden, K., Fugita, S., Bae, H., et al. (1992). A cross-cultural study of self-report depressive symptoms among college students. *Journal of Cross-Cultural Psychology, 23*(2), 163-178.

Czarra, F., & Kaltsounis, T. (1988). Introduction: helping U.S. students learn about South Korea. *The Social Studies, 79*(4), 135-136.

Dodd, C. (1987). *Dynamics of intercultural communication* (ed. 2). New York: W.C. Brown.

Eshleman, J. (1992, Nov.). Death with dignity: significance of religious beliefs and practices in Hinduism, Buddhism, and Islam. *Today's OR Nurse,* 19-20.

Fisher, N.E. (1996). *Cultural and ethnic diversity: a guide for genetics professionals.* Baltimore: Johns Hopkins University Press.

Giger, J., & Davidhizar, R. (1990). Transcultural nursing: implications for nursing practice. *International Congress of Nursing Review, 37*(1), 199-202.

Giger, J., Davidhizar, R., & Wieczorek, S. (1993). In Bobak, I., & Jensen, M. (Eds.), *Maternity and gynecological care* (ed. 5) (pp. 43-67). St. Louis: Mosby.

Hall, E.T. (1966). *The silent language.* New York: Doubleday.

Hurh, W., & Kim, K. (1990). Adaptation and mental health of Korean male immigrants. *International Migration Review, 24*(3), 456-470.

Information please almanac (1998). Boston: Houghton-Mifflin.

Kaltsounis, T., & Shin, S. (1988). South Korea: a country on the move. *The Social Studies, 79*(4), 137-139.

Kim, S.K. (1992). Korean elderly women in America: every day life, health, and illness. *The Journal of Asian Studies,* 402-404.

Klatsky, A., & Armstrong, M. (1991). Cardiovascular risk factors among Asian Americans living in Northern California. *American Journal of Public Health, 81*(11), 1423-1428.

Kudzma, E. (1992, Dec.). Drug interactions: all bodies are not created equal. *American Journal of Nursing, 92,* 48-50.

Lamba, S. (1993, April 15). Be careful with herbal medicines. *Tallahassee Democrat*, Section D, p. 4.

Lee, J.H. (1988). Features of Korean history. *The Social Studies, 79*(4), 147-152.

Levins, R., Epstein, P.R., Wilson, M.E., et al. (1993, Nov. 20). Hantavirus disease emergency [NEWS]. *Lancet, 342*(8802), 1292.

Lew, S. (1988). Life in South Korea today. *The Social Studies, 79*(4), 161-164.

Lin, K. (1983). *Hwa-byung*: a Korean cultural bound syndrome? *American Journal of Psychiatry, 140,* 105-107.

Lin-Fu, J.S. (1988). Population characteristics and health care needs of Asian Pacific Americans. *Public Health Report, 103*(1), 18-27.

Manderson, L. (1987). Hot-cold food and medical theories: Overview and introduction. *Social Science and Medicine, 25*(4), 329-330.

Messaris, P., & Woo, J.S. (1991). Image vs. reality in Korean Americans' responses to mass-mediated depictions of the United States. *Critical Studies in Mass Communication, 8,* 74-90.

Miller, J.K. (1990). Use of traditional Korean health care by Korean immigrants to the United States. *Sociology and Social Research, 75*(1), 38-48.

Molnar, S.C. (1983). *Human variations: races, types, and ethnic groups* (ed. 2). Englewood Cliffs, N.J.: Prentice Hall.

Moon, S., & Pearl, J. (1991). Alienation of elderly Korean American immigrants as related to place of residence, age, years of education, time in U.S., living with or without children, living with or without a spouse. *International Journal of Aging and Human Development, 32*(2), 115-124.

Ott, S.M. (1991). Bone density in adolescents. *The New England Journal of Medicine, 325*(23), 1646-1647.

Overfield, T. (1995). *Biological variations in health and illness: race, age, and sex differences* (ed. 7). New York: CRC Press.

Pang, K.Y. (1989). The practice of traditional Korean medicine in Washington, D.C. *Social Science and Medicine, 28*(8), 875-884.

Pang, K.Y. (1990). *Hwa-byung:* the construction of a Korean popular illness among Korean elderly immigrant women in the United States. *Culture, Medicine, and Psychiatry, 14,* 495-512.

Park, Y. (1988). The geography of Korea. *The Social Studies, 79*(4), 141-145.

Siegal, R.K. (1979). Ginseng abuse syndrome: problems with the pancreas. *Journal of the American Medical Association, 24*(15), 614.

Simmons, C., Klopf, D., & Park, M. (1991). Loneliness among Korean and American university students. *Psychological Reports, 68*(3), 754.

Tien-Hyatt, T.L. (1987, May). Keying in on the unique care needs of Asian clients. *Nursing and Health Care, 8*(5), 268-271.

Uchigata, Y., Kuwata, S., Tokunaga, K., et al. (1992). Strong association of insulin autoimmune syndrome with HLA-DR4. *Lancet, 339,* 393-94.

U.S. Department of Commerce, Bureau of the Census (1993a, June 12). *News release,* Commerce News.

U.S. Department of Commerce, Bureau of the Census (1993b). *Population Profile of the United States, 1993* (Publication No. 23-185). Washington, D.C.: Government Printing Office.

U.S. Department of Commerce, Bureau of the Census (1993c, Sept.). *We the Americans . . . Asians.* Washington, D.C.: Government Printing Office.

Van Decar, P. (1988). Teaching about Korea in secondary school. *The Social Studies, 79*(4), 177-193.

Voegelin, C.F., & Voegelin, F.M. (1997). *Classification and index of the world's languages.* New York/Amsterdam: Elsevier.

World almanac (1997). Mahwah, N.J.: World Almanac Books.

Yano, K., MacLean, C., Reed, D., et al. (1988). A comparison of the 12-year mortality and predictive factors of coronary heart disease among Japanese men in Japan and Hawaii. *American Journal of Epidemiology, 127,* 476-487.

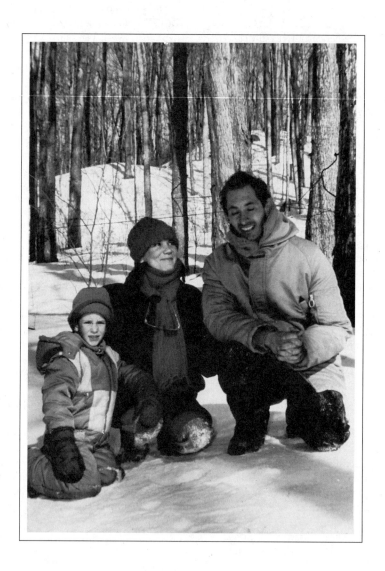

CHAPTER 23 French Canadians of Quebec Origin

Mary Reidy and Marie-Elizabeth Taggart

BEHAVIORAL OBJECTIVES

After reading this chapter, the nurse will be able to:

1. Understand the communication patterns and the dialectal variations of the French-Canadian people of Quebec.
2. Describe the spatial needs, distance, and intimacy behaviors of the French-Canadian people of Quebec.
3. Describe the time orientation and effects on treatment regimes of the French-Canadian people of Quebec.
4. Describe the social organization of family systems among the French-Canadian people of Quebec.
5. Identify the illness, wellness, and health-seeking behaviors of the French Canadians of Quebec.
6. Identify folk beliefs, folk practices, and folk healers unique to the health value systems of the French Canadians of Quebec.
7. Identify susceptibility of the French-Canadian people of Quebec to specific disease or illness conditions.

OVERVIEW OF QUEBECKERS

Conflict concerning French Canadians is an integral part of Canadian history. The history of the White man began in Canada in 1497, when John Cabot, an Italian in the service of Henry VII of England, reached Newfoundland. However, Canada was taken for France in 1534 by Jacques Cartier. The actual settlement of New France, as it was then called, began in 1604 in Nova Scotia. In 1608 Quebec was founded. By the seventeenth century French explor-

This chapter was prepared with the financial support of ESSPOIR-FRSQ and with the collaboration of research assistant Louise Mercier, master's student at the Faculty of Nursing, University of Montreal, and Stéphanie Simard, library assistant, master's degree student, Library Science, University of Montreal.

ers had penetrated beyond the Great Lakes to the western prairies. However, conflict for possession by England and France continued. The conflict climaxed in the Seven Years' War (1756-1763), which ended in a conquest by England. Nevertheless, at that time the population of Canada was almost entirely French. In the next few decades, thousands of British colonists emigrated to Canada (Information Please Almanac, 1998). Over the years, the rivalry between the French and the British in Canada has been ongoing.

Despite the vastness of Canada, some two thirds of the population is concentrated in the southeastern part of the country (southern areas of Ontario and Quebec provinces), especially in the highly industrialized areas of Toronto, Hamilton, London,

Windsor, and Montreal. Other densely populated areas include the Edmonton-Calgary axis in the plains of the eastern slope of the Rocky Mountains, the Pacific harbor of Vancouver, the region around Ottawa and the St. Lawrence lowlands with the historic city of Quebec (Information Please Almanac, 1998). Today, some 24.4% of the Canadian population are French speaking (Bailey & Bailey, 1995). However, because these individuals are spread throughout Canada and have a profoundly different history, French Canadians across Canada differ significantly. This chapter focuses on the French Canadians whose origin is the province of Quebec. Although Canadians pride themselves on tolerance toward diverse ethnic cultures in the country, the uniqueness of native and ethnocultural groups requires that health care knowledge of specific groups be utilized to provide culturally appropriate care (Ntetu & Fortin, 1996).

QUEBEC PROVINCE

Quebec (English /kwuh-bek′/, French /kay-bek′/, from Micmac *kepek* 'narrows') is a province of Canada that reaches almost to the Artic Circle. Geographically, Quebec borders on Labrador, Newfoundland, and New Brunswick in the east: the United States states of Vermont and New York in the south and southeast; and Ontario province and Hudson Bay in the west. The border with Labrador remains a matter of dispute. Quebec encompasses the Canadian land mass north of the Ottawa and the St. Lawrence Rivers. To the south of the St. Lawrence it takes in the lowlands as far as the United States border as well as the Gaspé Peninsula projecting into the gulf of St. Lawrence. In the west, an artificial line divides Quebec from Ontario (Bailey & Bailey, 1995).

Quebec is a vast province about one sixth of the whole of Canada. Quebec is so vast that it could accommodate the United Kingdom five times over, but it has a population of only 7.4 million (Statistiques Canada, 1996) with most of the people living in the two largest cities, its capital, the city of Quebec (645,500), and Montreal (3,127,242) (Statistics Canada, 1991). The lifeline of this province is the St. Lawrence River, which is almost 750 miles long. The St. Lawrence River along the St. Lawrence Seaway

has been the direct link between the Atlantic Ocean and the Great Lakes since 1959.

Quebec is the largest of the 10 Canadian provinces. Because of its geographical location, Quebec is divided into three climate zones: humid continental in the central southern areas (warm summers, cold winters), subartic farther to the north, and arctic in the far northern regions (long, intensely cold winters; short, cool summers). The greater part of Quebec's territory is covered by forests; only 2.5% is agricultural or urban.

The people and the culture of French Quebec

Quebec traces its cultural origins to approximately 500 Catholic colonists who came from Normandy and West Central France to the land called "New France" in 1604 (Laberge, 1992; Information Please Almanac, 1998). These colonists along with other immigrants to follow formed the cornerstone of a distinct sociocultural entity. A cholera epidemic and a poor potato crop in Ireland that caused a widespread famine prompted a later wave of immigrants. The trip to Quebec took many lives, resulting in many Irish children arriving as orphans. Although they were adopted by French-speaking families, they often kept their own names, which explains family names such as McNeill and Ryan among the current French-speaking population of Quebec. Their assimilation was such that the culture acquired a high degree of homogeneity while becoming rapidly differentiated from the French culture from which it was derived (Rioux, 1974).

Today, the descendants of these French colonists call themselves "*Québecois*" or, in popular speech, *nous autres* ('we others'), which one might translate as 'our people'. The term "French Canadians" has been largely replaced by *Québecois de souche* designating 'old-stock Quebeckers', or the Quebec people of French origin. Other colonists from France who emigrated to the United States became known as "Franco-Americans" and settled mainly in the Lake Champlain valley and in the states of New York, Vermont, Connecticut, and Massachusetts. In Canada other, though distinctively different, French-speaking communities developed in New Brunswick, Ontario, and Manitoba. In the United States, the Cajuns of Louisiana are descended from forced immigration of the Acadians from the maritime provinces of Canada. Historical and geographical factors caused each of these groups to evolve into very different cultural communities.

Many factors have contributed to the distinct character of the French-speaking people of Quebec. After the Treaty of Paris in 1763, which recognized English authority over former French possessions, the urban centers of Montreal and Quebec City became predominantly English speaking. However, until the mid-nineteenth century, agriculture, law, and medicine proved to be, almost exclusively, the professions of the French in Quebec. This historical and political evolution reinforced the isolation and homogeneity of the French-speaking community (Rioux, 1974).

From its beginning, Quebec society has been characterized by a fierce nationalism intent on preserving the French language and culture. This process has led to the creation of various movements in favor of political independence for Quebec, separate from Canadian provinces. These political tendencies are responsible for certain tensions in relations between Quebec's citizens and those in the rest of Canada. A charged emotional climate exists between those for and those against separatism.

Tensions exist between provincial and federal governments, between separatists and nonseparatists, between old immigrants and new, and between white Quebeckers and the native peoples who were the first inhabitants of this land. The recent massive arrival of immigrants has added a further dimension to the political and human problems of Quebec. This has caused population increase despite a declining birth rate (Labrie, 1990; Tétu de Labsade, 1990). During the eighteenth and nineteenth centuries, immigration came primarily from English-speaking countries (such as Scotland, Ireland) and to a certain extent from Eastern Europe (such as Poland, Czechoslovakia). More recently, Quebec has received French-speaking North Africans, Chileans, Vietnamese, Cambodians, Italians, Greeks, and Haitians.

The issue of separatist sentiments in French-speaking (or *francophone*) Quebec flared most recently in the Quebec referendum on succession of French-speaking Quebec in October of 1995. Although the referendum yielded a narrow rejection, the separatists vowed to try again (Information Please Almanac, 1998).

POLITICAL DEVELOPMENT

After the English conquest, the political system of Canada took on the form of a parliamentary democracy. In 1867, the British North America Act established Canada as a federal state, with strong central powers, uniting several dependent provinces. This system is, in fact, a constitutional monarchy: the Queen of England remains the Queen of Canada and holds the title of head of state. Each province has its own government and parliament. In Quebec, the parliament is known as the National Assembly. The federal government shares legal, fiscal, and social powers with the provinces. Criminal and international law are under federal jurisdiction in conformity with the British Common Law tradition, whereas the provinces retain the power to enact civil legislation affecting private property, family affairs, social welfare, and health. The Quebec civil code is unique to Canada because it was inspired by French legal tradition.

Health care

Before 1970, Canadian and Quebec health services were privately organized and funded. In 1969, Quebec put into place a medical insurance program guaranteeing free and universal access (Anctil & Bluteau, 1986). This program was followed in 1970 by the development of a network of social services for those in need of social or financial assistance.

Education

During the nineteenth and most of the twentieth centuries, free schooling to the eighth grade was provided. For Canadian students, high schools and colleges were private, maintained for the most part by religious orders who charged tuition. In 1943, attendance became compulsory in the Canadian school system (Gagnon, 1992). School systems were still organized according to religion. The Catholic School Commission and the Protestant School Board operated schools for French-speaking and English-speaking children in their denominations.

In 1960 and 1961, a series of laws that provided free universal education through the eleventh grade and compulsory education to 15 years of age was enacted (Audet & Gauthier, 1967). This Parent Report led to a reorganization of the educational system with free schooling up to the university level. A system of postsecondary junior colleges was established, replacing the last year of high school and first year of university. Universities provide 3-year undergraduate programs as well as graduate and professional education.

In June 1993, the Supreme Court of Canada upheld the constitutionality of a 1988 law that reorganized school boards along linguistic lines rather than religion. Reorganization of these new school boards is presently underway (Authier, 1993). Today, private schools, at all levels, coexist with the public system.

"Quiet Revolution"

In the years after World War II, Quebec underwent a rapid transition from a rural to an urban technological society. This pattern of change did not correspond to the classical steps of the industrial revolution seen in the urban centers of England and Europe. Until the 1960s, Quebeckers were very traditionally oriented. The so-called "Quiet Revolution" resulted in social, political, and behavioral transformations as profound and permanent as those produced by armed and violent revolution. The state progressively replaced the church in most of its functions. The school, health care, and social welfare systems were now controlled by the Quebec government. A widespread movement against the clergy resulted in a newfound sexual liberty. The divorce rate increased dramatically. Individuals became more interested in business. Women acquired a place in the work force (Bouchard, 1992, Lanthier & Rousseau, 1992). The social classes in Quebec evolved to the current four classes: nonspecialized workers, cyclically employed workers and welfare recipients make up the lower or disadvantaged class; specialized

workers, small business owners, and merchants are included in the middle class; executives, industrialists, professionals, and technocrats form the upper middle class; and intellectuals and artists are the intelligentsia (Lacroix & Simard, 1984).

Economy

Starting in the 1950s the control of political institutions and business enterprises shifted into the hands of French-speaking Quebeckers. Closely related to the change in the world economy during the 1980s, Quebec experienced a slowing of economic growth, a decrease in industrial jobs, and the deterioration of the economic climate (Langlois, 1992). Under these conditions, more families needed two sources of income to maintain living standards. Women with higher education began to pursue demanding careers, and underprivileged women worked longer hours for less pay. By 1990, the decline in the birthrate, the increase in the number of women in the work force, and the increase in the number of elderly persons produced a profound change in the Quebec economy.

COMMUNICATION
Language and culture

The French-Canadian people of Quebec are a linguistic minority in North America and as such fear the eventual loss of their cultural identity. Despite their ongoing efforts to preserve the distinct nature of the French-speaking culture, they are bombarded by pervasive American political and cultural influences exerted through various media, including film, radio, television, magazines, and recordings (Lamonde, 1991).

A Charte des Droits et des Lois was established to protect Quebec's language, culture, and identity (Bills 178, 101, 86, and so forth). These laws established French as Quebec's official language and enabled the French-speaking people to live and prosper. In addition, the laws promote the use of French among newly arrived immigrants and within commercial enterprises and public institutions. Several organizations have been created to monitor and encourage the use of French. The Commission for the Protection of the French Language handles complaints concerning the unavailability of health or social services by French-speaking professionals. Another task of this commission is to handle violations of the French sign law. Another organization, the Office de la Langue Française, administers French competency tests to individuals entering health and other professions and maintains the quality of the French language.

French

French is the everyday language of most of the people of Quebec and the foundation of their cultural identity. However, maintaining purity of one language is difficult in this era of mass communication when opinions, attitudes, values, and world views are constantly formed, reformed, and influenced by the flood of images, advertisements, and slogans of the mass media (Labrie, 1990). The language brought from the old country was shaped and refined for 2 centuries from an amalgam of accents and expressions of various regions of France with the assimilation of American Indian words designating places, lakes, flora, and fauna. In speaking this language, the *r*'s can be rolled, and long vowels, *t*'s, and *d*'s can slide into certain front vowels with a postconsonantal *s* sound (Tétu de Labsade, 1990).

Normative values of certain prosodic parameters of French-speaking persons has been evaluated to provide acoustic data to assist French-speaking subjects with communication disorders (Le-Dorze, Lever, Ryall, & Brassard, 1995).

With the migration of rural populations to the cities and the common use of English in the work place, a popular level of language often referred to as *joual* (literally 'stock of an anchor') was created. This type of speech, reserved for oral communication, incorporates English words into a syntax and grammatical system that is essentially French (Tétu de Labsade, 1990). The resulting speech patterns are, at times, quite remote from the standard French used by intellectuals, writers, and those in the media. *Joual* belongs, for the most part, to the poorly educated and economically underprivileged class (Tétu de Labsade, 1990). Some 83% of the population of Quebec are French-speaking descendants of the French (Bailey & Bailey, 1995). En-

glish is the language of 12% of the people. Although the English-speaking population has decreased and appears to be decreasing, 30% of the urban population is bilingual, speaking both French and English. Another 35 languages are spoken in the province, including Italian, Greek, Chinese, Native Indian, Inuit, Slavic, Spanish, Chinese, Vietnamese, Persian, and Tamil (Statistiques Canada, 1989). These immigrants usually learn French as a second language and frequently learn English as a third language.

COMMUNICATION BEHAVIOR

As the French language evolved in Quebec, so did the behavioral patterns of its speakers. For example, in Quebec there is a tendency to use the familiar pronoun *tu* ('you' or 'thou') very soon after a first meeting or being introduced to someone, a habit frowned on in France (Tétu de Labsade, 1990). Native French Quebeckers are warm-hearted people who express their thoughts and opinions openly. They are quite expressive and use their hands for emphasis when speaking. However, they do not use as many nonverbal movements as the Italians, Spaniards, or the continental French. They enjoy social gatherings and celebrating important dates. They have a quick sense of humor and are very resourceful.

With the older and more rural French Quebec population, conversation tends to center on subjects having to do with farm work and day-to-day life. Within the home, discussions take place between women in the kitchen about subjects of mutual concern such as children. Men appear to talk less; however, when they do converse, they prefer speaking to other men in the barn, the garage, the club, or the tavern. Little use is made of the living room of the home except on very special occasions.

Young people of both sexes discuss politics, art, or world events. When they are married and have young children, they tend to associate with others in similar life situations. Family and friends enjoy meals together, but the women soon leave for the kitchen and the men retire to the balcony or another room to watch sports on television.

Women tend to be well aware of feminist concerns and are increasingly vocal concerning issues of status, needed services, and treatment by various government agencies. French Quebec women demand respect and heatedly discuss the right to "freedom of choice" versus the "right to life."

The problem of illiteracy can be found in Quebec among those who have dropped out of school as well as in the immigrants from certain third world countries. The problem of illiteracy has become more apparent now that the computer has become a part of daily life. Consequently government efforts to retrain unemployed workers and to help the young workers enter the workforce through job development and placement programs are under way.

Implications for nursing care

In Canada as elsewhere the nurse must respect the client's choice of language. This respect is necessary not just to ensure clear communication and out of concern for the individual, but also to meet the requirements of Quebec law. The nurse should be familiar with the popular expressions used to designate parts of the body (such as *passage* 'vagina') or certain infections (such as *chaude pisse* 'gonorrhea'). A Quebecker will say that if a person is able to resist illness, that person is as "strong as an ox" or "able as a bear." However, if illness occurs, an expression such as "weak constitution" is used. If someone faints, he or she "falls into the apples" or "falls into the plums," and someone who is unconscious is said to "hit the canvas" or "hit the floor" (Dulong & Bergeron, 1980). When interacting with the older generation, the nurse should avoid using the familiar *tu* form because such usage is considered to show lack of respect.

The ethnic mosaic that exists in Quebec requires that the nurse be sensitive to the style, mode, and context of the communication patterns of different ethnic groups. For example, although the native Quebecker will not hesitate to ask for a pain medication, the Asian client, who does not manifest pain in the same way, may continue to suffer silently, waiting for someone to bring relief instead of requesting it. Because certain immigrant groups have high rates of illiteracy or are not comfortable with

written information, communication should be tailored to the client's ability to understand.

SPACE
Interpersonal space

In public, Quebeckers tend to avoid physical contact and to maintain a certain physical space. At work they may be in closer contact than that in public, but individuals generally attempt to maintain a distance of 18 to 30 inches between themselves and others (Hall, 1966). Among friends and close relations, greater intimacy is permitted: men may pat each other on the back or shake hands when they meet; women of the same family may embrace but seldom walk arm in arm down the street. Normally, physical contact in public is limited to young lovers, between adults and young children, or between adults at emotional or difficult moments when they require support. However, when family members are in public, the norms of interpersonal space are present. Although the kitchen used to be the key area for social interaction, today social interaction, beyond the immediate family, tends to occur in sidewalk cafés, restaurants, shopping centers, bars, and taverns.

Physical space

Families generally live in apartments, condominiums, or single-family dwellings in the suburbs, or in single-family dwellings in rural areas. Housing is plentiful in Quebec, and, except in the poorest parts of the inner cities, overcrowding is not a problem. However, some older, poorer, chronically mentally ill or alcoholic persons of French-Canadian descent live in poorly maintained rooming houses. In 1986, 83.8% of French Canadians living in Quebec lived as part of a family, with an average of 3.1 persons, of whom 1.2 were under 25 years of age. The majority of those living alone are women (Shirley & Duchesne, 1989).

In 1901, the rural population of Quebec formed 60% of the total population. However, by 1961 this number had decreased to 25% and continues to decrease. Today, the urban population of Quebec totals some 7,366,883 million people (Information Please Almanac, 1998). Nearly half of the population lives in 0.7% of Quebec. Thus the population is concentrated mainly in Montreal and Quebec City, the regions of Sherbrooke and Trois-Rivières, and along the St. Lawrence River Valley (Thibault, 1989).

Implications for nursing care

French Canadians generally maintain their distance when speaking with other individuals. The nurse should avoid overly familiar attitudes and respect the privacy needs of the client. Some French Canadians tend to be rather modest, particularly when receiving intimate care. It is important for the nurse to remember to draw the bed curtains or use the drawsheet to cover certain parts of the body to maintain the client's sense of dignity.

SOCIAL ORGANIZATION
Family and church

In early colonial days in French Quebec, families were large and stable and family members felt a sense of belonging. They attached great importance to the traditional values of "Holy Mother the Church" and accepted her dominance in health care, education, and population management (Fahmy-Eid & Dumont, 1983). During the period preceding the world wars, rural Quebeckers practiced what was known as the "Revenge of the Cradle." In other words, families had many children to provide additional help with farm work and out of respect for the teachings of the church.

With the advent of the Quiet Revolution of the 1960s, the state assumed responsibility for the Quebec family (health and social resources and services) (Fahmy-Eid & Dumont, 1983). From 1971 to 1976, changes in social and political attitudes, coupled with the introduction of a contraceptive pill, destroyed one of the fundamental values of Quebec society: the role of the family as a generous lifegiver. In the 1970s young Quebec women learned to control their fertility through contraceptives. They no longer accepted the birth of eight or more children. Most wanted only one or two, as they strove for a higher standard of living and a greater degree of personal liberty (Henripin, Huot, Lapierre-Adamcyk, & Marcil-Gratton, 1981). Consequently, during the

past 30 years, the family has undergone radical and disruptive changes (Rapport de la Commission d'Enquête sur les Services de santé et les Services sociaux, 1988).

Evolution of the family

In the past, family roles were well defined. The father was head of the family and responsible for its material well-being. The mother had specific household duties and was caregiver and religious educator. In addition to these duties, rural mothers also had specific farm duties. These roles remained relatively unchanged until women, in great numbers, began to join the work force and to become the heads of single-parent families. Amidst social change, the mother has remained the principal health care giver in the Quebec family (Thibaudeau & Reidy, 1985). From colonial times through the 1950s, the mother would depend on her eldest daughter, usually unmarried, who shared and later, if necessary, would assume this caregiver role. In her role as natural caregiver, the mother took responsibility for the maintenance of the health of all family members. She instilled and supervised the practice of healthy habits within the family.

With the transition to the new generation of families of the seventies, eighties, and nineties, men and women began to reevaluate their familial roles. However, the new model of family functioning has not evolved smoothly. Often the mother has maintained a double burden, still encumbered with her former tasks while assuming the obligations that come with outside employment. Meanwhile, the two-parent family remains the ideal in Quebec, and the fathers of young children today are beginning to play a larger role in the care of their children and in maintaining their home environment. The increase in the number of single-parent families has brought about the formation of new family units composed of the woman and her children, the man and his children, and, ultimately, their children.

Statistics confirm the seriousness of the breakup of the nuclear family. In 1985, Quebec had the lowest birthrate in Canada and one of the lowest in the world (Dandurand, 1990; Rapport de la Commission d'Enquête sur les Services de santé et les Services sociaux, 1988). Unmarried couples living together represent 10.8% of families (Shirley & Duchesne, 1989). Approximately 40% of Quebeckers over 18 years of age live with a child or adolescent under 18 years of age, many of whom are single parents, making a ratio of approximately one single-parent family per eight families (Rapport de la Commission d'Enquête sur les Services de santé et les Services sociaux, 1988). Nearly 80% of single-parent families are headed by women, with over half of these living in poverty (Lazure, 1990).

New models of interdependence

Quebec society has evolved in such a way as to seriously undermine the traditional network of support built around family and relatives, the neighborhood, and various religious institutions (Rapport de la Commission d'Enquête sur les Services de santé et les Services sociaux, 1988). However, the changes that have occurred over the last few years have stimulated the creation of new models of interdependence, founded on changing cultural options, emerging life-styles, or shared problems. This regrouping of individuals and communities into new networks of mutual or self-help is particularly significant. Community and volunteer organizations have assumed many social functions within Quebec society; they have become essential in providing support to individuals and services to the citizens. These models of informal social support and care are often inspired by needs no longer met by traditional means or by emerging social and health needs (such as those for persons with AIDS).

Aging of the population

Profound demographic changes of the last 20 years leave Quebec with a higher percentage of older citizens and fewer children. The number of persons over 65 years of age is increasing rapidly and now totals more than 650,000 (Rapport de la Commission d'Enquête sur les Services de santé et les Services sociaux, 1988). This general aging of the population entails an increase in the number of elderly women in relation to men of the same age and an increase in the number of the very old (Rapport

de la Commission d'Enquête sur les Services de santé et les Services sociaux, 1988). These persons often experience chronic illness and serious financial difficulties.

Youth

Unemployment is one of the most pressing concerns of Quebec's youth. Although the general unemployment rate in Quebec is currently at 12.8%, it is 18.3% for persons 18 to 24 years of age. This untapped work force, in great part untrained for Quebec's increasing technological demands, presents a considerable drain on the province's resources.

Religion

With the British military conquest, the Catholic Church became a social and political force defending faith, language, and culture. Until the Quiet Revolution of the sixties, the church was actively involved in financial, educational, and health affairs. In the sixties, however, the "Quiet Revolution" brought about greater separation of church and state. At this time, attendance at church declined greatly, and religious affiliations became more diversified (Orr, 1992). By 1981, 132,000 Quebeckers stated that they "had no religious preference." Despite the decline in religious influence and practice in Quebec, many individuals continue to conform to a model whereby one not only calls oneself "Catholic" and marks certain important events in life by a church ceremony (baptism, marriage, funeral, and so forth), but also continues to support both a school system organized on religious grounds and, in general, Catholic religious instruction in the schools (Laperrière, 1992).

The population of Quebec supports a wide variety of religions, including Catholicism, Protestantism, Judaism, Buddhism, Islam, Sikhism, Hinduism, and Seventh-Day Adventism.

Implications for nursing care

Despite Quebec's complex social problems, the social canvas of the province appears to be held together through the influence of the older generation, sense of family, and sharing and mutual aid between generations.

In working with single-parent families headed by women with limited financial means, the nurse may work with families whose members suffer from a variety of health problems and behavioral or learning difficulties. Problems unique to children often require prolonged interaction with the health and social welfare system as well as the intervention of several specialists. As the feelings of powerlessness increase among the single mothers of Quebec, self-confidence is undermined. The nurse must help the mother understand her situation, participate in the care process, and deal with the health system. With an increase in feelings of confidence as a parent and of self-esteem as an individual, the single mother may be able to function in her role as principal health agent in the family.

Because of economic conditions and widespread poverty, malnutrition and hunger have resurfaced among children. Children may fall asleep at their desks from hunger and from tiredness because of watching television into the early hours of the morning. These children have an increased likelihood of suffering from repeated respiratory infections and increased absenteeism.

It is necessary to develop or reinforce family support networks both for exchange of services and for stimulation of a sense of empowerment (that is, to help maintain neighborhoods free from drugs and prostitution). Within the family itself, efforts must be made to improve functioning in health matters, whether improving competencies, direct support, information, and advice, or arranging access to resource people. The nurse may also be asked to become an advocate for these families so that they may obtain the social and health services to which they are entitled (Thibaudeau & Reidy, 1985; Thibaudeau, Reidy, d'Amours, & Frappier, 1984).

An aging population and a diminishing national health budget require that more community services be available to enable elderly people to remain in their own homes. "Day" hospitals and centers, staffed by multidisciplinary teams, that offer various social and health services are increasing in numbers. Cossette, Levesque, & Laurin (1995) note that both gender and kinship should be considered with respect to support when the nurse is assisting French-speaking primary caregivers who provide care for aging and disabled relatives in the home. However, to attain the ultimate goal of health and autonomy of the aged, additional innovative nursing approaches must be created.

The extreme diversification of ethnic and cultural groups concentrated in Quebec's cities constitutes a challenge for the practice of nursing. The nurse must determine cultural attitudes of the client toward health, human reproduction, illness, and health care to be assured of the client's participation in the care. The client and the family caregiver must be included in planning, carrying out, and evaluating health interventions. Adaptation of a health care approach to cultural realities must consider a variety of factors, including behavioral patterns (verbal and nonverbal), use of health services, types and availability of family and group support networks, cultural attitudes toward health, illness and health services, degrees of assimilation into society, and sociodemographic characteristics (Schoolcraft, 1984).

TIME
Past and present

The people of Quebec tend to attach primary importance to day-to-day affairs and to living in the present (Paquet, 1989). Decisions are often made on a short-term basis; pleasure and sorrow are generally accepted as they occur; life goes on from one day to the next. However, climatic and historic conditions have prompted planning to survive long and cold winters and a context of stability that provides structure for these values and attitudes.

Although time is determined by the flow of the successive seasons for rural populations, urban life is characterized by variations in the relationship of time devoted to work, to family, and to leisure (Pronovost, 1989). For older Quebeckers, time is intimately associated with religion. They envision the future with the hope of life after death. Anniversaries of the death of family members are often commemorated by masses. However, younger urban Quebec people tend not to follow these traditions because they tend to reject traditional institutions. Time, for women in modern Quebec society, has taken on a new meaning. Working women assume a variety of roles (wife, mother, professional person). Many children wear a house key around their necks and spend the time between 4 and 6 o'clock alone at home. In such households, mothers are often exhausted when they get home from work and can provide little parental nurturance.

Implications for nursing care

The nurse must consider the present-time orientation, often demonstrated by the importance attributed to short-term goals, in interacting with families and individuals and in the approach and content of health education and information. A verbal "contract" between health professional and client often proves advantageous in increasing client self-care and in promoting compliance with prescribed medical regimens. The school nurse must support parents' and teachers' efforts in establishing study periods or activities during the after-school hours for children whose time is unsupervised.

ENVIRONMENTAL CONTROL
Attitudes toward health

The practice of medicine has always held a place of prestige and political power in Quebec. The Quiet Revolution, however, saw changes in nursing care and nursing services. The religious orders, responsible for hospitals and the care of the sick since colonization, began to withdraw their services. Their withdrawal left a vacuum within hospitals that professional nurses often have not seemed to recognize or fill. Consequently, medical dominance within the health system further increased.

The older generation has complete confidence in their doctors for the preservation of life and the restoration of health. With the advent of consumerism, the people of Quebec began to participate more directly in health care decision making. The ideology of the powerful medical establishment is now being questioned by both ordinary citizens and government health administrators (Saint-Arnaud & Pomerleau, 1995). The latter have increased responsibilities for health services, particularly with the control of health costs and with encouraging the medical profession to practice a greater degree of efficiency and economy.

In Quebec, having adequate financial resources or at least a regular job is often seen as more important than health itself. In intellectual circles, health is perceived as being in complete possession of one's physical and mental capacities and as a way of improving one's status, professional or otherwise. A global notion of health is found more frequently among the well-to-do, but even here the concept remains abstract (Paquet, 1989).

For financially secure families, health is seen as an ideal state in which illness is absent. These individuals view illness as a slow and insidious degradation of health that occurs over time. In the lower classes, health is defined as the ability to work, to be self-sufficient, and to satisfy primary needs. The disadvantaged often attach less value to a general state of good health than the well-to-do because they tend to seek the satisfaction of immediate needs rather than engage in the pursuit of long-term goals (Paquet, 1989). Illness is seen as accidental, causing a momentary rupture in one's normal state of health, or as a chance stroke of bad luck. The popular French phrase "to catch an illness" supports this perception (Rapport de la Commission d'Enquête sur les Services de santé et les Services sociaux, 1988). Religion has greatly encouraged the perception of illness as a necessary evil brought on by sins committed by the individual and therefore as a form of divine punishment.

In the last 10 years, various "alternative medicine" approaches have appeared on the Quebec health scene. For some people, alternative forms of medicine have apparently answered a need for therapies that allow for greater control of the bodily functions (Laforest, 1985). Such practices have gained ground in Quebec: 14% of individuals over 18 years of age use alternative treatments (Rapport de la Commission d'Enquête sur les Services de santé et les Services sociaux, 1988). However, this relatively low proportion, in relation to international rates, is a partial result of their recent introduction and because they are generally administered in Quebec by nonmedical therapists (Rapport de la Commission d'Enquête sur les Services de santé et les Services sociaux, 1988; Renaud, Jutras, & Bouchard, 1987). The usual pattern of behavior is consultation with practitioners of alternative medicine only when ordinary medicine has failed to bring about a cure or to avoid chemically derived treatments. Also consulted are certain individuals with the reputation of having the "gift" of healing or stopping the flow of blood by the laying on of hands (Renaud, Jutras, & Bouchard, 1987). These folkhealers and bonesetters are still quite popular in rural areas. They have learned through knowledge passed from generation to generation and are often experts in the massage of strained muscles and ligaments or in the setting of certain bones (Desautels, 1984).

The people of Quebec seek long and prosperous lives, and death is perceived as the ultimate failure. They usually withdraw from the reality of death and avoid speaking of it. With earlier generations, death was formalized and dealt with by adherence to the symbols and ceremonies of the Catholic Church and by a strong belief in an afterlife. Today, death is more often treated as taboo because it cannot be mastered or controlled by technology. The inherent repulsiveness of the final agony of death and all the emotions it provokes are concealed from public view because death usually occurs in an institution. Although many hospitals have palliative care units, the practice of caring for the chronically ill at home is increasing.

Physical environment

Problems of pollution and waste management constitute a serious challenge to the environment in terms of costs, contamination, and health. A water-purification program, under way in Quebec since 1981, involves water-processing plants and greater control of industrial waste. Effective pollution control has been estimated between 3.2 and 5 billion Canadian dollars per year, or 600 dollars per person per year (Thibault, 1989).

A new partnership is evolving in Quebec between the environment and the people. Not only has the government enacted laws specifying serious penalties in case of infringement, but public awareness programs have also been created concerning recycling, composting, using natural products, cleaning up lakes and rivers, disposing of dangerous household wastes, and so on. Cities, towns, and villages have organized projects for beautifying their settings. In sum, Quebeckers are taking concrete steps to protect their environment and reduce the effects of toxic elements and other pollution on health.

Illness and wellness behavior

Since 1969, when free access to health care was instituted in Quebec, user satisfaction has been at a high level (80%), and heavy use has been made of the health care network (Renaud, Jutras, & Bouchard, 1987). Clients belonging to the middle or upper classes usually consult private doctors, outpatient clinics in hospitals, or community centers. Underprivileged people of Quebec often wait until a physical or psychological crisis occurs before consulting a doctor. When these individuals do seek treatment, it is often at a hospital emergency department. These visits for nonemergency situations often cause crowded conditions in units that should theoretically be reserved for accidents, heart attacks, or other actual emergencies. Distrust of the system plays a particular role in reluctance and hesitancy seen in clients who delay seeking treatment. Many of these individuals will consult family members or close friends as to whether they should see a doctor. In disadvantaged environments, state services are often viewed with distrust as a menace to privacy.

Women in Quebec make greater use of preventive services than men do. Women's groups have been formed both for and against abortion and home birth. Women seek favorable work conditions, daycare facilities, and support for health-promotion and illness-prevention programs. They also tend to pay more attention to symptoms than men do. In addition, women tend to seek treatment in health centers, where they submit to more radical treatments than men do in terms of medication, hospitalization, and surgery (Conseil du Statut de la Femme, 1981). Upper-class women engage more often in health-promotion activities such as aerobics, aesthetic treatments, and cosmetic surgery than lower-class women do (Chanlat, 1985).

According to Taggart (1983), French Canadians are weak in compliance with medical treatment at all social levels. Some French Canadians will stop medication use and medical consultation as soon as they feel better. When they are admitted to hospitals, French Canadians are generally cooperative clients.

Exercise

The importance of exercise in relation to health and general well-being has been widely recognized (Rapport de la Commission d'Enquête sur les Services de santé et les Services sociaux, 1988). The physical condition of the people of Quebec is estimated to be equal or slightly inferior to that of other North American populations (Roy, 1985). Between 40% and 50% are estimated to be quite active, whereas 15% to 20% may be classified as sedentary. Nevertheless, no more than one third of the population engage in a physical exercise to a degree that is potentially beneficial to health. Therefore the Quebec government has inaugurated programs designed to increase public awareness of the importance of exercise on one's overall health.

Married persons exercise less than unmarried persons, men more than women, and well-educated individuals more than less-educated (Paquet, 1989; Roy, 1985). Sports and health clubs that provide aerobic dance classes and fitness exercises are the privilege of prosperous Quebeckers. In Quebec, ice hockey has the widest appeal for both spectators and participants (Paradis, 1992).

Implications for nursing care

In the larger cities, nurses are likely to encounter clients who are suffering from the harmful effects of polluted air and water or soil contamination. Air pollution is responsible for such problems as asthma, bronchitis, and allergies affecting the skin, eyes, and respiratory systems and is seasonal as well as situational. For example, parents should avoid exposing infants to automobile fumes during the rush hour and should minimize use of possible allergy-producing substances found in rugs and humidifiers in homes in which there are young children, older people, or individuals with symptoms of acquired immunodeficiency. The problem of eliminating symptoms caused by stagnant air in large buildings or factories also falls within the domain of the nurse concerned with the work environment and the reduction of worker absenteeism.

Hunting and fishing are popular activities in Quebec. However, both of these activities can be detrimental to an individual's health because of the pollution present in fresh water and soil. Therefore, pregnant women should be advised against consuming freshwater fish or game during pregnancy. Even when women are not pregnant, the federal government recommends that fish from contaminated lakes be consumed no more than once a week, to prevent accumulation of polychlorinated biphenyls (PCBs) in body tissues. The nurse's role includes participation in awareness campaigns, in short-term and long-term preventive measures, and in research to determine possible interrelation between such aspects as pollution, health, life-style, and heredity.

The low level of physical activity observed in members of Quebec's less educated classes should stimulate the community health nurse to participate in educational campaigns in various community sectors. Because women are usually the principal health agents in the family, nursing interventions should be directed toward encouraging their collaboration in fostering healthful living habits.

The nurse should participate in setting up and maintaining programs designed to reduce malnutrition in schools serving underprivileged children. School nurses are in a good position to assess needs and seek ways to foster healthful living habits among children and to act as liaison between parents and teachers.

BIOLOGICAL VARIATIONS
Genetic factors

The various social, economic, and cultural practices of a given population influence the eventual formation of a genetic "pool" that determines the biological characteristics of a community (Bouchard & DeBraekeleer, 1991a). Quebeckers of French origin have a specific genotype inherited from the original group of 5000 colonists. Such phenomena as migrations, successive waves of immigration, family inbreeding, and concentration of certain groups in specific areas have directly contributed to reducing or increasing the frequency of certain genes in the Quebec population. For example, the genetic abnormalities found in the populations of the Saguenay and Charlevoix regions of Quebec represent an important public health problem in these areas. The most striking example is that of muscular dystrophy, a disorder of genetic origin characterized by a progressive increase of muscular debility (Bouchard, 1991). Its worldwide frequency is approximately 1 in 25,000 individuals. In the Saguenay region, the frequency is estimated to be 1 in 514 (DeBraekeleer, 1991). Familial hypercholesterolemia has a worldwide frequency of 1 in 500 in the general population; in eastern Quebec its frequency is estimated to be 1 in 150 (DeBraekeleer, 1991). Familial hypercholesterolemia has probably been the most carefully studied of dominant chromosome abnormalities. The principal complication of this disease is coronary thrombosis in the young adult, which is often fatal (Bouchard & DeBraekeleer, 1991b). Cystic fibrosis is the most common fatal hereditary illness among White French Canadians. Its frequency of 1 in 895 births in the Saguenay region is higher than that in most populations. Tay-Sachs disease also seems to occur frequently in Quebec. No treatment has been discovered for this condition, which occurs in infants from 2 to 6 months of age (DeBraekeleer, 1991).

Life expectancy

During the past 30 years, the life expectancy of Quebeckers has increased: women now live, on average, to 80.2 years of age and men to 72.8 years of age (Côté, 1992). However, after 70 years of age a rapid deterioration of quality of life occurs, accompanied by various chronic illnesses associated with aging. It is also important to understand that wide differences in mortalities exist between the sexes, socioprofessional categories, and urban and rural areas of Quebec (Rapport de la Commission d'Enquête sur les Services de santé et les Services sociaux, 1988).

The most important cause of death in Quebeckers is heart disease, with cardiac malfunction responsible for 40% of all deaths. Recognized risk factors for heart disease include smoking, hypertension, and hypercholesterolemia. It is estimated that 70% of the population between 18 and 74 years of age have at least one of these risk factors. Poor eating habits and lack of physical exercise compound risk of heart failure (Rapport de la Commission d'Enquête sur les Services de santé et les Services sociaux, 1988). A new cause of death appeared in the eighties, and the possibility exists that by the next century AIDS may

replace heart failure as the primary cause of mortality in Quebec. At present, the second cause of death is cancer, accounting for approximately 30% of all deaths. The most typical forms are lung cancer in men and breast cancer in women, the latter occurring especially after 25 years of age (Côté, 1992).

Although Quebec has a very low rate of perinatal and infant mortality (6.9 and 6.3 out of 1000 births respectively), premature birth (weight less than 2500 g) remains a serious health problem with rates of 5.7 per 1000 in 1980 and 6.6 per 1000 in 1990. Rates for low birth weight are 6.5 per 1000 in 1980 and 5.9 per 1000 in 1990. The unsatisfactory health status of these infants may be the result of lack of resources among very young mothers, unsatisfactory nutrition caused by poverty, and lack of or poorly applied contraceptive practices, particularly among adolescent girls in disadvantaged environments (Côté, 1992).

Premature death among French Canadians has two primary causes: highway accidents and suicide. Trauma and accidents account for 60% of these deaths and are the major cause of death for persons 30 years of age or younger. Each year, there are 60,000 highway accident victims and 1200 of these victims die from injuries received (Côté, 1992; Rapport de la Commission d'Enquête sur les Services de santé et les Services sociaux, 1988). Each year, more than 1000 suicides occur in Quebec. Most suicide attempts and suicidal tendencies occur in persons 15 to 24 years of age. Quebec's suicide rate exceeds that of the United States, Japan, and Sweden (Rapport de la Commission d'Enquête sur les Services de santé et les Services sociaux, 1988). Family breakup (divorce, reconstitution of family units, lack of attachment), upheaval of traditional values, social isolation, and the current depressed economic climate contribute to the high suicide rate among these young people.

Susceptibility to disease

Osteoarthritic disorders Because of Quebec's harsh climate and its very low temperatures and high humidity in winter, approximately 19% of the population suffers from some form of osteoarthritic condition, which hampers them in their occupational or personal activities (Pampalon, Gauthier, Raymond, & Beaudry, 1990).

Allergies An estimated 13.3% of the population suffers from one or more allergies. This occurrence is primarily an urban phenomenon caused by smog, pollen, and lack of air circulation in buildings. Women and children are the principal groups affected (Pampalon, Gauthier, Raymond, & Beaudry, 1990).

Sexually and intravenously transmitted diseases Diseases transmitted sexually and through the bloodstream constitute a serious public health problem in Quebec. It is estimated that 12,500 persons annually contract genital herpes (Steben, 1985). Every year in Canada 125,000 cases of chlamydiosis and 50,000 cases of gonorrhea occur (Soumis, 1987). Both are widespread in adolescent girls and adult women. In Quebec, half the cases of these diseases occur in persons 15 to 24 years of age (Côté, 1992; Rapport de la Commission d'Enquête sur les Services de santé et les Services sociaux, 1988). The repercussions of these sexually transmitted diseases are particularly critical in relation to feminine reproduction, causing pelvic inflammation, which in turn results in salpingitis producing infertility (Bryant, 1990; Lavoie-Roux, 1989).

Among Canadian provinces, Quebec currently has the second highest number of cases of AIDS: 2192 cases reported up to 1993. Bisexual and homosexual men 25 to 39 years of age and intravenous drug users account for 89% of all AIDS cases (Côté, 1992). Women infected with HIV and their children infected by vertical transmission constitute a growing group in Quebec. They are concentrated in the Montreal area, and the women contract the disease either from infected male sexual partners or through intravenous drug use.

In Quebec, an individual's knowledge about AIDS increases with degree of education and socioeconomic status. However, the level of knowledge is inferior to that of persons in other Canadian provinces. Women are more knowledgeable than men on this subject (Ornstein, 1989). Unfortunately a commonly held view of AIDS is that it is a problem that concerns only homosexuals and intravenous drug users. The population of Quebec demonstrates a generally negative attitude toward the adoption of preventive behavior patterns such as the use of condoms. In Montreal, 51.6% of adults having occasional partners and 75% having a regular partner report that they never use a condom (Dupras, 1989).

Lévy-Marchal, Karjalainen, Dubois, et al. (1995) studied diabetes in relation to evaluated BSA antibody levels. They concluded that elevated IgC anti-BSA levels are associated with the low incidence of insulin-dependent diabetes mellitus (IDDM) in the French population studied. Thus their results support an immunological role of BSA in diabetic autoimmunity.

Nutritional preferences

For some French Canadians, food constitutes a whole system of meanings. There is "language of food," which includes how society views eating and how it designates foods into categories of normal and healthful. In addition, there is the personal adaptation that an individual or group makes concerning eating habits. Although socioeconomic and cultural factors influence the way these two concepts function, both must be considered when attempts are made to improve living habits.

From early colonial times, because of the harsh climate, the diet of French Canadians has been rich in starchy foods and fat. The people of Quebec have consistently continued to devote a considerable portion of their family budget to food. Fish has been a favorite food because it is much less costly than red meat. In the sixties and seventies the practice of eating in restaurants became more frequent and "fast foods" became popular because of their low price and convenience. Unfortunately these foods are rich in fatty substances and salt and poor in fibers and vitamins.

A portion of the population of Quebec is reported to have improved their eating habits over the last 10 years (Rapport de la Commission d'Enquête sur les Services de santé et les Services sociaux, 1988). In a study conducted by Renaud, Jutras, and Bouchard (1987), a majority of respondents claimed to have made a particular effort to balance their diets. Although they consume less fatty foods, they still consume too much sugar and too few milk products, fruits, and vegetables. Since the economic recession, there have been experiments such as the "community kitchen," where women buy healthful foods in large quantity. Because of the high cost of living and rampant unemployment, students and people out of work are often undernourished. To combat the problem of undernourishment in schools and in disadvantaged neighborhoods, cafeterias are subsidized by the government and free milk is regularly distributed.

In Quebec, men are more likely than women to be prone to poor eating habits (Renaud, Jutras, & Bouchard, 1987; Rapport de la Commission d'Enquête sur les Services de santé et les Services sociaux, 1988). Women of all ages attempt to control their weight. The perceived social requirement of staying slim, coupled with the burdens of motherhood and outside employment, causes many women to be undernourished and to fall victim to "miracle diets." Given the importance of the relationship between nutrition, the health of newborns and adolescents, and osteoporosis in older women, much remains to be accomplished in the area of proper diets for women. In Quebec, women have a predominant role in the choice and preparation of food. Consequently the way women nourish themselves and their families is of vital importance to the health of the community.

Psychological characteristics

Alcoholism and drug abuse Alcoholism and the abuse of psychotropic and illegal drugs are serious problems in Quebec. More than 6% of Quebeckers over 15 years of age have dependency problems with alcohol, with the highest proportion of drinkers being males 20 to 24 years of age (Côté, 1992; Moisan, 1991). Women have a tendency to abuse antidepressants and sleeping pills. Older people tend to abuse psychotropic drugs, which are often routinely prescribed.

Users of illegal drugs, such as cocaine, crack, and hallucinogenics, are becoming younger and younger. The current drug-use curve is different from that of the seventies, when addiction tended to be progressive, beginning with "soft" drugs such as marijuana and ending with "hard" drugs such as heroin. To-day's drug users often go right to hard substances and intravenous drugs as they make contact with the world of illegal drugs. However, the use of heroin in Quebec is restrained by its limited availability, even in urban centers.

Smoking is another behavior with an unfavorable effect on health. Although there has been a recent decrease in the number of smokers, approximately 35% of men and 31% of women still smoke. Each year, tobacco use is responsible for 8000 deaths occurring as a result of cardiovascular and respiratory diseases and lung cancer (Lavoie-Roux, 1989; Rapport de la Commission d'Enquête sur les Services de santé et les Services sociaux, 1988).

Mental health One member of the Quebec population in five will suffer a mental health problem at some point during his or her life. Women suffer more psychological distress than men and consult health professionals three times more frequently (Gouvernement du Quebec, 1989; Perreault, Légaré, & Boyer, 1988-1989).

Chronic mental illness, deinstitutionalizing, and drug and alcohol abuse problems have combined with the depressed economy to produce a new subpopulation: the homeless. It has been estimated in Montreal that, during a 1-year period, between 10,000 and 15,000 people have no fixed address and roam the streets. These individuals include adult men and women, young people who have run away from home, and families with young children. Many of these individuals are former psychiatric patients who are no longer taking their medications (Côté, 1992; Lavoie-Roux, 1989).

Implications for nursing care

Regardless of the biological variations, the nurse needs to consider the relationship between social integration, social support, and health. Mortalities and morbidities, in different cultural communities, are partially determined by the degree of an individual's integration in a society and the social support supplied by the community. Social support has a preventive value if it is associated with networks that are stable, homogeneous, and dense and that provide for a variety of links between individuals (Bozzini & Tessier, 1985).

Given the ethnic variety in Quebec society, the nurse should include the following three differentiating factors in health care assessment. First, note should be made of the meaning of health and illness in terms of the underlying significance of these concepts in the cultural group. Second, consideration must be given to the social class of the individual requiring care. Descriptions of symptoms, compliance with treatment, and reaction to pain will differ according to social level and ethnic origin. Third, the client's gender must be considered because gender influences how individuals view their bodies and the adoption of dependent or independent behavior patterns with regard to health (Dorvil, 1985). These three factors have a dominant influence on one's representation of illness. French-Canadian people tend to adopt terms of reference of one of the various subcultural groups (French-speaking, English-speaking, and so on) as the "dominant" or reference group in the creation of these representations. These terms influence the way the clients explain their illness and participate in care and the degree to which they comply when following the advice of health professionals.

Bellavance and Perreault (1995) interviewed eight French-Canadian homosexual men living with AIDS in Quebec and noted that Herzlich's framework of health and illness as socially constructed concepts can be utilized to assist individuals with AIDS to make behavioral changes that will generate health throughout the course of the illness.

Perinatal, physical, and mental health services for women exposed to venereal disease should be promoted in parallel with preventive and health programs. These programs should be designed to educate the public concerning the dangers of sexually transmitted diseases, especially AIDS, and the part played by illegal drugs in the transmission process. Nurses are also subject to the influence of these fears and prejudices. However, nurses need to maintain open, nonjudgmental attitudes in their interactions with clients suffering from AIDS (Taggart, Reidy, & Grenier, 1992).

The particular mortality and morbidity curves occurring in the Quebec population, combined with severe budget limitations placed on health services, call for the creation of new approaches in the care of those affected by illness. Target populations include those who suffer from chronic illnesses or are infected by viruses (such as AIDS) or other agents (such as tuberculosis). The evolution of these latter illnesses follows a pattern in which brief hospitalizations occur periodically, followed by long periods of time when the client must learn to function at home within the limits imposed by the condition. As the periods of allowed hospitalization become shorter, nurses must develop home care approaches facilitating the participation of the client's family caregiver. The participation of client and caregiver enables individuals to make those decisions that will maintain a quality of life at an acceptable level.

With the aging of the population and the subsequent increase in the incidence of chronic illnesses has come an intensification in the use of various drugs and medicines in the community. It is the nurse's responsibility to help clients maintain their medical regimen and to inform them about the dangers of uncontrolled and irrational use of prescription or nonprescription drugs, of accidental or intentional intoxication, of teratogenic and iatrogenic effects, and of physical and psychological dependency. It is also important for the Canadian nurse to be active in administrative boards that play a strategic role in making decisions about health and social service establishments. The public-centered approach is at the heart of health and social service reform in Quebec. Nursing input is being welcomed as new public policy is being designed (Trudel, 1995). Additionally, Dumas, Plouffe, Boutin, & Desaulniers (1995) describe the important role the nurse can serve in providing interdisciplinary care.

SUMMARY

The people of Quebec have a long, colorful past. It is essential for the nurse to remember that the people of Quebec represent a multicultural, heterogeneous, pluralistic society. Thus the illness or wellness behaviors of these people are difficult to characterize as unique to a specific cultural group. To understand the cultural significance of behaviors noted among Quebec people, it is essential that the nurse develop an understanding of the different cultural, ethnic, and racial groups who blend to make Quebec society.

Case Study

Marguerite Tremblay (born McNeill) married in 1929 at 16 years of age. Her husband, Théophile Tremblay, worked at a farm in the Laurentians. They were for the most part self-sufficient, with cows, a few sheep, and a market garden. They traded for certain goods and had a small cash crop. Life was hard, with a day that began before dawn and continued until bedtime.

In 1960, at the death of Théophile, the eldest son, Étienne, took over running the family farm, where he had continued to live with his wife, Estelle, and their children. Several years later, the land was expropriated to make room for a highway. The family, now composed of Mrs. Tremblay, Rose (her unmarried daughter), and Étienne and his children, moved to a small farm property in Ste-Rose. Mrs. Tremblay, with the help of Rose, raised Étienne's children after their mother died in childbirth.

Mrs. Tremblay, a good Catholic and farm wife, had 15 children between 1930 and 1956, eight of whom survived to maturity (see Tremblay Family Tree, Fig. 23-1). Two of these children were born dead, two died after premature births, one died of meningitis, one died of polio, and one did not survive a hard winter. One son died in an automobile accident, when drunk, at 18 years of age.

The life situation of the surviving family members demonstrates how the family structure and religious practices have changed within the life span of one family.

Rose
Age 63; unmarried; lives with mother; suffers from obesity, diabetes, and osteoporosis; attends church and receives the sacraments regularly.

Étienne
Age 62; widower; farmer and truck driver; father of seven children, five of whom survived to maturity, all of whom have left home; suffers from severe arthritis.

Philippe
Age 59; notary; father of six children, five of whom lived to maturity; smoker; suffers from hypertension and hypercholesterolemia; wife has recovered from breast cancer.

Line
Age 56; married a farmer; worked as a volunteer for the parish church; mother of four children, all of whom survived to maturity.

Victor
Age 55; missionary in Africa; smoker; suffers from certain chronic parasitical infections.

Marie-Madeleine
Age 45; was a nun in a nursing order; after leaving the convent, has worked with adolescents with drug problems; does not practice her religion.

Catherine
Age 43; former teacher; divorced from a doctor; mother of two children; suffers from chronic anxiety and mild abuse of tranquilizers; has become a Christian Scientist.

Denise
Age 34; former commercial artist; unmarried; mother of one child whose father, an actor, died of AIDS; mother and child HIV positive; activist in AIDS self-help group; very interested in spiritual renewal but refuses her mother's pleas to return to the Church.

Mrs. Tremblay has remained active and involved in the life of her children and grandchildren. At 80 years of age, she suffered a cerebrovascular accident that left her with a left-sided hemiplegia. She has made only moderate recovery. She requires help with transfer but can stand with a walker. She requires help with many activities of daily living and spends much of her time in a wheelchair. She speaks slowly but is lucid, if somewhat anxious.

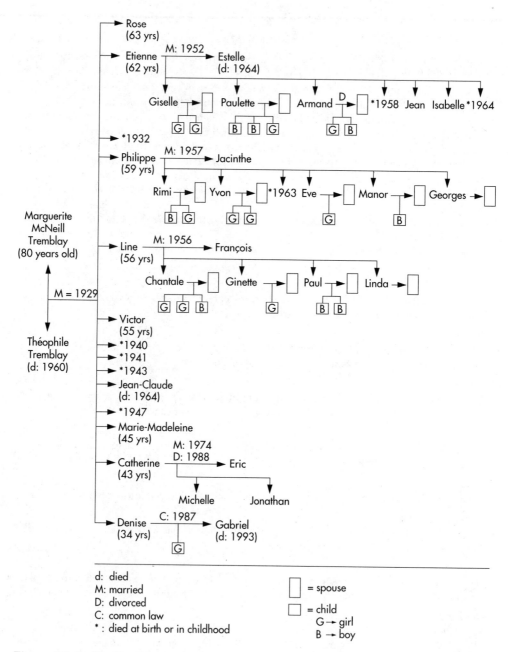

d: died
M: married
D: divorced
C: common law
* : died at birth or in childhood

☐ = spouse

☐ = child
G → girl
B → boy

Figure 23-1 The Tremblay family tree.

Mrs. Tremblay has been admitted to a long-term care unit because of her physical limitations and her immediate family's inability to care for her at home. She alternates between understanding the need for long-term care and fear that her family no longer needs her. Her family, particularly her eldest son and daughter, with whom she lived, feel guilty and fear that they are not doing their "duty," despite their own health problems and physical limitations.

CARE PLAN

 Nursing Diagnosis   Anxiety, related to situational crises (Adapted from Sparks & Taylor, 1993; p. 41)

Client Outcomes

1. Client will identify the factors in the situation that provoke anxiety (such as strange room, room shared with other resident).
2. Client will identify those activities, feasible in the new situation, that have helped her relax in the past.
3. Client will begin to accept the limits imposed by stroke and to control the anxiety provoked by life in a long-term care setting.

Nursing Interventions

1. Take the time, daily, to talk personally with client in an informal setting such as the lounge or kitchen.
2. When talking about client's stroke, as much as possible, use the language and words she uses. Verify client's comprehension of new or technical language.
3. Use the techniques of reminiscence therapy to remind client of past strategies for dealing with anxiety.
4. Identify those strategies appropriate to new environment that have previously helped control anxiety.

 Nursing Diagnosis   Powerlessness, related to the health care environment (Adapted from Sparks & Taylor, 1993; p. 221)

Client Outcomes

1. Client will understand and express her feelings of powerlessness.
2. Client will understand that her powerlessness is not universal.
3. Client will identify factors she can learn to control in the current situation.
4. Client will succeed in learning to control these factors.
5. Client will learn to use her interpersonal skills to exercise some control over her social environment.

Nursing Interventions

1. Help client arrange her room and equipment such as telephone, radio, and call-bell so that she is comfortable in using them.
2. Arrange with client's family to have a telephone with memory for frequently called numbers and remote control for television (both with "user-friendly" boards).
3. Develop with client daily routine that incorporates, as much as possible, strategies that give client control in current situation.
4. Develop with the client a prosthetic and secure environment where she compensates for her physical limits and maintains some control on her physical environment.
5. Encourage client to participate in social and recreational activities such as group singing and bingo.
6. Encourage client's interest and sense of responsibility in building the morale of other residents whom she seems to like.

 Nursing Diagnosis   Role performance, altered, related to ineffective coping (Adapted from Sparks & Taylor, 1993; p. 515)

Client Outcomes

1. Client will maintain and strengthen those aspects of her former social and familial roles that are possible within the current situation.
2. Client will identify, with the participation of her family, modified social roles within the family.

Nursing Interventions

1. Encourage the client to express her feelings and wishes concerning the roles she would like to play and the activities she would like to do.
2. Help client's daughter to aid the client to explore the sustainable aspects of her former roles and to develop new roles within the family.

3. Client will identify a role, within the long-term unit, that takes into consideration her limits but makes use of her abilities and the prosthetic environment.

3. Help the client to understand and play her role in maintaining effective interrelationships between the generations of her family.
4. Develop a "caring" relationship with the client and explore with her the relationships she can develop and the roles she can play in interacting with other staff members, volunteers, and other residents.

 Nursing Diagnosis   Self-esteem, (situational) low, related to hospitalization and forced dependence on health care team (Adapted from Sparks & Taylor, 1993; p. 515)

Client Outcomes

1. Client will express opinions and her preferences to both staff and family.
2. Client will participate in the various aspects of her care process (such as decision making, physical care, assessment).
3. Client will experience and express, through her body language, an increase in self-esteem.

Nursing Interventions

1. Address the client by her name, Madame Tremblay, never "Mama" ("*Maman*") or other diminutives.
2. Respect the client's privacy and her physical space and go slowly in manifesting a physical display of affection. Permit client to set the parameters of her social space.
3. Listen to the client, encourage her to use "I" in her conversation, respect her opinion, encourage her to make decisions, and respect these decisions.
4. Encourage the family to help client maintain her personal appearance by providing clothes that fit and are attractive, personal grooming equipment, and the like. Compliment her on any improvements in appearance.
5. Work with occupational and physiotherapy personnel to develop appropriate but practical and worthwhile projects (such as weaving, food preparation).

 Nursing Diagnosis   Sensory or perceptual alteration (kinesthetic), related to sensory reception, transmission, or integration (Adapted from Sparks & Taylor, 1993; p. 256)

Client Outcomes

1. Client will understand the relationship between her neurological pathology ("stroke") and the sensory and perceptual changes she has experienced.
2. Client will begin to compensate for inability to identify position of body parts by developing other senses (sight, sensations of unaffected members, and so on).
3. Client will learn to master prosthetic aids to compensate for diminished motor coordination.
4. Client will understand the importance of practicing preventive and safety measures (such as skin care and proper shoes).

Nursing Interventions

1. Validate with the client that she understands the effect of the "stroke" on her ability to function and that she realizes that certain false perceptions can occur because of this condition.
2. Work with the client so that she learns to use her "good" hand routinely and to use visual inspection to verify the position and location of her affected limbs.
3. Develop with the client compensatory routines such as turning her head to improve her visual field or repositioning items in her physical environment.
4. Show the client how to inspect her skin for pressure points and help her develop a routine for turning and relieving these pressure points.

 Nursing Diagnosis   Coping, ineffective family, related to caring for dependent, aging family member (Adapted from Sparks & Taylor, 1993; p. 496)

Client Outcomes

1. Family will improve communications leading to clarification of needs and expectations and to evolution of the roles of family members.

Nursing Interventions

1. Clarify with the daughter the mutual affiliative role of mother and daughter.

2. Family will maintain and strengthen those aspects of existing family roles appropriate to the current situation.
3. Family will develop appropriate involvement of all family members in the client's current situation (such as involvement that encourages both affiliation and autonomy).
4. Family will mutually accept new roles of the client and the principal caregiver in the family.
5. Family will experience reduction in destructive feelings, such as guilt, on the part of family members.

2. Clarify with the daughter, in terms of her limits and abilities, her new role as principal health care giver in the family, emphasizing the essential nature of this new role.
3. Clarify with family members (especially the eldest son) the importance of visits, family celebrations, development of relationships with grandchildren, and keeping client informed of family events.
4. Include the daughter in the planning of the client's care.
5. Encourage family members to develop joint family projects such as a family photo album.

References

Anctil, H., & Bluteau, M.A. (1986). *La santé et l'assistance publique au Québec, 1886-1986* [Quebec health and social welfare, 1886-1986]. Québec: Ministère de la Santé et des Services sociaux, Direction des Communications.

Audet, L.P., & Gauthier, A. (1967). *Le système scolaire du Québec: organisation et fonctionnement* [Quebec educational system: structure and function]. Montréal: Librairie Beauchemin Limitée.

Authier, P. (1993). New rules allow bilingual signs for all stores. *The Montreal Gazette, A3,* (June 15).

Bailey, E., & Bailey, R. (1995). *Discover Canada*. Oxford, England: Berlitz Publishing Company, Ltd.

Bellavance, M., & Perreault, M. (1995). [Concepts of AIDS in relation to health and illness in homosexual men living in Québec with AIDS. *Canadian Journal of Nursing Research, 27*(1),57-75.

Bouchard, G. (1991). Pour une approche historique et sociale du génome québécois [Historical and social approach to the Quebec genome]. In Bouchard, G., & DeBraekeleer, M., (Eds.), *Histoire d'un génome: population et génétique dans l'est du Québec* [History of a genome: population and genetics in eastern Quebec] (pp. 3-18). Québec: Les Presses de l'Université de Québec.

Bouchard, G. (1992). Sur les perspectives de la culture québécoise comme francophonie nord-américaine [On the perspectives of Quebec culture as a French-speaking community in North America]. In Lanthier, P., & Rousseau, G. (Eds.), *La culture inventée, stratégies culturelles aux XIXe et XXe siècles.* [Cultural tendencies and cultural strategies of the nineteenth and twentieth centuries] (pp. 319-328). Québec: Institut Québécois de Recherche sur la Culture.

Bouchard, G., & DeBraekeleer, M. (Eds.). (1991a). *Histoire d'un génome: population et génétique dans l'est du Québec* [History of a genome: population and genetics in eastern Quebec]. Québec: Les Presses de l'Université de Québec.

Bouchard, G., & DeBraekeleer, M. (1991b). Mouvements migratoires, effets fondateurs et homogénéisation génétique [Migratory shifts, founders effects and genetic homogenization]. In Bouchard, G., & DeBraekeleer, M. (Eds.), *Histoire d'un génome: population et génétique dans l'est du Québec* [History of a genome: population and genetics in eastern Quebec] (pp. 281-321). Québec: Les Presses de l'Université de Québec.

Bozzini, L., & Tessier, R. (1985). Support social et santé. [Social support and health]. In Dufresne, J., Dumont, F., & Martin, Y. (Eds.), *Traité d'anthropologie médicale* [Medical anthropology treatise] (pp. 905-939). Québec: Les Presses de l'Université du Québec.

Bryant, H. (1990). *L'infertilité à l'heure de la procréatique. . .et la prévention?* [Infertility in the age of artificial reproduction . . .and prevention?]. Ottawa: Conseil consultatif canadien sur la Situation de la Femme.

Chanlat, J. F. (1985). Types de sociétés, types de morbidités: la socio-génèse des maladies [Types of societies, types of morbidities: Sociogenesis of illness]. In Dufresne, J., Dumont, F., & Martin, Y. (Eds.), *Traité d'anthropologie médicale.* [Medical anthropology treatise] (pp. 293-304). Québec: Les Presses de l'Université du Québec.

Conseil du Statut de la Femme. (1981). *Pour les Québécoises: égalité et indépendance* [For the women of Quebec: equality and independence]. Québec: Éditeur officiel.

Cossette, S., Lévesque, L., & Laurin, L. (1995). Informal and formal support for caregivers of a demented relative: do gender and kinship make a difference? *Research in Nursing and Health, 18*(5), 437-451.

Côté, M.Y. (1992). *La politique de la santé et du bien-être* [Health and welfare policy]. Québec: Le Ministère.

Dandurand, R.B. (1990). Peut-on encore définir la famille? [Can we still define the family?]. In Dumont, F. (Ed.), *La société québécoise après 30 ans de changements* [Quebec society after 30 years of change] (pp. 49-66). Québec: Institut Québécois de Recherche sur la Culture.

DeBraekeleer, M. (1991). Les gènes délétères [Deleterious genes]. In Bouchard, G., & DeBraekeleer, M. (Eds.), *Histoire d'un génome: population et génétique dans l'est du Québec* [History of a genome: population and genetics in eastern Quebec] (pp. 343-363). Québec: Les Presses de l'Université de Québec.

Desautels, Y. (1984). *Les coutumes de nos ancêtres* [Customs of our ancestors]. Montréal: Édition Paulines.

Dorvil, H. (1985). Types de sociétés et représentations. [Types of societies and representations]. In Dufresne, J., Dumont, F., & Martin, Y. (Eds.), *Traité d'anthropologie médicale* [Medical anthropology treatise]. Québec: Presses de l'Université du Québec.

Dulong, G., & Bergeron, G. (1980). Le parler populaire du Québec et de ses régions voisines [Popular language of Quebec and its neighboring regions]. *La documentation québécoise, 8*, 3124-3655.

Dumas, L., Plouffe, M., Boutin, D., & Desaulniers, M. (1995). University and community service center (CLSC) and collaboration. *Canadian Nurse, 91*(8), 45-49.

Dupras, A. (1989). *La sexualité des montréalais et le sida* [Sexuality of Montrealers and AIDS]. Longueuil: Éditions IRIS.

Fahmy-Eid, N., & Dumont, M. (1983). *Maîtresses de maison, maîtresses d'écoles: femmes, familles et éducation dans l'histoire du Québec* [Housewives, school mistresses: women, Families, and education in Quebec history]. Montréal: Boréal Express.

Gagnon, S. (1992). L'École élémentaire québécoise au XIXe siècle [Quebec elementary school in the nineteenth century]. In Lanthier, P., & Rousseau, G. (Eds.), *La culture inventée, stratégies culturelles aux XIXe et XXe siècles* [Cultural tendencies and cultural strategies of the nineteenth and twentieth centuries] (pp. 135-153). Québec: Institut Québécois de Recherche sur la Culture.

Gouvernement du Québec. (1989). *Politique de santé mentale* [Mental health policy]. Québec: Le Ministère.

Hall, E.T. (1966). *The hidden dimension.* New York: Doubleday & Co., Inc.

Henripin, J., Huot, P.M., Lapierre-Adamcyk, E., & Marcil-Gratton, N. (1981). *Les enfants qu'on n'a plus au Québec* [Children that we no longer have in Quebec] Montréal: Les Presses de l'Université de Montréal.

Information please almanac (1998). Boston & New York: Houghton Mifflin Company.

Laberge, H. (1992). Culture nationale et cultures ethniques: l'interculturalisme à la québécoise [National and ethnic cultures: interculturalism in Quebec]. *Action Nationale, 82* (7), 897-906.

Labrie, N. (1990). La question linguistique et les communautés culturelles au Québec [Quebec linguistic issue and cultural communities]. In Guilbert, L. (Ed.), *Identité ethnique et interculturalité: état de la recherche en ethnologie et en socio-linguistique.* [Ethnic identity and interculture: State of research in ethnology and in sociolinguistics] (pp. 33-46). Sainte-Foy: CELAT (Centre d'Études sur la Langue, les Arts, et les Traditions populaires des Francophones en Amérique du Nord), Université de Laval.

Lacroix, B., & Simard, J. (1984). Religion populaire, religion de clercs [Popular religion and clergymen]. Collection: *Culture Populaire,* No. 2. Québec: Institut Québécois de Recherche sur la Culture.

Laforest, L. (1985). Pratiques médicales et évolution sociale [Medical practices and social evolution]. In Dufresne, J., Dumont, F., & Martin, Y. (Eds.), *Traité d'anthropologie médicale* [Medical anthropology treatise] (pp. 267-280). Québec: Les Presses de l'Université du Québec.

Lamonde, Y. (1991). *Territoires de la culture québécoise* [Quebec cultural territories]. Québec: Les Presses de l'Université de Laval.

Lanthier, P., & Rousseau, G. (Eds.). (1992). *La culture inventée, stratégies culturelles aux XIXe et XXe siècles* [Cultural tendencies and cultural strategies of the nineteenth and twentieth centuries). Québec: Institut québécois de Recherche sur la Culture.

Laperrière, G. (1992). La place du catholicisme [The place of Catholicism]. Dossier: Catholicisme et société distincte [Catholicism and distinct society]. *Présence, 2*(5), 21-23.

Lavoie-Roux, T. (1989). *Pour améliorer la santé et le bien-être au Québec: orientations* [Improving health and well-being in Quebec: orientations]. Québec: Le Ministère.

Lazure, J. (1990). Mouvance des générations. Condition féminine et masculine [Generational sphere of influence. Female and male status]. In Dumont, F. (Ed.), *La Société québecoise après 30 ans de changements* [Quebec society after 30 years of change] (pp. 27-40). Québec: Institut québécois de Recherche sur la Culture.

Le-Dorze, G., Lever, N., Ryalls, J., & Brassard, C. (1995). Normative values of certain prosodic parameters obtained with French-speaking persons without a communication disorder. *Folia Phoniatrica et Logopaedica, 47*(1), 39-47.

Lévy-Marchal, C., Karjalainen, J., Dubois, F., et al. (1995, Aug.). Antibodies against bovine albumin and other diabetes markers in French children. *Diabetes Care, 18*(8), 1089-94.

Moisan, C. (1991). *Portrait de la consommation d'alcool et de drogues au Québec: principales données de l'Enquête nationale sur l'alcool et les autres drogues* [Portrait of alcohol and drug consumption in Quebec: principal data of the national survey on alcohol and other drugs]. Collection: Données statistiques et Indicateurs. Québec: Ministère de la Santé et des Services sociaux.

Ntetu, A., & Fortin, J. (1996). Reconsidering nursing interventions among Native people. *Canadian Nurse, 9*(3), 42-46.

Ornstein, M. (1989). *AIDS in Canada: knowledge, behavior and attitudes of adults.* Ontario: Institute for Social Research, York University.

Orr, R. (1992). Notre héritage Catholique. [Our Catholic heritage]. Translated by Serge Gagnon. Dossier: Catholicisme et société distincte [Catholicism and distinct society]. *Présence, 1* (5), 11-13.

Pampalon, R., Gauthier, D., Raymond, G., & Beaudry, D. (1990). *La santé à la carte: une exploration géographique de l'Enquête Santé Québec* [Health map: a geographic exploration of the Quebec Health Survey]. Québec: Ministère de la Santé et des Services sociaux.

Paquet, G. (1989). *Santé et inégalité sociales: un problème de distance culturelle* [Health and social inequality: cultural gap]. Québec: Institut Québécois de Recherche sur la Culture.

Paradis, J.M. (1992). La pratique du sport en Mauricie: du fair play britannique à la compétition nord-américaine. [Sport practices in Mauricie: British fair play in North American competition]. In Lanthier, P., & Rousseau, G. (Eds.), *La culture inventée, stratégies culturelles aux XIXe et XXe siècles* [Cultural tendencies and cultural strategies of the nineteenth and twentieth centuries] (pp. 87-97). Québec: Institut québécois de Recherche sur la Culture.

Perreault, C., Légaré, G., & Boyer, R. (1988-1989). La santé mentale des Québécois [Mental health of Quebeckers]. *Santé et Société, 2*(1), 50-53.

Pronovost, G. (1989). Les transformations des rapports entre le temps de travail et le temps libre [Transformation in work time and leisure time]. In Pronovost, G., & Mercure, D. (Eds.), *Temps et sociétés* [Time and societies] (pp. 37-61). Québec: Institut québécois de Recherche sur la Culture.

Rapport de la Commission d'Enquête sur les Services de santé et les Services sociaux (1988). *Commission d'Enquête sur les Services de santé et les Services sociaux* [Inquiry commission on health and social services]. Québec: Les Publications du Québec.

Renaud, M., Jutras, S., & Bouchard, P. (1987). *Les solutions qu'apportent les Québécois à leurs problèmes sociaux et sanitaires* [Solutions brought forth by Quebeckers concerning social and health problems]. In *Commission d'Enquête sur les Services de santé et les Services sociaux* [Inquiry Commission on Health and Social Services]. Québec: Les Publications du Québec.

Rioux, M. (1974). *Les Québécois* [The Quebeckers]. Paris: Seuil.

Roy, L. (1985). *Le point sur les habitudes de vies: l'activité physique* [Focusing on health patterns: physical activity]. Québec: Gouvernement du Québec.

Saint-Arnaud, J., & Pomerleau, J. (1995). [Consent for organ transplantation]. *Canadian Nurse, 91*(11), 33-38.

Schoolcraft, V. (1984). *Nursing in the community.* Toronto: Wiley & Sons.

Shirley, J., & Duchesne, L. (1989). Population et ménage [Population and household]. In Asselin, R. (Ed.), *Le Québec statistique 1989* [1989 Quebec's statistics] (ed. 59) (pp. 293-323). Québec: Les Publications du Québec.

Soumis, L. (1987, Aug.). La guerre aux MTS et au sida [The war on STD and AIDS]. Commercial: Radio-Canada refuse diffuser les messages au Québec. *Le Devoir, 1*(25).

Sparks, S.M., & Taylor, C.M. (1993). *Nursing diagnosis reference manual: an indispensable guide to better patient care* (ed. 2). Springhouse, Pa.: Springhouse Corporation.

Statistics Canada (1991). *Statistics Canada, 1991 census: metropolitan areas.* Ottawa: Ministère des Approvisionnements et Services, Canada.

Statistiques Canada (1989). *Annuaire du Canada 1990* [1990 Canadian annual]. Ottawa: Ministère des Approvisionnements et Services, Canada.

Statistiques Canada (1996). *Annuaire du Canada 1996* [1996 Canadian annual]. Ottawa: Ministère des Approvisionnements et Services, Canada.

Steben, M. (1985). Les maladies transmises sexuellement: l'épidémie catastrophique [Sexually transmitted diseases: a catastrophic epidemic]. In Dupras, A., & Lévy, J.J. (Eds.), *La sexualité au Québec: perspectives contemporaines* [Sexuality in Quebec: contemporary perspectives]. Longueuil: Éditions IRIS.

Taggart, M.E. (1983). *Acquisition de connaissances et de comportements chez les primipares à la suite de deux types de programmes èducatifs postnatals* [Acquisition of knowledge and behaviors in primiparas after two types of postnatal educational programs]. Doctoral thesis in Education (not published). Montréal: Université de Montréal.

Taggart, M.E., Reidy, M., & Grenier, D. (1992). Attitudes d'infirmières francophones face au sida [French-speaking nurses' attitudes toward AIDS]. *Infirmière canadienne/Canadian Nurse, 88*(1), 48-52.

Tétu de Labsade, F. (1990). *Le Québec: un pays, une culture* [Quebec: a country, a culture]. Montréal: Boréal.

Thibaudeau, M.F., & Reidy, M. (1985). A nursing care model for the disadvantaged family. In Stewart, M. (Ed.), *Community health nursing in Canada* (pp. 269-286). Toronto: Gage Publishing Co.

Thibaudeau, M.F., Reidy, M., d'Amours, F., & Frappier, G. (1984). *La santé de la famille défavorisée: évaluation de l'application d'un modèle de soins infirmiers auprès de familles défavorisées qui utilisent les services du CLSC* [Health of the disadvantaged family: Assessment of the application of a nursing care model in disadvantaged families using community health clinics]. Montréal: Faculté des Sciences infirmières, Université de Montréal.

Thibault, M.T. (1989). Environnement [Environment]. In Asselin, R. (Ed.), *Le Québec statistique 1989* [1989 Quebec statistics] (ed. 59) (pp. 261-291). Québec: Les Publications du Québec.

Trudel, A. (1995). Nurses as members of administrative boards. *Canadian Nurse, 91*(5), 37-40.

INDEX